Joyce Semradek

490
OHSU
MED/NSG BKST
34.00

D1773361

IMMUNOLOGY
A SYNTHESIS

IMMUNOLOGY
A SYNTHESIS

EDWARD S. GOLUB
DIRECTOR OF RESEARCH
ORTHO PHARMACEUTICAL

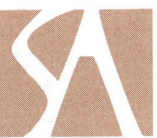

SINAUER ASSOCIATES, INC. • PUBLISHERS
Sunderland, Massachusetts 01375

THE COVER

Computer graphic view of insulin showing that antigenic determinants cluster at highly flexible regions. The alpha carbon backbone is shown with purple lines. The molecular surface is indicated with dots, color-coded from most mobile to most rigid in the order red, yellow, green, cyan, blue. Residues forming antigenic determinants are labeled in pink (contiguous) and yellow (discontiguous) and can be seen to correspond with the more mobile regions (see pages 28 and 29). [Image created by John A. Tainer and Elizabeth D. Getzoff, Research Institute of Scripps Clinic]

PART-OPENING ELECTRON MICROGRAPHS

Part One, p. 15: Antibody–hapten complex (purified rabbit anti–2,4-dinitrophenyl antibody and a bivalent hapten). [From R. C. Valentine and N. M. Green (1967), *J. Mol. Biol.* 27, 615]

Part Two, p. 155: A resting lymphocyte, probably a T cell, ×21,840. [Courtesy of D. Zucker-Franklin, New York University Medical Center]

Part Three, p. 437: Immune complexes, seen as electron-dense, hump-shaped deposits in the upper third of the photo, along a capillary wall in a glomerulus following streptococcal glomerulonephritis (×17,250). [Courtesy of M. N. Yum, Indiana University Medical Center]

IMMUNOLOGY: A SYNTHESIS

Copyright © 1987 by Sinauer Associates Inc. All rights reserved. This book may not be reproduced in whole or in part for any purpose whatever, without permission from the publisher. For information address Sinauer Associates Inc., Sunderland, Massachusetts 01375.

Library of Congress Cataloging-in-Publication Data

Golub, Edward S., 1934–
 Immunology, a synthesis.

 Bibliography: p.
 Includes index.
 1. Immunology. 2. Immunologic diseases. I. Title.
[DNLM: 1. Immunity. 2. Immunologic Diseases.
QW 504 G629i]
QR181.G66   1987   616.079   86-26079
ISBN 0-87893-268-2

Printed in U.S.A.

7 6 5 4 3 2

To the two most important women in my life,
My MOTHER *and my* WIFE, CONSTANCE,
and to the memory of two important men in my life,
My FATHER *and my* FRIEND, GOOCH

Brief Contents

1 The Clonal Nature of the Immune Response   1

Part One Immunochemistry   15

Section I Antigens and Antibodies   16

2 The Nature of Antigens   17
3 The Basic Immunoglobulin Monomer   36
4 Heterogeneity of Immunoglobulins   54
5 Organization of Immunoglobulin Genes   73
6 Monoclonal and Hybrid Antibodies   92

Section II The Antigen-Antibody Reaction   102

7 The Antigen-Antibody Complex   103
8 Measuring Antigen-Antibody Reactions   112
9 Complement   137

Part Two Cellular Immunology   155

Section I The Origins and Organization of Lymphoid Tissue   156

10 Hemopoiesis   157
11 Lymphocytes   179
12 Organization and Structure of Lymphoid Tissue   196
13 The Major Histocompatibility Complex   208

Section II Cell Cooperation   234

14 The Division of Labor   235
15 Helper and Effector Cells   250
16 Helper and Effector Determinants   267
17 MHC Restriction   280
18 Acquisition of the Restriction Repertoire   299

Section III Receptors and Signals   316

19 Antigen-Specific Receptors on Lymphocytes   317
20 Genetic Organization of Receptors   338
21 Interleukins   354

Section IV Regulation of the Immune Response   378

22 The Network   379
23 Suppressor Cells   393
24 Immune Tolerance   415

Part Three Immunity and Immunopathology   437

25 Immunity, Infections, and Tumors   439
36 Hypersensitivity   461
27 Autoimmunity   481
28 Transplantation   497
29 Immunodeficiency and Immunoproliferative Diseases   509

Appendix I The Immunological Orchestra   531

Appendix II Chromosome Locations of Some Genes of Immunological Importance   536

Contents

Preface xvii

A Note to the Reader xxi

1 THE CLONAL NATURE OF THE IMMUNE RESPONSE 1

Immunity and Disease 2
Instructive Versus Selective Theories of Antibody
    Formation 4
    Paul Ehrlich and the Side-Chain Theory 4
    Karl Landsteiner and Artificial Antigens 6
    Felix Haurowitz and the Template Theory 7

Niels Jerne, David Talmage, and Macfarlane
    Burnet: Clonal Selection 9
Thomas Kuhn and the Notion of the
    Paradigm 11
The Modern Era 11

PART ONE IMMUNOCHEMISTRY 15

Section I Antigens and Antibodies 16

2 THE NATURE OF ANTIGENS 17

Antigenicity and Immunogenicity 18
Studies with Haptens 18
    Haptens and Carriers 18
    The Specificity of Serological Reactions 19
    Cross Reactivity 22
Antibodies to Proteins 24
INFORMATION BOX 1: BLOOD GROUP
    ANTIGENS 25
    The Roles of Conformation and Amino Acid
    Sequence in Antigenicity 26

The Role of Segmental Mobility 28
The Multideterminant Hypothesis 29
Molecular Mapping of Antigenic
    Determinants 29
Antibodies of Predetermined Specificities 32
    Antibodies to Products of Nucleotide
    Sequence 33
    Antibodies to Predetermined Amino Acid
    Sequences 34

3 THE BASIC IMMUNOGLOBULIN MONOMER 36

Antibodies and Immunoglobulins 37
The Chain Structure of Ig 37
    Early Studies Using Antiserum: Treatment with
    Proteolytic Enzymes 37
    The Use of Myeloma Proteins 39

Chain Dissociation Studies 39
The Hinge Region and Interchain Disulfide
    Bonds 40
Three-Dimensional Structure 40
Domains of the Immunoglobulin Molecule 41

CONTENTS

The Structural Basis of Antibody Diversity 42
    Constant and Variable Regions 42
    Hypervariable Regions 44
Synthesis: The Strategy of Antibody Diversity 45
    Sequence Homology of C_H Regions 47

Nature of the Antigen-Combining Site 48
    Electron Microscopic Studies 48
    Size of the Combining Site 48
    Shape of the Combining Site 49
    X-Ray Diffraction Studies 51

4 HETEROGENEITY OF IMMUNOGLOBULINS 54

Physical Heterogeneity 55
Class (or Isotype) of Immunoglobulins 55
    Definition of Class 55
    Classes, or Isotypes 55
    Subclasses 56
    Common Origin of Immunoglobulin Classes 56
INFORMATION BOX 1: Ig CLASSES AND SUBCLASSES IN SOME VERTEBRATES 58
Properties of Immunoglobulin Classes 59
INFORMATION BOX 2: HUMAN IMMUNOGLOBULINS 60
    Immunoglobulin G 61
    Immunoglobulin M 61
    Immunoglobulin A 62

Immunoglobulin D 64
Immunoglobulin E 65
Genetic Variation in Immunoglobulins (Allotypes and Idiotypes) 66
    Allotypic Variation 66
INFORMATION BOX 3: HUMAN ALLOTYPES 66
INFORMATION BOX 4: RABBIT ALLOTYPES 67
    Idiotypic Variation 67
INFORMATION BOX 5: ALLOTYPES ON C_H REGIONS OF MOUSE Ig 68
    Idiotypes as Markers of Antigen-Combining Sites 69
    Inheritance of Idiotypes 69

5 THE ORGANIZATION OF IMMUNOGLOBULIN GENES 73

The Generation of Diversity 74
    Germ Line versus Somatic Mechanisms 74
    Two Genes, One Polypeptide Chain 75
    Genetic Reorganization 75
METHODS BOX 1: CLONING AN ANTIBODY GENE 77
Mechanisms of Gene Reorganization 79
    V–J Joining Forms the Light Chain Variable Region 79
    V–D–J Joining Forms the Heavy Chain Variable Region 80
    Gene Reorganization Results in Diversity 81
    Combinatorial Diversification 82

    Junctional Site Diversity 83
Constant-Region Genes 86
    Organization of Constant-Region Genes 86
    Formation of a Complete Immunoglobulin Heavy Chain 86
    Class Switching 87
Transcription Enhancement of Immunoglobulin Genes 88
    Enhancer Sequences 88
    Switch and Enhancement in Malignant Transformations 89
Allelic Exclusion 89

6 MONOCLONAL AND HYBRID ANTIBODIES 92

Monoclonal and Polyclonal Antibodies 93
The Principle of Monoclonal Antibody Production 94
    Cell Fusion 94
    Screening the Hybridomas 97

INFORMATION BOX 1: PRINCIPLE OF HAT SELECTION 97
The Production of Hybrid Antibody Molecules 98
Production of Hybrid Immunoglobulin Genes 99

CONTENTS

Section II The Antigen–Antibody Reaction 102

7 THE ANTIGEN–ANTIBODY COMPLEX 103

The Antigen–Antibody Complex 104
Affinity of the Antigen–Antibody Reaction 104
Determining Affinity 105
Antibody Affinity and Valence 107
Heterogeneity of Binding 109
Kinetics of Antigen–Antibody Reactions 110

8 MEASURING ANTIGEN–ANTIBODY REACTIONS 112

The Antigen–Antibody Complex 113
The Precipitin Reaction 113
METHODS BOX 1: QUANTITATIVE PRECIPITIN REACTION 115
Reactions in Gels 116
    The Ouchterlony Assay 116
    The Mancini Assay 116
    Immunoelectrophoresis (IEP) 118
    Western Blotting 120
Agglutination Reactions 112
METHODS BOX 2: RBC TYPING 122
Labeled Antibody Techniques 123
    Primary and Secondary Antibody Methods 123
    Radioactive Labels (RIA) 125
    Enzyme Labels (ELISA) 125
METHODS BOX 3: RADIOIMMUNOASSAYS 126
    Fluorescent labels 127
    Electron-Dense Labels 127
METHODS BOX 4: ENZYME-LINKED IMMUNOSORBANT ASSAYS (ELISA) 128
    Nonspecific Binding to Immunoglobulin 134
    Flow Cytometry 134

9 COMPLEMENT 137

Discovery of the Complement System 138
METHODS BOX 1: THE COMPLEMENT FIXATION TEST 138
The Classical Pathway 142
    The Recognition Unit 142
    The Activation Unit: C4 and C2 144
The Alternate Pathway 147
Activation of the Alternate Pathway 148
Stabilization of the C3bBb Complex 149
The Common Complement Pathway 149
    The Membrane Attack Unit: C5b, C6, C7, C8, C9 149
INFORMATION BOX 1: COMPLEMENT COMPONENTS 151

PART TWO CELLULAR IMMUNOLOGY 155

Section I The Origins and Organization of Lymphoid Tissue 156

10 HEMOPOIESIS 157

Hemopoiesis 158
Assay of Colony Forming Units 159
Single-Cell Origin of Colonies 160
Multipotency of the CFU-S 161
Characteristics of the Hemopoietic Stem Cell 165
Commitment and Differentiation 166
Differentiation of Stem Cells into Progenitor Cells 168
Hemopoietic Inducing Factors 169
INFORMATION BOX 1: MYELOID INDUCING FACTORS 170
Hemopoietic Inducing Microenvironments 172
Mutant Mice and Cloned Tumor Lines 173
Introduction of New Genes into Stems Cells 173
INFORMATION BOX 2: SOME MOUSE MUTANTS OF HEMOPOIETIC DEVELOPMENT 174

CONTENTS

11 LYMPHOCYTES 179

The Origins of Lymphocytes 180
   Derivation of Lymphocytes from the Multipotent Stem Cell 180
   Primary and Secondary Lymphoid Organs 181
B Cells and T Cells 183
   The Concept of Differentiation Antigens 183
Differentiation Antigens on Murine T Cells 184
INFORMATION BOX 1: STUDYING DIFFERENTIATION ANTIGENS WITH ALLOANTIBODIES AND MONOCLONAL ANTIBODIES 185
   Differentiation Antigens on Human T Cells 186
INFORMATION BOX 2: PROPERTIES OF MURINE T CELL DIFFERENTIATION ANTIGENS 187
INFORMATION BOX 3: PROPERTIES OF HUMAN T CELL DIFFERENTIATION ANTIGENS 189
INFORMATION BOX 4: CLUSTERS OF DIFFERENTIATION 190
   Surface Markers on B Cells 191
The Introduction of Lymphocyte Differentiation 192
   T Cell Inducing Factors 192
   Induction of B Cell Differentiation 193
Mitogen Responses of T Cells and B Cells 193

12 ORGANIZATION AND STRUCTURE OF LYMPHOID TISSUE 196

Structure of Lymphoid Organs 197
   The Thymus 197
   The Spleen 200
Lymphatic Vessels and Lymph Nodes 202
Circulation of Lymphocytes 203
B and T Cell Regions of Lymphoid Organs 206

13 THE MAJOR HISTOCOMPATIBILITY COMPLEX 208

The Discovery of the Major Histocompatibility Complex 209
Traits Controlled by the Major Histocompatibility Complex 211
Mapping the MHC Genes by Function and Gene Product 213
Polymorphism of the Major Histocompatibility Complex 214
   MHC, Multigenic and Multiallelic 214
INFORMATION BOX 1: CLASS I DETERMINANTS OF SOME COMMONLY USED MOUSE STRAINS 215
   The Notion of the Haplotype 216
   Public and Private Specificities 216
INFORMATION BOX 2: CLASS II DETERMINANTS OF SOME COMMONLY USED MOUSE STRAINS 217
INFORMATION BOX 3: NEW AND OLD NOMENCLATURE FOR HUMAN LYMPHOCYTE ANTIGENS 218
   Congenic Mice 220
   Production of Congenic Mice 220
Structure of MHC Molecules 222
   Class I Molecules 222
   Class II Molecules 223
Organization of the MHC Genes 224
Recombinant Class I–Class II Molecules 225
Expression of MHC Molecules 226
The Immunoglobulin Superfamily 227
   Sequence Homology between MHC, Immunoglobulin, and Thy 1 227
The T Locus 228
INFORMATION BOX 4: CONTROL OF IMMUNE RESPONSES BY Ir GENES 229

CONTENTS

Section II Cell Cooperation 234

14 THE DIVISION OF LABOR 235

Humoral and Cell-Mediated Immune Responses 236
  The Immunocompetent Cells 236
  Cell-Mediated Responses Defined 237
METHODS BOX 1: DELAYED-TYPE HYPERSENSITIVITY 237
METHODS BOX 2: ALLOGRAFT REJECTION 238
Division of Labor among Cells in the Immune Response 238
  Effect of Neonatal Thymectomy 239
METHODS BOX 3: GRAFT-VS-HOST REACTION 240
METHODS BOX 4: CYTOTOXIC LYMPHOCYTE REACTION 242
METHODS BOX 5: MIXED LYMPHOCYTE REACTION 243
  Effect of Bursectomy 243
The Role of the Macrophage 245
  Antibody Responses In Vitro: The Mosier Experiment 245
  Cytotoxic T Cells 247
  Proliferative Responses to Mitogens 248

15 HELPER AND EFFECTOR CELLS 250

Evidence of Cooperating Cell Populations 251
  Bone Marrow–Thymus Reconstitution: The Claman Experiment 252
  Cell Cooperation in Graft-versus-Host Reaction 254
Evidence for Effector and Helper Cells 255
  Reconstitution after Neonatal Thymectomy: The Mitchell–Miller Experiment 255
The Failure of Allogeneic Bone Marrow–Thymus Reconstitution 259
Varied Nature of Cell-Mediated Responses 261
T Cells are the Effector Cells in Cell-Mediated Responses 261
Evidence for Cell Cooperation in the Generation of CTL 262
Helper and Effector Cells 263

16 HELPER AND EFFECTOR DETERMINANTS 267

Antibody Formation 268
  The Carrier Effect 268
  Adoptive Transfer of the Carrier Effect 270
  Overcoming the Carrier Effect by Carrier Priming 270
  Hapten-Reactive and Carrier–Reactive Lymphocytes: The Raff Experiment 273
  Overcoming the Carrier Effect with Allogeneic Cells: The Allogeneic Effect 275
Cell-Mediated Responses 275
  MLR and CTL Responses and MHC Antigens 276
  The "Three-Cell Experiment" 278

17 MHC RESTRICTION 280

MHC Restriction in Antibody Formation 281
  Mitchell–Miller Revisited: The Need for Syngeneic Cells 281
  Population Failure in Nude Mice 281
  Claman Revisited: The Need For I Region (Class II) MHC Identity 282
MHC Restriction in Cell–Mediated Responses 284
The Zinkernagel-Doherty-Shearer Phenomenon 285
Site of Restriction 286
Compatibility between Responder and Stimulator 286
Lyt Phenotype and Recognition of MHC Class 288

CONTENTS

Cell Interaction Molecules 289
Studies Using Chimeras 290
   Allophenic Chimeras 290
   Bone Marrow Chimeras 292
Experiments Using $P_1 + P_2 \rightarrow F_1$: Evidence for Histoincompatible Cooperation 293
Experiments Using $F_1 \rightarrow P_1$ Adaptive Differentiation 295

18 ACQUISITION OF THE RESTRICTION REPERTOIRE 299

MHC-Restriction and Accessory Cells 300
   Macrophage Activation of T Cells 300
   Role of MHC Haplotype of Macrophages and T Cells 300
   Two Populations of T Cells in the F_1 302
   MHC Restriction is for an Accessory Cell 304
Synthesis: MHC Restriction is Self:Anti-Self 307
The Thymus as a Site of Acquistion of MHC Restriction 309
   Studies with Thymus Chimeras 309
   Studies with Nude Mice 310
   Intrathymic and Extrathymic Acquisition of Class I and Class II MHC Restriction 313
Synthesis: Selection versus Education in the Thymus 314

Section III Receptors and Signals 317

19 ANTIGEN–SPECIFIC RECEPTORS ON LYMPHOCYTES 318

The B Cell Receptor 319
   Surface Ig Receptors on B Cells 319
   Isotypes of Surface Immunoglobulin 320
   Mobility of sIg: Patching and Capping 321
The T Cell Receptor 321
   Absence of sIg on T Cells 323
   MHC Molecules and Antigen Binding T Cells 325
Models for the T Cell Receptor 327
   Single Receptor versus Dual Recognition 327
   Ruling Out the Two Independent Receptors Model 327
   Unanswered Questions 328
An Immunological Approach to the Nature of the T Cell Receptor 329
   Anti-Idiotypic Antibody against the Receptor: The Classical Approach 329
   The Use of T Cell Clones 331
   Monoclonal Antibody against the Receptor: The Modern Approach 332
   Two-Chained T Cell Receptor 334
   Resemblance of β Chain to Immunoglobulin 335
   T3, A Differentiation Antigen 336

20 GENETIC ORGANIZATION OF RECEPTORS 338

Organization of Receptor Genes in B Cells 339
   Synthesis of Surface Immunoglobulin and Secreted Immunoglobulin 339
Organization of the T Cell Receptor Genes 340
   Isolation of cDNA Clones: The Subtraction Method 341
   Evidence of Gene Rearrangement 343
   V, C, J, and D Regions in the β Chain 343
   Three Classes of T Cell Receptor Genes 345
   Chromosome Locations of T Cell Receptor Genes 346
Generation of Diversity in T Cell Receptor Genes 346
   The Generation of Diversity 348
   A Caution to the Reader and a Disclaimer from the Author 348
   Developmental Expression of the Genes 348
   Structure of the Receptor in the Membrane 349
   Some Alternative Views 349

CONTENTS

21 INTERLEUKINS 354

T Cell Activation 355
    Factors Produced by T Cells and Macrophages: Lymphokines and Monokines 355
INFORMATION BOX 1: THE MANY NAMES OF CYTOKINES 355
INFORMATION BOX 2: PROPERTIES OF IL-1 AND IL-2 356
    The Discovery of IL-1 357
    Production of IL-1 by Macrophages 357
    The Discovery of IL-2 359
    Production of IL-2 by T Cells 360
    Roles of Adherent and Nonadherent Cells in IL-2 Release 360
    The Interleukin Cascade 362
    IL-2 Receptors 362
    Induction of IL-2 Receptors by Antigen or Mitogen 363
INFORMATION BOX 3: THE IL-2 RECEPTOR 364
Synthesis: Interleukins and T Cell Proliferation 366
INFORMATION BOX 4: THE CELL CYCLE 367
B Cell Activation 368
    Need for Receptor Cross-Linking 368
    B Cell Growth Factor 369
    Interleukin 4 370
The Consequences of Activation 372
    B Cell Activation 373
    T Cell Activation 375

Section IV Regulation of the Immune Response 378

22 THE NETWORK 379

Epitopes, Paratopes and Idiotypes: The Language of the Network 380
The Internal Image 381
    Cross-Reactivity Between Paratopes and Epitopes: The Generative Grammar of the Network 383
Testing the Network Theory 384
The Production of Auto–Anti-Idiotype Antibodies 385
The Regulatory Role of Anti-Idiotype Antibody 386
The Ability of Anti-Idiotype to Mimic Antigen 388

23 SUPPRESSOR CELLS 393

The Discovery of Suppressor T Cells 394
    Nonspecific Suppression 396
    Allotype-Specific and Idiotype-Specific Suppressor Cells 397
    Antigen-Specific Suppressor Cells 398
Properties of Suppressor T Cells 400
    Lyt Profile 400
    The I–J Enigma 400
    Antigen Binding by T_s 403
    Suppressor T Cell Receptor 404
Suppressor and Helper Determinants 404
    Induction of Suppressor and Helper Cells 405
    Need for a Triad of Determinants 407
Soluble Suppressor Factors 409
    Antigen-Specific Suppressor Factors 409
    Nature of Antigen-Specific Suppressor Factors 410
Regulatory Circuits 411
    Cell Interactions in the Induction of Suppressor T Cells 411
    Soluble Factors in the Regulatory Circuit 411
    Contrasuppressor Cells 411

CONTENTS

24 IMMUNE TOLERANCE: THE PROBLEM OF SELF-NONSELF DISCRIMINATION 415

Self and Nonself 416
    The Concept of the Self-Marker 416
    The Experimental Induction of Tolerance in the Newborn 417
    The Triplett Experiment 419
    Naturally-Occurring Self-reactivity 420
Induction of Tolerance in the Adult 421
    Immunological Paralysis 421
    Induction of Adult Tolerance 422

Mechanisms of Immune Tolerance 426
    Induction of Tolerance in B Cells and T Cells 426
    Clonal Deletion, Clonal Abortion, Clonal Anergy, or Tolerant Cells? 429
    The Veto Concept 432
    Suppressor Cells in Tolerance 433
Synthesis: Recognition and Response in MHC Restriction and Tolerance 433

PART THREE IMMUNITY AND IMMUNOPATHOLOGY 437

25 IMMUNITY, INFECTIONS, AND TUMORS 439

The Response to External Invaders: Host–Parasite Relationships 440
    Factors Affecting the Host-Parasite Relationship 441
The Inflammatory Response 442
    The Cardinal Signs of Inflammation 442
    Granulocytes in Inflammation 443
    Phagocytosis 444
The Interplay Between Nonspecific and Specific Immunity 446
Opsonization 447
    Complement–Mediated Cytolysis 448
    Antibody-Dependent, Cell-Mediated Cytotoxicity (ADCC) 449

Responses to Viral Infections 449
    Interferon 449
    Antibodies and Cytotoxic Cells 450
Responses to Parasite Infections 451
The Response to Internal Invaders: The Response to Tumors 451
    Immune Surveillance 451
    Tumor-Specific Antigens 452
INFORMATION BOX 1: CANCER TERMINOLOGY 453
    Immune Suppression and Cancer 455
    Natural Killer Cells in Tumor Immunity 456
    Tumor Immunotherapy 458

26 HYPERSENSITIVITY 461

The Nature of Hypersensitivity 462
    Origins of the Idea That an Immune Response Can Be Harmful 462
    The Need for Sensitization 463
    The Gell and Coombs Classification 464
Type I Reactions: Immediate Hypersensitivity 465
    Atopic Diseases 465
    Atopy 466

    Mast Cell Degranulation 466
    The IgE Receptor and Its Regulation 471
Type II Reactions: Cytolytic Reactions 474
Type III Reactions: Antigen–Antibody Complex Diseases 475
METHODS BOX 1: DETERMINING IgE LEVELS 476
Type IV Reactions: Delayed-Type Hypersensitivity 478

CONTENTS

27 AUTOIMMUNITY 481

Horror Autotoxicus Revisited 482
    Recognition versus Reaction 482
    Organ-Specific and Non–Organ-specific
        Autoimmune Diseases 483
Antibody-Mediated, Organ-Specific Autoimmune
    Diseases 483
    Anti-Receptor Diseases 483
    Autoimmune Thyroiditis 489
    Hemolytic Anemia 489
Non–Antibody-Mediated, Organ-Specific
    Autoimmune Diseases Associated with
    Antibody 490

Systemic Lupus Erythematosus 490
    Animal Models of SLE 491
    Rheumatoid Arthritis 492
T Cell-Mediated Autoimmunity: Autoimmune
    Demyelinating Diseases 493
    Multiple Sclerosis 493
    Experimental Autoimmune Encephalitis 494
Self-Reactivity in the Absence of Pathology 494

28 TRANSPLANTATION 497

Graft Rejection as an Immune Phenomenon 498
The Laws of Transplantation 499
Problems in Human Transplantation 501
    Matching Donor and Recipients and
        Immunosuppression 501

Pretreatment of the Recipient 504
The Mechanism of Graft Rejection 505
Types of Transplants 505

29 IMMUNODEFICIENCY AND IMMUNOPROLIFERATIVE DISEASES 509

Immunodeficiency Diseases 510
Congenital Immunodeficiency Diseases 510
    Immunodeficiency Diseases as Defects in
        Differentiation 510
    Defects of Stem Cells and Progenitor Cells 510
    Deficiencies of B Cell Origin 513
    Deficiencies of T Cell Origin 514
    Disorders of Granulocytes 515
Acquired Immunodeficiencies 515
    Common, Variable Unclassifiable
        Immunodeficiency (Acquired
        Hypogammaglobulinemia) 516
Acquired Immune Deficiency Syndrome: AIDS 516

The First Appearances of AIDS 516
    Immunology of AIDS 518
    Risk Groups and Modes of Transmission 520
    Etiology 521
    Some Important Questions 522
Therapy for AIDS 522
Lymphoproliferative Diseases 524
    Leukemias and Lymphomas 524
    Leukemias 524
    Lymphomas 527
    Non-Hodgkins Lymphomas: T Cell Tumors 528
    Non-Hodgkins Lymphomas: B Cell Tumors 529

Appendix I: The Immunological Orchestra 531

Appendix II: Chromosome Locations of Some Genes of Immunological Importance 536

Index 537

Preface

This book is an extension of both my earlier book, *The Cellular Basis of the Immune Response*, and my personality. My aim is to convey to the nonimmunologist the complexity, logic, and above all the beauty of the immune system. The purpose of any textbook in the sciences should also be to teach the mode of thinking of the discipline and to convey the excitement that the participants in the field feel as they attempt to uncover the beauty, logic, and complexity. As I did in *The Cellular Basis*, and as I do in all of my teaching, I have attempted to define the problems of the field and then to lead the student through the reasoning that led to the solution. This means that it will be very difficult to go through this book with a Hi-liter marking pen to cram for a machine-scored exam. This method of teaching requires active participation because, God knows, the doing of science is not a passive activity. As I mention in the Note to the Reader, I have made every attempt to help organize the reader's thoughts by breaking the book into manageable sections, so little energy has to be expended in trying to figure out where one is.

This book, though covering a much wider range of material than *The Cellular Basis*, like its predecessor is not a compendium of facts. It is meant to prepare the reader to read the immunology literature so that he/she can follow the continuing progress in the field. It most certainly is not meant to be used only by immunologists. The mode of thought that immunologists use is not unique. Each discipline solves its problems with different tools, but the practice is the same: defining the problem, designing the experiment, and interpreting the results in order to ask the next question.

In *Chance and Necessity*, Jacques Monod says that anyone who does not use an analytic or reductionist view to approach systems as complex as living beings "is doomed to fail in (the) attempt to reduce the properties of a very complex organism to the 'sum' of the properties of its parts." I have taken a reductionist view of the teaching of immunology, attempting to break the subject down into concepts, then describing the concepts in such a way that the whole picture emerges. When a complex subject is divided into its component parts, the viewpoint of

PREFACE

the author always comes through. With this come all of the ambiguities, redundancies, and deficiencies of that viewpoint. A case in point is quoted by Borges in *Other Inquisitions 1937–1952*:

> These ambiguities, redundancies, and deficiencies recall those attributed by Dr. Franz Kuhn to a certain Chinese encyclopedia entitled *Celestial Emporium of Benevolent Knowledge*. On those remote pages it is written that animals are divided into (a) those that belong to the Emperor, (b) embalmed ones, (c) those that are trained, (d) suckling pigs, (e) mermaids, (f) fabulous ones, (g) stray dogs, (h) those that are included in this classification, (i) those that tremble as if they were mad, (j) innumerable ones, (k) those drawn with a very fine camel's brush, (l) others, (m) those that have just broken a flower vase, (n) those that resemble flies at a distance.

Because this book is not a compendium of facts I have ordered the subject of immunology in what I think is the clearest sequence for approaching the major questions of immunology. Others, like the author of the *Celestial Emporium*, will have other viewpoints.

Contrary to the generally held belief, I am not an expert in all aspects of immunology. My own work has been in cell interactions and surface molecules and is currently in the differentiation of stem cells. I needed help from many, many people to attempt this expanded book. The following are some of the people who, over the last three years, have been of great help to me in preparing this book. I have relentlessly and sometimes cruelly picked their brains to find their views on a field, get preprints, have drafts read, and find my way out of an occasional morass. I apologize to the many people whose names I have neglected to include in this list; if the book stinks, you will be relieved not to have been associated with it.

> Joe Albright, David Asai, Don Bailey, Dave Benjamin, Eli Benjamini, Jay Berzofsky, John Cambier, Henry Claman, Carol Cowing, Harvey Cantor, Dick Dutton, Marc Feldman, Doug Green, Gene Goldwasser, Allison Hall, Lee Hood, Richard Hodes, Chris Henney, Niels Jerne, Jack Johnson, Dave Katz, John Kappler, Rich Lerner, Av Mitchison, Pippa Marack, John Najarian, Judith Owen, Martin Raff, Yvonne Rosenberg, Osias Stutman, Eli Sercarz, Liz Simpson, Kendall Smith, George Snell, Susie Swain, Al Singer, Don Shreffler, Ed Simon, Irwin Tessman, Leon Weiss, Dorothea Zucker-Franklin, Maurizio Zanetti.

I am especially indebted to Larry Draper and Lee Metcalf for their thorough critical readings of the entire manuscript, which caught so many inelegancies and stupidities. In the last book I blamed any faults on other people; Larry and Lee must be excused from any blame because I did not always take their advice. As usual, the staff of the Jackson

PREFACE

Laboratory in Bar Harbor were wonderfully helpful, as were the librarians at Case Western Reserve University Medical Schools.

This book was harder for me to write than *The Cellular Basis of the Immune Response*, partly because the field has changed, and partly because I included so much more of immunology in this book. But to a large degree I must admit the difficulty was because both immunology and I have entered middle age and we both are more difficult to deal with than we used to be. Others had to bear the burden of this condition and, while the reader may not be interested in my problems, I feel honor-bound to tell those who suffered that I am aware of their kindness, devotion, and anger:

The expanded crew at Sinauer Associates, who have had to deal with a bigger book and a more crotchety author (especially Joe Vesely, who I finally pushed to the edge of not smiling), and, of course, that surehanded shortstop and trusted friend, Andy Sinauer, who charted the course of this adventure and only appeared to be coming close to abandoning ship. I hope the case of scotch will put me back in the good graces of this beleaguered group.

And, of course, my family: my wife, Constance, who put aside the galley proofs of her own first book and the manuscript of her second to listen to my woes and never hesitated to comfort, humor, or correct egregious solecisms; my son Jon, who had the good sense to leave home during the ordeal; and my son Mark, who wished he could have followed his brother but, finding himself stuck, was a constant source of joy and occasional editorial help; my mother, who naturally thinks that her genius son deserves all of this devotion; and, finally, Terasita Pagan, who ran the lab and delivered Deborita as if all were normal.

But even with this difficulty, in retrospect it has been a joy to do this book, because it has given me a chance to rethink the field I have worked in all my scientific life and love so much. Twenty years ago neither I nor any of my contemporaries could have predicted the wonderous twists and turns the field would take, and I don't think that many of us could have guessed the real beauty of the immune system that has been revealed. If the reader comes away from this book feeling half the wonder and joy about the immune system that those of us who have been participants feel, then my little problems in writing the book will seem as nothing.

E. S. GOLUB

A Note to the Reader

> I don't know what's the matter with people: they don't learn by understanding; they learn by rote or something. Their knowledge is so fragile.
> —Richard Feynman, *Surely You're Joking, Mr. Feynman*, p. 23.

The reader of this book should be aware at the outset that I feel very strongly that the way to learn science is not to learn a bunch of facts. Science is a process of solving problems to figure out how the world works. And the way to really learn science so that the knowledge is not fragile is to immerse oneself in the process. I have tried to fashion this book according to that passion. Certainly, one needs to know facts in science. But I strongly believe that we need them only to carry the process further. Because our understanding of the world changes, every scientist gets only a temporary view of what we think the world is like. To master the facts of the current view of the world is, to me, a rather futile pastime if one is not also gaining the ability to follow future changes in a given field.

As much as possible I have tried to organize immunology along *conceptual* lines. The pattern of this approach will become obvious as the reader moves through the text. In order to maintain the continuity of thought, I have included Methods Boxes and Information Boxes along the way. The Methods Boxes will give the reader who needs it an understanding of the method being used in an experiment described in the text. The Information Boxes are for reference if the reader needs or wants more facts.

I have tried to organize the book into conceptual blocks, which are clearly marked by typography. The plan is that every reader should know where he/she is in the unfolding saga. For as much of the material as I could I have begun by stating the problem as it was viewed in the last decade, which for immunologists is the distant past, and then following the path of experiments that have lead us to the present view. But as I said, the present view is temporary, and my hope is that by following the flow of the ideas and experiments the student will be able to understand the next phase as it unfolds.

A NOTE TO THE READER

Of course, one can choose to read only the "bottom line" and buy the next edition of the book to see how things have developed. That will please me, as I use the royalties to pay my sons' college tuitions. It will not, however, please the people who pay the tuition of students who use this book in a course. If you won't learn the process for me, do it for them!

CHAPTER 1
THE CLONAL NATURE OF THE IMMUNE RESPONSE

Overview In his book *The Structure of Scientific Revolutions*, Thomas Kuhn elaborated the notion of the paradigm. A paradigm is a concept or fact that is an underlying assumption in a scientific field. Therefore, when experiments are designed, it is not the paradigm, but rather some hypothesis consistent with the paradigm, that is being tested. The underlying assumption of modern immunology is that the cells that carry out the reactions leading to specific immune responses are preprogrammed to respond to the material (called antigen) that induces the response. Antigen does not instruct the immune system in what specificity to generate; rather, it selects those cells displaying a receptor of the appropriate specificity and induces them to proliferate and differentiate, resulting in expansion of specific clones of reactive cells. This process is called clonal selection.

All the experiments designed to ask how the immune system works are designed with this understanding, which is so ingrained in immunological thought that we will not refer to it as the clonal selection theory (because a theory is something that is still being tested), but merely as Clonal Selection. Throughout this book we will assume its validity and follow its development from the origin of immunology in folk medicine to the modern era of molecular biology. And although this chapter does not convey scientific "facts" in the manner usual in textbooks, the reader is urged to read it because of the importance of the idea of clonal selection to the understanding of immunology.

CHAPTER ONE

Immunity and Disease

The study of immunology is to a great extent the study of the cell biology of lymphocytes. It is a discipline that, using the tools of cell and molecular biology, asks questions about self:nonself discrimination, cellular recognition, and genetic organization. As the reader will soon learn, it requires an interest in and a knowledge of many aspects of modern biology and biochemistry. Yet the beginnings of immunology are to be found in the ancient folk observation that people, having once recovered from a disease, do not get the disease again.[1]

> Yet still the ones who felt most pity for the sick and the dying were those who had had the plague themselves and had recovered from it. They knew what it was like and at the same time felt themselves to be safe, *for no one caught the disease twice*, or, if he did, the second attack was never fatal. Such people were congratulated on all sides, and they themselves were so elated at the time of their recovery that *they fondly imagined that they could never die of any other disease in the future*. [Thucydides, *The Peloponnesian War* (italics added)]

The fortunate few who recovered from the plague conceived of this *immunitas* as a boon from the gods. If a benevolent deity spared you from one plague, they reasoned, it was only natural to assume that you were to be spared from *all* diseases. Of course, people learned, over a period of time, that this was not the case. Immunity from one disease did not grant you immunity to another; the immunity was *specific*, whatever (or whoever) was responsible for it.

Because the concept of specific immunity came to be firmly implanted in folklore, it is not surprising that eventually it was given a practical application in some societies. (It is equally inter-

---

[1] Even the name immunology comes from this experience. The Latin words *immunitas* and *immunis* derive from the Roman notion of being exempt from service (usually military) to the state. Art Silverstein, who has arguably become the foremost historian of immunology, points out that the word was probably first used in the context in which we use it today by the Roman Marcus Annaeus Lucanus (A.D. 39–65) in his poem "Pharsalia" to describe the resistance to snakebite of the Psylli tribe of North Africa [Silverstein, A. M. and A. A. Bialasiewicz (1980) *Cell. Immunol.* 51: 151].

THE CLONAL NATURE OF THE IMMUNE RESPONSE

esting to ask why it was *not* put into practice in others.) We know that the Chinese inoculated healthy people with material removed from a pustule of a person suffering from smallpox. According to a letter from an English trader of the East India Company in 1700, the method involved "opening the pustules of one who has the Small Pox ripe upon them and drying up the Matter with a little Cotton, ... and afterwards put it up the nostrils of those they would infect." The letter was communicated to the Royal Society that same year; but the members of this august body failed to follow the suggestion of their compatriot even though smallpox was then a scourge in England.

Lady Mary Montagu, the wife of the British ambassador to Constantinople in the early 1700s, is usually credited with introducing the practice of inoculation against smallpox into "civilized" society. In a much-quoted letter to her friend Sarah Chiswell in 1717, she wrote: "I am going to tell you a thing that I am sure will make you wish yourself here. The small-pox, so fatal, and so general amongst us, is here entirely harmless by the invention of *ingrafting* ... I am patriot enough to take pains to bring this useful invention into fashion in England and I should not fail to write to some of our doctors very particularly about it, if I knew any one of them that I thought had virtue enough to destroy such a considerable branch of their revenue for the good of mankind!" In 1718, while still in Constantinople, the six-year-old Montagu son was inoculated by Charles Maitland, the surgeon to the embassy. Upon her return to London, Lady Montagu attempted to get the same Dr. Maitland, now retired and also returned to England, to inoculate her three-year-old daughter with pustules from people afflicted in the smallpox epidemic of 1721. But Maitland consented to perform the deed, which he had done in the East with no apparent reservations, only if outside physicians were present as witnesses. (Perhaps we see here not only the origins of vaccination but also an incident in the early history of malpractice suits.) Witnesses were found, and the child was successfully inoculated; in fact, one witness was so impressed that he had the only one of his children who had not died of the pox similarly inoculated. But the practice of inoculating healthy individuals with pustules from infected ones did not gain favor in England despite further testing.[2] Edward Jenner introduced a safer (and esthetically more pleasing) method of vaccination in 1798. It is part of medical lore that Jenner had noted that milkmaids had the scars of the pox on their hands and not on their faces. Milkmaids themselves knew that because they were infected with cowpox they did not get smallpox; and Jenner, reasoning from this experience, intentionally induced a mild case of cowpox in his patients in order to protect them from from smallpox.[3]

The turn of the century is considered the Golden Era of microbiology. Through the work of Pasteur, Koch, and their schools, the germ theory of disease became firmly established and the causative agents of many diseases were isolated. It was also the Golden Era of immunizations: these same people found that specific immunity could be developed in humans and animals to most of the organisms that cause disease. The agent responsible for the induced immunity was found to be a substance in the serum of the blood called ANTIBODY. Antibodies appeared in the serum after inoculation with the organisms. (Agents that induce the appearance of antibodies were called ANTIGENS.) The field of immunology arose first to develop these new immunization procedures, and it gradually became devoted to explaining the nature of the antibodies and the mechanism by which antigen induced their appearance.

Instructive Versus Selective Theories of Antibody Formation

Paul Ehrlich and the Side-Chain Theory

Because immunology was originally concerned with the prevention of disease, it is not surprising that the first theory to explain the phenomenon of specific

---

[2] The complex reasons for this are discussed in Silverstein and Miller (1981), The royal experiment on immunity: 1721–1722. *Cell. Immunol.* 61: 437.

[3] (Friends have urged me to include this, the most popular footnote from *The Cellular Basis of the Immune Response*.) The Dutch scientist–musician G. J. van den Engh has pointed out to me the likelihood that milkmaids were generally known to be something special. The number of milkmaids who are chased through fields singing "fa la la" in English folk tunes far exceeds that of scullery maids, nannies, or seamstresses.

5
THE CLONAL NATURE OF THE IMMUNE RESPONSE

antibody formation was fashioned with immunity to disease in mind. Paul Ehrlich (1854–1915), who was one of the great thinkers in all of biomedicine, presented the first theory of antibody formation in the Croonian Lecture of 1900. Ehrlich realized that the antibodies in the serum must come from cells and postulated the SIDE CHAIN THEORY as an explanation. According to the side chain theory, every cell capable of synthesizing antibody (the exact cells were not known at the time) has on its surface an array of "side chains," each of which is able to react with a different specific antigen (Figure 1). No doubt Ehrlich developed this theory with

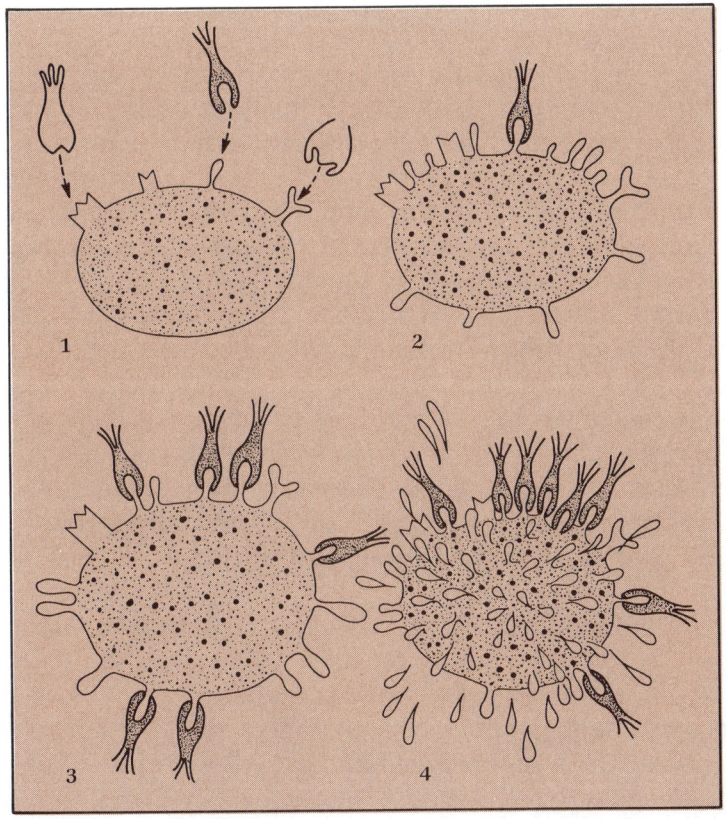

FIGURE 1   SIDE-CHAIN THEORY
Paul Ehrlich's side-chain theory for antibody production. [From Ehrlich (1900) *Proc. Roy. Soc. B.* 66, 424]

infectious microbes in mind. He assumed that each cell has a side chain for the array of microbial antigens to which the individual can produce antibody: for example, tetanus toxin, and the organisms that cause whooping cough, syphilis, and tuberculosis. When the specific agent (antigen) infected the body, it reacted with the *specific* side chain on the cell. This interaction between side chain and infectious agent (which in modern terms would be described as an interaction between a receptor and a ligand) somehow caused the cell to cease producing all of the other side chains and initiate production of only the specific side chain with which the agent had interacted. Eventually, however, the cell overproduced this side chain and the excess appeared in the serum as antibody.

Note, first of all, that the essential part of the theory is that all of the side chains the cell can produce are *predetermined*. The infectious agent *selects* the specific side chain; it has no role in instructing the cell how to make that side chain. Obviously, this theory requires that all of the agents to which the organism can make antibody are represented on the surface of each antibody-producing cell. This theory is tenable if there are a reasonably small number of agents to which the animal makes antibody.

But at about the same time that Ehrlich was formulating his theory, others were showing that animals made perfectly fine antibody responses to nonpathogenic substances such as foreign red blood cells. In fact, it was soon learned that the easiest way to study the immune response was with these innocuous agents because they could be used with no harm to investigator or animal and provided a perfect surrogate for the infectious agents.

Karl Landsteiner and Artificial Antigens

The side chain theory was the dominant (and virtually the only) theory for many years. It fell out of favor for many reasons, but in retrospect the work of Karl Landsteiner ought to have been the most significant. Landsteiner (1868–1943) was a pathologist–chemist who won the Nobel prize for his work on red blood cell antigens. In Chapter 2 we will discuss his work with haptens—small molecules which can initiate an immune response when they are attached to carrier molecules. Landsteiner was able to raise antibodies against simple

THE CLONAL NATURE OF THE IMMUNE RESPONSE

compounds such as nitrophenyl. But he found that an alteration in the position of the nitro group resulted in unique antibodies. Thus he could get specific antibodies to ortho-, meta-, or para-nitrophenyl. Moreover, he could get antibodies to arsenate as well as to a vast array of other groups conjugated to carriers. If one can go into the laboratory and synthesize almost any compound, conjugate it to a carrier protein and get antibodies against it, at some point one must realize that there will not be enough side chains to react with all possible antigens.

Felix Haurowitz and the Template Theory

In 1931 a new theory appeared on the scene. Its authors were Friedrich Breinl and Felix Haurowitz, both working in Prague. Breinl was a young virologist who had spent a few years at the Rockefeller Institute in New York, where he became fascinated with Landsteiner's work. Haurowitz was a protein chemist who worked on hemoglobin. When Breinl returned to Prague, he interested Haurowitz in the antibody problem.[4]

They immunized rabbits with hemoglobin and attempted to analyze the amino acid composition of the antibodies that were produced. In 1930 this was a tedious and inexact procedure, but they concluded that there was no difference between the amino acid composition of the protein molecules in serum before or after immunization. They reasoned that the difference between a normal molecule and an antibody molecule must be in the arrangement of the amino acids or the shape of the molecule. They reasoned further that, because the difference between a molecule with antibody activity and one without it was the fact that antigen had been introduced into the animal with the antibody mol-

---

[4] In an interview that I conducted with Haurowitz on his eighty-first birthday in 1976, he described the start of the short collaboration. "His [Breinl's] enthusiasm was infectious and, well, he declared he would introduce me to immunological matters. He would immunize animals... inject some of the antigens which I would supply him. He would bleed the animals, send me serum and I would try to isolate the antibodies. I remember he said, 'Haurowitz, we *must* find out what antibodies are!' Well, I said, I will try my best." Breinl died a few years later in a laboratory accident, and Haurowitz went on to devote his entire career to the study of antibody molecules. At 91 he still comes to his laboratory every day and still ponders the nature of the mechanism of antibody formation.

ecules, antigen must *instruct* the cell about the specificity of the antibody.

Breinl and Haurowitz postulated that the antigen acts as a *template*; for example, each acidic amino acid in the antigen will be reflected as a basic group in the antibody molecule, and vice versa. This theory is fundamentally different from the selective theory because in it the cell that synthesizes the antibody molecule is not preprogrammed to make the antibody; rather, it makes "blank" molecules whose specificity is imposed by the antigen. Rather than a selective theory, the template theory is an *instructive* theory of antibody formation.

The publication in German of the paper of Breinl and Haurowitz coincided with the formulation of a very similar theory by two Americans, Alexander and Mudd. The great chemist Linus Pauling also became interested in the problem and made the theory more accessible to a wider scientific audience (Figure 2). It quickly supplanted the side-chain theory and even influenced the development of early theories that attempted to explain regulatory phenomena in microbial systems. It was only when modern molecular biology began, with the understanding of the "trin-

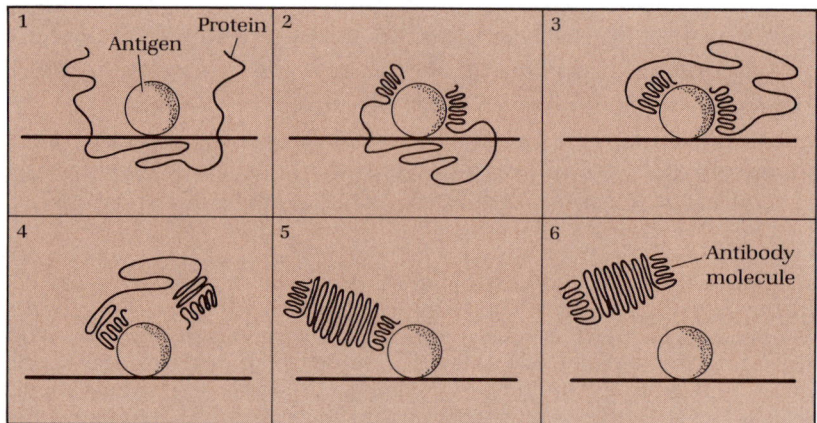

FIGURE 2 DIRECT TEMPLATE THEORY
Linus Pauling's direct template theory. [From Pauling (1940) *J. Amer. Chem. Soc.* 62, 2643]

THE CLONAL NATURE OF THE IMMUNE RESPONSE

ity" (DNA, RNA, peptide), that the instructive theories had to be abandoned.

Niels Jerne, David Talmage, and Macfarlane Burnet: Clonal Selection

With the realization that the amino acid sequence and shape of proteins were the result of the nucleotide sequence of the genes in which they were encoded, the instructive model of antibody formation became difficult to defend. Niels Jerne, probably as a result of the influence of Max Delbrück and the Phage Group, evolved a new incarnation of the selective theory, which he called the NATURAL SELECTION THEORY. Here is Jerne's reminiscence about his insight.

> "Can the truth (*the capacity to synthesize antibody*) be learned? If so, it must be assumed not to pre-exist; to be learned, it must be acquired. We are thus confronted with the difficulty to which Socrates calls attention in Meno (Socrates, 375 B.C.), namely that it makes as little sense to search for what one does not know as to search for what one knows; what one knows one cannot search for, since one knows it already, and what one does not know one cannot search for since one does not even know what to search for. Socrates resolves this difficulty by postulating that learning is nothing but recollection. The truth (*the capability to synthesize an antibody*) cannot be brought in, but was already inherent."

> The above paragraph is a translation of the first lines of Soren Kierkegaard's "Philosophical Bits or a Bit of Philosophy" (Kierkegaard, 1844). By replacing the word "truth" by the italicized words, the statement can be made to present the logical basis of the selective theories of antibody formation. Or, in the parlance of Molecular Biology: synthetic potentialities cannot be imposed upon nucleic acid, but must pre-exist.

> I do not know whether reverberations of Kierkegaard contributed to the idea of a selective mechanism of antibody formation that occurred to me one evening in March 1954, as I was walking home in Copenhagen from the Danish State Serum Institute to Amaliegade. The train of thought went like this: the only property that all antigens share is that they can attach to the combining site of an appropriate antibody molecule; this attachment must, therefore, be a crucial step in the sequence of events by which the introduction of an antigen into an animal leads to antibody formation; a million structurally different antibody-combining sites would suffice to explain structural specificity; if all 10^{17} gammaglobulin molecules per ml of blood are

antibodies, they must include a vast number of different combining sites, because otherwise normal serum would show a high titer against all usual antigens; three mechanisms must be assumed: (1) a random mechanism for ensuring the limited synthesis of antibody molecules possessing all possible combining sites, in the absence of antigen, (2) a purging mechanism for repressing the synthesis of such antibody molecules that happen to fit to auto-antigens, and (3) a selective mechanism for promoting the synthesis of those antibody molecules that make the best fit to any antigen entering the animal. The framework of the theory was complete before I had crossed Knippelsbridge. I decided to let it mature and to preserve it for a first discussion with Max Delbrück on our freighter trip to the U.S.A., planned for that summer. [Niels K. Jerne, 1966. The natural selection theory of antibody formation: ten years later. In *Phage and the Origin of Molecular Biology*, Cold Spring Harbor Laboratory, New York, p. 301.]

The natural selection theory Jerne devised was based upon the fact that all animals have detectable levels of antibody to a wide array of antigens in their serum despite the fact that they have not been intentionally immunized to these antigens. Jerne postulated that antigen enters the system and reacts with one of these "natural antibody" molecules in the serum. The complex of antigen and antibody is then transported to a cell, and this cell is induced to produce more of the antibody. The important point here is that Jerne has returned to a selective theory: antigen is the selective agent.[5]

In Denver in 1957, David Talmage pointed out that Jerne's theory was a modification of the side-chain theory and suggested that it would be improved if the selective elements were cellular. In Melbourne, F. M. Burnet, who had been at work on a similar theory at the time, then introduced what he called the CLONAL SELECTION THEORY. He found that the "major objection [to the Jerne theory] is the absence of any precedent for, and the intrinsic unlikelihood, of the suggestion, that a molecule of partially

---

[5] "The crucial point of the natural-selection theory is the postulate that the introduction of antibody molecules into appropriate cells can be the signal for the production of more of their kind. This notion is unfamiliar." [N. K. Jerne, (1955) The natural-selection theory of antibody formation. *PNAS* 41: 849.] Even though the theory is a return to *selection* explanations, Jerne apparently didn't know of the Ehrlich theory because it is not quoted in his paper.

11
THE CLONAL NATURE OF THE IMMUNE RESPONSE

denatured antibody could stimulate a cell, into which it had been taken, to produce a series of replicas of the molecule." He modified the natural selection theory by having the selection occur between the antigen and the cell that produces the antibody. The role of antigen was to select the proper clone of lymphocytes. In his theory, a given lymphocyte has the ability to produce antibodies of one (or at most a few) specificities. In addition, it expresses antibody on its surface which acts as a receptor so that the reaction between the antigen and the surface antibody causes the cell to proliferate. In this way a "clone" of the cells is generated and produces more antibodies of that specificity.

Thomas Kuhn and the Notion of the Paradigm — With only slight modification, clonal selection has passed from the status of theory to paradigm. According to Thomas Kuhn in *The Structure of Scientific Revolutions*, a paradigm is a commonly held belief among scientists of a given discipline. It need not be correct, only accepted. Scientific progress, according to Kuhn, comes from the changing of the paradigm. Paradigms are not changed lightly, but when they do change there is a revolution—hence the title of his book. Kuhn also argues that, because the paradigm is assumed to be correct, all experiments are carried out within the confines of the paradigm. In this book we will be assuming the correctness of clonal selection and the reader will see that the explanations of the immune response are all fashioned around this paradigm.

The Modern Era

The acceptance of clonal selection as the underlying paradigm of immunology allowed the phenomena observed by generations of immunologists to be put into a framework that had the promise of giving it coherence. It was fortunate that this new paradigm came at a time when technical and conceptual advances in biochemistry and cell biology allowed the generations of immunologists who followed to begin to solve the problems of the immune response.

In the following chapters we will examine the fascinating story of the attempt to determine what cells are involved in the

CHAPTER ONE

immune response; the way they interact with each other; the nature of the antibody molecule; and the organization of the genes responsible for the generation of the great diversity in the immune response. We will also see the first successful attempts at the application of what we know in designing new vaccines, using immunological techniques in diagnosis and in the modulation of the immune response.

The picture is complex and the solutions have not come easily. Embarking on an attempt to understand the immune system is a bit like starting to work your way through a labyrinth. In this case, by following the flow of the experiments the reader will emerge at the other end with an understanding of the picture as a whole.

"How do you know that? Are you an expert on labyrinths?"
"No, I am citing an ancient text I once read."
"And by observing this rule you get out?"
"Almost never, as far as I know. But we will try it, all the same."

Umberto Eco, *The Name of the Rose*[6]

Additional Readings

Breinl, F., and F. Haurowitz. 1930. Chemical investigation of the precipitate from hemoglobin and anti-hemoglobin serum and remarks on the nature of antibodies. *Z. Physiol. Chem.* 192: 45 (in German).

Burnet, F. M. 1957. A modification of Jerne's theory of antibody production using the concept of clonal selection. *Aust. J. Sci.* 20: 67.

Burnet, F. M. 1959. *The Clonal Selection Theory of Immunity*. Vanderbilt University Press, Nashville, Tenn.

Ehrlich, P. 1900. The Croonian lecture: On immunity. *Proc. R. Soc. London* 66: 424.

Golub, E. S. (1980) Paradigms lost. *Immunol. Today* 1: v; (1981) Shadows, stepping stones and the nature of scientific truth. *Immunol. Today* 2: v; (1982) Paradigms regained. *Immunol. Today* 3: v.

---

[6] It has been pointed out to me by Professor Constance Jordan that Eco is a poststructuralist semiotician and that this passage is really an infinite regress and an invitation to deconstructive analysis. I have assured Professor Jordan that all immunologists will be aware of this obvious fact but will still find the quote amusing.

13
THE CLONAL NATURE OF THE IMMUNE RESPONSE

Jerne, N. K. 1955. The natural selection theory of antibody formation. *PNAS* 41: 849.

Landsteiner, K. 1936. *The Specificity of Serological Reactions*. Thomas, Springfield, Ill.

Lederberg, J. 1959. Genes and antibodies. *Science* 129: 1669.

Pauling, L. 1940. A theory of the structure and process formation of antibodies. *J. Am. Chem. Soc.* 62: 2643.

Silverstein, A. M. Papers on the history of immunology. In *Cellular Immunology* (1979) 48: 208; (1982) 67: 396; 71: 183; (1983) 78: 174; 80: 416; (1985) 91: 263.

Talmage, D.W. 1957. Allergy and immunology. *Annu. Rev. Medicine* 8: 239.

PART ONE

IMMUNOCHEMISTRY

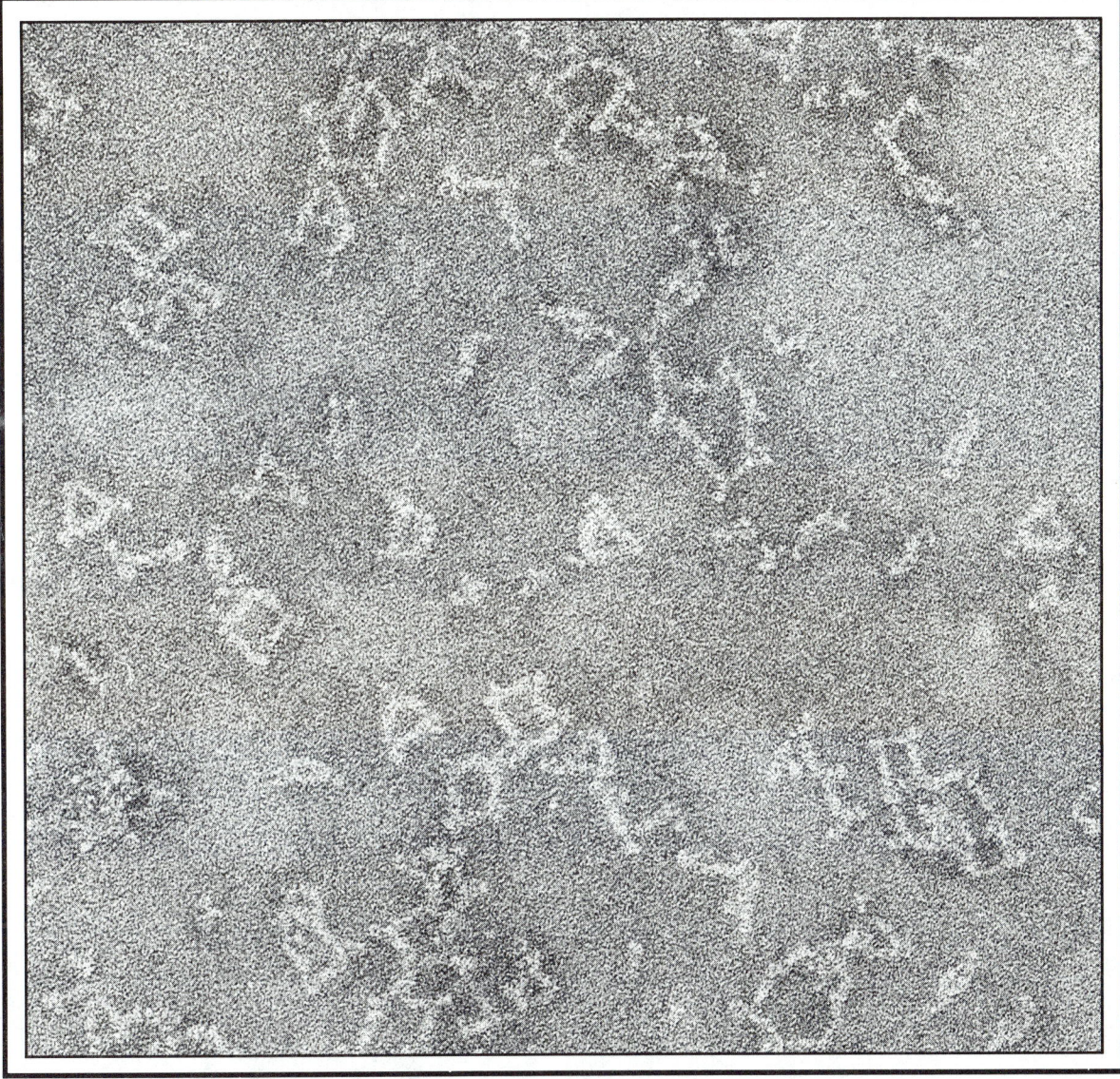

SECTION I

ANTIGENS AND ANTIBODIES

> The sciences are divided by Aristotle into the theoretical, the practical, and the productive; the immediate purpose of each kind is to know, but their ultimate purposes are respectively knowledge, conduct, and the making of beautiful or useful objects.
>
> Sir David Ross, *Aristotle*

In these six chapters we will examine the nature of antigens and antibodies. The purpose of these chapters is to give the reader the theoretical understanding of both antigens and antibodies so that the application of monoclonal antibodies and vaccines constructed to order can be fully appreciated. This section relates the solution to the problem of antibody diversity, one of the most elegant and exciting stories in modern biology.

CHAPTER 2

THE NATURE OF ANTIGENS

Overview The immune response begins with the introduction of antigen into the system, so we will begin our discussion by examining the nature of antigens.

The properties of a molecule that enable it to induce a response are called immunogenicity; and the properties that allow it to react with antibodies are called antigenicity. Even though the factors that make a molecule immunogenic are not as yet clearly defined, advances in protein chemistry, computer-generated graphics, and monoclonal antibody techniques have allowed the nature of antigenicity to be addressed at molecular and even atomic levels. We will see that almost any stretch of amino acids can be antigenic if it is in the proper conformation. Even small stretches of peptides that have been synthesized and added to a proper carrier can in some cases induce the production of antibodies and react with those induced by the molecule in its natural configuration. This technique has brought us to the threshold of constructing vaccines from synthetic peptides that have been synthesized on the basis of either the protein sequence as analyzed or the sequence deduced from the DNA code.

CHAPTER TWO

Antigenicity and Immunogenicity

The introduction of antigen into an animal initiates a series of events culminating in either effector cells or antibody formation. In this chapter we will deal only with antibody formation and the reaction of these antibodies with that antigen. By convention, the property of a molecule that allows it to INDUCE the formation of antibody is called IMMUNOGENICITY. The property of being able to REACT with the antibody that has been induced is called ANTIGENICITY. Of course, in most cases an antigen molecule has both properties—both immunogenicity and antigenicity. The hapten–carrier systems to be described in this chapter enable us to make a clear distinction between these two properties.

Studies with Haptens

Haptens and Carriers

The theme of specificity runs through the study of the immune response. Resistance to disease was known to be specific long before immunity and the immune system was studied scientifically. Karl Landsteiner (1868–1943), the great pathologist and immunologist, was the first to systematically study specificity using a chemically defined system. Landsteiner studied the reaction of antibodies directed against HAPTENS, which are traditionally defined as small molecules that of themselves do not *induce* the production of antibody but are capable of *reacting* with antibodies. At first glance the last statement appears to be a contradiction—after all, how can something react with antibody but not induce its formation? The critical clause in the statement is "of themselves." Haptens injected by themselves into an animal do not induce the production of antibody (Figure 1). But when the hapten is conjugated to a CARRIER (a large immunogenic molecule such as a protein), the animal responds by producing antibodies both to the hapten and to the carrier. Anti-hapten antibody, once it is induced by the hapten–carrier conjugate, is able to react with free hapten. In general, carriers are molecules that are of themselves immunogenic. Hence we may think of the hapten as an added determinant on an already immunogenic molecule. The study of hapten–

19
THE NATURE OF ANTIGENS

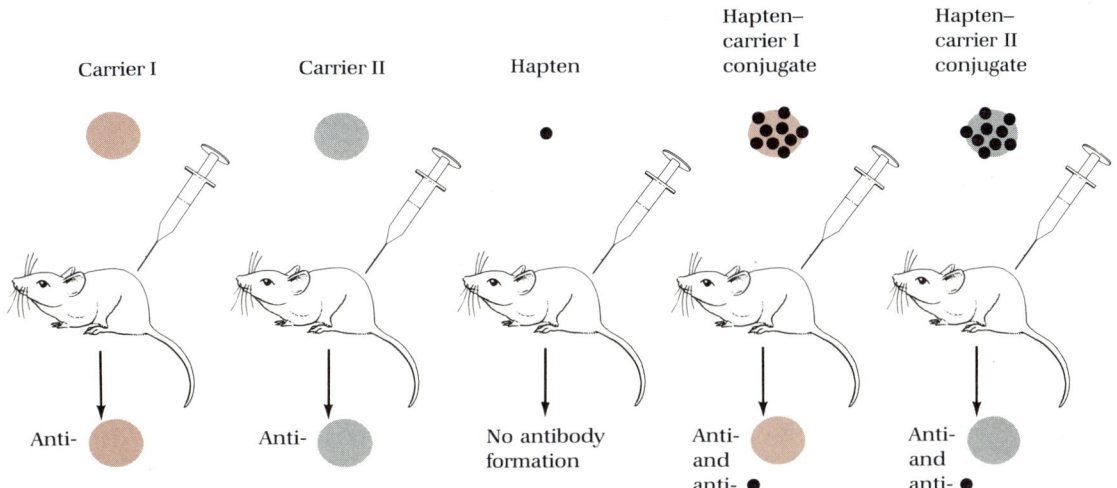

FIGURE 1 ANTIBODY RESPONSES

The injection of immunogenic carrier alone results in formation of carrier-specific antibody. The injection of hapten alone does not result in formation of anti-hapten antibody. When the hapten is conjugated to an immunogenic carrier and injected, however, the animal responds by producing both anti-carrier and anti-hapten antibodies.

carrier systems has given us much information about the nature of antigens and the antigen–antibody interaction but it has also been one of the keys to understanding the cellular events in the immune response (see Chapter 16).

The Specificity of Serological Reactions

Landsteiner set out to study haptens and carriers in an attempt to work out the rules that govern antigenicity. The compilation of these studies appeared in his classic treatise, *The Specificity of Serological Reactions*. As we will see, no universal rules governing antigenicity came out of this work, but what did emerge was the realization that the chemical properties of the antigen molecule determined the specificity of the immune system. SPECIFICITY is defined as the ability of antibodies produced in response to an antigen to react with that antigen and not with others. The thoroughness of Landsteiner's approach and the elegance of his thought make browsing in this volume, which is available in paperback, a worthwhile experience for any scientist.

Landsteiner immunized a rabbit with a hapten–carrier conjugate. This injection led to both anti-hapten and anti-carrier responses. He then conjugated the hapten to a different carrier and reacted it with the antiserum to test for the presence of *anti-hapten* antibodies. Because he had changed carrier molecules for the test, there was no anti-carrier reaction; the reaction observed was between the anti-hapten antibodies and the hapten. He then varied the properties of the hapten in order to study, for example, the effect of acidic or ionic groups on the ability of the antibody raised against the original hapten to react with the modified hapten. Although no general rules emerged, it is instructive to look at some of Landsteiner's conclusions (Landsteiner, 1962):

> The principal results of numerous precipitin tests with azoproteins were the following...
> 1. First of all, the nature of the acidic groups was of decisive influence. [p. 163]

Data from Landsteiner's experiments are shown in Tables 1–4. Antibody is raised against aminobenzene or aminobenzene with

TABLE 1 Acidic groups and specificity.

Antiserum against	Reactivity with			
	Aminobenzene (Aniline)	p-Aminobenzoic acid	p-Aminobenzene sulfonic acid	p-Aminobenzene arsenic acid
Aminobenzene	+++	0	0	0
p-Aminobenzoic acid	0	++++±	0	0
p-Aminobenzene sulfonic acid	0	0	++++±	0
p-Aminobenzene arsenic acid	0	0	0	+++±

Source: From Landsteiner (1962). Modified by Klein.

21
THE NATURE OF ANTIGENS

TABLE 2 Non-ionic groups and specificity.

Antiserum against	Reactivity with			
	Aminobenzene (Aniline)	p-Chloroamino-benzene	p-Toluidine	p-Nitroamino-benzene
Aminobenzene	+ + ±	+	+ ±	+
p-Chloroaminobenzene	± + + +	+ +	+ +	+ ±
p-Toluidine	+ ±	+ +	+ +	+
p-Nitroaminobenzene	+	+ +	+ ±	+

Source: From Landsteiner (1962). Modified by Klein.

acidic groups substituted at the para position (Table 1). In each case the antibody induced by one of the haptens reacts with *only* that hapten and none of the others.

    2. In contrast to acid groups, substitution of the aromatic nucleus by methyl, halogen, methoxyl and nitro groups was of less influence on specificity. [p. 163]

Antibody raised against any hapten is likely to react with all of the haptens (Table 2). From this we see that the nature of the added group is critical in determining the effect on the ability to react.

    3. Another rule, seen from the very distinctive reactions of the three isomeric aminobenzoic acids and aminocinnamic acids, is that the relative position of the acid radical to the azo group has a pronounced effect on specificity and the occurrence of cross reactions. [p. 167]

Moving the carboxyl group from ortho to meta to para results in different specificities (Table 3).

Another example deals with subtle differences between two molecules, such as the interchange of H and OH on one carbon

TABLE 3 Group position and specificity.

Antiserum against	Reactivity with			
	Aminobenzene (Aniline)	o-Aminobenzoic acid	m-Aminobenzoic acid	p-Aminobenzoic acid
Aminobenzene	+++	0	0	0
o-Aminobenzoic acid	0	+++	0	0
m-Aminobenzoic acid	0	0	++++	0
p-Aminobenzoic acid	0	0	0	+++±

Source: From Landsteiner (1962). Modified by Klein.

atom. These data (which are actually from the work of Avery and Goebel and are quoted by Landsteiner) are shown in Table 4. The presentation of the aminophenyl group in either the α or β configuration from glucose has a slight effect on the reaction. However, rotation of the H and OH on the sugar to form galactose has a profound effect.

These experiments clearly demonstrate that subtle changes in the molecule have profound effects on the ability of the molecule to react with an antibody directed against a similar molecule, a fact that must be kept in mind throughout the text when the nature of specificity of the immune response is discussed.

Cross Reactivity

Antibody molecules can exhibit great specificity, but there are CROSS REACTIONS—cases in which antibody to antigen A also reacts with antigen B. This reaction can be due to the presence of the same molecular configuration of ANTIGENIC DETERMINANT on the two antigens, or to properties of a determinant that allow it to be recognized as though it were another group. We can conceive of molecules that have similar

23
THE NATURE OF ANTIGENS

TABLE 4 Glycoside bonds and specificity.

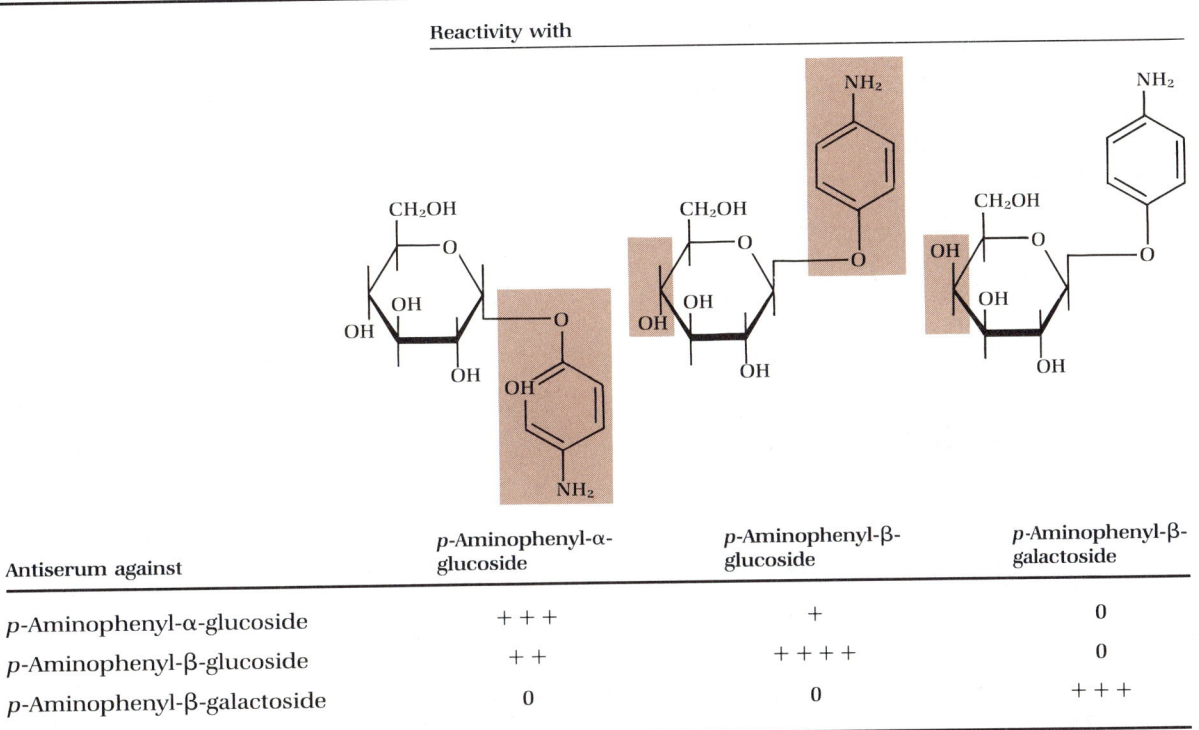

Antiserum against	Reactivity with		
	p-Aminophenyl-α-glucoside	p-Aminophenyl-β-glucoside	p-Aminophenyl-β-galactoside
p-Aminophenyl-α-glucoside	+++	+	0
p-Aminophenyl-β-glucoside	++	++++	0
p-Aminophenyl-β-galactoside	0	0	+++

Source: From Landsteiner (1962). Modified by Klein.

but not identical structures and appear in closely related species. These molecules may have enough similarity to allow antibodies against one to react with the other.[1]

Table 5 shows the percentage of cross reactivity between albumins of different species. The antibody is made against bovine serum albumin (BSA), and the extent of the ability of albumins from other species to react with the anti-BSA is then determined. This cross reactivity is probably due to the presence of common determinants on the different albumins. To determine this, however, each of the determinants must be isolated and studied chemically. Even then, as we will see later in this chapter, we

[1] The neurobiologist A. K. Hall has suggested the term "immunofrequent" for such determinants.

CHAPTER TWO

TABLE 5 Cross-reaction between BSA and other albumins.

Albumin source	Percentage of cross-reactivity with BSA[a]	Albumin source	Percentage of cross-reactivity with BSA[a]
Human	15	Mouse	10
Pig	32	Rat	13
Sheep	75	Hamster	13
Horse	13	Cat	25
Guinea pig	5	Vallaroo	6
Dog	13		

Source: Data from Weigle (1961), *J. Immunol.* 87: 599.
[a]Rabbit anti-BSA as absorbed with one of the albumins and the antiserum tested for its ability to precipitate BSA.

cannot be quite certain of the causes of the cross reactivity because factors such as conformation and amino acid sequence are also involved.

Antibodies to Proteins

As elegant and informative as the hapten–carrier studies were, they were meant to be the groundwork for the study of the more complex protein and carbohydrate antigens found in nature. Landsteiner, in contemplating the vast array of natural antigens in the world concluded that an antigenic determinant in a naturally occurring molecule would not be a simple structure.

> Clearly the highly selective action of the immune sera precludes specificity being determined by simple structures as single amino acids, and even reacting groups composed of di- or tripeptides could not furnish a sufficient number of combinations ... the specificity of proteins must be referable to complicated structures—possibly multiple, like groups in one molecule—or to several groupings whose affinities have to be satisfied before a visible reaction can occur, in which event the spatial arrangement of the reacting groups may be significant. [Landsteiner, quoted in Lerner (1984) *Adv. Immunol.* 36: 4.]

THE NATURE OF ANTIGENS

INFORMATION BOX 1

Blood Group Antigens

There are over 20 blood groups in humans, the most common being the ABO system. The ABO system was discovered in 1901 by Landsteiner, who noted that serum from some individuals agglutinated the red blood cells from some other individuals. We now know that type A individuals have antibody to type B cells in their serum. Because the blood group antigens are oligosaccharides that occur commonly in nature, type A people become immunized to type B antigen present on ingested foods, although they remain tolerant to A antigen. The reverse is true for type B individuals.

The ABO antigens are a good example of how a small change in chemical structure results in a unique and drastic change in antigenic structure under natural conditions. The A and B structures differ at the terminal sugars on a common "stem." The genes that determine A and B encode enzymes called transferases—an N-acetylgalactosamine transferase for A and a galactose transferase for B. These transferases add either N-acetylgalactosamine or galactose to the "stem" (see Figure).

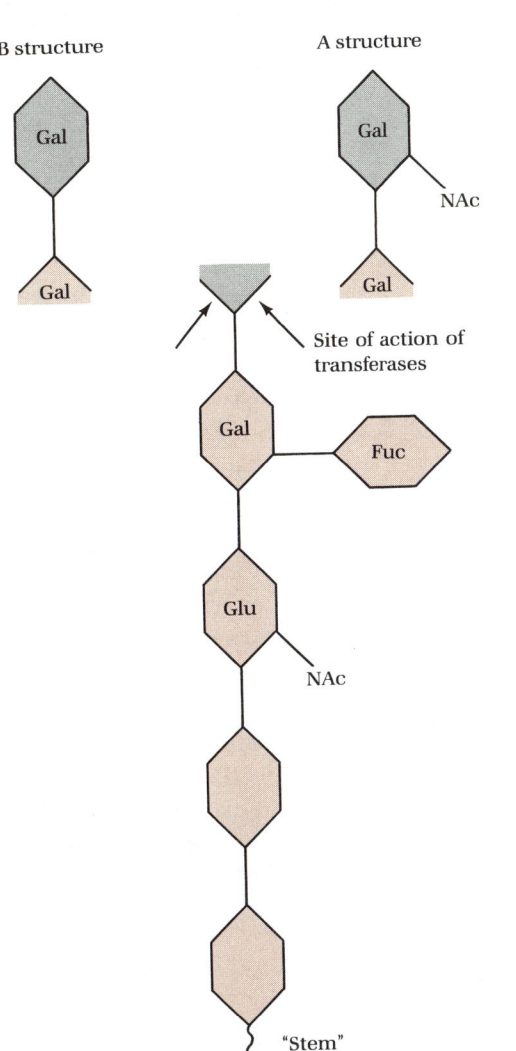

CHAPTER TWO

The Roles of Conformation and Amino Acid Sequence in Antigenicity

True to Landsteiner's prediction, early studies on proteins did show that the *conformation* of a molecule could be important to its antigenicity. For example, when antibody was raised against a native protein, the antibody would not react with the protein after the protein had been denatured. In studies of controlled denaturation, for example, antibody against ribonuclease did not react with ribonuclease after its four disulfide bonds had been oxidized and the *shape* of the ribonuclease molecule changed.

Arnon, Sela, and their colleagues in Israel carried out a particularly lovely series of experiments in the 1970s to examine the role of conformation in the antigenicity of lysozyme. In the lysozyme molecule (Figure 2A) residues 64–80 form a loop through the formation of a disulfide bond between Cys 64 and Cys 80. These investigators synthesized the amino acids that constitute the loop (Figure 2B) and found that antibodies against either the intact molecule or the isolated but still closed loop reacted with both the whole molecule and the closed loop. However, when the disulfide bond forming the loop was oxidized so that the loop was no longer present even though the sequence of the amino acids was unchanged, there was a dramatic reduction in the ability of the antibody to bind to the intact molecule (Figure 2C).

Studies of this kind showed that the conformation of the protein was crucial for its antigenicity. But, as we will see, conformation need not be an absolute requirement. At about the same time that the experiments showing the importance of conformation were being done, other evidence showed that the requirement for complex structure was not absolute. These studies showed that *amino acid sequence* was important to antigenicity.

FIGURE 2 EFFECT OF CONFORMATION ON ANTIGENICITY

(A) Amino acid sequence of hen egg-white lysozyme. The shaded area forms the "loop." (B) Diagrammatic representation of the synthetic open and closed loops. (C) Reacting the anti-loop antiserum with lysozyme, natural loop, or synthetic loop inhibits the reaction between loop:anti-loop. However, reaction with open loop does not. These results show that the specificity of the anti-loop antibody is for the conformation of the loop. [After Arnon and Sela (1969) *PNAS* 62, 164; Arnon et al. (1971) *PNAS* 68, 1450]

27
THE NATURE OF ANTIGENS

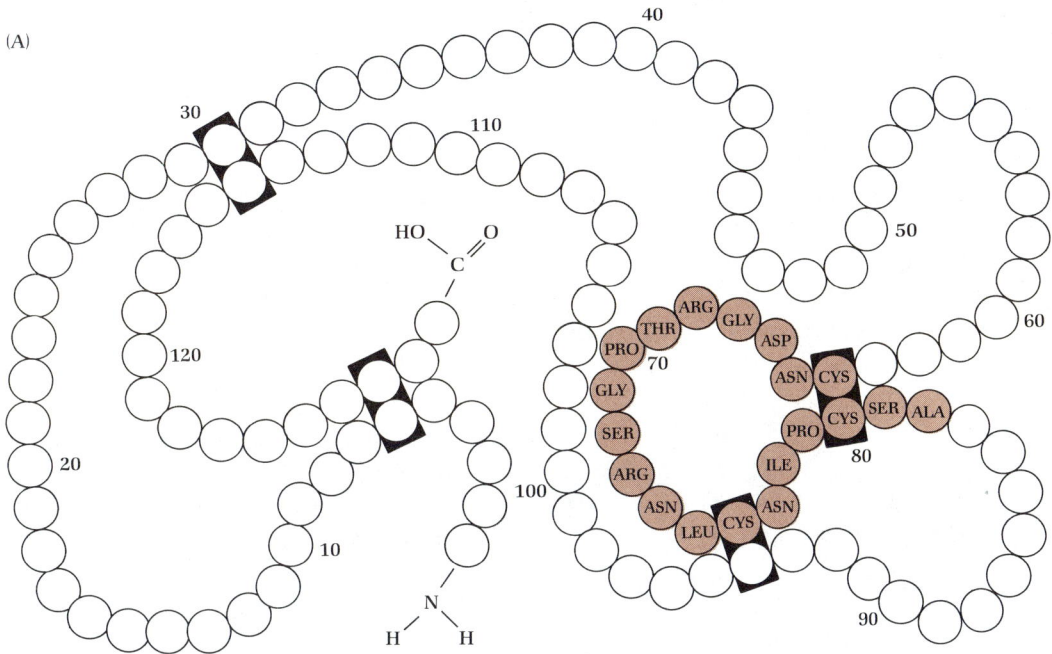

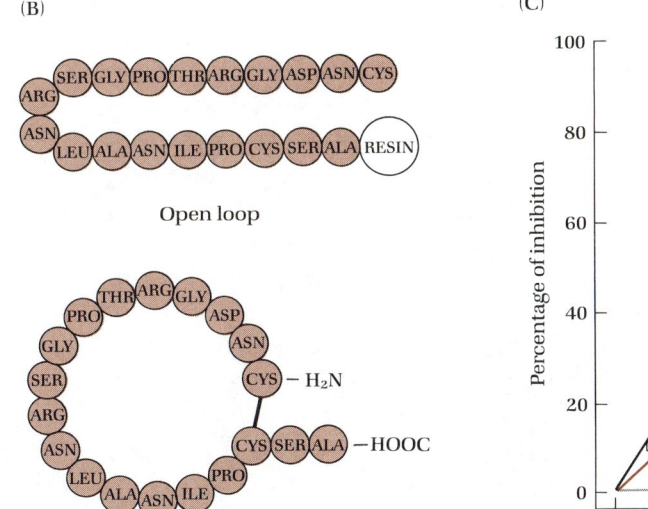

Studies with the protein of the tobacco mosaic virus (TMV) provide a good example.

Tobacco mosaic virus is a large virus composed of a spiral series of protein subunits around a nucleic acid core. In the early 1960s Anderer and his co-workers in Germany produced antibody against TMV and tested the ability of fragments of TMVP (tobacco mosaic virus protein), produced by enzymatic digestion, to inhibit the reaction of anti-TMV with TMVP. They found that several peptides efficiently inhibited the reaction. Some of these peptides were very short and did not have significant three-dimensional conformation; thus the dependence of antigenicity on conformation was shown not to be absolute.

Benjamini and his colleagues in California pursued these findings and demonstrated that the antibody to TMVP that reacted with the intact molecule was directed against one of the TMVP tryptic peptides. The specificity of the reaction was in the terminal five amino acids of the peptide, further demonstrating that a small stretch of amino acids with no apparent complex structure can serve as an antigen.

The Role of Segmental Mobility

Recent work from the laboratories of Klug in England and Lerner in La Jolla have shown that the *mobility* of the segment of an antigen molecule influences whether it will be antigenic. Klug and van Regenmortel have identified in TMV seven antigenic determinants, each of which consists of between five and ten amino acids. Because TMV can be crystallized and analyzed by X-ray diffraction, they were able to show that six of the seven determinants had high temperature factors along the polypeptide backbone. This means that the determinants had high SEGMENTAL MOBILITY (that is, they could move about 1 angstrom from the mean backbone position).

Lerner and his colleagues analyzed several proteins and found that mobile peptide segments were more likely to be antigenic than nonmobile segments were. Figure 3A is a computer-generated view of the protein backbone in which the labeled amino acids are the antigenic determinants. It can be seen that the antigenic determinants are clustered in the more mobile segments. Figure 3B shows a computer-generated "glowing coal" model of insulin; the lighter areas have greater mobility than the dark ones.

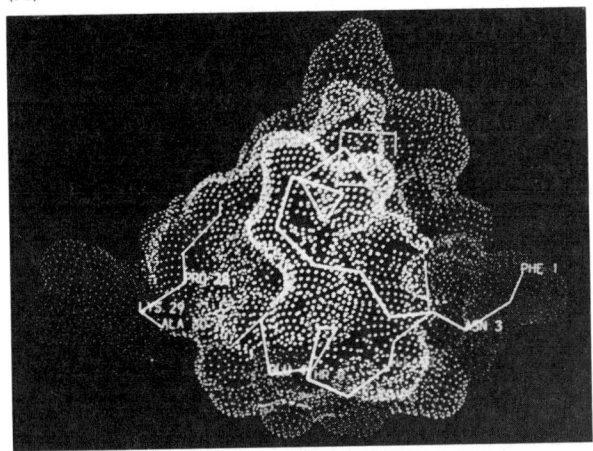 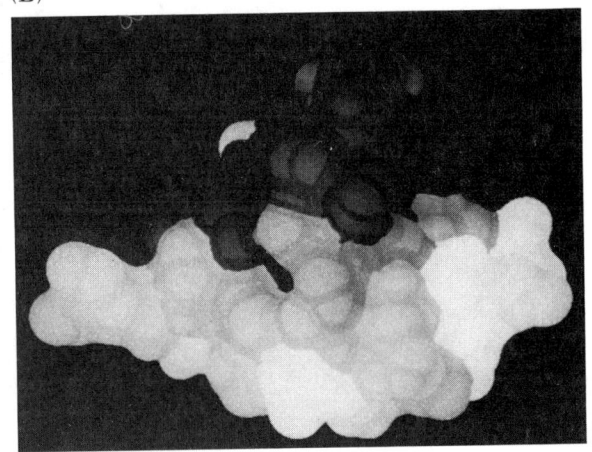

FIGURE 3 COMPUTER GRAPHIC VIEWS OF INSULIN
Computer graphics show that the antigenic determinants cluster at flexible regions. (A) In this view (which is shown in color on the cover), the alpha carbon backbone (lines) and the molecular surface (dots) are displayed with residue labels indicating the contiguous and discontiguous antigenic determinants. (B) The "glowing coal" model illustrates the correspondence of antigenic sites with the more mobile regions of insulin, which are highlighted with the lightest colors. [Adapted from Tainer et al. (1985), *Annu. Rev. Immunol.* 3, 501, with permission]

The Multideterminant Hypothesis
We have seen so far that both amino acid sequence and conformation are important to the antigenicity of a molecule and that the segmental mobility of the determinant is crucial. These observations have led to the hypothesis that the surface of a protein is a continuum of *potential* antigenic sites. Or, in other words, almost any sequence of amino acids can be antigenic if it is located in the larger molecule in such a manner that it has a conformation allowing segmental mobility.

Molecular Mapping of Antigenic Determinants
It would be interesting and useful to understand the nature of antigenicity and to determine which parts of molecules are antigenic. Indeed, these determinations have been made by using monoclonal antibodies alone and monoclonal antibodies in conjunction with X-ray crystallography. Before the advent of monoclonal antibodies, it was very difficult to map the antigenic determinants of a molecule (that is, to determine which sites on the molecule were immunogenic and

CHAPTER TWO

antigenic) because the antisera that were used had antibodies to all of the determinants. But monoclonal antibodies react with a single determinant; hence they can be used in conjunction with sequence studies, computer-generated graphics, and crystallography to determine the fine structure of determinants. (Monoclonal antibodies are described in Chapter 6.)

A very instructive example of the combined use of these methods can be seen in the work which determined the antigenic sites on the human rhino virus (HRV; the virus that causes the common cold). Rueckert and his colleagues in Madison studied this virus by producing monoclonal antibodies against it and selecting variants of the virus that were not neutralized by a given antibody. In this way they were able to identify four antigenic groups which they called NIm (for neutralizing immunogen) IA, IB, II and III. The RNA of the variants was sequenced so that the positions of the amino acids responsible for each of the variants could be identified. Some of these data appeared to be anomalous, however, because some of the variants seemed to have substitutions that were located far from the clusters that were thought to be the antigenic determinants. This anomaly was cleared up when Rossmann and his colleagues at Purdue and Hogle and his colleagues in La Jolla worked out the three-dimensional structures of HRV and polio by X-ray crystallography. They found that picorna viruses, of which HRV and polio are examples, have the same basic structure: several "beta barrels." The individual strands of these barrels are connected by chains of peptides (Figure 4A), which protrude from the virus surface and are likely candidate structures for antigenic determinants because they are accessible to antibody and have relatively high flexibility. It is of

FIGURE 4 DIAGRAMMATIC REPRESENTATIONS OF "BETA BARRELS" AND POLYPEPTIDE CHAINS

(A) "Viral protein 1" of human rhino virus (HRV). Note that antigenic deteterminant NIm-IB is on two separate strands but NIm-IA is contiguous. (B) shows that a plant virus, soybean mosaic virus (SBMV), has the same organization but smaller polypeptide chains. [Diagrams from Rossmann et al. (1986) *Nature*. Similar structural data for polio virus can be seen in Hogle et al. (1985) *Science* 229, 1358]

31
THE NATURE OF ANTIGENS

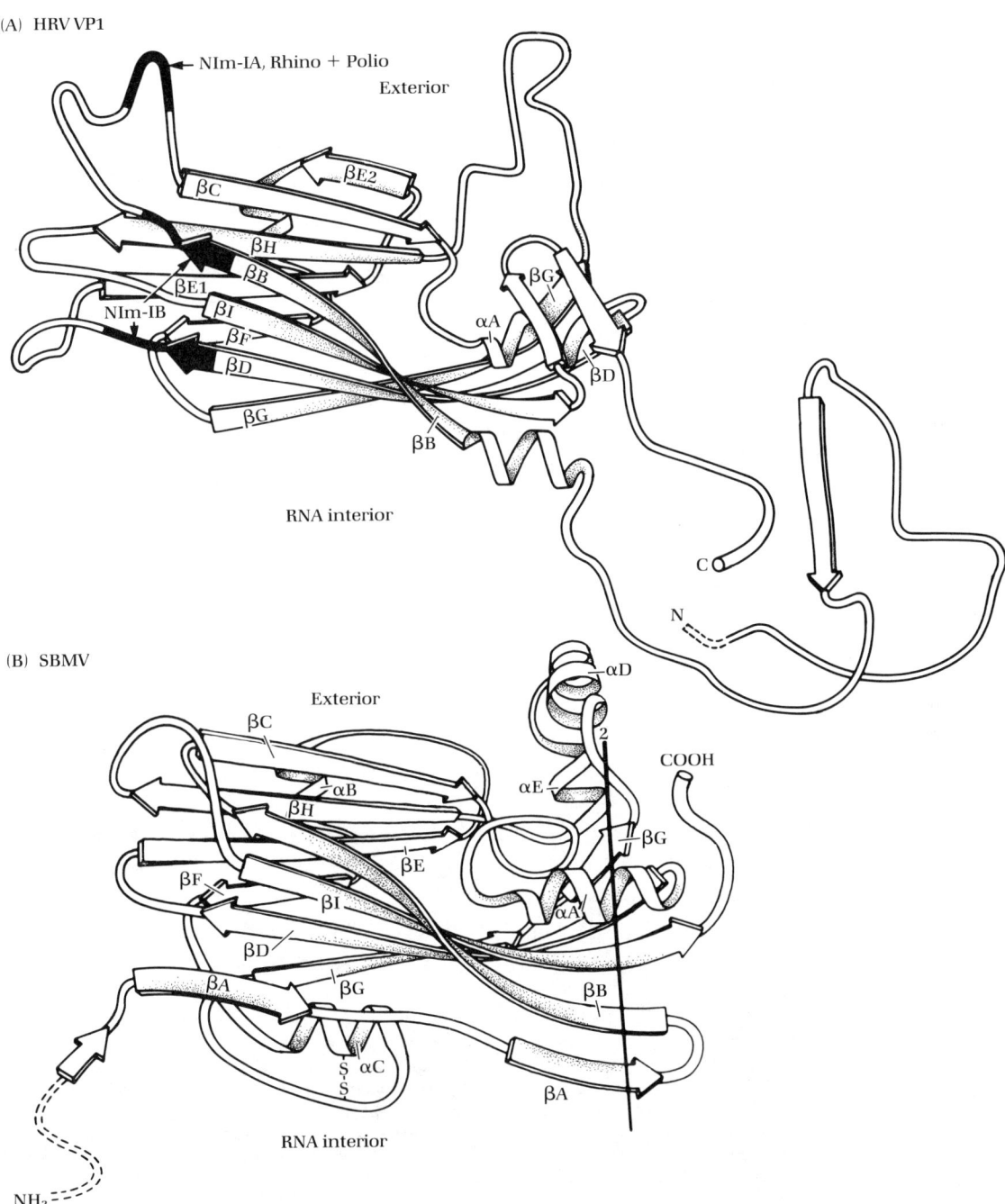

(A) HRV VP1

(B) SBMV

interest that a plant virus whose three-dimensional structure had been worked out earlier has the same basic construction (see Figure 4B). When the three-dimensional structure of HRV was compared to its amino acid sequences, it was found that the antigenic determinants (NIm) were in fact located on the protruding peptides that connect the strands of beta sheets (which compose the barrels) and that the anomalous data now made sense because some of the antigenic determinants were made up of amino acids that are distant from each other on a *linear* representation of the amino acid sequence, but are adjacent to each other in the three-dimensional structure. In other words, the determinant can be formed by amino acids that are in close association by virtue of spatial orientation of the viral peptides. This finding is shown in Figure 4A; the black areas form the antigenic determinant.[2] Similar studies are being carried out by several groups around the world and will give us greater insight into the structure–function relationship of antigenic determinants in their natural setting so that we may better modify them for our own purposes.

Antibodies of Predetermined Specificities

A protein immunogen[3] is usually composed of a large number of antigenic determinants. Hence, immunizing with a protein results in the formation of antibody molecules with different specificities, the number of different antibodies depending on the number of antigenic determinants and their inherent immunogenicity. On the basis of the pioneering work of immunochemists who studied the responses to fragments of proteins and peptides, a new technology that allows us to produce antibodies of predetermined specificity against protein antigens is developing.

[2] One additional point of interest is that the protruding area in the plant virus is very small; but in both the HRV and polio virus the protruding chains occupy a much larger space. Crystallographer Jack Johnson has suggested that the plant virus has evolved in the absence of pressure from the immune response (plants do not make antibody), whereas the polio and cold viruses have developed ways of evading the immune response by introducing variation into their antibody-accessible parts.

[3] "Immunogen" is the term used when the immunogenic properties of an antigen are discussed.

THE NATURE OF ANTIGENS

One of the revolutionary changes in biology in the past few years is the ability to sequence DNA. In fact, it is often easier to clone a gene, sequence it, and infer the amino acid sequence of the protein that it encodes than it is to purify the protein and sequence it. Consequently, immunologists have been able to synthesize the protein from the inferred sequence and use the synthetic protein as an immunogen.

Antibodies to Products of Nucleotide Sequence The power of the new technology is evident in the following example. In examining the nucleotide sequence of the Moloney leukemia virus, Lerner and his colleagues at La Jolla found that there was a stretch of nucleotides that could not be explained. This reading frame was part of the envelope gene and predicted a protein that was not known to exist in the virus. The predicted protein was synthesized, conjugated to a carrier, and used to immunize rabbits. The resulting antibody precipitated two previously unidentified proteins from infected and transformed cells. The proteins had not been isolated earlier because during the process of viral budding from the cell, the C-termini of these two proteins are cleaved. The antibody had detected the cleaved portions of the proteins, which were part of previously unknown precursor proteins. Their discovery allowed the synthesis and assembly of the virus to be studied in more detail.

Another example of the use of antigens synthesized from nucleotide sequences is seen in the work of Sutcliffe and his colleagues. There is a large amount of messenger RNA in the brain that is not accounted for in known brain proteins. These workers approached the problem of identifying the proteins by producing complementary DNA (cDNA) from messenger RNA of the whole brain. The cDNA was then hybridized to messenger RNA from different regions of the brain; and when a message coding for a product unique to an area of the brain was found, the corresponding cDNA was sequenced and the amino acid sequence of the protein inferred. Several regions of the predicted peptide were then synthesized and injected into animals to produce antibodies. The antibodies were used to search for the predicted protein in brain slices. Using this technique a protein was found which may be a precursor to a new neurotransmitter.

CHAPTER TWO

Antibodies to Predetermined Amino Acid Sequences

The amino acid sequences of many antigens, including those on pathogens that may be of importance in immunization strategies, have been determined since their genes have been sequenced. This advance should facilitate the production of vaccines because the immunogenic portion of the agents can be synthesized and used for immunization. One strategy for doing this has recently been worked out. Monoclonal antibodies to a feline leukemia virus have been found to protect cats from infection with the virus. To determine which of the viral antigens are responsible for the protection, advantage has been taken of the techniques of molecular biology. The gene for the immunogenic protein was cloned and then cut at random by DNase I. These fragments were then inserted individually into a phage so that they could be expressed in infected host bacteria. Colonies of bacteria that contained the gene for the antigen were plated and identified by treating the colonies with the monoclonal antibody. In this way, the fragment actually containing the antigenic determinant was identified. Because the DNA sequence of each fragment can be easily determined in the laboratory, the amino acid sequence was deduced and synthesized and the synthetic peptide used as immunogen. This elegant strategy can be used, in principle, for almost any pathogen.

Another interesting advance in immunization has also come about through the use of the methods of molecular biology. It is possible to put the DNA sequence for a desired antigenic determinant into the vaccinia virus genome so that when an individual is immunized with vaccinia he/she is also immunized with the desired antigen. One can foresee the construction of genomes containing DNA sequences for several antigenic determinants of several pathogens and the expression of these determinants in a single organism, which is then used for immunization.

In some cases, even though the genes are cloned, the selection of antigen for the vaccine is hampered by the complexity of the natural history of the host and the parasite. Malaria is a good example. It is known that antibodies against the sporozoite stage of the disease protect the host. The gene for the sporozoite antigen of several species has been cloned and monoclonal antibodies against the antigen have been developed. Unfortunately, it may turn out that vaccines will have to be developed to antigens

THE NATURE OF ANTIGENS

expressed during the merozoite and the gametocyte stages as well. In other parasitic diseases the parasite actually changes its antigenic profile during the course of the disease, a fact that will make the task of choosing the antigens for immunization very difficult.

Summary

1. Immunogenicity is the property of a molecule that allows it to induce an immune response. Antigenicity is the ability of a molecule to react with antibody.
2. Haptens are molecules that are not immunogenic unless conjugated to a carrier but that are able to react with anti-hapten antibody. Using hapten:anti-hapten systems, Landsteiner showed that the chemical nature of the hapten affected its antigenicity.
3. The antigenicity of a protein is determined by its sequence of amino acids as well as by its conformation. Peptide sequences with high segmental mobility are frequently antigenic.
4. The combined use of monoclonal antibody, computer-generated graphics, and X-ray crystallography is making molecular–antigenic mapping of complex structures possible.
5. Antibodies of predetermined specificity can be made by immunizing an animal with synthetic peptides. In this manner vaccines of desired specificity should be able to be made in the future.

Additional Readings

Benjamin, D. C., J. A. Berzofsky, I. J. East, F. R. N. Gurd, C. Hannum, S. J. Leach, E. Margoliash, J. G. Micheal, A. Miller, E. M. Prager, M. Reichlin, E. E. Sercarz, S. J. Smith-Gill, P. E. Todd, and A. C. Wilson. 1984. The antigenic structure of proteins: a reappraisal. *Annu. Rev. Immunol.* 2:51.

Landsteiner, K. 1962. *The Specificity of Serological Reactions*, Rev. Ed. New York, Dover Publications.

Lerner, R. A. 1984. Antibodies to predetermined specificity in biology and medicine. *Adv. Immunol.* 36:1.

Silverstein, A. M. 1982. Development of the concept of immunological specificity. *Cell. Immunol.* 67:396.

Sutcliffe, J. G., R. J. Milner, T. N. Shennick, and F. E. Bloom. 1983. Identifying the protein products of brain-specific genes with antibodies to chemically synthesized peptides. *Cell* 33:671.

Tainer, J. A., E. D. Getzoff, Y. Paterson, A. J. Olson, and R. A. Lerner. 1985. The atomic mobility component of protein antigenicity. *Annu. Rev. Immunol.* 3:501.

CHAPTER 3
THE BASIC IMMUNOGLOBULIN MONOMER

Overview The body can produce antibodies to what may be a limitless array of antigens, each antibody reacting specifically with the antigen that caused its induction. Determining the structure of the molecule that can impart so much diversity and the structural basis for the specificity of the antibodies has been one of the profound problems of biology. During the past two decades, however, this problem has come very close to being solved, and the solution is one of the more thrilling episodes in modern biology—one that reads almost like a detective story. The next three chapters will discuss the ways in which these problems were defined, attacked, and solved. At each stage the problem was defined through an advance in immunology, although the solution required advances in other areas such as protein chemistry and molecular biology.

The antibody molecule should be thought of as a monomer composed of four chains: two identical heavy chains and two identical light chains held together by disulfide bonds. There are several classes of immunoglobulin molecules, and they differ in size and number of monomers; but all are composed only of immunoglobulin monomers. The specificity in the antibody molecule comes from varying amino acid sequences of the variable portion of the immunoglobulin molecules while the structure of the remainder of the molecule remains constant.

THE BASIC IMMUNOGLOBULIN MONOMER

Antibodies and Immunoglobulins

It has been known from the prehistoric days of immunology that antibody activity was found in the SERUM, the fluid portion of blood after it has been allowed to clot.[1] Serum contains many proteins but antibodies are found almost exclusively in the globulin fraction. In a classic experiment, Tiselius and Kabat in 1939 showed that after reacting serum from an immune animal (called ANTISERUM) with specific antigen and collecting the immune precipitate, the γ-globulin fraction of the serum was diminished, indicating that the γ-globulins contained the antibody activity (Figure 1).

Later it appeared that the only function of the γ-globulins was antibody activity, and this group of molecules was called IMMUNOGLOBULINS (IG).

The Chain Structure of Ig

Early Studies Using Antiserum: Treatment with Proteolytic Enzymes

It had been known from physiochemical studies done a very long time ago that the antibody molecule had two antigen-binding sites. The early research leading to our understanding of the *chain structure* of the basic Ig monomer earned Nobel prizes for the two prime movers in the field, R. R. Porter and G. M. Edelman.[2] Porter, working in England, treated rabbit antibody with the proteolytic enzyme papain and separated the products on a carboxymethylcellulose column. This treatment produced three fragments. Two of the fragments were of equal molecular weight (ca. 50,000) and could bind antigen. These two were called FAB fragments (FRAGMENT with ANTIGEN BINDING). The third fragment, which had a molecular weight of ca. 80,000, did not bind antigen, but it crystallized and therefore was called FC. Treatment of the antibody molecule (which had a sedimentation coefficient of 7 S) with another proteolytic enzyme, pepsin, by Nisonoff and his colleagues gave different results. In contrast to papain, pepsin treatment produced a single 5 S fragment and many small pieces.

It became clear after further work that the different proteoly-

---

[1] Plasma is the fluid portion containing unreacted clotting factors.
[2] Rodney Porter died on September 6, 1985, in a tragic auto accident.

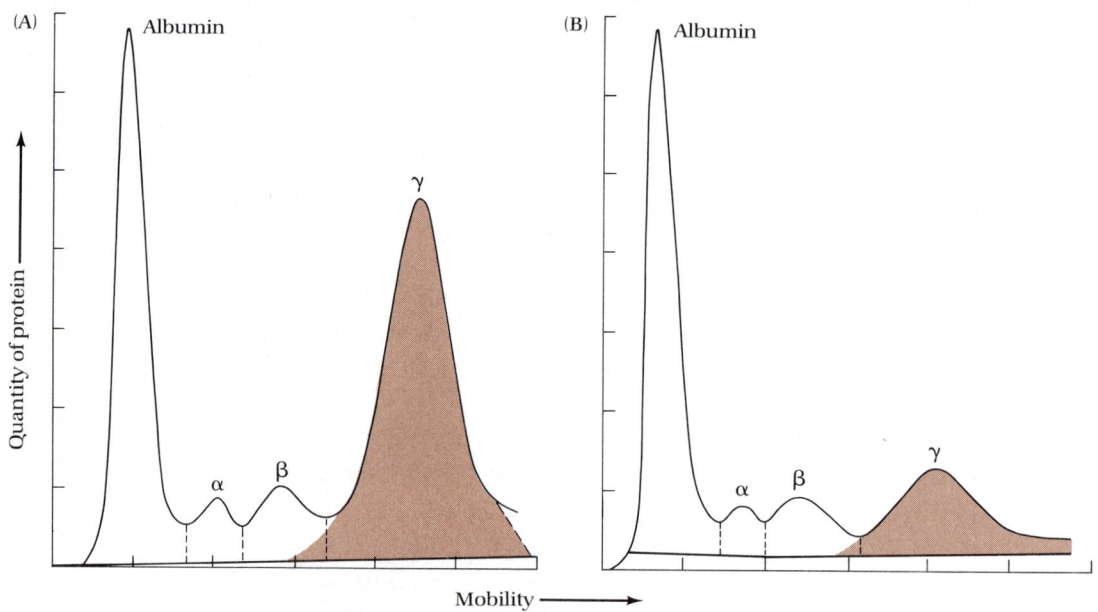

FIGURE 1 ELECTROPHORETIC ANALYSES OF RABBIT ANTI-EGG ALBUMIN ANTISERUM

Analyses were made before (A) and after (B) reaction of the antiserum with antigen. Note that the γ-globulin fraction is selectively reduced after reaction with antigen. [Redrawn from Tiselius and Kabat (1939) *J. Exp. Med.* **69**, 119]

tic enzymes cleaved the molecule at different sites, thus accounting for the different sizes of the fragments. To activate papain, reducing agents must be used; and it was shown that these agents were reducing disulfide bonds in the Ig molecule. The two antigen-binding fragments were produced by papain treatment because the reducing agents broke a disulfide bond that held the fragments together in the intact molecule. Pepsin activation, in contrast, did not require reducing agents; and pepsin cleaved in a manner that left the disulfide bond intact. In short, the two binding portions of the antibody molecule were separated after papain treatment (producing two Fab fragments) but remained united by a disulfide bond after pepsin treatment (producing an (Fab$_2$) fragment).

THE BASIC IMMUNOGLOBULIN MONOMER

The Use of Myeloma Proteins

The antibodies in serum (antiserum) are extremely heterogeneous because they reflect antibody specificities to every antigen the individual has recently come in contact with. This heterogeneity is one of the stumbling blocks in the study of the chemistry of antibodies (this will be covered in detail in Chapter 4). The use of *myeloma protein*, however, has overcome this difficulty. Multiple myeloma is a disease in which there is a malignant transformation in a single cell that normally produces antibody. The transformed cell, now a cancer cell (in this case a myeloma cell), multiplies in an uncontrolled manner while continuing to secrete its immunoglobulin product into the serum. The result is a very high concentration of only one kind of immunoglobulin (the MYELOMA PROTEIN) in the serum of the patient.[3] The myeloma protein molecules are physically homogeneous, being the products of the progeny of a single clone of cells. This unfortunate "experiment of nature," however, gives us access to high concentrations of identical immunoglobulin molecules.

The late Henry Kunkel at Rockefeller University in New York introduced the use of homogeneous myeloma proteins for studying the structure of normal antibody molecules. His was a very creative move because he made the assumption that the product of the myeloma cell was normal even though the cell itself was abnormal, having lost its growth control. We will see that this assumption was correct.

Chain Dissociation Studies

The other Nobel prize winner for work on immunoglobulin structure, G. M. Edelman of Rockefeller University, worked out the chain structure of the antibody molecule. His approach was to allow the molecule to unfold in $6\,M$ urea and then reduce the disulfide bonds with mercaptoethanol. The reduced disulfides were then alkylated so that the chains of the molecule could not reform. He found that there were two kinds of reduced and alkylated chains in each Ig molecule. One of the chains had a molecular weight of approximately 20,000 and one a molecular weight of approximately 50,000. They

---

[3] It will be recalled that one of our basic assumptions from clonal selection is that a single antibody-producing cell produces a single kind of antibody.

CHAPTER THREE

were named LIGHT CHAINS and HEAVY CHAINS (L and H CHAINS). From the relative concentrations of each it was determined that the monomeric Ig molecule contained four chains, two H and two L, held together by disulfide bonds.

By combining the data from the two approaches, it became clear that the L chains and part of the H chains were located in the Fab portion of the molecule. The remainder of the H chains were contained in the Fc portion. The picture which emerged from this pioneering work is seen in Figure 2.

The Hinge Region and Interchain Disulfide Bonds

The region of the immunoglobulin molecule in which papain and pepsin cleavages occur is called the HINGE REGION. This region, which is rich in half-cysteines and prolines, probably serves several functions: the half-cysteines contribute to the INTERCHAIN DISULFIDE BRIDGES (Chapter 4), and the prolines may keep the two combining sites of the molecule separated in space.

Three-Dimensional Structure

From the voluminous work that followed these pioneering studies, we now have a reasonably complete picture of the overall shape and structure of the immunoglobulin molecule. X-ray crystallographic analysis is now beginning to reveal the three-dimensional picture of the mole-

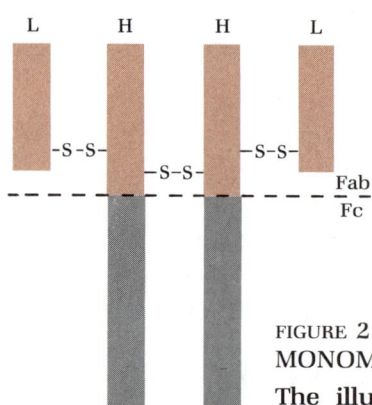

FIGURE 2 MODEL OF THE BASIC IMMUNOGLOBULIN MONOMER

The illustration combines information from the proteolytic digestion studies and reduction and alkylation studies and shows the relationship between the H and L chains and the Fab and Fc portions.

THE BASIC IMMUNOGLOBULIN MONOMER

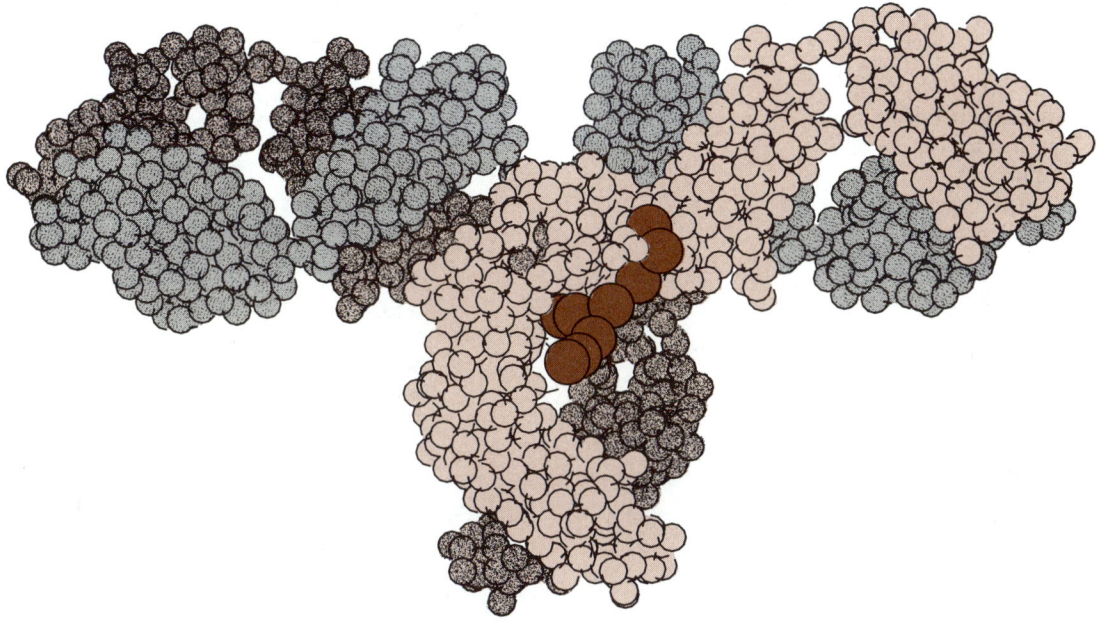

FIGURE 3 THREE-DIMENSIONAL STRUCTURE OF HUMAN IgG MOLECULE

The schematic drawing is based on an early X-ray crystallographic analysis. The heavy chains are represented by tan and dark brown. The light chains are gray. The large brown spheres are the carbohydrate moieties that lie between the C_H2 domains of the two heavy chains. [From Silverton et al. (1977) *PNAS* 74, 5140; reprinted with permission]

cule. Figure 3 shows the orientation in space of an entire human Ig.

Domains of the Immunoglobulin Molecule

Analysis of the disulfide bonds in the basic Ig molecule revealed that there are regularly spaced half cysteines which result in INTRACHAIN (as compared to interchain) DISULFIDE BONDS. These disulfide bonds give the molecule shape and result in clear structural domains (conserved units of which the protein is composed) of the molecule (Figure 4).

These structural domains reflect exon–intron relationships at the DNA level and are in fact functional domains.

CHAPTER THREE

FIGURE 4 HUMAN IgG2 MOLECULE

The domains are defined by intrachain disulfide bonds. The intrachain disulfide bonds are indicated by ○ and the interchain disulfides, which hold the chains together, are indicated by ●. [Based on an illustration from Turner, in Glynn and Steward (1981) *Structure and Function of Antibodies*]

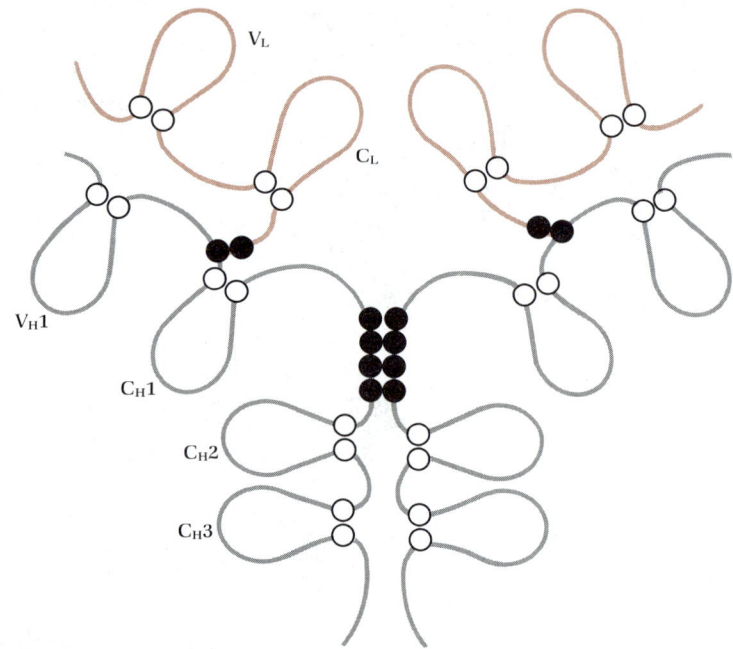

The Structural Basis of Antibody Diversity

Constant and Variable Regions

The chain structure of the basic immunoglobulin molecule explains neither the structural basis for diversity of the antibody molecule nor how the molecule functions to combine with antigen. The discovery that was crucial to solving these problems was the finding that there are *constant* and *variable* regions of amino acid sequence in the immunoglobulin molecule. The announcement of the discovery was one of those rare moments in science when everyone is aware of an important advance. Russell Doolittle describes the moment:

> Early in 1965 a meeting of the Antibody Workshop was held at Warner Springs, California, a small resort community about 60 miles east of San Diego. The meeting, with about 80 persons in attendance, was unique on several counts. Largely organized by Melvin Cohn (of the Salk Institute), a determined effort had been made to infiltrate the immunologic ranks with a galaxy of stellar molecular biologists, including James Watson, Francis Crick, Christian Anfinsen, Max Delbrück, Seymour Benzer, and a

THE BASIC IMMUNOGLOBULIN MONOMER

dozen other nonimmunologists of high repute. The program was simple enough—a few talks on immunologically competent cells, immunogenetics, antibody structure, and the like. For the first two days everything went according to schedule, predictable progress—but not much more—being reported, and the sessions were only slightly lengthened by the presence of the imported Brain Trust. On the third morning, however, the assemblage was electrified by the unexpected announcement from Norbert Hilschmann, reporting on work he had done in Lyman Craig's laboratory, that he had virtually completed the amino acid sequences of two very different Bence-Jones proteins (the equivalent of antibody light chains) and, with one quite explicable exception, had found that all the many amino acid replacements had occurred in the amino-terminal half of the molecules. Clearly, immunoglobulin light chains had a variable half and a constant half.

The impact on the meeting was instantaneous, something very close to pandemonium ensuing. Francis Crick made his way to the chalkboard and drew a flurry of twisted loops, implying that simple DNA rearrangements could now explain antibody diversity; Seymour Benzer declared that at last immunology had become a science. It was one of those rare moments when an entire group senses that a solution to a major problem is directly at hand, but no one is quite sure of how to put the last piece in the puzzle, or even how to find it. Surely, if only a few more sequences were obtained the pattern would become absolutely clear. [R. Doolittle (1974), *Science* 183: 190, review of Smith, *The Variation and Adaptive Expression of Antibodies.*]

In other words, when the first amino acids from the amino-terminal end of Bence-Jones protein A and protein B are compared, they are found to be different. Similarly, when the second, third, and following amino acids are compared, the amino acids at each of these positions in one protein are different from those in the other protein. This difference at each position continues until roughly the midpoint of the light chain. From that point on there is almost complete correspondence of amino acids, position for position (except for the genetically controlled allotypic variation which will be discussed in Chapter 4). Thus the first amino acid beyond the midpoint in proteins A and B is identical in both proteins, and this correspondence continues through to the carboxy-terminal end of the chain. The light chain can therefore be divided into a variable half and a constant half. The VARIA-

BLE REGION, or V REGION, starts at the amino-terminal end of the light chain and comprises the first 100 or so amino acids. The CONSTANT REGION, or C REGION, begins at about residue 100 and continues to the carboxy-terminal end of the chain. Analysis of the H chains soon showed that they too were divided into C and V regions.

The chains of the immunoglobulin molecule can thus be divided into V_L and V_H (variable region of light chain and variable region of heavy chain) and C_L and C_H (constant region of light and heavy chains). The importance of this discovery cannot be understated. For the first time the structural basis for the diversity of the antibody molecule could be visualized. If each antibody molecule can differ from other antibody molecules at a large number of amino acid positions, we can then see how the basic four-chain structure can give rise to an astronomical number of different functional molecules. Clearly, the variation of a few amino acids in the V region of an immunoglobulin must be responsible for antibody diversity and specificity.

Hypervariable Regions   With the realization that the immunoglobulin molecule contained variable and constant regions, it became clear that these regions could be the structural basis for diversity. If there were total variability at all of the 100 or so amino acids in the V region, the permutations of possible antigen-binding structures would be astronomical. However, as more light chains were sequenced, it became clear that there was not total variability in the V regions. Comparisons of sequences of light chains revealed that there were large stretches that were invariant even within the V region.

In 1970 Wu and Kabat compared all of the then-known V_L sequences and came to the conclusion that there were "hot spots" of variability in the V regions. They defined the VARIABILITY RATIO, V, as:

$$\text{Variability} = \frac{\text{number of different amino acids at a given position}}{\text{frequency of the most common amino acids at that position}}$$

Wu-Kabat plots for H and L chains are shown in Figure 5. The

THE BASIC IMMUNOGLOBULIN MONOMER

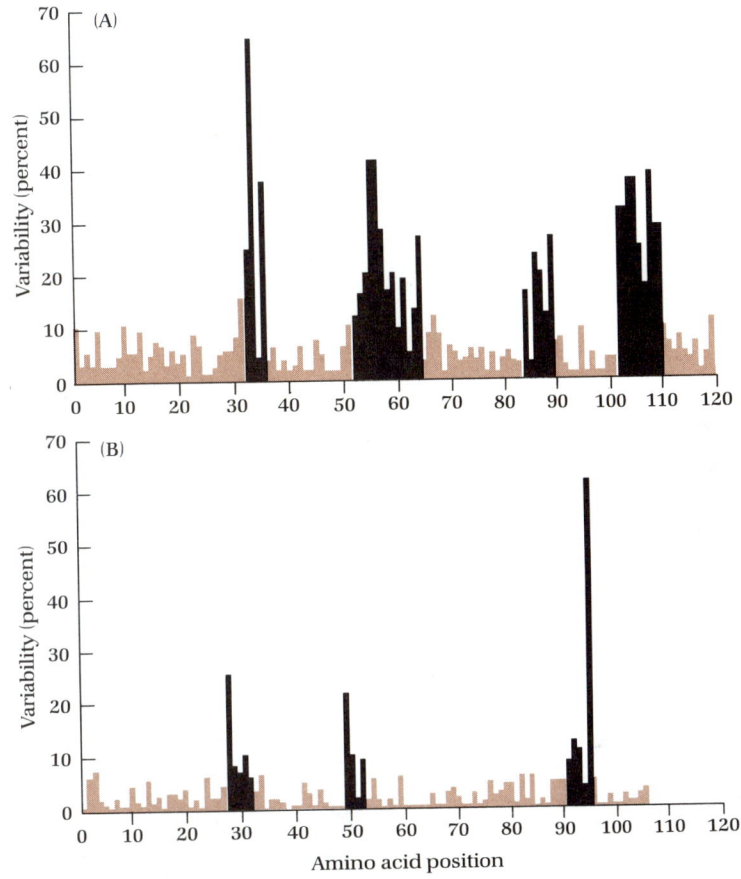

FIGURE 5 WU AND KABAT VARIABILITY PLOTS

Plots of amino acid positions of immunoglobulin heavy chains (A) and light chains (B). The method of calculating variability is described in the text. The hypervariable regions are indicated in black. [Redrawn from Kindt and Capra (1983) *The Antibody Enigma*, p. 83, with permission]

areas of variability are called the HYPERVARIABLE REGIONS and the areas with little variability are called the FRAMEWORK REGIONS.

Synthesis: The Strategy of Antibody Diversity

The basic strategy of antibody diversity is now apparent. Portions of the amino acid sequence of the Ig molecule remain constant but they do not determine the antigen-binding capacity of the antibody molecule. Rather, antigen-binding ability resides in the portions of the molecule that are variable. Compare this strategy with that of the enzyme cytochrome *c*. Figure 6A shows Wu-

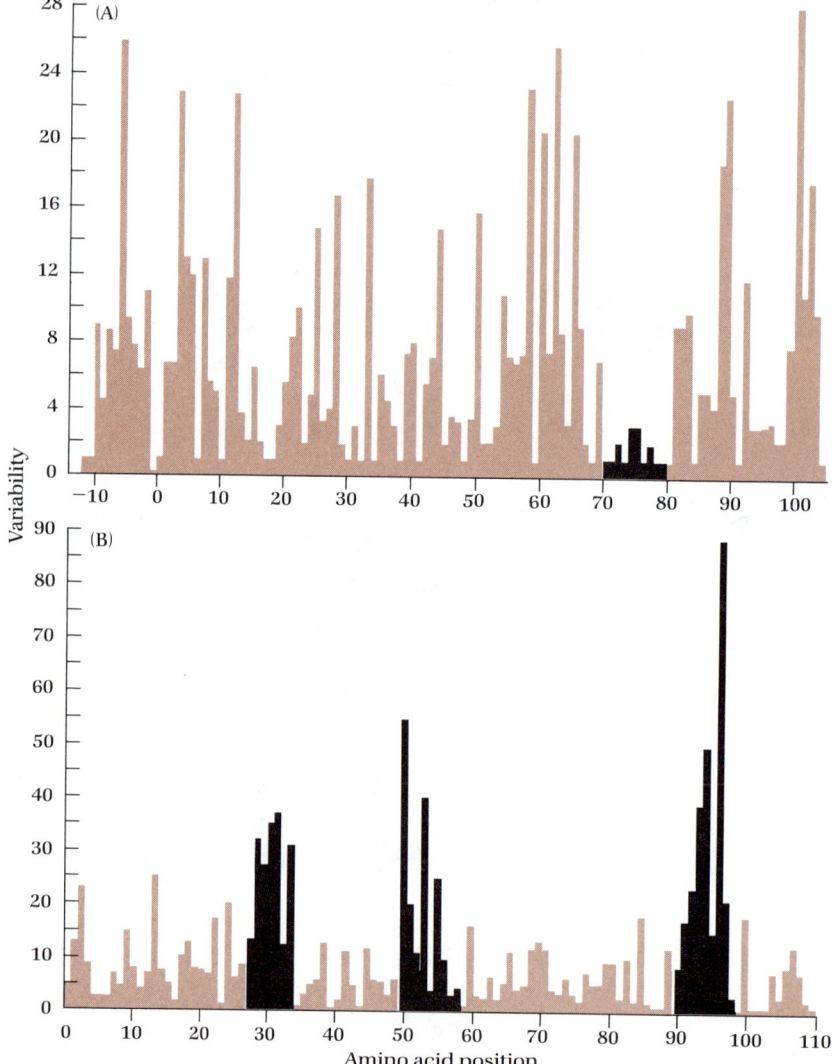

FIGURE 6 WU AND KABAT VARIABILITY PLOTS

Plots of cytochromes *c* of various species (A) and human light chains (B) illustrate the different evolutionary strategies for conserving or generating variation. The active site of the cytochromes is located near residues 70–80, which are the invariant residues. The antigen-binding sites for the light chain are near residues 28–34, 50–58, and 90–98, which are the variable residues. [After Kabat, Wu, and Bilofsky (1979) *Sequence of Immunoglobulin Chains*. U.S. Dept. Health, Education, and Welfare, PHS, NIH, p. 121]

THE BASIC IMMUNOGLOBULIN MONOMER

Kabat variability plots of cytochrome *c* from various species. Note that there is variability everywhere *except* in residues 70–80. These are the residues that constitute the active site of the enzyme. So, in contrast to immunoglobulin (Figure 6B), the active site is maintained as an invariant or constant region and the rest of the molecule is variable. This makes sense because all cytochrome *c* molecules in all species must carry out only one function and the sequence required for that function is maintained. Antibodies, in contrast, must be able to bind with an enormous number of antigens, so the active site varies to allow this to happen. (The genetic mechanism for this variability will be discussed in Chapter 5.)

Sequence Homology of C_H Regions

In 1969 Edelman reported the amino acid sequence of an entire immunoglobulin molecule. He noted that on each H chain the C_H region, which is approximately 330 amino acids long, can be divided into three domains of 110 amino acids each on the basis of *sequence homology*.

HOMOLOGOUS SEQUENCES of amino acids are those sequences that show more similarity (not identity) than could occur by chance. By using a computer analysis that was developed for comparing sequences of different chains of a molecule, investigators can compare the parts of the Ig molecule to determine whether the chains have similarities in sequence composition greater than that expected by chance. As Edelman showed, when parts of the C_H of the Ig molecule are compared this way, they are found to be homologous. This finding implies that they arose from a common gene that underwent tandem duplication and subsequent independent mutation of each new gene. For example, the chains of hemoglobin have different amino acid sequences, but it is known that there once was a single ancestral gene that underwent duplication, yielding two peptides of the same amino acid sequence. During evolutionary time, each of the two genes underwent different mutations; hence the peptides encoded by the two genes are different at the present time. If we know the dictionary of nucleic acid sequences for each amino acid, we can determine the number of mutations needed to go from one amino acid to another. By determining the minimal number of mutations required to change one amino acid to another, it has been possible to show that the three homologous C_H regions probably arose in this manner. The regions are called C_H1, C_H2, and C_H3 (see Figure 4).

These three areas constitute the three STRUCTURAL DOMAINS of the molecule. Their structural similarity has been maintained because each has an intrachain disulfide bond that forms a loop. The basic domain structure and conserved sequences appear in many structures involved in the immune response and have been called the IMMUNOGLOBULIN SUPERFAMILY (Chapter 13).

Nature of the Antigen-Combining Site

Electron Microscopic Studies

The structural studies discussed earlier indicated that the monomeric antibody molecule has two combining sites. This conjecture was confirmed in 1967 when electron micrographs were made of antigen–antibody complexes. In these studies a bivalent hapten of 2,4-dinitrophenyl was constructed and reacted with anti-2,4-dinitrophenyl antibody. Figure 7A is a micrograph in which clear Y-shaped structures can be seen. Figure 7B is the diagrammatic interpretation of this picture, showing the Fab portions of the molecule bound to the hapten.

Size of the Combining Site

Some of the earliest attempts to determine the *size* of the combining site were experiments involving inhibition of antigen–antibody reactions, experiments logically similar to those involving competitive inhibition of enzyme–substrate interactions. In the classic studies by Kabat and his co-workers, a dextran : anti-dextran system was used. Dextran is a large molecule of repeating sugar subunits. Smaller subunits of dextran (3, 4, 5, . . . sugar subunits) were added to the anti-dextran antibody to determine whether they could *inhibit* the binding of the antibody to the dextran. If the small molecule could react with the combining sites on the antibody molecule, then, when the large dextran molecule was added, the combining site would be filled with the small molecules and the large molecules would be prevented from reacting. By using a graded series of sizes of dextran subunits, it was found that in general each site

THE BASIC IMMUNOGLOBULIN MONOMER

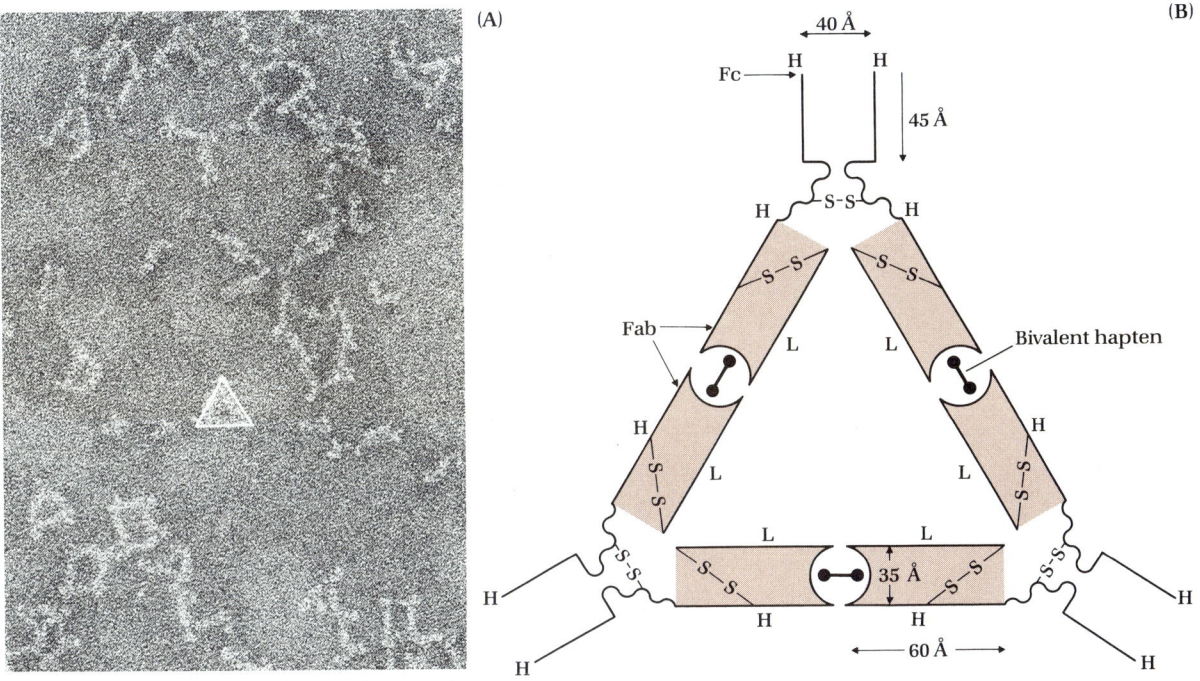

FIGURE 7 RABBIT ANTI-2,4-DINITROPHENYL ANTIBODY AND BIVALENT HAPTEN

(A) Electron micrograph of mixture. Note the Y shapes, which indicate binding of antibody to hapten. (B) Schematic diagram of bound molecules. [From Valentine and Green (1967) *J. Mol. Biol.* 27, 615]

was fully occupied (inhibition approached maximum) by a molecule containing seven sugar moieties. Similar experiments with other antigen–antibody systems using small subunits of the various antigens showed that the combining sites had dimensions of about 30 Å × 10 Å × 6 Å.

Shape of the Combining Site

Figure 8A depicts the antibody molecule, 8B depicts a Fab fragment, and 8C the polypeptide backbone of an immunoglobulin molecule. The brown areas in Figure 8C are the hypervariable regions. Figure 9 shows a schematic of one of the combining sites of an anti-vitamin K antibody with

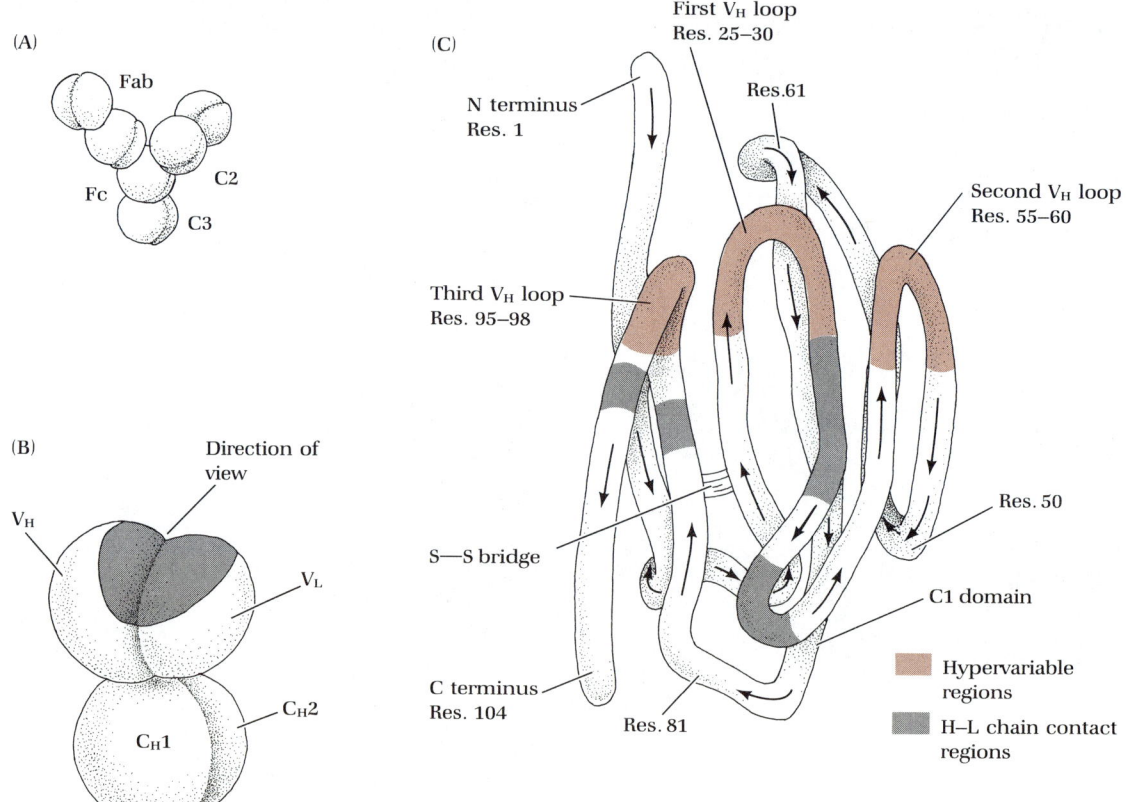

FIGURE 8 COMBINING SITE OF THE ANTIBODY MOLECULE
(A) Ig monomer. Arrangement of the six domains of the antibody molecule with respect to each other. (B) Fab fragment. A diagram of the variable domain showing the V_L–V_H contact surface (shaded area). (C) The folded polypeptide backbone of the heavy chain. The areas of contact with the light chain and the hypervariable regions are highlighted. [From Richards, Varga, Rosenstein and Konigsberg, in Glynn and Steward (1981) *Structure and Function of Antibodies*]

the antigen bound. The message these illustrations carry is that the combining site must be a trough or cavity composed of parts of the hypervariable regions of both an H and an L chain.

THE BASIC IMMUNOGLOBULIN MONOMER

X-Ray Diffraction Studies   Studies of the three-dimensional configuration of the antigen-combining sites of antibodies comes primarily from X-ray diffraction studies of Fab fragments. Antigen appears to combine with antibody in the IMMUNOGLOBULIN FOLD, which is formed by both an H and an L chain. The combining sites for different specificities will of course be slightly different, but it appears that the basic nature of the site is now known.

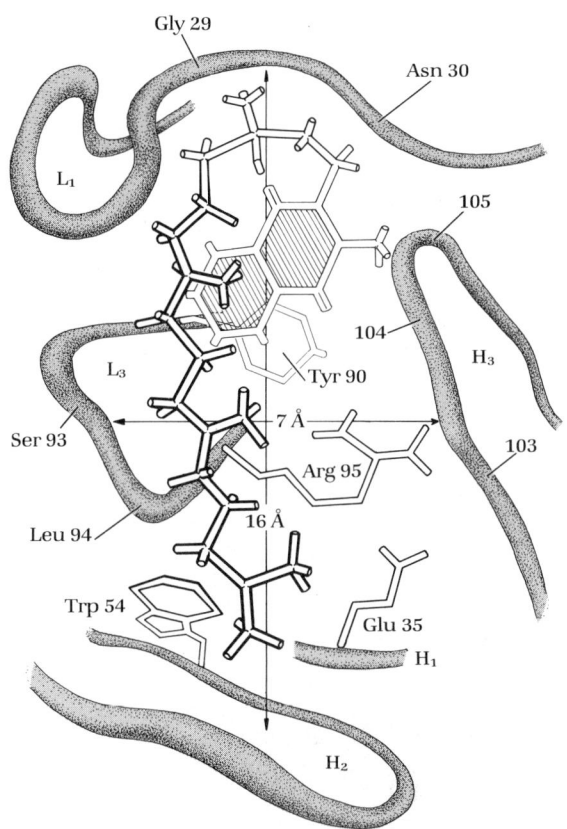

FIGURE 9   ANTIGEN-COMBINING SITE OF AN ANTIBODY MOLECULE

The haptenic site interacts with the variable regions of the heavy (brown) and light (gray) chains. [From Amzel et al. (1974) *PNAS* **71**, 1427]

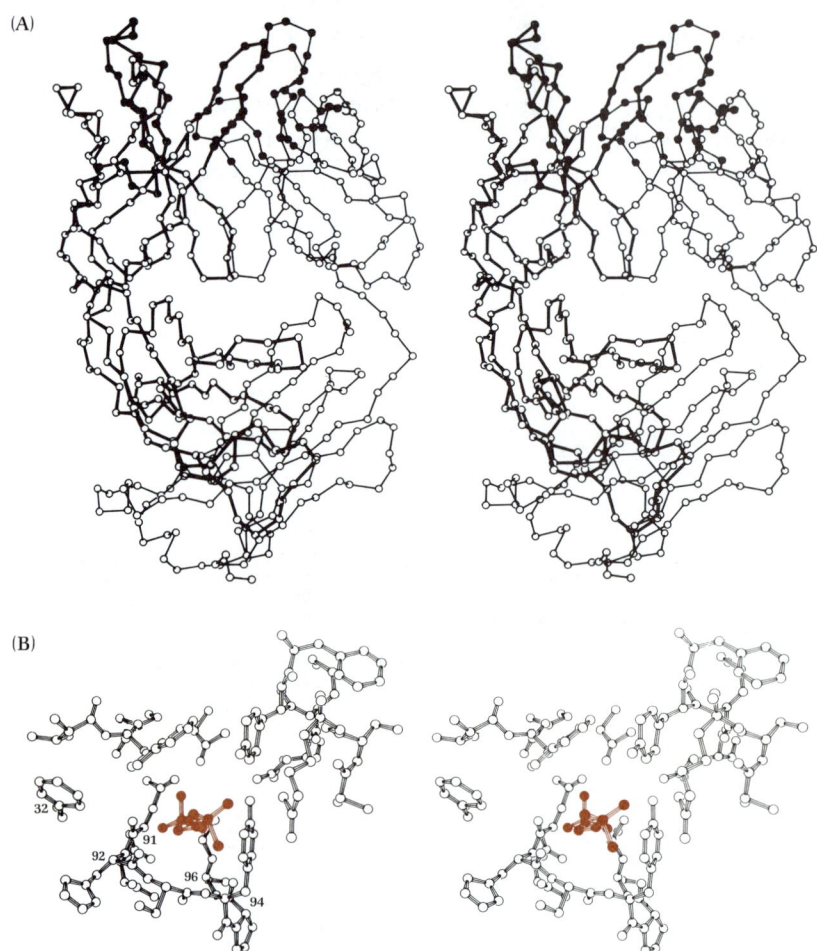

FIGURE 10 α-CARBON BACKBONE OF A PHOSPHOCHOLINE-BINDING MYELOMA PROTEIN

(A) In this stereo drawing the heavy chain is represented by the thick line. The two variable domains are at the top and the constant domains are at the bottom of the figure. The complementarity-determining residues (CDR) are shown as filled circles. (B) The combining site of the phosphocholine-binding myeloma protein shown in (A). The lower residues 91–96 and 32 are from the light chains. The remaining residues belong to the three CDR of the heavy chain. The phosphocholine (in brown) has the phosphate group in front, with the choline moiety buried in a pocket. [From Davies and Metzger (1983) *Annu. Rev. Immunol.* 1, 87; with permission]

THE BASIC IMMUNOGLOBULIN MONOMER

Figure 10A shows the α carbon backbone of a Fab that binds the hapten phosphocholine (PC). In the figure the antigen binding surface, or COMPLEMENTARITY-DETERMINING SURFACE, is indicated by closed circles. Figure 10B is a stereo drawing of the combining site for PC, with the PC bound. The choline is attached at the bottom of the pocket located between hypervariable regions H3 and L3. The phosphate contacts residues of the H chain.

Summary

1. Antibodies are found in the γ-globulin fraction of serum and are called immunoglobulins (Ig). Because serum Ig is so heterogeneous, myeloma proteins (which are homogeneous) are used to study Ig structure.
2. Treatment of Ig with the proteolytic enzyme papain results in Fab and Fc fragments. Fab has the antigen-binding capacity of the molecule and Fc binds complement.
3. The basic Ig monomer is composed of two heavy (H) and two light (L) chains which are joined by interchain disulfide bonds.
4. H and L chains are composed of variable and constant regions. Within the variable regions are hypervariable regions, which are also called complementarity-determining regions (CDR). Antibody diversity is generated by amino acid substitutions that occur within the hypervariable regions and result in unique antigen-binding structures.
5. The antigen-combining site is located in a trough formed by the interaction of H and L chain hypervariable regions.

Additional Readings

Davies, D.R. and H. Metzger. 1983. Structural basis of antibody function. *Annu. Rev. Immunol.* 1: 87.

Glynn, L.E. and M.W. Steward (eds.). 1981. *Structure and Function of Antibodies*. Wiley, Chichester.

Kindt, T.J. and J.D. Capra. 1984. *The Antibody Enigma*. Plenum, New York.

Wall, R. and M. Kuehl. 1983. Biosynthesis and regulation of immunoglobulins. *Annu. Rev. Immunol.* 1: 393.

CHAPTER 4
HETEROGENEITY OF IMMUNOGLOBULINS

Overview Immunoglobulin molecules are extremely heterogeneous, a fact that has made the detailed study of the basic monomer of the molecule very difficult. But the introduction of myeloma proteins allowed homogeneous products to be isolated and studied. When referring to the heterogeneity of the immunoglobulin molecule, we mean not only the variations in the antigen-binding site (the multitude of different hypervariable regions that make up the repertoire of reactions of antibody molecules), but also the physical heterogeneity among antibody molecules. There are five classes of immunoglobulin molecules, called isotypes. Each class has unique physical characteristics, but the antigen-combining property is present in all of the classes. A second kind of physical heterogeneity involves the allelic distribution of antigens on the immunoglobulin molecules within a class. These subgroups are called allotypes and are of great use in studying the genetics of the Ig molecule. Finally, a third kind of physical heterogeneity involves individual differences between Ig molecules, differences identified as idiotypes.

This chapter contains information that the reader will perhaps want to refer back to at various times as the text proceeds. Only practicing immunologists have this kind of information at their fingertips; the student should learn about the various kinds of heterogeneity and properties of the various classes so that he/she can appreciate the uses made of this heterogeneity in experiments designed to understand how the immune system functions.

HETEROGENEITY OF IMMUNOGLOBULINS

Physical Heterogeneity

Antibody activity is found in a broad spectrum of immunoglobulins. When analyzed by ultracentrifugation, antibody activity is found in molecules with sedimentation coefficients ranging from 7 S to 19 S. This indicates great heterogeneity in *size* since these sedimentation coefficients correspond to molecular weights ranging from approximately 150,000 to 1,000,000. Heterogeneity is also seen when antibody molecules are analyzed by electrophoresis, indicating there is also great heterogeneity in *charge*.

When immunoglobulins of one species are injected into an animal of another species, they act as antigens. The antibodies raised against the immunoglobulins can be used as reagents to study the *antigenic heterogeneity* of the Ig. This antigenic heterogeneity has proved very important in the study of the immunoglobulins because it defines their *class*—the most useful means of categorizing the immunoglobulins.

Class (or Isotype) of Immunoglobulins

Definition of Class

The immunoglobulins are classified according to their antigenic properties. Antibodies against the immunoglobulins of a species (human, for example) can be raised in a rabbit. Because there is great heterogeneity among Ig molecules, such an antiserum will contain antibodies against all the classes of Ig in the serum. Because the classes also differ in charge, the different reactivities can be visualized by immunoelectrophoresis (see Chapter 8). In a typical electrophoretic pattern there are several bands of precipitate, each representing a class of Ig. All normal individuals have molecules of each class in their serum.

Classes, or Isotypes

The CLASS of an immunoglobulin is determined by its unique antigenic properties. The antigenic determinants that define class are located on the heavy (H) chain and are called ISOTYPIC DETERMINANTS. The five classes of Ig are designated by capital Roman letters: IgG, IgM, IgA, IgD, and IgE. The H chain of each class is designated by the small Greek letter corresponding to the Roman letter of the class. Thus the H

CHAPTER FOUR

chain of IgG is a γ chain, and the H chain of IgM is a μ chain; IgA has an α chain, IgD has a δ chain, and IgE has an ε chain.

Some of the Ig classes are composed of polymers of the basic four-chain structure described in Chapter 3. Different classes have different molecular weights and diverse biological properties in addition to antigen binding. None of these other qualities, however, defines class. The class of an immunoglobulin is always determined by its H chain antigens.

There are two antigenic varieties of the LIGHT (L) CHAINS of immunoglobulin molecules, called KAPPA (κ) and LAMBDA (λ). All classes of Ig have these two types of L chains. Each monomeric immunoglobulin molecule, it will be recalled, has two L chains that are linked to the two H chains by disulfide bonds. A given immunoglobulin molecule has two identical L chains, either κ or λ, and never contains one κ chain and one λ chain. The monomeric form of any immunoglobulin can therefore be described by its chain structure. An IgG molecule, for example, will always have two γ chains and either two κ chains or two λ chains. It would thus be $\gamma_2\kappa_2$ or $\gamma_2\lambda_2$.

We said earlier that the molecular weights of the immunoglobulins varied from 150,000 to 1,000,000. This variation in molecular weight is due to *polymerization* of the basic monomeric unit. An IgM molecule, for example, has a molecular weight of approximately 1,000,000. IgM is a pentamer, but it is *not* a polymer of five IgG monomers. Because the monomer of IgM is $\mu_2\kappa_2$ or $\mu_2\lambda_2$, IgM is described as $(\mu_2\kappa_2)_5$ or $(\mu_2\lambda_2)_5$. IgA can have a variable number of monomeric units polymerized into a large molecule and would be designated $(\alpha_2\kappa_2)_n$ or $(\alpha_2\lambda_2)_n$, where n can range from 2 to 5.

There is variation in the number and position of disulfide bridges in the monomeric form of each class and subclass of Ig (Figure 1). The Ig classes and subclasses in various vertebrates are given in Information Box 1.

Subclasses

Antisera that distinguish between molecules within a class can be made. For example, antisera that have been produced to detect differences *within* the IgG class will detect differences in the γ chains. These differences define SUBCLASSES of H chains and thus subclasses of immuno-

HETEROGENEITY OF IMMUNOGLOBULINS

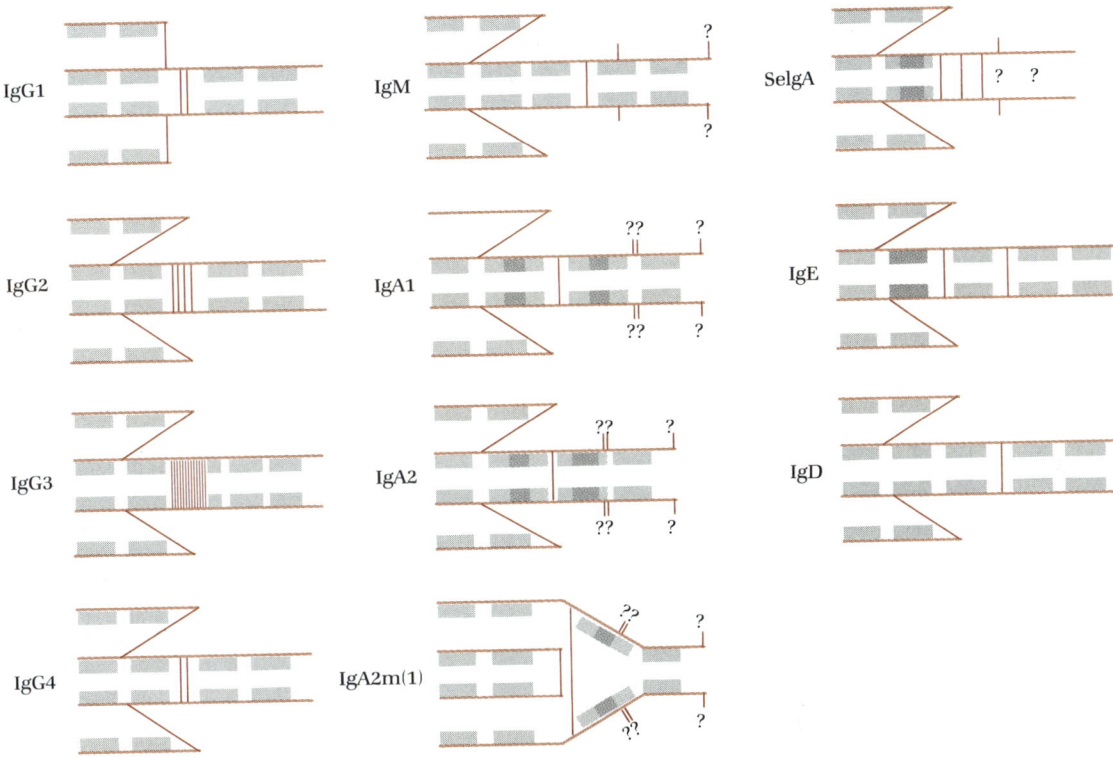

FIGURE 1 INTERCHAIN AND INTRACHAIN DISULFIDE BRIDGES IN HUMAN IMMUNOGLOBULINS

globulins. Two molecules may both contain two γ chains, but the H chains of the two IgG molecules may differ in antigenic properties as well as in biological properties. In all cases where subclasses of immunoglobulin molecules have been found, the antigenic differences have been located on the H chain in the Fc portion.

In humans there are four known γ chain subclasses, cleverly called IgG1, IgG2, IgG3, and IgG4. All subclasses of immunoglobulin are found in the serum of every normal individual.

Common Origin of Immunoglobulin Classes

Figure 2 shows the amino acid sequences of the Fc regions of all five classes of human immunoglobulin. There are seventeen positions at which all five classes have an identical amino acid. This homology between the

INFORMATION BOX 1

Ig Classes and Subclasses in Some Vertebrates

Species	Class and subclass				
Human	IgG1, IgG2, IgG3, IgG4	IgA1, IgA2	IgM1, IgM2	IgD	IgE
Ape	IgG	IgA	IgM	IgD	IgE
Monkey	IgG	IgA	IgM	IgD	IgE
Mouse	IgG2a, IgG2b, —[a], IgG1	IgA1, IgA2	IgM	IgD	IgE
Rat	IgG2a, IgG2b, IgG2c, IgG1	IgA	IgM	?	IgE
Guinea pig	IgG2, —, —, IgG1	IgA	IgM	?	IgE
Rabbit	IgG2, —, —, IgG1	IgA1, IgA2	IgM	?	IgE
Dog	IgG2a, IgG2b, IgG2c, IgG1	IgA	IgM	?	IgE
Cow	IgG2, —, —, IgG1	IgA	IgM	?	?
Horse	IgGa, IgGb, IgGc, IgGT	IgA	IgM	?	?
Fowl	IgG	IgA	IgM	?	?
Reptile	IgG	?	IgM	?	?
Amphibian	IgG	?	IgM	?	?
Fish	?	?	IgM	?	?
Lamprey	?	?	IgM	?	?

Source: From Wang, (1976), in Fudenberg et al. (eds.), *Basic and Clinical Immunology.*
[a]Absence of an additional subclass corresponding to that in humans.

classes has been used as an argument for the common evolutionary origins of the chains.[1]

There is approximately 95% homology between subclasses (e.g., IgG1 and IgG2) and 30% homology between any two Ig classes. The areas of homology are found clustered in areas of β-

---

[1]These same 17 invariant residues are shared by β_2-microglobulin, Thy-1, and MHC antigens, all of which are members of the immunoglobulin "superfamily" (see Chapter 5).

HETEROGENEITY OF IMMUNOGLOBULINS

```
δ  H T Q P L G V Y L L T P A V Q D - L W L R D K A T F T C F V V G S D L K D A - - - - H L T W E V A G K V P T G
μ  Q D T A I R V F A I P P S F A S - I F L T K S T K L T C L V T - - D L T Y D S - - V T I S W T R Q D G E A V K
γ  L L G G P S V F L F P P K P K D T L M I S R T P E V T C V V V - - D V S H E D P Q V K F N W Y V - D G V Q V H
α  S C C H P R L S L H R P A L Q D - L L L G S E A N L T C T L T - - G L R D A S G - V T F T W P S T S G K - - -
ε  N P R G V S A Y L S R P S P F D - L F I R K S P T I T C L V V - - D L A P S K G T V N L T W S R A S G K P V -

δ  G V E E G L L E R H S N G S Q S Q H S R L T L P R S L W N A G T S V T C T L N H P S L P P Q R L M A L R E P A
μ  T H T B - I S E S H P B A T F S A V G E A S I C E B B W N S G E R F T C T V T H T D L P S P L K Q T I S R P K
γ  N A K T K P R E Q Q Y B S T Y R V V S V L T V L H Q N W L D G K E Y K C K V S N K A L P A P I E K T I S K A K
α  S A V Q G P P E R D L C G C Y S V S S V L P G C A E P W N H G K T F T C T A A Y P E S K T P L T A T L S K - S
ε  N H S T R K E E K Q R N G T L T V T S T L P V G T R D W I E G E T Y G C R V T H P H L P R A L M R S T T K T S

δ  A Q A P V K L S L N L L A S S D P P E A A S - - - W L L C E V S G F S P P N I L L M W L E D Q R - E V N T S G
μ  G V A L H R P D V Y L L P P A R E Q L N L R E S A T I T C L V T G F S P A D V F V Q W M Q R G Q P L S P E K
γ  G Q P R E - P Q V Y T L P P S R E E M T K N Q - V S L T C L V K G F Y P S D I A V E W E S N D G E - - - P E N
α  G - N T F R P Q V H L L P P P S Z Z L A L B Z L V T L T C L A R G F S P K D V L V R W L - Q G S Q E L P R E K
ε  G - P R A A P E V Y A F A T P E W P G S R D K - R T L A C L I Q N F M P E D I S V Q W L H N E V Q - L P D A R

δ  F - - A P A R P P P Q P G S T T F W A W S V L R V P A P P S P Q P A T Y T C V V S H E D S R T L L N A S R S L
μ  Y V T S A P M P E P Q - A P G R Y F A H S I L T V S E E E W N T G E T Y T C V V A H E A L P N R V T - E R T V
γ  Y K T T P P V L D - S D G S - - F F L Y S K L T V D K S R W Q Q G N V F S C S V M H E A L H N H Y T - Q K S L
α  Y L T W A S R Q E P S Q G T T T F A V T S I L R V A A E D W K K G D T F S C M V G H Z A L P L A F T - Q K T I
ε  H S T T Q P R K - - T K G S G - F F V F S R L E V T R A E W Q E K D E F I C R A V H E A A S P S Q T V Q R A V

δ  E V S Y V T D H G P M
μ  D K S T G K P T L Y B V S L V M S B T A G T C Y
γ  S L S P G
α  D R L A G K P T H V N V S V V M A E V D G T C Y
ε  S V N P G K
```

FIGURE 2 COMPARISON OF THE AMINO ACID SEQUENCES OF Fc REGIONS

The Fc regions of the five classes of human immunoglobulins are compared; the one-letter notations are for amino acids. The positions in gray boxes are those at which the same amino acids appear in all classes; the positions in brown boxes are those positions at which at least two classes have the same amino acid. This great homology is used as an argument for the common evolutionary origin of the heavy chains. [Redrawn from Lin and Putnam (1981) *PNAS* 78, 504; with permission]

pleated sheets, especially around the two cysteines that form the intrachain disulfide bond.

Properties of Immunoglobulin Classes

Each class of immunoglobulin has the ability to carry out the primary function of antibody molecules—the combination with antigen—but they each have specialized functional ways of acting as EFFECTOR MOLECULES. These effector functions will be dis-

INFORMATION BOX 2

Human Immunoglobulins

	IgG1	IgG2	IgG3	IgG4	IgM	IgA1	IgA2	IgA$_{sec}$	IgD	IgE
H chain	γ1	γ2	γ3	γ4	μ	α1	α2	α1, α2	δ	ε
Sedimentation constant(s)	7	7	7	7	19	7	7	11	7	8
Molecular weight (in thousands)	146	146	170	146	970	160	160	385	184	188
Mol. wt. of H chain (in thousands)	51	51	60	51	65	56	52	52–56	70	73
Number of H chain domain	4	4	4	4	5	4	4	4	5	5
Carbohydrate (%)	2–3	2–3	2–3	2–3	12	7–11	7–11	7–11	9–14	12
Serum conc. (mg/ml)	9	3	1	0.5	1.5	3	0.5	0.05	0.03	0.00005
Classical C fixation	++	+	+++	−	+++	−	−	−	−	−
Alt. pathway C activity	−	−	−	−	−	+	+	−	−	−
Placental transfer	+	+	+	+	−	−	−	−	−	−
Binding to mononuclear cells	+	−	+	−	−	−	−	−	−	−
Binding to mast cells and to basophils	−	−	−	−	−	−	−	−	−	+++
Reaction with Staph A	+	+	−	+	−	−	−	−	−	−
Half-life (days)	21	20	7	21	10	6	6	—	3	2
Distribution (% intravascular)	45	45	45	45	80	42	42	—	75	50
Fractional catabolic rate (% intravascular pool catabolized/day)	7	7	17	7	9	25	25	—	37	71
Synthetic rate (mg/kg/day)	33	33	33	33	3.3	24	24	—	0.4	0.002

Source: From many sources, but heavily from Turner (1981), in Glynn and Steward (eds.), *Structure and Function of Antibodies.*

HETEROGENEITY OF IMMUNOGLOBULINS

cussed at appropriate points in the chapter. The different properties of the classes are listed in Information Box 2.

Immunoglobulin G

IgG is a monomer and has the properties of the basic immunoglobulin monomer described in Chapter 3. It consists of two γ chains and two L chains. Human IgG has a sedimentation coefficient of 7 S and a molecular weight of approximately 150,000. In normal human adults, it is the major class of immunoglobulin, constituting approximately 75% of the total Ig.

There are four subclasses of IgG, each with a slight structural variation. These are shown in Figure 3. IgG1 constitutes 70% of the IgG and IgG2 20%; IgG3 and IgG4 make up only 8 and 2% respectively. IgG3 has a rapid *catabolic rate* (the rate at which it is catabolized in the serum), with a half-life of one week; the other classes have half-lives of three weeks.

IgG is the only class of immunoglobulin that is able to cross the placenta; it is therefore the class of maternal antibodies that protects the newborn. IgG2, however, crosses more slowly than do the other subclasses.

Immunoglobulin M

IgM makes up approximately 10% of normal human serum immunoglobulin. It has a sedimentation coefficient of 19 S, which corresponds to a molecular weight of approximately 850,000 to 1,000,000. The molecule is rich in carbohydrate, which constitutes approximately 12% of its weight.

IgM is a pentamer of monomeric units with μ chains (Figure 4). Each monomer has a molecular weight of approximately 180,000. IgM, unlike all other Ig classes except IgE, has a fourth C_H domain. The monomers are joined together through disulfide bridges in this C_H4 domain. The entire pentamer assumes the circular shape seen in Figure 4. It was not known for some time what is responsible for this configuration. One alternative was that the entire circle is composed of the monomers joined together by disulfide bonds to form a bracelet. Another alternative, called the CLASP MODEL, was that four of the monomers are attached to each other by disulfide bonds but the start and the end

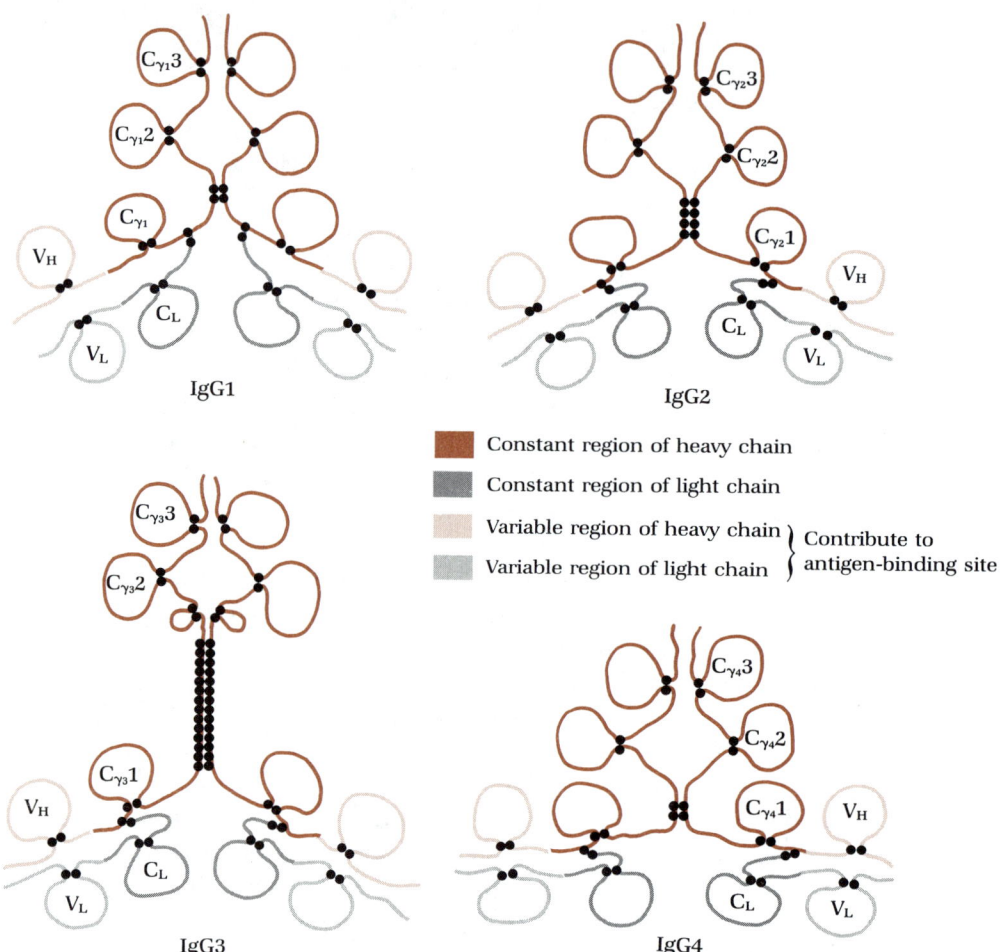

FIGURE 3 STRUCTURES OF THE FOUR SUBCLASSES OF HUMAN IgG

of the ring are attached to a structure called the J PROTEIN, which acts as a clasp. Data favors the clasp model and the J chain clasp can be seen holding the circle of monomers together in Figure 4.

Immunoglobulin A

Serum IgA. IgA constitutes 20% of the serum immunoglobulin. Of this, 80% is in the form of monomer of molecular weight 160,000. The remaining 20% are polymers that can be two, three, four, or five monomers held

HETEROGENEITY OF IMMUNOGLOBULINS

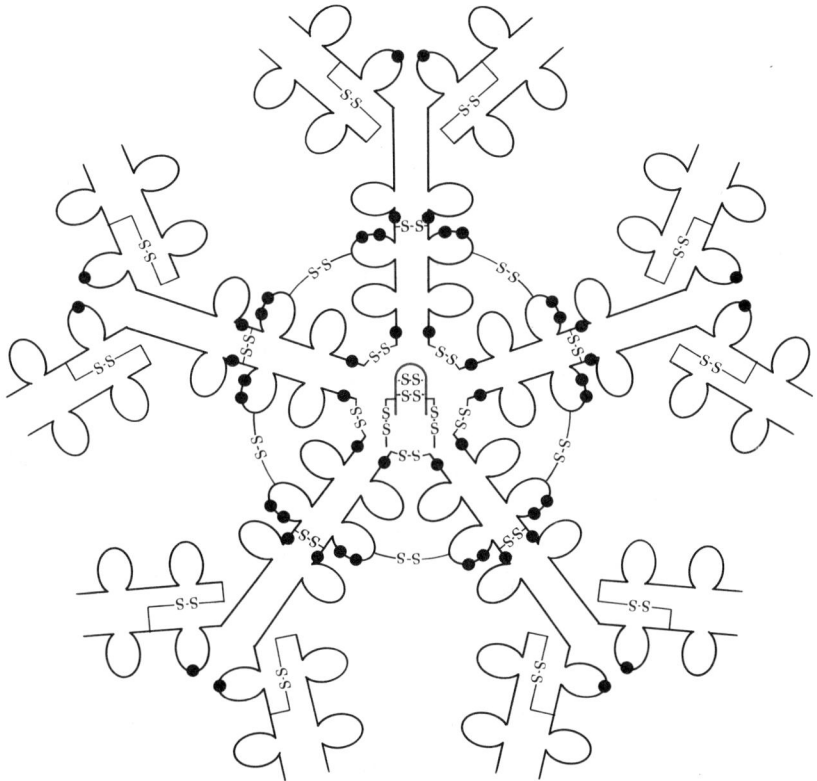

FIGURE 4 POSSIBLE LOCATION OF J CHAIN IN HUMAN IgM
Black circles represent carbohydrate side chains. [From Turner, in Glynn and Steward (1981) *Structure and Function of Antibodies*]

together by disulfide bridges and a single J chain. The polymers have sedimentation coefficients of 10, 13, and 15 S, with the 10 S form predominant.

Secretory IgA. Secretory IgA is the predominant immunoglobulin in *seromucous secretions* and is found in external secretions such as saliva, tracheobronchial secretions, colostrum, milk, and genitourinary secretions. (The IgA in internal secretions such as synovial, amniotic, pleural, and cerebrospinal fluids is the serum type rather than the secretory type.)

Secretory IgA consists of four components: a dimer of two

CHAPTER FOUR

monomeric molecules, a 70,000-dalton SECRETORY COMPONENT, and a 15,000-dalton J CHAIN. The J chain is produced by the same cells that produce the IgA and is probably linked in the same manner as in IgM (see Figure 4). The secretory piece, in contrast, is synthesized by epithelial cells and is covalently linked to the Fc of the IgA:J chain dimer as it passes through the epithelial cells of the mucosa. A schematic diagram of the association of secretory components and J chain with the IgA molecule is shown in Figure 5.

Immunoglobulin D

The concentration of IgD in the serum is very low, approximately 0.03 mg/ml. Because the concentration of IgD is so low, study of the molecule is very difficult and is complicated even further by the fact that the molecule is extremely labile. It is much more sensitive to proteolysis and heat than are other immunoglobulin classes, and proteolytic enzymes in serum may be sufficient to fragment the molecule during isolation procedures.

The molecular weight of IgD is approximately 180,000. The δ chain has a molecular weight of 60,000 to 70,000, with approximately 12% carbohydrate associated with this chain.

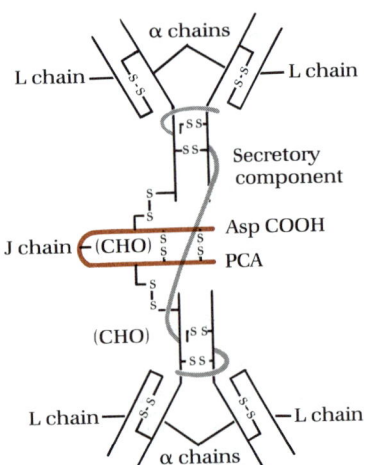

FIGURE 5   HUMAN SECRETORY IgA

Diagram showing the possible arrangement of the two IgA monomers in relation to the secretory component and the J chain. The secretory component is synthesized by epithelial cells and is linked covalently to the Fc of the α chains (which are joined by the J chain) as it passes through the epithelial cells of the mucosa. [From Turner, in Glynn and Steward (1981) *Structure and Function of Antibodies*]

HETEROGENEITY OF IMMUNOGLOBULINS

The apparent biological function of IgD has recently been established. IgD is found to be present in association with IgM on the surface membranes of B lymphocytes. A cell that expresses both IgM and IgD is a mature but "virgin" B cell. The IgM and IgD molecules on the same cell have the same antigen-binding specificity.

Immunoglobulin E

IgE is the HOMOCYTOTROPIC, or REAGINIC ANTIBODY, involved in immediate hypersensitivity and allergy (see Chapter 26). It has the lowest concentration in serum, approximately 0.00005 mg/ml; yet it has profound effector function.

IgE was discovered in 1966 in an ingenious experiment done by the Ishizakas in Baltimore. They produced a reaginic rich fraction of serum from an allergic (atopic) patient and injected the fraction into a rabbit to produce anti-reaginic antibody. At the time, the known classes of immunoglobulin were IgG, IgM, IgA, and IgD. The antiserum was reacted with myeloma proteins of each of the known classes in an attempt to determine the class of the reaginic antibody by removing its activity. The antiserum against the human reaginic serum, now depleted of antibody to all *known* immunoglobulin classes, should have been devoid of any reactivity. However, this "empty antiserum" was able to form a precipitate with the reaginic-rich fraction of the patient's serum. In this way, they showed that an as yet unknown class of immunoglobulin was responsible for allergic reactions; but it was in such low concentration in the serum that it had been previously unidentified. It was not until IgE-producing myelomas became available that structural work became possible.

The IgE molecule exists as a monomer ($\epsilon_2\kappa_2$, $\epsilon_2\lambda_2$) with a molecular weight of 180,000. The ϵ chain is 72,000 and, like IgM, has four C_H domains. The Fc portion binds strongly to a receptor on mast cells and in this manner carries out the molecule's effector function. The consequences of this binding are allergies due to mast cell degranulation and release of pharmacologically active substances. This whole fascinating story is covered in detail in Chapter 26.

CHAPTER FOUR

Genetic Variation in Immunoglobulins (Allotypes and Idiotypes)

Allotypic Variation

ALLOTYPIC VARIATION is the variation between Ig molecules due to genetically controlled antigenic determinants (allotypic determinants). Ig molecules that exhibit allotypic variation are called ALLOTYPES. The name derives from the fact that these antigens are products of *allelic* forms of a gene that are inherited in a Mendelian fashion. Although every normal individual of a species has all immunoglobulin classes, each individual has only one form of each of the allotypes on

---

INFORMATION BOX 3

Human Allotypes

Chain and Allotype	Determinant	Location	Chain and Allotype	Determinant	Location
γ_1, G1m	G1m (1)	C_H3	α_3, G3m (continued)	(21)	C_H2
	(2)	C_H3		(24)	C_H
	(3)	C_H1		(25)	C_H
	(7)	C_H		(26)	C_H
	(17)	C_H1		(27)	C_H
	(18)	C_H	γ_4, G4m	G4m(4a)	C_H2
	(20)	C_H		(4b)	C_H2
γ_2, G2m	G2m(23)	C_H2	α2m, A2m	A2m (1)	C_H
	(5)	C_H2		(2)	C_H
γ_3, G3m	G3m (6)	C_H3	μ, Mm	Mm (1)	C_H
	(11)	C_H3	κ, Km[a]	Km (1)	C_κ
	(13)	C_H3		(2)	C_κ
	(14)	C_H3		(3)	C_κ
	(15)	C_H2			
	(16)	C_H2			

[a] Formerly Inv

HETEROGENEITY OF IMMUNOGLOBULINS

INFORMATION BOX 4

Rabbit Allotypes

Chain and Allotype	Determinant	Location
γ, de	d11, d12 e14, e15	C_H1 hinge C_H1 Fc
α_1, f	f69 to f73	C_H
α_2, g	g74 to g77	C_H, Fc and Fab
μ, n	n80 to n87	C_H

Chain and Allotype	Determinant	Location
V_H, a	a1-3, a100-103	V_H
V_H, x	x32	V_H
V_H, y	y33	V_H
κ, b	b4, 5, 6, 9	?
λ, c	c7, c21	?

their immunoglobulins. Allotypes are codominantly expressed, but an individual B lymphocyte secretes only one of the parental forms, a phenomenon known as ALLELIC EXCLUSION (see Chapter 5).

Both human and rabbit allotypes were discovered in 1956, and because they have such a long history their nomenclature has become very complicated. The nomenclature of allotypes and the chain locations of human, rabbit, and mouse allotypic determinants are given in Information Boxes 3, 4, and 5.

Allotypes are useful in studying the genetics of immunoglobulins and have served as useful markers in linkage studies in cellular immunology. They have also been useful tools to anthropologists and population geneticists because they have unique distributions among ethnic groups.

Idiotypic Variation

So far in this chapter we have seen that there are antigenic determinants on H chains which are unique to each class of immunoglobulins and are called isotypic determinants. Each normal member of a species has all of the immunoglobulin classes in its serum. In addition to

INFORMATION BOX 5

Allotypes on C_H Regions of Mouse Ig[a]

Haplotype	Prototype strain	Locus and chain						
		Igh-1 γ_{2a}	Igh-2 α	Igh-3 γ_{2b}	Igh-4 γ_1	Igh-5 δ	Igh-6 μ	Igh-7 ϵ
a	BALB/c	a	a	a	a	a	a	a
b	C57BL	b	b	b	b	b	b	b
c	DBA/2	c	c	a	a	a	—[c]	—
d	AKR	d	d	d	a	a	—	a
e	A	e	d	e	a	e	e	a
f	CE	f	f	f	a	a	—	—
g	RIII	g	c	g	a	a	—	—
h	SEA	h	a	a	a	a	—	—
j	CBA	j	a	a	a	a	a	a[d]
k	KH-1[b]	k	c	a	a	—	—	—
l	KH-2[b]	l	c	a	a	—	—	—
m	Ky[b]	m	b	b	b	—	—	—
n	NZB	e	d	e	a	a	e	—

Source: From Nisonoff (1983), *Introduction to Molecular Immunology*, Second Edition.

[a]In compiling the mouse allotypes, strains were grouped into 12 haplotypes based on the allotype of their γ_{2a} chain. The genetic loci which control the allotypes on the various chains are determined as: Igh-1 for γ_{2a}; Igh-2 for α; Igh-3 for γ_{2b}; etc.

[b]Wild mice.

[c]Not determined.

[d]One member of this group of strains, C3H, expresses the α allele in its IgE. The prototype, CBA, has not been tested.

HETEROGENEITY OF IMMUNOGLOBULINS

isotypic determinants, each member of a species has allotypic determinants, individually specific allelic variants of certain antigenic determinants which are inherited in a Mendelian fashion.

There is yet another kind of antigenic determinant on Ig molecules which is unique to particular molecules of an individual. These are called IDIOTYPIC DETERMINANTS. (The word *idiotypic* derives from the Greek *idio*, which means "individual.")

Like isotypic and allotypic determinants, idiotypic determinants are identified by the ability to raise antibody against them. For example, an animal is injected with an antigen, and the resulting antibody is reacted with the antigen in vitro to form an antigen–antibody complex (Figure 6). When the purified antibody or even the antigen–antibody complexes are injected into another animal, an antiserum will be produced and will contain antibodies against many parts of the first antibody molecule, including the antigen-combining site. By judicious absorption from the antiserum of all antibodies to isotypic and allotypic determinants, one is left with an antibody to unique determinants on the first antibody molecule. These are the idiotypic determinants.

Idiotypes as Markers of Antigen-Combining Sites

The anti-idiotype antibody raised in this way (with rare exception) will not react with any other immunoglobulins in the donor other than those that have antibody activity against the antigen used. This suggests that the anti-idiotype antibody is directed against the antigen-combining site of the antibody molecule. In fact, one test of the idea that the activity is directed against the antigen-combining site is to react the antibody used to raise the anti-idiotype antiserum with specific antigen and show that when the combining site is occupied there is no reaction with the anti-idiotype antibody.

In most cases, response to an antigen results in a mixture of antibody molecules with several idiotypes. This is another way of saying that there are many idiotypes (id) for a given antigen specificity, which in turn indicates that there is heterogeneity in the composition of the combining site. In some strains of mice, however, the response to certain antigens results in a predominant idiotype on the antibody molecule. Because this idiotype is seen in all members of the strain in response to the same antigen, it is

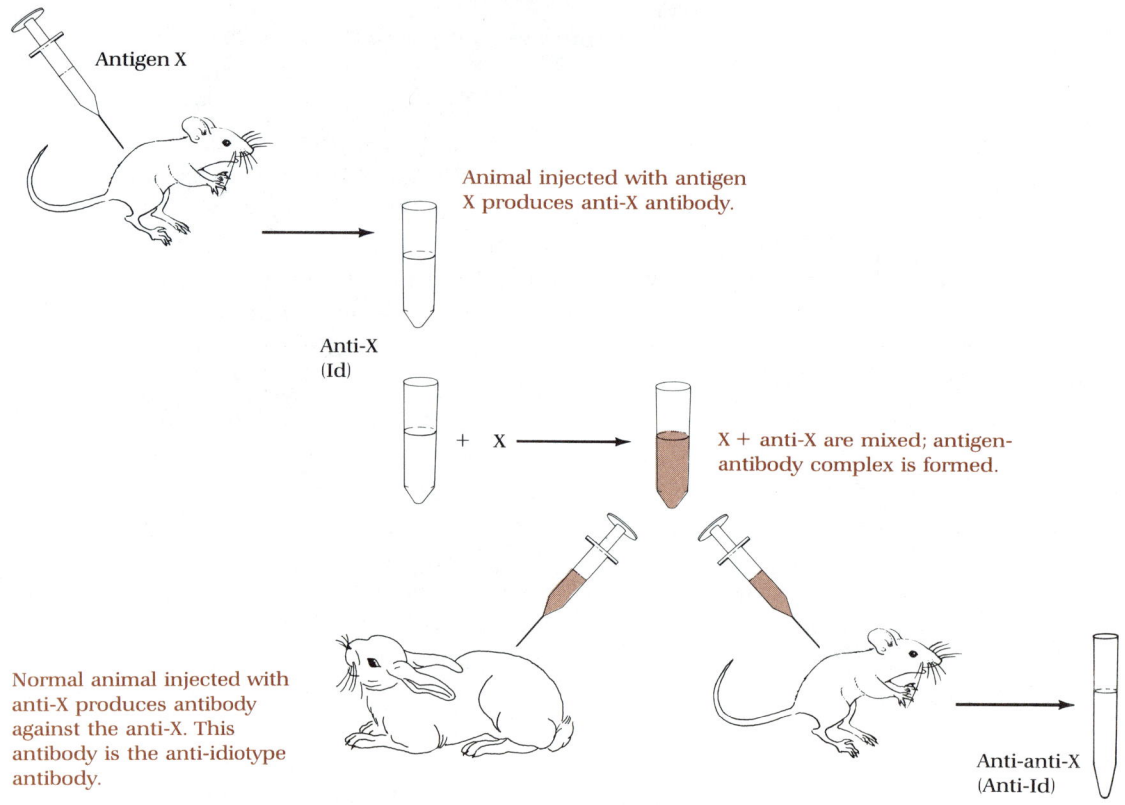

FIGURE 6 PRODUCTION OF ANTI-IDIOTYPE ANTIBODY

an inherited quality. These inherited idiotypes are called MAJOR, CROSS REACTIVE, or PUBLIC idiotypes.

Inheritance of Idiotypes   Some major idiotypes are inherited from generation to generation and are genetically linked to allotypes. The arsonate (Ars) system, introduced by Nisonoff and his colleagues, is a well-studied system that illustrates some basic concepts of the genetics of idiotypy. In the original system, A/J and BALB/c mice were immunized with the Ars hapten conjugated to an appropriate carrier. The anti-Ars antibodies were purified and used as antigen to immunize rabbits. The rabbit anti-Ars antibodies are therefore ANTI-IDIOTYPE (anti-id) ANTIBODIES. The

HETEROGENEITY OF IMMUNOGLOBULINS

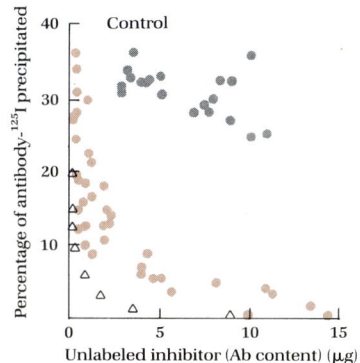

FIGURE 7   BINDING INHIBITION

Binding of anti-id [rabbit anti-mouse anti-Ars] with ^{125}I-labeled id (mouse anti-Ars) is inhibited by individual Id from A/J but not C57BL/6 mice. Triangles: Control inhibition of labeled reference A/J Id by unlabeled reference A/J id (autologous antiserum) showing optimal inhibition. Brown circles: Ten individual A/J mice cause inhibition of the reference antiserum, a result indicating that they all share the id with the reference antiserum. Gray circles: Ten individual C57BL/6 mice do not cause inhibition, indicating that they do not share the id. [Redrawn from Kuettner, Wang, and Nisonoff (1972) *J. Exp. Med.* 135, 579]

question then was asked, "Will the anti-id react with anti-Ars antisera from all A/J mice?" It was answered by determining whether an aliquot of anti-Ars antiserum from an individual A/J mouse could *inhibit* the reaction between id and anti-id. As seen in Figure 7 (the brown circles represent antiserum from 10 individual A/J mice), every A/J mouse tested is able to inhibit the reaction, a result indicating that each individual mouse has the idiotype. In contrast, the gray circles in Figure 7 are anti-Ars from individual C57BL/6 mice. Even though these mice are producing anti-Ars antibodies, their antibody molecules do not have the same idiotype as do those of the A/J mice. Thus we see that A/J mice have a major, or cross-reactive, idiotype to the Ars hapten that BALB/c mice do not.[2]

Summary

1. Immunoglobulins (Ig) are extremely heterogeneous molecules, differing in size, charge, and antigenicity.
2. There are five Ig classes, or isotypes, called IgG, IgM, IgA, IgD, and IgE.
3. Allotypes are antigens found on Ig molecules. These antigens are coded by genes that have several alleles.
4. Idiotypes are antigenic determinants on an individual Ig molecule, usually at the antigen-combining site.

[2]The reader is urged to think through the idiotype:anti-idiotype system because it will appear again in the chapter on regulation of the immune response by the network.

CHAPTER FOUR

Additional Readings

Ishizaka, K. 1983. Structure and biological activity of immunoglobulin E. In F. J. Dixon and D. W. Fisher (eds.), *The Biology of Immunologic Disease*. Sinauer Associates, Sunderland, MA. p. 13.

Janeway, C., E. E. Sercarz, and H. Wigzell (eds.). 1981. *Immunoglobulin Idiotypes*. Academic Press, New York.

Koshland, M. E. 1985. The coming of age of the immunoglobulin J chain. *Annu. Rev. Immunol.* 3: 425.

Metzger, H. 1970. Structure and functions of IgM immunoglobulins. *Adv. Immunol.* 12: 57.

Nisonoff, A. 1984. *Introduction to Molecular Immunology*, 2nd ed. Sinauer Associates, Sunderland, MA.

Tomasi, T. B. Jr. 1976. *The Immune System in Secretions*. Prentice-Hall, Englewood Cliffs, NJ.

CHAPTER 5

THE ORGANIZATION OF IMMUNOGLOBULIN GENES

Overview By the time the molecular basis of specificity was worked out, cellular immunologists had fairly well established the validity of the clonal selection hypothesis. It was known that a lymphocyte synthesized antibody of only one specificity and was preprogrammed for this specificity. The importance of this fact cannot be overemphasized, because it means that the events responsible for the synthesis of antibody of a certain specificity have occurred *before* the introduction of antigen. The path to the molecular solution to the generation of antibody diversity is one of the most fascinating stories in recent biology.

The problem was conceptualized as having two general explanations. Either the genes for the entire repertoire of the response were carried in the germ line (sperm and egg) and passed on to each member of the species, or a few crucial antibody genes were transmitted through the germ line and the bulk of the generation of diversity was carried out in the somatic cells by some kind of somatic reorganization of the germ-line genes. In fact, both explanations are correct. The discovery of variable and constant regions was the clue that led to the two gene–one polypeptide hypothesis. Germ-line genes are reorganized in somatic cells to give a complete variable region gene. These reorganized variable region genes are then associated with a constant region gene to generate the message for a complete immunoglobulin molecule.

CHAPTER FIVE

The Generation of Diversity

Germ Line versus Somatic Mechanisms

Before advances in molecular biology made it possible to directly answer the question of how V regions and C regions were generated, one of those seemingly interminable arguments in which immunologists specialize was raging over how much information for antibody specificity could be carried in the germ line (sperm and egg) and how much was generated in somatic cells. The two sides were divided into germ-line and somatic variation camps.

The germ-line side argued that the genes for every antibody specificity are transmitted via the germ line, so that each cell has all the genes for the entire antibody repertoire. Each cell would thus have all of the variable regions for H and L chains but by some unknown means would use only one.

The somatic diversification camp argued that, given the fact that there must be at least 10^6–10^8 specificities and that most of the response repertoire is under no selective pressure for survival (the responses to such diverse antigens as DNP and camel erythrocytes are intact in all members of the species but have no obvious survival value), there should have been genetic drift resulting in the loss of some specificities in some individuals. This does not occur. Furthermore, they argued, if the repertoire of responses exceeded 10^9 (which is certainly possible), the amount of DNA required to be conserved and transmitted would be too great to make biological sense. They argued that there must be a small number of germ-line genes that are highly conserved because of their survival value to the species and are transmitted from generation to generation via the germ cells. This number, they argued, must be far too small to account for the entire repertoire; so during differentiation into lymphocytes these genes must undergo some sort of somatic variation. This variation in the somatic cells would result in the enormous diversity of the response.

With the discovery that there are variable and constant regions (Chapter 3), each of the models had to explain how the V regions attained (or retained, depending on your persuasion) such a high level of diversity while the C-region genes retained such constancy.

THE ORGANIZATION OF IMMUNOGLOBULIN GENES

Two Genes, One Polypeptide Chain

It was known from studies of human allotypes that C-region genes were inherited in a simple Mendelian fashion. This finding presented a paradoxical situation: How could the same molecule have a C region inherited as a single gene and any one of 10^8 variable regions? In 1965 Dreyer and Bennett proposed that in light of these facts V regions and C regions must be products of two genes. In other words, there are *two genes for one polypeptide chain* in antibody formation. To quote from their paper:

> These facts rule out the possibility that each of the complete polypeptide chains is synthesized under the genetic control of a separate and independent gene contained in the germ line. It appears that immunologically competent cells have evolved a pattern of somatic genetic behavior which is radically different from anything normally found in modern molecular biology.

The idea of two genes for one polypeptide chain ran counter to the dictum of one gene–one enzyme or one gene–one polypeptide chain and was met with a good deal of resistance. In retrospect, however, it provided the framework for further thinking about the problem.

Shortly after the discovery of the V and C regions, experiments showed that there is only one "growing point" on the L chain as it is being synthesized, thus demonstrating that the mRNA for the chain is a continuous molecule. If this is so, then how do the two genes code for a single RNA molecule? The test of the two-gene model must somehow show that this mRNA can be coded for by two separate genes but be read as a single gene.

Genetic Reorganization

The discovery that the V and C regions are indeed coded for by two separate genes was made be Tonegawa and his associates in Basel and is one of the most elegant and definitive series of experiments in the history of immunology. This seminal discovery came at a time when the idea and definition of a gene was changing. Work on adenovirus-infected cells had shown that the genes of eukaryotic cells, unlike those of bacteria, are not uninterrupted sequences coding in a sequential manner for the amino acids of the peptide. Surprisingly, the coding sequences in a stretch of DNA were found to be interspersed among noncoding sequences, results of interrup-

CHAPTER FIVE

tions of informational material in the gene. The sequences that are used for coding are called EXONS (because they are *ex*pressed), and the noncoding *inter*vening sequences between them are called INTRONS.

The first step in the experimental process of testing the two gene–one polypeptide hypothesis was to isolate mRNA from a κ chain-producing myeloma cell line (Methods Box 1). The full-length κ mRNA contained the coding information for both the V and C regions. The 3′ half of the mRNA contained the coding information for the C region only (Figure 1).

When radiolabeled, RNA can serve as a probe in hybridization experiments to detect and isolate DNA fragments containing sequences that are complementary to the RNA used. Hozumi and Tonegawa treated DNA obtained from the myeloma cells or from whole mouse embryos with restriction nuclease and then reacted the fragments with either the probe for V–C or for C alone. They found (Figure 2) that both probes reacted with DNA fragments of the same size in the DNA obtained from the myeloma. However, the two probes reacted with different DNA segments in the DNA

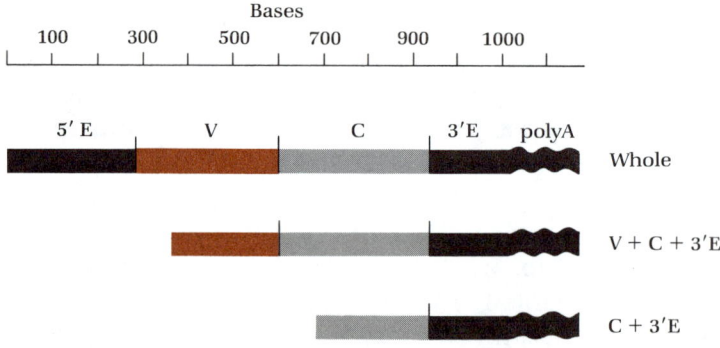

FIGURE 1 LIGHT-CHAIN mRNA AND ITS SPECIFIC FRAGMENTS

Light-chain mRNA is about 1250 nucleotides long. It consists of five regions, including the poly(A) sequence at the 3′ end. These regions are designated by 5′E (external region at the 5′ end), V (variable region, colored brown), C (constant region, colored gray), and 3′E (external region toward the 3′ end). [From Tonegawa et al. (1976) *Cold Spring Harbor Symp. Quant. Biol.* 41, 877]

METHODS BOX 1

Cloning an Antibody Gene

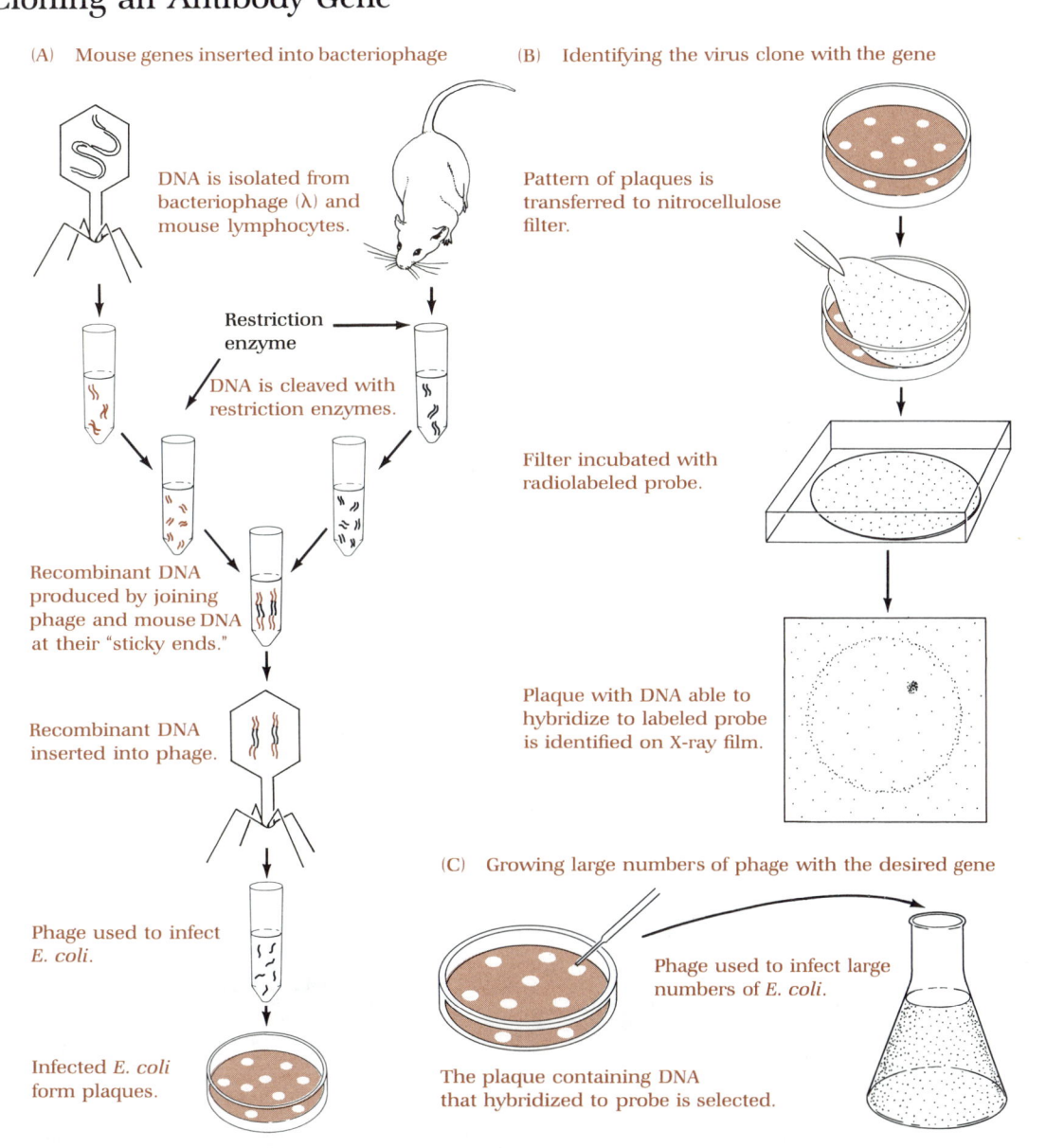

(A) Mouse genes inserted into bacteriophage

DNA is isolated from bacteriophage (λ) and mouse lymphocytes.

Restriction enzyme

DNA is cleaved with restriction enzymes.

Recombinant DNA produced by joining phage and mouse DNA at their "sticky ends."

Recombinant DNA inserted into phage.

Phage used to infect *E. coli*.

Infected *E. coli* form plaques.

(B) Identifying the virus clone with the gene

Pattern of plaques is transferred to nitrocellulose filter.

Filter incubated with radiolabeled probe.

Plaque with DNA able to hybridize to labeled probe is identified on X-ray film.

(C) Growing large numbers of phage with the desired gene

Phage used to infect large numbers of *E. coli*.

The plaque containing DNA that hybridized to probe is selected.

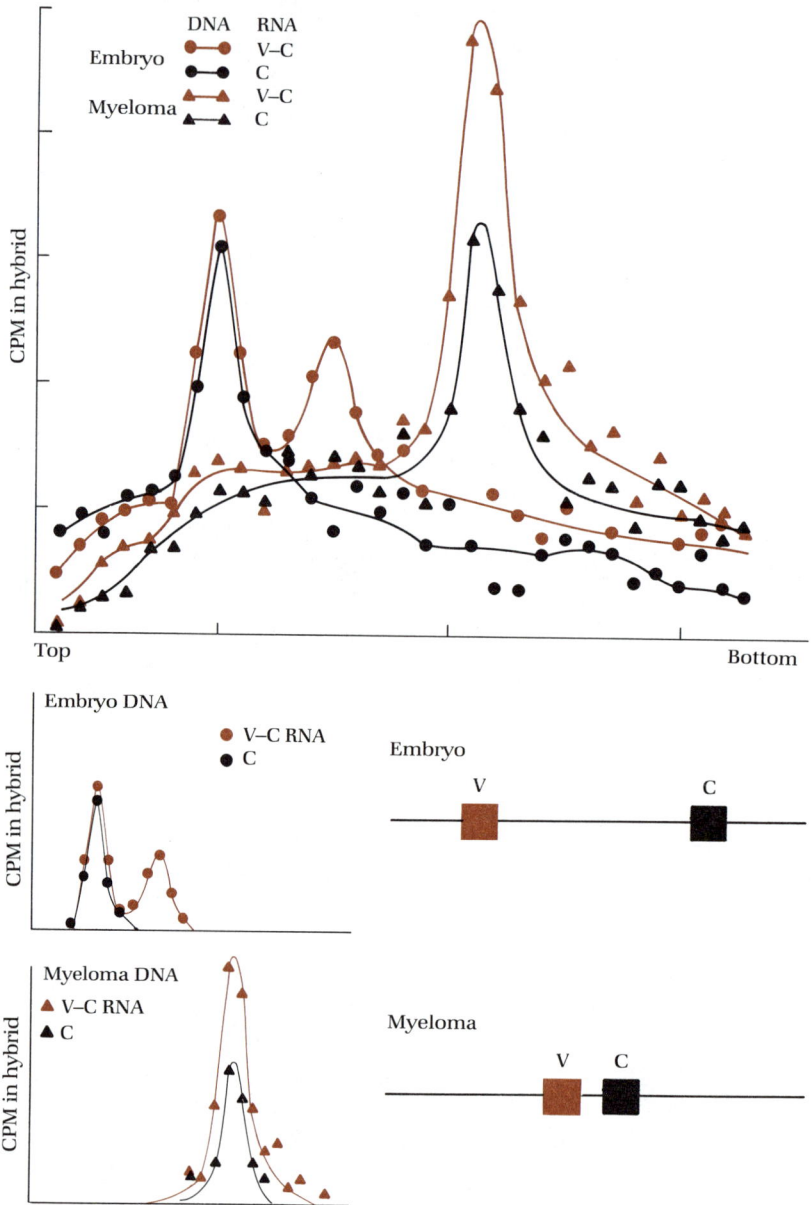

THE ORGANIZATION OF IMMUNOGLOBULIN GENES

FIGURE 2   HYBRIDIZATION OF ^{125}I-LABELED mRNA TO DNA FRAGMENTS
Gel electrophoresis patterns of restriction endonuclease-treated mouse embryo DNA or myeloma DNA hybridized to ^{125}I-labeled mRNA are different, a result indicating gene rearrangement. RNA is either whole myeloma (V–C) or the 3′ end (C) from Figure 1. Note that the two probes obtained from myeloma bind to the same fragment of DNA, but the two RNA probes bind to two fragments of embryonic DNA. CPM, counts per minute. [Redrawn from Tonegawa et al. (1976) *Cold Spring Harbor Symp. Quant. Biol.* 44, 877]

obtained from the embryo. This finding implies that in the myeloma cell there is one gene that codes for the V and C regions, and in the embryo there are two genes, one coding for V and one coding for C.

The Dreyer-Bennett prediction was correct: There are two separate genes that code for a single chain of an antibody molecule. In the undifferentiated, or germ-line, form the DNA for the V region is separated from the DNA that codes for the C region. In differentiated cells able to produce antibodies (the B lymphocytes), the two segments are brought together to form a V–C segment. This is diagrammed in Figure 2; the V and C regions are seen to be separated in the embryo but are joined in the myeloma cell.

Mechanisms of Gene Reorganization

V–J Joining Forms the Light Chain Variable Region

Analysis of the DNA in the V region of the L chain gene showed that the situation was more complex than it had at first appeared. A set of genes called J SEGMENT (for joining), separated from the germ-line V genes by a segment of DNA of unknown length, was discovered. The V segments and J segments are rearranged to form the functional V region of a light chain.

Figure 3 shows the organization of the light chain genes. The κ and λ gene sequences contain LEADER SEQUENCES which are transcribed and translated but excised from the protein before it is secreted from the cell. This leader sequence may be used for the transport of the molecule within the cell, because the light and

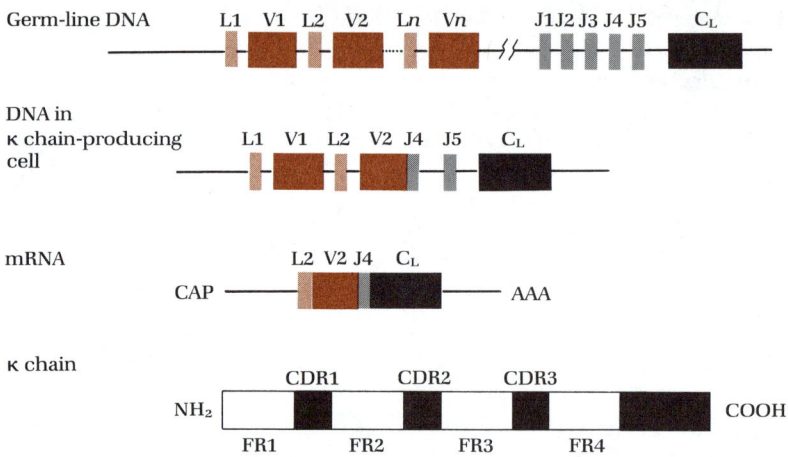

FIGURE 3   ORGANIZATION OF κ CHAIN GENES

The germ-line DNA is rearranged in a κ-producing cell so that one V region is brought together with one J region. The mRNA that encodes the protein has the C region adjoined to the V–J region and yields a complete κ chain. L1, L2, Ln are leader sequences. [Based on Kindt and Capra (1985) *The Antibody Enigma* p. 191; and Tonegawa (1983) *Nature* 302, 575]

heavy chains are encoded and synthesized on different chromosomes. The chromosomal locations of these genes in both human and mouse are given in Table 1.

V–D–J Joining Forms the Heavy Chain Variable Region

The H chain gene, like that of the L chain, has a tandem array of V segments, each separated by 5–15 kilobases (kb) of DNA. At an undetermined distance from the V segments of the H chain gene, however, there are 5–15 segments of DNA that are not present on the L chain gene; each of these segments codes for only 10 amino acids. These additional elements of variation are the D SEGMENTS (for diversity). Each of the D segments is separated from its neighbors by about 10 kb of DNA. In the formation of an H chain V region, a V-D segment is formed and transposed to the vicinity of a J gene. Thus, to form a functional V_H region, there is a V-D-J joining, as depicted in Figure 4.

THE ORGANIZATION OF IMMUNOGLOBULIN GENES

TABLE 1 Chromosomal locations of κ, λ, and H chain genes.

	Located on chromosome		
	κ	λ	Heavy
Mouse	6	16	12
Human	2	22	14

Gene Reorganization Results in Diversity

The variable regions of both H and L chains are formed by the rearrangement of gene segments. The reader must keep in mind that V–J and V–D–J joining can occur in many combinations, thereby producing an enormous number of V-region genes from a small number of V, D, and J segments. The actual number of specificities that can be generated in this way depends, of course, on the number of V segments in the germ line.

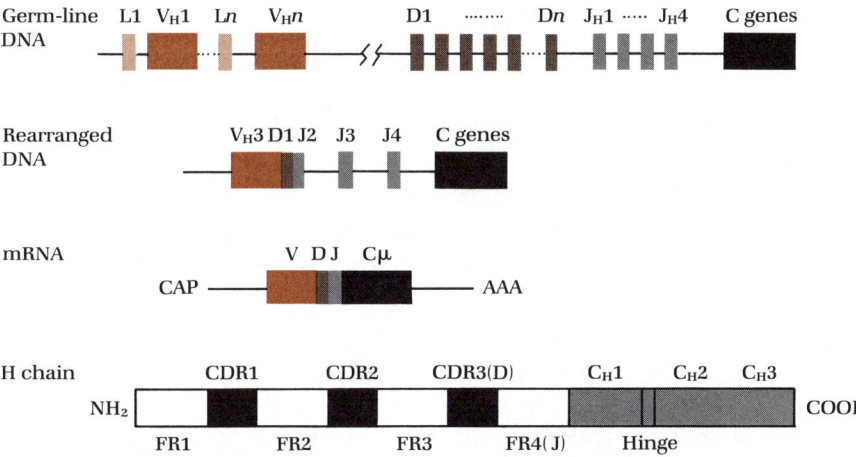

FIGURE 4 ORGANIZATION OF HEAVY CHAIN GENES
The germ-line DNA is rearranged so that V–D–J joining results in a V region. In the mRNA this is joined to one of the Cμ genes, which encodes a complete H chain. L1 and Ln are leader sequences.

CHAPTER FIVE

Variable-region genes, formed by the rearrangement of gene segments described above, join with C regions from three *families* of genes: heavy chain genes, κ chain genes, and λ chain genes. Recall that the germ-line proponents had argued that all of the V regions should be encoded in the DNA of each cell. The somatic variation proponents had argued that there were only a few germ-line V genes. RNA–DNA hybridization techniques have been used to estimate the number of germ-line V gene segments in each of these families. The numbers, although still very imprecise, are approximately 300 V_κ, 2 V_λ, and 200 V_H. Clearly there are not enough germ-line V genes for the complete repertoire of the antibody response, so there must be some other mechanism for generating diversity. This mechanism is somatic diversification.

A large number of combinations of genes can arise in this manner. For example, if there were in the genome 2 Vλ, 3 Jλ, 300 Vκ, and 4 Jκ segments, approximately 10^3 V_L regions [(2 × 3) + (300 × 4) = 1,206] would be available through somatic generation. Similarly, if there were 200 V_H, 12 D, and 4 J_H segments, approximately 10^4 V_H regions (200 × 12 × 4 = 9,600) would be available. If the 10^3 V_L were able to associate with the 10^4 V_H, there would be 10^7 possible antigen-combining sites. Of course, all of the possible combinations may not occur, but it is still clear that the combinatorial mechanism allows 725 gene segments to be combined into 10^7 genes.

Neither the germ-line nor the somatic diversification camps were completely correct or completely wrong, and there has been an amicable coming together of the two sides to study the possible genetic mechanisms for somatic diversification. We will discuss three of them: combinatorial and junction site diversification and somatic mutation.

Combinatorial Diversification

Because the V_L and V_H regions are coded for by two or three gene segments (V–J and V–D–J), with each segment existing in multiple forms, they can join in many combinations. The coming together of these gene segments to form the complete V-region gene introduces a level of diversity called COMBINATORIAL DIVERSITY.

The mechanism for the joining of one V and one J segment

THE ORGANIZATION OF IMMUNOGLOBULIN GENES

follows the *heptamer–nonamer and 12/23 rule*. In the λ light chain family, for example, each V region contains a palindromic seven-nucleotide thymine-rich sequence (the heptamer) on the 5' side and a nine-nucleotide adenine-rich sequence (the nonamer) 23 bases away from the heptamer (Figure 5). Note that the palindrome is really a "Chargaff" palindrome, in which T and G become A and C at the opposite end.

The J-region DNA has an inverted repeat of the palindrome and a thymine-rich sequence comparable to the adenine-rich sequence on the V segment. As shown in Figure 5, the V and J regions can be joined together and the noncoding sequences, which are looped out, can be excised by appropriate enzymes. From the diagram it is easy to see why this is called the heptamer–nonamer and 12/23 base pair rule. A form of this rule applies to κ, λ, and H chain gene segments, as shown in the inset in Figure 5.

Junctional Site Diversity If there are 200 V_κ gene segments that encode to amino acid 95 and 4 J_κ gene segments encoding positions 96 through 108, then there could be 800 sequences for the light chain variable region. But when the amino acid sequences of κ chains were compared with the germ-line DNA sequences of J1, J2, J4, and J5, one amino acid in the protein —number 96—showed variability. In fact this diversity, called JUNCTIONAL SITE DIVERSITY, may account for a very significant amount of the diversity in the system because it results in the generation of new codons at the variable joining region.

A possible mechanism for junctional site diversity is seen in Figure 6. At stage I the two gene segments are lined up for joining. Presumably this is done with the help of DNA-binding proteins. The four strands are cut at the signal heptamer adjacent to the coding sequences (dark areas). In stage II the two heptamers are joined tail-to-tail, but the coding sequences do not join. Instead they are held by protein and retain their proximity. At stage III exonucleases remove some nucleotides from the ends of the coding sequences. In stage IV it is hypothesized that terminal transferase (which is found in bone marrow where this rearrangement is going on) adds one or more nucleotides to these

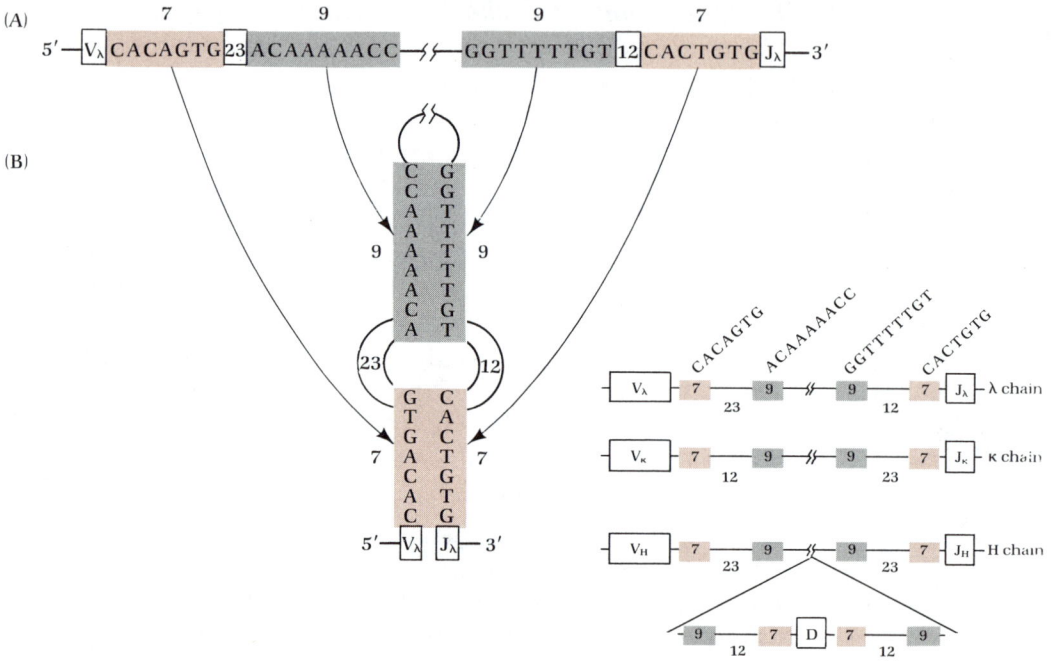

FIGURE 5   V–J JOINING IN λ CHAIN

V–J joining in λ chain by the heptamer–nonamer and 12/23 base pair rule. The shaded DNA segments in A separate the Vλ and Jλ segments that are to be rearranged by joining. Because they are "Chargaff" palindromes, they can associate (as in B) to bring the V and J regions together. Inset: The heptamer–nonamer and 12/23 base pair rule in heavy and light chains. [After Tonegawa (1983) *Nature* 302, 575]

ends. Stage V is the final joining process. DNA polymerase replicates the added bases and a ligase seals the structure. The new codon(s) are represented by N in the figure.

Junctional site diversity introduces additional variability into the third hypervariable region (CDR3). But another mechanism must account for the variability seen in the first two hypervariable regions (CDR1 and CDR2). This added diversification has come from *somatic mutation*.

Tonegawa showed that there was a single λ V-region gene for each of the two λ V-region subgroups. Others then compared the

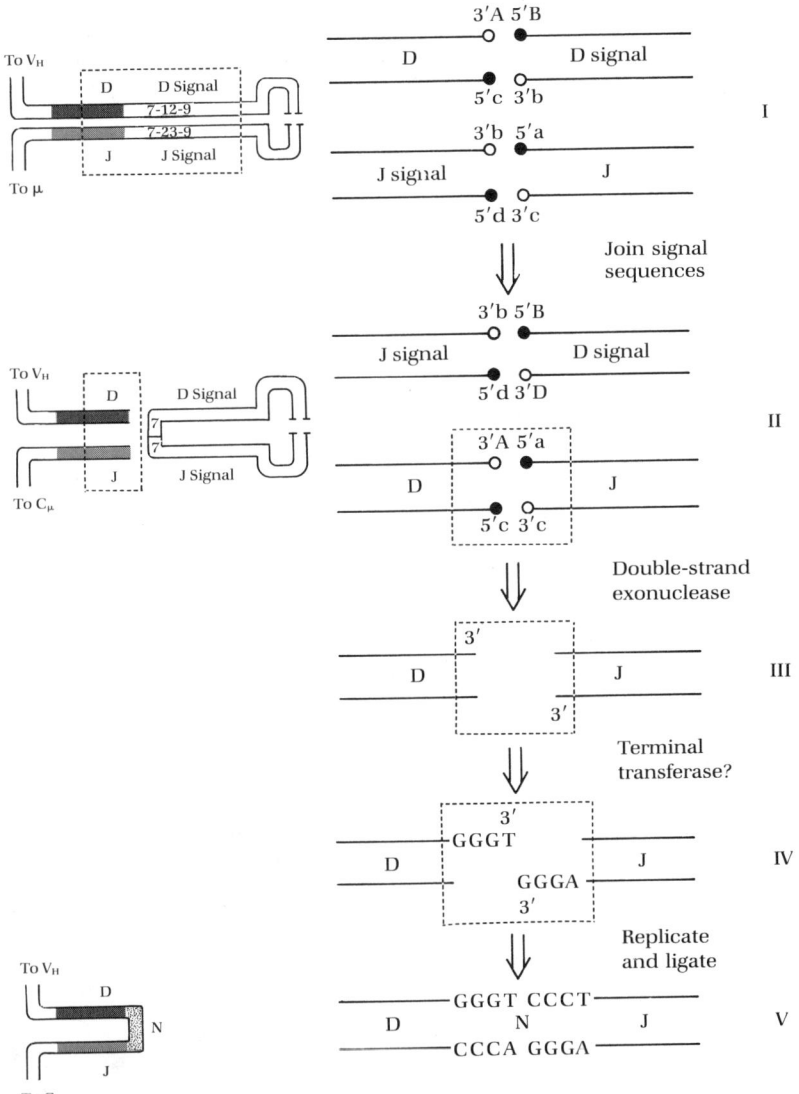

FIGURE 6 HYPOTHETICAL MODEL FOR THE D–J RECOMBINATION IN H CHAINS

Stage I. The D and J segments are lined up for joining and cut at the signal heptamer adjacent to the coding sequences (dark circles). Stage II. The heptamers that form the signal sequences are joined, but the coding sequences are held by a protein. Stage III. An exonuclease excises the coding sequences. Stages IV and V. A terminal transferase adds bases to the 3' ends, which are joined by a ligase. [From Alt and Baltimore (1982) *PNAS* 79, 4118]

CHAPTER FIVE

sequence of known Vλ proteins with the germ-line DNA. This analysis showed that somatic mutation must have occurred in CDR1 and CDR2.

And so we see that in addition to combinatorial and junctional site diversity there is also somatic mutation. Together these mechanisms generate the enormous diversity seen in the immune response.

Constant-Region Genes

Organization of Constant-Region Genes

The C-region genes (designated by C) are located on the 3' side of the V, D, and J regions. Light chains of both human and mouse are encoded by one C_κ and four C_λ genes (corresponding to the number of κ and λ families). Obviously, there are as many C_H genes as there are classes and subclasses of immunoglobulins, because isotype is determined in the constant region. All of the C regions are coded in a single stretch of DNA. This is shown for both human and mouse in Figure 7.

Formation of a Complete Immunoglobulin Heavy Chain

To form a complete immunoglobulin chain, which is of course composed of a V region and C region, the V-region genes (made up of the rearranged V–J or V–D–J segments) is brought into association with one of the C-

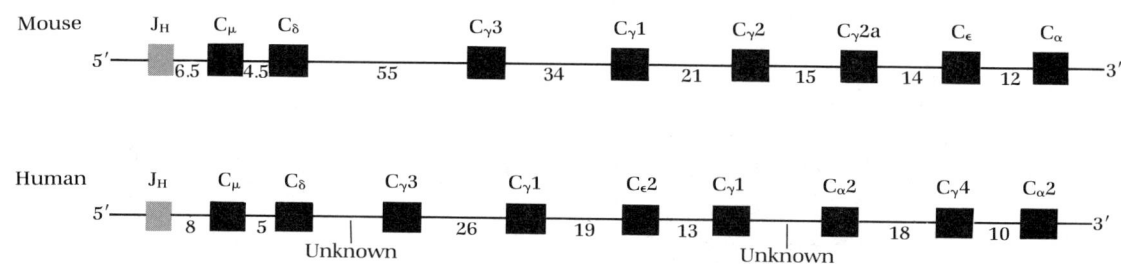

FIGURE 7 ORGANIZATION OF CONSTANT REGION GENES OF THE HEAVY CHAIN

The constant region genes of the heavy chain are encoded in a single stretch of DNA located 3' of the V, D, and J genes. The distances in kilobases between the genes is indicated. [Based on Shimizu et al. (1982) *Cell* 28, 499; and Flanagan and Rabbitts (1982) *Nature* 300, 709]

THE ORGANIZATION OF IMMUNOGLOBULIN GENES

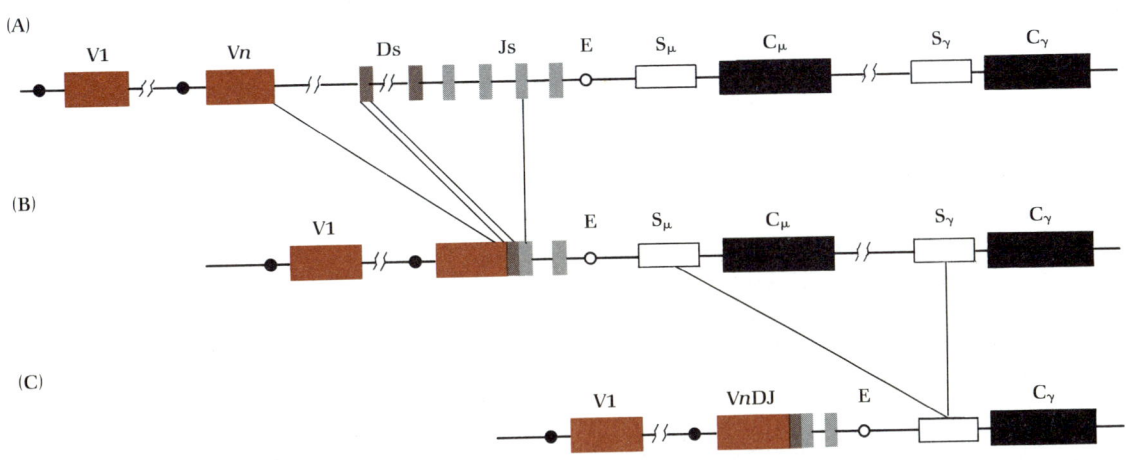

FIGURE 8 ORGANIZATION OF Ig H-CHAIN GENES AND THE ENHANCER
(A) Germ-line DNA of μ chain in preswitch DNA. Sμ and Sγ are areas in which switch recombination occurs. (B) Rearranged DNA in preswitch DNA. Note that the enhancer sequence (E) is located between the J regions and the μ gene. (C) Rearranged DNA in postswitch DNA. Note that the same enhancer sequence is now between the rearranged V gene and the Cγ region. The Sμ and Sγ refer to the regions in which switch recombination occurs. E is the enhancer sequence. [From Gillies et al. (1983) *Cell* 33, 717; with permission]

region genes located downstream on the 3' side. The V region associates with the μ C_H gene, which is closest to the J_H segments (Figure 8). Thus the first complete heavy chain produced is a μ chain.

Class Switching

During the proliferation of lymphocytes in an immune response there is usually a class switch (see Section II for the cellular events). CLASS SWITCHING refers to the phenomenon by which the class, or isotype, of an antibody changes from μ to one of the other classes. This class switch is mediated by yet another DNA rearrangement. In the DNA rearrangement involved in class switching, the V region that was associated with the Cμ becomes associated with another C_H gene segment—for example Cγ1 or Cα. The V region remains the same during this switch.

CHAPTER FIVE

The recombination required for class switching takes place in an intervening sequence between the V_H and C_H genes (Figure 8). These stretches of DNA, called the S REGION (for switch), are the 5' flanking regions of each C_H gene (except C_δ).

A most interesting fact is that a DNA fragment with a nucleotide sequence almost identical to that of the mouse S_μ but with unknown function has been isolated from *Drosophila* DNA. This could mean that Ig genes have used a system already in place in other biological systems.

Transcription Enhancement of Immunoglobulin Genes

Enhancer Sequences
The unrearranged V segment has 0.1 RNA transcript copy per gene in the cell. This concentration is four orders of magnitude less than that of the rearranged V_κ segment in the same cell. On the other hand, C-gene segments are transcriptionally active even in the unrearranged form. This suggests that there might be an enhancer sequence associated with the C-gene segment. ENHANCER SEQUENCES are DNA segments that increase the level of transcription when they are placed within several kilobases of some promoters. It is known that viral DNA segments can enhance viral or recombinant cellular gene transcription, and a similar ENHANCER ELEMENT has been found in the major intron of rearranged H chain genes. The sequence is located between the V-region J segment and the switch-recombination site of the C region (see preceding section). It is derived from sequences upstream of the germ-line C segment. The L chain also has an enhancer that is downstream from κ. The position of the enhancer during rearrangement is shown in Figure 8.

The enhancer has been shown to be tissue-specific; after transfection of enhancer DNA, it functions only in lymphocytes and not in other cell types such as fibroblasts. For the H chain the enchancer sequence functions when it is on either the 5' or 3' side of the rearranged V_H gene, and it even functions when its base sequence is reversed.

THE ORGANIZATION OF IMMUNOGLOBULIN GENES

Switch and Enhancement in Malignant Transformations

The *myc* gene of the acute avian retrovirus MC29 (*v-myc*) induces tumors within weeks after injection into newly hatched chicks. Avian leukosis virus (AVL) transforms chicken B lymphocytes by integrating near and stimulating the transcription of *c-myc* (the normal cellular homolog of *v-myc*). In this manner a normal gene (*c-myc*) is overexpressed because the cell has acquired a new gene (*v-myc*).

The *c-myc* gene can also be activated by chromosome translocations. Many B cell tumors (lymphomas and plasmacytomas) have chromosomal translocations, and it has been shown that in the mouse the *c-myc* gene on chromosome 15 is translocated to chromosome 12, which contains the Ig H chain genes, or to chromosome 6, which has the κ chain genes. In human B cell tumors, translocation between chromosome 8, which contains *c-myc*, and chromosomes 2, 14, and 22, which contain H, κ, and λ genes, are also frequently seen.

The recombination site between *c-myc* and the H chain gene is in the μ switch region and joins the Ig H chain gene to the *c-myc* gene. Why the recombination occurs preferentially with Ig genes is not known but may be due to special switch enzymes. It appears that this oncogene rearrangement can cause the cell to lose the ability to regulate its own growth and thus become a cancer cell.

Allelic Exclusion

ALLELIC EXCLUSION is the phenomenon in which only one pair of genes coding for an immunoglobulin molecule in a cell is expressed. B lymphocytes—the cells that synthesize and secrete immunoglobulins—have two immunoglobulin genes on each of the two homologous chromosomes (one chromosome from each parent). Each of the genes can undergo independent rearrangement, and the cell would be expected to synthesize products from both pairs. Allelic exclusion prevents this from happening.

The mechanism for allelic exclusion is not known. One of the theoretical explanations holds that, because gene rearrangement is random, there is a probability that only one of the alleles will be functionally rearranged. This explanation is known as the STOCHASTIC MODEL. Analysis of κ-producing cells shows that the second allele is very often in its germ-line configuration, indicating that it has not undergone rearrangement. However, there have been some cases in which both alleles are rearranged, transcribed, and even translated. But when this happens, only one of the transcripts combines with H chain. To explain this, a REGULATED MODEL has been proposed. According to this model, as soon as an L chain able to combine with an H chain is produced, the cell generates a signal that stops further rearrangement on the other allele. The result is one rearranged gene and one germ-line gene. If the first product made is unable to combine, then the second allele will be rearranged.

Summary

1. Because both H and L chains of Ig molecules consist of variable and constant regions, it was proposed that the molecule is encoded by two genes. This model is known as the two gene–one polypeptide hypothesis.
2. Comparing the Ig genes of embryos and antibody-producing cells shows that the two gene–one polypeptide hypothesis is basically correct; that is, antigen specificity comes about through the joining of gene segments in the potential antibody-forming cell. One V segment of several carried in the germ line is joined with one of several J segments to form a complete L chain V-region gene. For H chains there is V–D–J joining to form a V region. The V-region gene is then associated with one of several C-region genes. Gene reorganization enables 725 gene segments to yield more than 10^7 different genes for antigen specificity.
3. The joining of gene segments that results in combinatorial diversification occurs at palindromic sequences in the DNA and follows the heptamer–nonamer and 12/23 rule. Junctional site diversity also introduces extra diversity into the third hypervariable region (CDR3). Somatic mutation in CDR1 and CDR2 is known to occur and is another source of diversity.
4. During an antibody response, the class of Ig switches, usually from IgM to IgG. This comes about by another form of gene rearrangement in which the μ DNA is excised and the V_H region is connected to the DNA of a C_H region of another class.
5. There are tissue-specific transcription enhancer sequences located between the J segment and the switch-recombination site of the C_H region. At least one oncogene, *c-myc*, is known to be associated with the Ig genes at the μ switch site.

THE ORGANIZATION OF IMMUNOGLOBULIN GENES

Additional Readings

Ephrussi, A., G. M. Church, S. Tonegawa and W. Gilbert. 1985. B lineage-specific interactions of an immunoglobulin enhancer with cellular factors in vivo. *Science* 227: 134.

Honjo, T. 1983. Immunoglobulin genes. *Annu. Rev. Immunol.* 1: 499.

Tonegawa, S. 1983. Somatic generation of antibody diversity. *Nature* 302: 575.

Wall, R. and M. Kuehl. 1983. Biosynthesis and regulation of immunoglobulins. *Annu. Rev. Immunol.* 1: 393.

CHAPTER 6
MONOCLONAL AND HYBRID ANTIBODIES

Overview Because most antigens contain several antigenic determinants, when an antigen is introduced into an animal a separate clone of antibody producing cells is generated for each of the antigenic determinants. The individual clones can be separated and cultured, so it is possible to produce antibody against a specific determinant. Recent advances in technology have led to the production of these "monoclonal antibodies."

The ideal that immunologists had dreamed of was to be able to grow pure clones of antibody-forming cells in vitro. But there was no way to propagate normal antibody-producing cells in vitro, and there was no way to separate the cells producing antibody to a given antigenic determinant from the bulk of cells producing antibodies to all other determinants. The introduction of the method of fusing an antibody-forming cell to a myeloma cell (which is able to grow in vitro) by Köhler and Milstein and the selection of those fused cells that synthesize the antibody of the desired specificity has revolutionized the way we can use antibodies. The method, in short, captures the specific antigen-binding property of the antibody-forming cell and joins it with the ability to grow in vitro of the myeloma cell. Once the clones are produced, they are screened to determine which of them is producing antibodies of the desired specificity.

Thus problems that seemed insurmountable a decade ago have been solved, and monoclonal antibodies have become a routine part of immunology and cell biology.

MONOCLONAL AND HYBRID ANTIBODIES

Monoclonal and Polyclonal Antibodies

We learned from clonal selection (Chapter 1) that the repertoire of immune responses is distributed clonally among the lymphocytes. In other words, a given B cell is preprogrammed to respond to a single antigenic determinant. We will see in Part Two that the reaction of antigen with a cell-surface receptor on a lymphocyte leads to proliferation and clonal expansion that results in a large number of cells producing antibodies of the same specificity. But, as we saw in Chapter 2, most immunogens have multiple antigenic sites and therefore induce the expansion of several clones of antigen-reactive cells (one clone for each determinant). The response of the animal to the whole antigen is therefore POLYCLONAL, but the response to each antigen determinant is MONOCLONAL. A "conventional" antiserum, one raised by injecting antigen into an animal or immunizing cells in vitro, therefore almost always has antibodies directed against many antigenic determinants on the antigen molecule. In other words, conventional antiserum are multispecific because they are polyclonal.

Immunologists have spent countless hours attempting to make multispecific antisera monospecific by *adsorbing* out as many of the unwanted specificities as possible. This is done by mixing with the antiserum all of the antigens except the one to which antibody is desired; hence each antigenic determinant forms an antigen–antibody complex with its specific antibody, which can then be removed. In theory this leaves an antiserum with antibody to only one determinant. The reader can imagine that this ideal situation was almost never achieved, even after exhaustive attempts to adsorb out all of the unwanted specificities. If we could separate out those antibody-forming cells that were synthesizing and secreting antibody to the desired antigenic determinant and grow them in tissue culture, we could have antibodies of only that specificity. We would have, in other words, MONOCLONAL ANTIBODIES. Unfortunately, even if there were a means available for selecting out those few cells producing the antibody to the desired determinant, no tissue culture methods exist for the long-term cultivation of normal antibody-producing cells.

CHAPTER SIX

This technical problem seemed insurmountable until Georges Köhler and Cesar Milstein in 1975 introduced a method for generating antibodies that are known to be monospecific because they are monoclonal. This monoclonal methodology has revolutionized the uses of antibody in all of biology and medicine, and in 1984 Köhler and Milstein were awarded the Nobel Prize for their work. The prize was shared with Niels Jerne, who introduced the concept of clonality of the immune response—the theoretical foundation upon which the method is based. Again we see a case where the question was formulated in terms of immunology but the solution required methodological advances.

The Principle of Monoclonal Antibody Production

The principle of monoclonal antibody production is elegant. By applying it we can capture the specific synthesis of a single antibody-forming cell and "immortalize" it in tissue culture. Whereas normal antibody-forming cells cannot be grown and perpetuated in culture, tumors of the antibody-forming system, called MYELOMAS (Chapter 3), can be grown indefinitely in culture. In the jargon, they are immortal. What is needed, then, is a method for bringing together in one cell the separate abilities to synthesize a specific antibody and to grow forever in culture. Köhler and Milstein achieved this by fusing the antibody-forming cell with a myeloma cell. The resulting hybrid cell is called a HYBRIDOMA. The problem of *selecting* the antibody-forming cell of the desired specificity is solved by fusing large numbers of antibody-forming cells and myeloma cells and then examining (or selecting) the resulting hybridomas for those that are synthesizing the antibody of the desired specificity.

Cell Fusion

Monoclonal antibodies are achieved by fusing an antibody-forming cell (usually a spleen cell) with a myeloma cell (myelomas are tumors of B cells) in the presence of one of a variety of agents; polyethylene glycol (PEG) is the most commonly used agent (Figure 1). The resulting hybrid of the two cells is called a hybridoma. The problem of separating

MONOCLONAL AND HYBRID ANTIBODIES

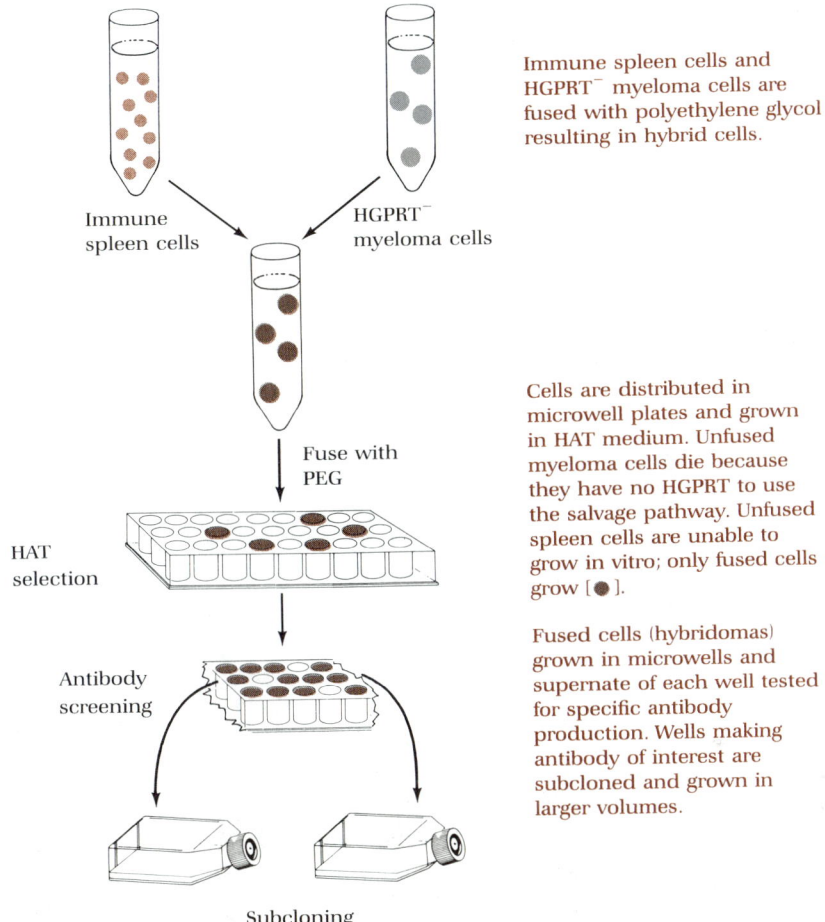

FIGURE 1   PRODUCTION OF MONOCLONAL ANTIBODIES

the fused hybridoma cells from the normal spleen cell population is easily solved because the spleen cells die off in culture after a short period of time. But both the unfused myeloma cells and the hybridoma cells are immortal, so a method is needed to get rid of the unfused myeloma cells. This result is achieved by using myeloma cells that are killed in the presence of the drug aminopterin.

CHAPTER SIX

Myeloma cells, like most cells, use two pathways of DNA synthesis: the major synthetic pathway and a salvage pathway (Figure 2). Normal cells synthesize DNA using both pathways. When the drug 8-AZAGUANINE is added to normal cells, it is incorporated into DNA through a reaction catalyzed by the enzyme HYPOXANTHINE–GUANINE PHOSPHORIBOSYLTRANSFERASE (HGPRT) via the salvage pathway. Such cells die because they cannot function with the altered base. A variant cell that cannot carry out the salvage pathway because it lacks HGPRT would be 8AzG RESISTANT and would therefore not be killed by the drug. These HGPRT⁻ mutants are used in selecting for fused myeloma cells.

The drug AMINOPTERIN acts on the major synthetic pathway by interfering with the conversion of tetrahydrofolate to dihydrofolate and preventing a series of one-carbon transfers. Thus in the presence of aminopterin the cell cannot synthesize DNA via the main synthetic pathway, and so must use the salvage pathway. A normal cell can still grow in the presence of aminopterin, but a

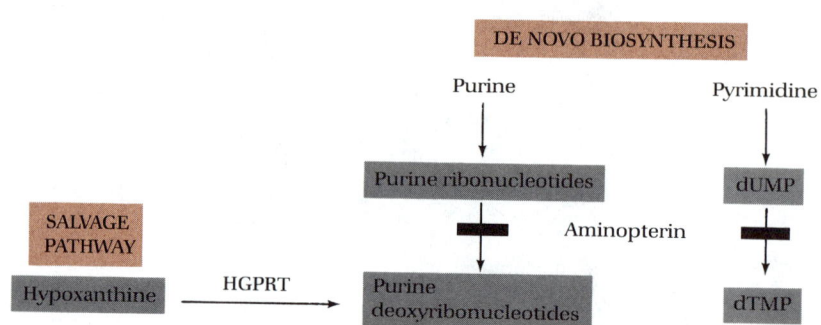

FIGURE 2 AMINOPTERIN WORKS BY BLOCKING THE REDUCTION OF DIHYDROFOLATE TO TETRAHYDROFOLATE

In pyrimidine biosynthesis $CoFH_4$ is oxidized to FH_2 thus using up FH_4. In purine biosynthesis $CoFH_4$ is converted to FH_4 nonenzymatically so that FH_4 can be reconstituted to $CoFH_4$. Aminopterin blocks the conversion of FH_2 to FH_4 so that no more FH_4 can be generated. As soon as it has depleted the existing FH_4 it can no longer function. As a consequence of the pyrimidine pathway now using up all of the FH_4 the purine pathway also stops; however, the cell still carries out DNA synthesis via the salvage pathway.

MONOCLONAL AND HYBRID ANTIBODIES

HGPRT⁻ cell cannot because HGPRT⁻ mutants cannot carry out the salvage pathway; HGPRT⁻ cells are therefore killed in the presence of aminopterin.

When HGPRT⁻ myeloma cells are fused with normal cells, the resulting hybridomas are able to grow in the presence of aminopterin because the normal cell contributes functional HGPRT. When hypoxanthine and adenine, which are the precursor molecules used by the enzyme HGPRT in the salvage pathway, are added to the medium, the hybridoma is able to use the alternate pathway to synthesize DNA. The unfused normal spleen cells die because they are unable to grow for long periods of time in tissue culture, and the unfused myeloma cells are killed by the aminopterin. Thus only the fused hybridomas are able to grow. This process is called HAT SELECTION (see Information Box 1).

Screening the Hybridomas But we still need a means of identifying and isolating those hybridomas that are producing the antibodies of the desired specificities. Single hybridoma cells are distributed into micro wells and grown. The supernatant fluid

---

INFORMATION BOX 1

Principle of HAT Selection

1. When the main synthetic pathways are blocked by the folic acid analogue AMINOPTERIN, the cell must use the salvage pathway. This pathway contains the enzyme HGPRT.

2. HGPRT⁻ myeloma cells can be selected because they can grow in the presence of 8-azaguanine. HGPRT⁺ cells incorporate 8-azaguanine into DNA. HGPRT⁻ cells do not incorporate the toxic molecule. Thus, HGPRT⁻ cells can grow in its presence.

3. HGPRT⁻ cells die in the presence of HAT (HYPOXANTHINE, AMINOPTERIN, THYMIDINE) because both the main pathway and the salvage pathway are blocked.

4. Fusion of the HGPRT⁻ myeloma cells with HGPRT⁺ spleen cells allows growth in HAT by providing the missing enzyme for the salvage pathway.

CHAPTER SIX

over each of the wells containing growing hybridoma cells is sampled and tested for antibody of the desired specificity using any of the methods described in Chapter 8. The most commonly used method, however, is the ELISA assay because it is fast, accurate, and reasonably sensitive. Screening also requires a source of the antigenic determinant.[1]

Wells that contain cells producing antibody of the desired specificity are *cloned* so that the investigator is sure that there are cells of only one specificity present. The monoclonal antibody production method enables researchers to produce large amounts of antibody that is monospecific because it is monoclonal. It also opens up a whole new world of biological manipulation of the genes for antibody production.

The Production of Hybrid Antibody Molecules

With current technology it is possible to introduce DNA into cells and have it expressed as if it were part of the cell's own genetic apparatus. By this process, called DNA TRANSFECTION, Ig gene DNA can be introduced into myeloma cells. By the process of *in vitro mutagenesis* it is possible to introduce changes into DNA in vitro, so that when the DNA is introduced into an appropriate cell the altered DNA is expressed and a new product is obtained. In this manner, not only can we have myeloma cells producing monoclonal antibodies, but we can even custom-alter the DNA so that we can produce monoclonal-modified antibodies. For example, we could produce RECOMBINANT ANTIBODIES with the desired antigen-binding capacity fused to a portion of the molecule with enzymatic function. Such a molecule could be used in immunoassays, with no need of second-antibody techniques. Or the gene for the antigen-binding region could be coupled to the gene for a toxin so that the final molecule could be used as a specific toxin to kill tumor cells.

---

[1] These facts are often overlooked by investigators who want to use monoclonal antibodies. In fact, the reason for failure to be able to use the technology is almost always because no reasonable screening procedure is available. Most investigators find that with some effort this problem can be overcome.

MONOCLONAL AND HYBRID ANTIBODIES

An example of the merging of these powerful technologies is seen in the next section.

Production of Hybrid Immunoglobulin Genes

Suppose a certain plasmid consists of a complete mouse μ gene containing the antigen-binding specificity for the hapten NP and the complete C region for the μ chain (Figure 3A). The DNA of this plasmid can be

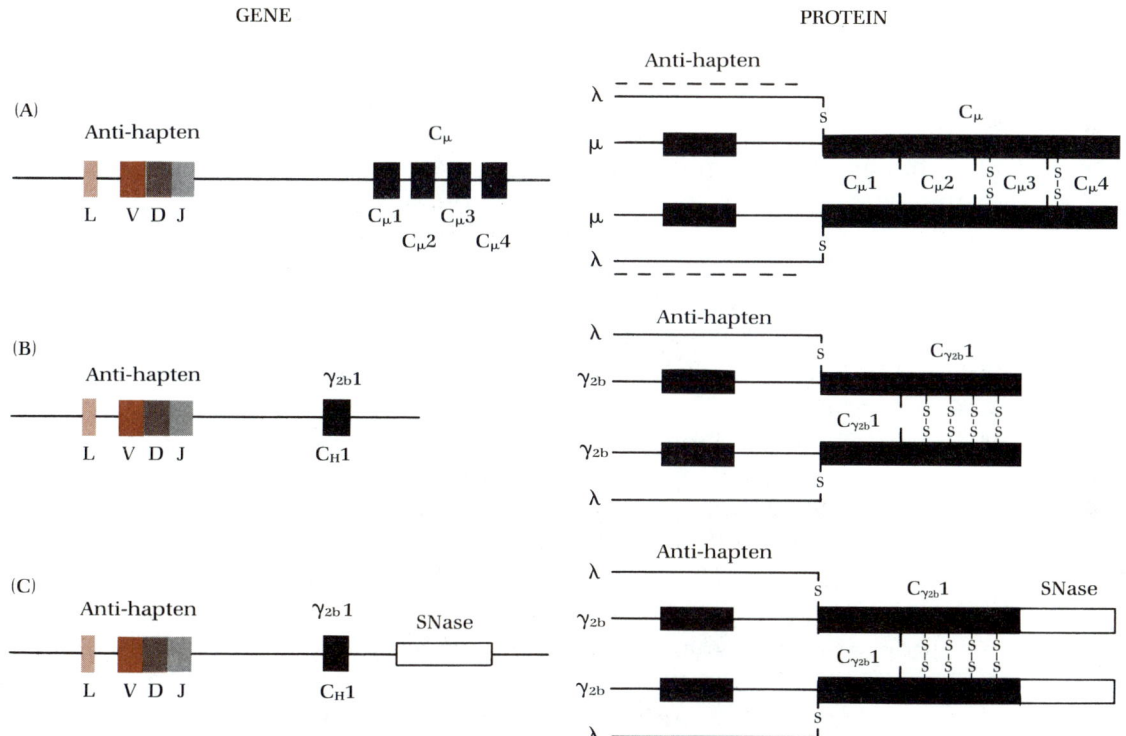

FIGURE 3 PRODUCTION OF HYBRID ANTIBODY MOLECULES
(A) Whole μ chain gene is transfected into a cell that expresses only λ genes. The secreted Ig is a complete antibody molecule. (B) Altered gene with the same V region as in A but with the C region gene altered so that it is the C_H1 of γ2b. The secreted immunoglobulin is an Fab with complete antibody activity. (C) DNase gene spliced to gene in B. The secreted molecule has both anti-hapten and DNase activity. [Redrawn from Neuberg, William, and Fox (1984) *Nature* 312, 604; with permission]

transfected into a myeloma cell that expresses light chains but not heavy chains, thereby converting the cell into one that synthesizes and secretes complete Ig molecules. The secreted Ig molecules are IgM with λ light chains and NP-binding capacity—that is, they are functional antibody molecules.

Next the portion of the plasmid encoding the Fc region of the molecule is removed and replaced with the DNA encoding the C_H1 and hinge region exons of a γ2b gene. If this in vitro manipulation of the heavy chain gene is successful, the resultant gene should still have the V region encoding anti-NP, but it should be joined to a C region encoding a small part of γ rather than all of μ. When the plasmid containing the altered gene is transfected into the myeloma cells, the antibody molecule shown in Figure 3B is obtained. This experiment shows that the V-region portion of the gene encoding the anti-hapten antibody can be joined to the new C-region gene and combine with the light chain in the myeloma to give an Fab that still retains the functional capacity to bind hapten.

Next the gene for *Staphylococcus aureus* nuclease (SNase) is inserted into the C_H2 exon of the γ2b gene. The gene now has the V region for anti-NP, a part of the C region for γ2, and, attached to this, the DNA for a gene from a bacterium (Figure 3C) that encodes an enzyme activity. This DNA construct, when transfected into the myeloma cells, can be shown to be expressed, because when the supernatant fluids from the myelomas transfected with the hybrid gene were tested, they were found to secrete molecules that had both anti-hapten *and* nuclease activities.

Using a similar methodology, investigators have generated monoclonal antibodies that are hybrids of mouse and human. In these molecules, the antigen-combining portion is from the mouse gene and the C-region is from the human gene. This methodology may be useful in cases where it is necessary to have human Ig molecules, but it is not possible to either immunize humans or to generate an in vitro antibody response with human cells.

MONOCLONAL AND HYBRID ANTIBODIES

Additional Readings

Goding, J. W. 1983. *Monoclonal Antibodies, Principles and Practice: Production and Application of Monoclonal Antibodies in Cell Biology, Biochemistry and Immunology.* Academic Press, New York.

Hurrell, J. G. R. 1982. *Monoclonal Hybridoma Antibodies: Techniques and Applications.* CRC Press, Boca Raton, FL.

Kennett, R. H., T. J. McKearn and K. Bechtol. 1980. *Monoclonal Antibodies. Hybridomas: A New Dimension in Biological Analyses.* Plenum, New York.

Köhler, G. and C. Milstein. 1975. Continuous cultures of fused cells secreting antibody of predefined specificity. *Nature* 256: 495.

Neuberger, M. S., G. T. Williams and R. O. Fox. 1984. Recombinant antibodies possessing novel effector functions. *Nature* 312: 604.

Yelton, D. E. and M. D. Scharff. 1981. Monoclonal antibodies: A powerful new tool in biology and medicine. *Annu. Rev. Biochem.* 50: 657.

SECTION II
THE ANTIGEN–ANTIBODY REACTION

Acta exteriora indicant interiora sereta.
Outward actions show inward intent.

LEGAL MAXIM

In the three chapters in this section we will cover some of the consequences of the union of antigen and antibody. These chapters will differ from the rest of the book because we will not be following the logical flow of ideas through experiments but will be examining the facts in a fairly traditional way. The practical application of what we know about antigens and antibodies is of great importance, and these chapters are to some extent an introduction to applied immunology.

CHAPTER 7

THE ANTIGEN–ANTIBODY COMPLEX

Overview Up to now we have discussed the nature of antigens and the structure of antibodies. In this chapter we will discuss the interaction between the two that leads to the formation of an antigen–antibody complex. It will become obvious that this reaction between antigen and antibody can be looked upon as a problem in physical chemistry in which reaction rates and affinities can be calculated and used to analyze the reaction. Our purpose is not to rigorously derive the equations that describe the reaction, but only to provide the average reader with enough detail about the reaction to be useful in understanding some of the methods that will be described, and as a starting point to understanding the discussion of the complement system.

All methods of quantifying the antibody response depend upon analyzing the formation of the antigen–antibody complex. The reaction leading to the formation of the complex can be treated as an interaction between any two ligands. We will apply the laws of mass action to show that both an equilibrium constant and an affinity constant can be derived. The strength of the reaction can thus be described in exact physical terms. We saw in an earlier chapter that antibodies are heterogeneous, and this heterogeneity is seen in the binding to antigen. For this reason we will derive the equation to determine a heterogeneity index.

CHAPTER SEVEN

The interaction of an antibody with an antigen is no different in principle from any other bimolecular reaction between a ligand and a molecule that specifically binds that ligand. The reaction between enzyme and substrate is a bimolecular reaction and follows the same rules of physical chemistry as do antigen–antibody reactions. The difference between the two is that the substrate is changed in an enzyme–substrate reaction, but not in an antigen–antibody reaction. A reaction in which one of the reactants is altered will be a one-way, or nonreversible, reaction. Antigen–antibody reactions are reversible because the interaction does not result in permanent change to either of the reactants.

The Antigen–Antibody Complex

The reaction of antigen with antibody results in the formation of an ANTIGEN–ANTIBODY COMPLEX (AgAb):

$$Ag + Ab \rightleftharpoons AgAb \tag{1}$$

AgAb is formed by *noncovalent* interactions such as hydrogen bonding, polar or hydrophobic bonding, ionic or coulombic interaction, and van der Waals forces. Because the reaction is noncovalent and neither reactant is altered, the reaction is in theory a reversible one. All of the methods used to quantify the antigen–antibody reaction depend upon the ability to measure AgAb.

We will see in the next chapter that the form taken by AgAb depends on the nature of the antigen. Soluble antigens such as proteins form complexes with antigen and become insoluble precipitates. Particulate antigens, such as cells, after reacting with antibody may form an AgAb that agglutinates. The reaction is analyzed by determining either the rate or quantity of precipitate or agglutinate.

Affinity of the Antigen–Antibody Reaction

Because the formation of AgAb can be treated as a chemical reaction between two ligands and because the reaction is reversible, the *affinity*, or strength, of the reaction can be determined. The law of mass action states that the rate of a reaction is propor-

THE ANTIGEN–ANTIBODY COMPLEX

tional to the concentration of the reactants. By applying the law of mass action to equation (1) we obtain

$$Ag + Ab \underset{k_d}{\overset{k_a}{\rightleftharpoons}} AgAb \tag{2}$$

$$k_a[Ab][Ag] = k_d[AgAb]$$

where [Ag] and [Ab] are the concentrations of free antigen and antibody; [AgAb] is the concentration of bound Ag and Ab, that is, the AgAb complex; and k_a and k_d are the association and dissociation constants.

From equation (2) we can arrive at the *equilibrium constant* for the reaction:

$$K = \frac{k_a}{k_d} = \frac{[AgAb]}{[Ag][Ab]} \tag{3}$$

AFFINITY is the sum of the noncovalent attractive and repulsive forces stabilizing the complex and is therefore the same as the EQUILIBRIUM CONSTANT K (which is expressed in liters/mole).

These reactions hold only for homogeneous binding sites (antibodies) and ligands (haptens). We know from the preceding chapters that antibodies are extremely heterogeneous; therefore these equations are only an approximation of the actual conditions. For monoclonal antibodies, however, these equations come very close to representing the actual interactions.

Determining Affinity

To determine the affinity of the reaction, we obviously need a means of determining the concentration of free antigen and bound hapten. This is most conveniently accomplished by EQUILIBRIUM DIALYSIS. This method is diagrammed in Figure 1. Antibody and hapten are separated by a semipermeable membrane. The hapten, with a suitable label (such as a radioisotope) is placed on one side of the membrane and the antibody is placed on the other. The pore size of the membrane is such that the hapten freely passes through; but the antibody, being of higher molecular weight, does not. Samples are then taken from each side at various times to determine the amount of hapten on each side.

CHAPTER SEVEN

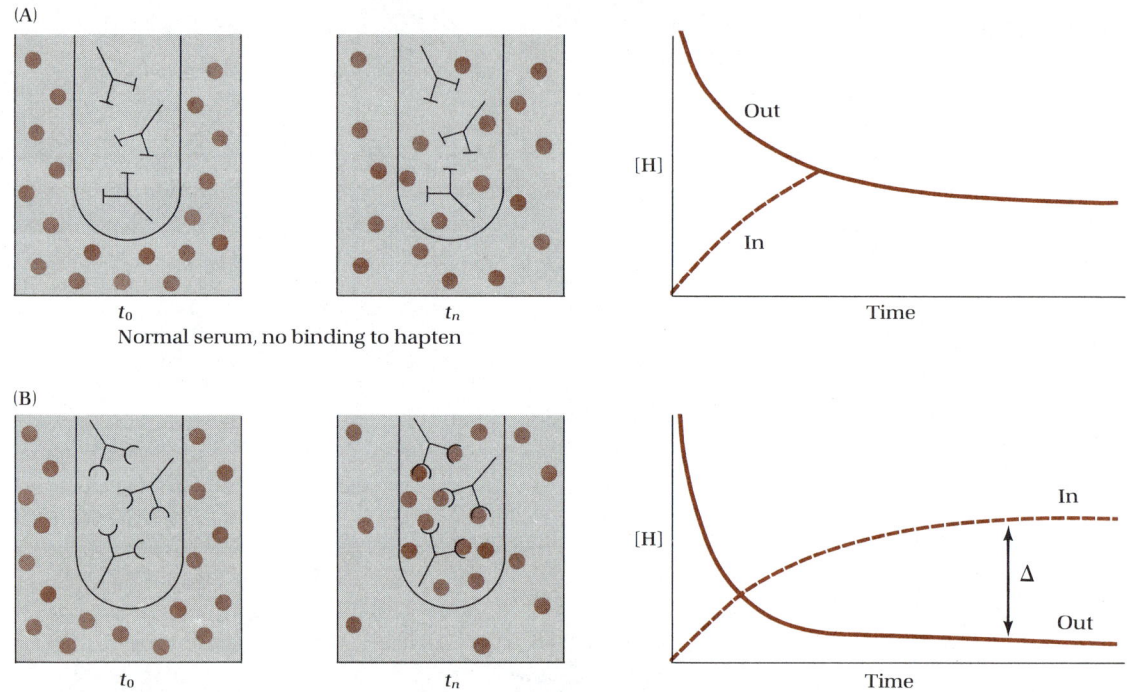

FIGURE 1   EQUILIBRIUM DIALYSIS

Anti-hapten antibody and labeled hapten are separated by a dialysis membrane. With time the hapten molecules diffuse across the membrane and reach equilibrium. (A) In normal serum no binding of the hapten occurs when it crosses the membrane. At equilibrium equal amounts of hapten are present on both sides of the membrane. (B) In immune serum the hapten is bound by the anti-hapten antibody, reducing the concentration of free hapten [H] inside. When the unbound hapten reaches equilibrium, there is a difference Δ between [H] in and [H] out. The difference Δ is the amount of hapten bound.

In Figure 1A the antibody is not directed to the hapten, so no AgAb forms and all of the hapten is unbound. This condition serves as a control because it tells the rate at which the concentration of the hapten reaches equilibrium on both sides of the membrane. In Figure 1B the antibody reacts with the hapten, so that some of the hapten moving into the antibody compartment

THE ANTIGEN–ANTIBODY COMPLEX

becomes bound and forms an AgAb complex. The system will still come to equilibrium, of course, but at equilibrium the concentration of free or *unbound* hapten will be lower than in A. This happens because the equilibrium is established by the unbound molecules, even though the *total* amount of hapten on the antibody side is greater than the amount of hapten on the other side.

Other methods, such as FLUORESCENCE QUENCHING, can also be used. This method takes advantage of the fact that tryptophan absorbs light at 280 nm and emits the absorbed light at 350 nm. (*Fluorescence* is defined as absorption of light at one wavelength and emission of it at another.) When a hapten is bound to an antibody, some of the tryptophan residues in the combining site are not accessible to absorb the ultraviolet light at 280 nm; hence emission at 350 nm will be reduced, or "quenched."

Antibody Affinity and Valence

The reader with knowledge of thermodynamics will see that from equation (3) a form of the Langmuir absorption isotherm may be derived.[1]

$$\frac{[AgAb]}{[Ab]} = r = \frac{nK[Ag]}{1 + K[Ag]} \tag{4}$$

where r is moles of Ag bound per mole Ab; [AgAb] is the concentration of bound Ab; [Ab] is the concentration of free Ab; [Ag] is the concentration of free Ag; and n is the valence of the antibody.

By algebraic manipulation one can convert equation (4) into equation (5).

$$\frac{r}{[Ag]} = nK - rK \tag{5}$$

By plotting $r/[Ag]$ versus r, we can derive the values of both K (which is the affinity) and n (which is the valence). Such a plot (Figure 2) is called a SCATCHARD PLOT. Figure 3 shows some actual data [taken from Eisen] plotted according to equation (5).

[1] For the reader without knowledge of thermodynamics, trust me. I have relied very heavily for this section on the clearest discussion I know of the subject, which is in M.W. Steward's chapter in Glynn and Steward, *Immunochemistry: An Advanced Textbook*.

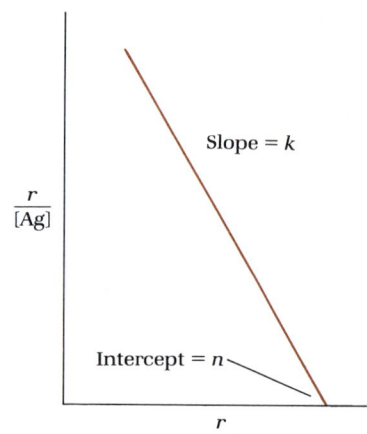

FIGURE 2 SCATCHARD PLOT OF IDEAL HAPTEN–ANTIHAPTEN BINDING

The values of r are obtained from equation (4) and $r/[Ag]$ from equation (5). In this plot the slope (k) is equal to the affinity, and the intercept (n) is equal to the valence.

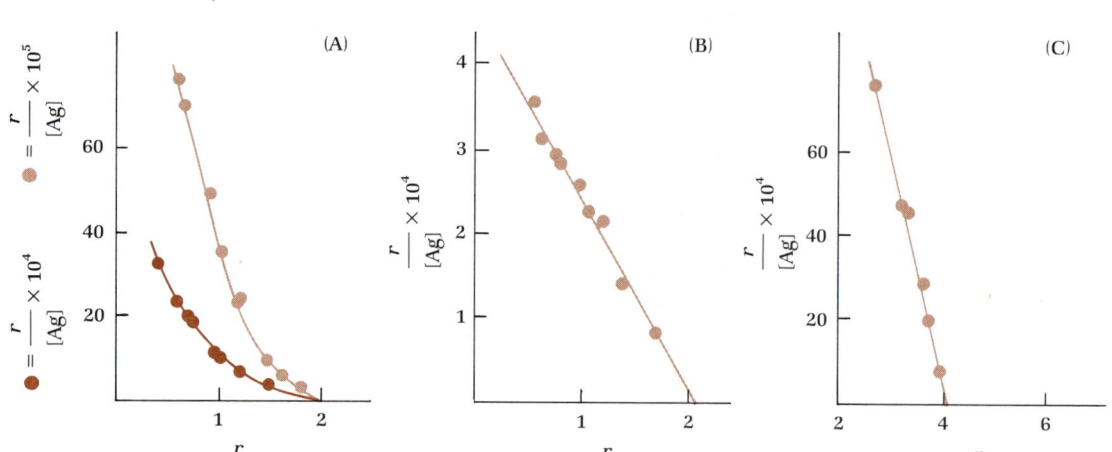

FIGURE 3 SCATCHARD PLOTS OF EXPERIMENTAL DATA

(A) Hapten–anti-hapten binding. Two antibody preparations (anti-DNP) which differ about 30-fold in affinity, react with dinitroanaline. (B) Hapten–anti-hapten binding. A myeloma protein with anti-DNP activity reacts with dinitroanaline. Because the population of molecules is homogeneous it gives a straight line plot. (C) Enzyme:substrate binding. Muscle phosphorylase *a* binds AMP. [Redrawn from Eisen (1974) *Immunology*]

THE ANTIGEN–ANTIBODY COMPLEX

For divalent antibody (i.e., where $n = 2$), the average intrinsic association constant (k_0) can be calculated from equation (5). Divalent antibody has two binding sites $(n = 2)$, so when half of them are bound to antigen, $r = 1$. In that case equation (5) becomes:

$$\frac{1}{[Ag]} = 2K - K = K_0 \qquad (6)$$

Affinity may also be calculated by the Langmuir plot by converting equations (4) and (5) into equation (7).

$$\frac{1}{r} = \frac{1}{n} \cdot \frac{1}{[Ag]} \cdot \frac{1}{k} + \frac{1}{n} \qquad (7)$$

Plotting the data in this form results in a curve like that shown in Figure 4.

Heterogeneity of Binding

Because (as we already know) antigens and antibodies are not homogeneous, the actual curves obtained are not linear. It has been shown, however, that the distribution of affinities can be described by the Sips distribution function:

$$\frac{r}{n} = \frac{[K_0 Ag]^a}{1 + [K_0 Ag]^a} \qquad (8)$$

where a is the HETEROGENEITY INDEX.

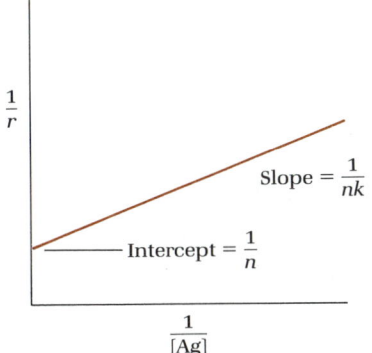

FIGURE 4 LANGMUIR PLOT OF IDEAL HAPTEN–ANTI-HAPTEN BINDING

This plot was obtained by using equation (7).

CHAPTER SEVEN

By using the logarithmic transformation of equation (8), we get

$$\log \frac{r}{n-r} = a\log K_0 + a\log[Ag] \tag{9}$$

Plotting $\log[r/(n-r)]$ versus $\log[Ag]$, we get a straight line where the slope is the heterogeneity index, a (Figure 5).

Kinetics of Antigen–Antibody Reactions

The combination of antigen and antibody is so rapid that it can only be studied with extremely sophisticated methods such as temperature-jump relaxation and stopped-flow techniques.[2] These methods show that the association rates for most hapten–anti-hapten systems studied are similar (ca. $10^8\ M^{-1}\text{sec}^{-1}$). In contrast, the dissociation rate constants show great variation, which means that the stability of the complex is determined to a great extent by the dissociation rate.

Summary

1. Antigen and antibody combine to form an antigen–antibody complex, AgAb, which is held together by noncovalent forces. This reaction obeys the laws of bimolecular reactions.

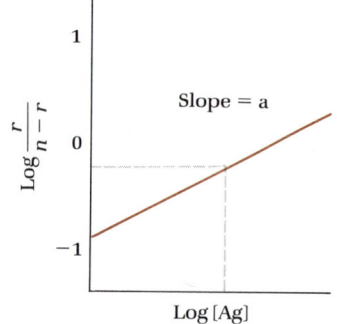

FIGURE 5 SIPS PLOT OF IDEAL ANTIGEN–ANTIBODY BINDING
Plot was obtained by using equation (9), in which a is the heterogeneity index.

[2] For the reader without knowledge of thermodynamics and advanced physical chemistry who trusted me on page 107, you are now on your own.

THE ANTIGEN–ANTIBODY COMPLEX

2. The concentration of free and bound hapten can be experimentally determined by equilibrium dialysis. Using these values and applying the law of mass action to the basic equation, we can determine the affinity of the AgAb reaction.

3. The valence of antibody molecules can be determined from Scatchard plots. By using the Sips distribution function, we can calculate the heterogeneity index.

Additional Readings

Day, E. D. 1966. *Foundations of Immunochemistry*. Williams and Wilkins, Baltimore.

Eisen, H. N. 1974. *Immunology*. Harper & Row, Hagerstown, MD.

Steward, M. W. 1977. Affinity of the antigen–antibody reaction and its biological significance. In L. E. Glynn and M. W. Steward, *Immunochemistry: An Advanced Textbook*. Wiley, Chichester.

CHAPTER 8
MEASURING ANTIGEN–ANTIBODY REACTIONS

Overview In this chapter we will discuss some of the methods used in immunochemistry. This chapter is not intended to be a substitute for a methods book but rather to give the reader a general notion of the methods of immunochemistry and, most important, a basis for understanding some of the results obtained using the methods.

The most important point to be made in this chapter is that all methods of identifying, localizing, or quantifying the antigen–antibody reaction rely on the study of the antigen–antibody complex. Very much like the biblical instruction "by their fruits you shall know them," the only way to know about the interaction is to know the product. This is true whether the purpose of measuring the reaction is to determine the amount of hormone in a solution by immunochemical methods or to localize an antigen in a section of tissue by immunohistochemical means.

The most impressive advances in measuring the antigen–antibody complex have come from advances in methods of labeling the reactants. Radioimmunoassays and enzyme-linked immunosorbant assays, which take advantage of these advances, offer exquisite sensitivity for the assay of compounds that were once thought to be outside the limits of assay. Uses of the labeling methods of immunohistochemistry have revolutionized our understanding of cellular structure and function. Virtually all areas of biology and biomedicine take advantage of these advances.

MEASURING ANTIGEN–ANTIBODY REACTIONS

The Antigen–Antibody Complex

The union of antigen and antibody results in the formation of an antigen–antibody complex (AgAb). All methods of measuring and quantitating antigen–antibody reactions take advantage of this fact and measure either the amount or the rate of formation of the complex. The complex takes one of several forms, depending upon the nature of the antigen. For example, soluble proteins react with antibody to produce an AgAb complex that forms a precipitate, whereas with particulate antigens such as cells the AgAb complex agglutinates. But whether one is localizing an antigen on a cell surface or within a cytoplasmic structure of a cell or determining the concentration of a hormone in a body fluid, the assay systems all rely on the same principle: assay of the amount or rate of formation of the antigen–antibody complex.

The Precipitin Reaction

When the antigen is soluble (a protein, for example) the reaction of antigen and antibody results in the formation of an insoluble precipitate.

$$Ag + Ab \rightleftharpoons AgAb \text{ (precipitate)}$$

For a precipitate to form, both the antigen and the antibody molecules must be at least *bivalent* (i.e., have a minimum of two combining sites). One combining site on an antibody molecule can react with an antigenic determinant on one antigen molecule and the other combining site can react with a determinant on another antigen molecule. If this happens often enough, a *lattice* will form, and will grow until it becomes insoluble and forms a precipitate (Figure 1). For historical reasons this is called the PRECIPITIN REACTION and is probably the assay with the most variations used in immunology.

Precipitin reactions can be quantitative or qualitative; they can be carried out in solution or in semisolid support medium such as a gel. Traditional texts and methods books cover the *quantitative precipitin reaction* and its many variations in detail. Even though the quantitative precipitin reaction was very important in the development of immunology into a quantitative sci-

114
CHAPTER EIGHT

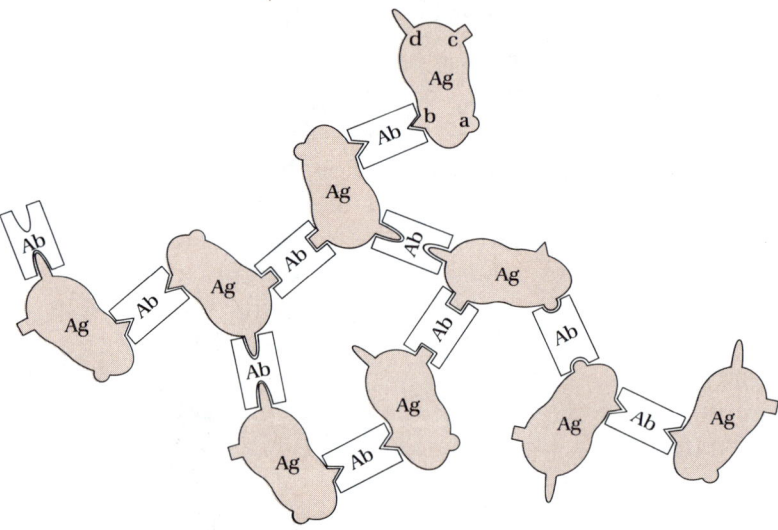

FIGURE 1 CROSS-LINKING OF ANTIGENIC DETERMINANTS AND ANTIBODIES

The soluble antigen has determinants a through d. Each determinant reacts with the specific antibody, which is bivalent. In this way the antigen molecules are cross-linked forming a large complex which precipitates. [Redrawn from Nisonoff (1984) *Molecular Immunology*, 2nd ed.]

ence, it has been supplanted by other methods. However, one very important theoretical point came out of this pioneering early work, and for this reason the reaction is described in Methods Box 1. The figure in that Box shows that the optimum amount of precipitate forms at the EQUIVALENCE ZONE. When either antigen or antibody is present in excess, less precipitate forms. This means that we cannot merely mix some antigen and some antibody together and get the maximum amount of precipitate. Nor can we add extra antigen to ensure that all the antibody will be bound into an AgAb complex and be part of the precipitate. While all of the antibody may indeed be bound into the complex, the complexes at any given ratio of antigen and antibody may not be the one that gives the maximum amount of precipitate.

METHODS BOX 1

Quantitative Precipitin Reaction

The quantitative precipitin reaction was developed by one of the most remarkable scientists of our age, Michael Heidelberger. Professor Heidelberger, who was born in 1888, is still active in his lab at NYU Medical School.

The purpose of the reaction is to *quantitate* the AgAb complex so that the exact amount of either reactant can be determined. The reaction was originally carried out with polysaccharide antigens that contain no nitrogen so that the amount of antibody nitrogen in the precipitate could be used as the measure of the quantity of antibody (because antibodies are proteins, they contain nitrogen). Subsequent modifications using radioisotopes now allow any antigen–antibody system to be quantified. When a constant amount of antibody is added to various concentrations of antigen and the precipitate is collected, washed, and analyzed, the curve shown in the accompanying figure is obtained.

The most striking thing about the curve is that it does not reach a plateau as expected; instead, as more antigen is added the amount of precipitate peaks and then *decreases*. When the supernatant fluid above the precipitate is tested for free antigen and free antibody, it is found that at the EQUIVALENCE POINT (the point of peak precipitation), neither can be detected. On either side of the equivalence point, either free antigen or free antibody is present. The results in the presence of excess antibody and at equivalence are easy to under-

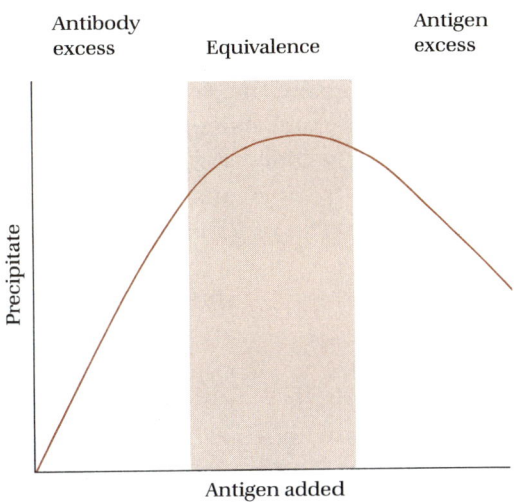

stand, but the result in the presence of antigen excess is not. The finding that even though all the antibody is bound to antigen the amount of precipitate decreases can be interpreted to mean that the complexes that form in the presence of antigen excess have different antigen:antibody ratios. As the "limiting complex" of $Ag:Ab_2$ is approached, less and less complex is in the form of a precipitate. Because the method quantifies only the precipitate, it gives the appearance of reduced reaction. The important point is that in antibody excess or in antigen excess we do not find the maximal quantity of precipitate; thus the exact quantity of antibody can only be determined at equivalence.

CHAPTER EIGHT

Reactions in Gels

In most precipitin reactions, there are many antigen and antibody reactions going on because most antigens have several antigenic determinants. For example, when we use human serum as the antigen, antibodies are generated against all of the components of the serum. Even when we use only one of the serum components (e.g., albumin) as antigen, it elicits the production of many different antibodies because it has many antigenic determinants. Fortunately, these complex reactions can be analyzed by carrying out the precipitin reaction in gels.

The Ouchterlony Assay In this assay—named after its inventor—the antigen and the antiserum are placed in wells that have been cut in agar. The reaction is conveniently done in a petri dish, but is often miniaturized and carried out on microscope slides. The antigen and antibody diffuse toward each other through the agar and at some point meet and react to form an AgAb complex. A precipitate forms where the reactants are close to the equivalence zone. Because the complex is too large to diffuse through the gel, it is immobilized. Each antigen diffuses at its own rate, depending on characteristics such as size and shape; and when it meets its specific antibody, a precipitate forms. The pattern of lines that form can be interpreted to determine whether the reactants are the same or different, as illustrated in Figure 2.

The Mancini Assay The Ouchterlony assay is qualitative. It tells us the minimum number of reactants involved but does not give information about the amount of the reactants present. A variant of the Ouchterlony assay that allows some quantitation of the antigen is called the MANCINI ASSAY. In this reaction the agar contains antibody, and antigen is placed in the well. As the antigen diffuses into the antibody-containing agar, the zone of equivalence is approached and a ring of precipitate is formed. The diameter of the ring is an indication of the concentration of antigen in the well, which is determined by comparing the diameter of the ring with the diameters of rings formed by a set of standards. The Mancini test is illustrated in Figure 3. This

MEASURING ANTIGEN–ANTIBODY REACTIONS

(A) Line of identity

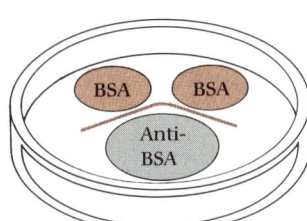

(B) Line of partial identity

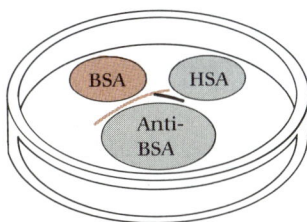

(C) No cross reaction

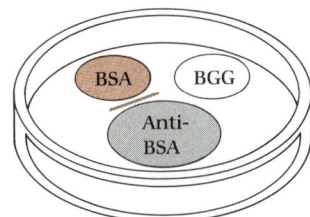

(D) No cross reaction

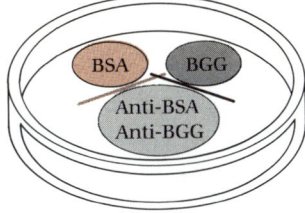

FIGURE 2 OUCHTERLONY GEL DIFFUSION PATTERNS
(A) Line of identity. The reactants (bovine serum albumin, BSA) are the same in both wells; hence a smooth line of precipitate forms. (B) Line of partial identity. The reactants are cross reactive, and the "spur" shows that there is some cross-reaction between human serum albumin (HSA) and anti-BSA. (C, D) Lines showing no cross reactions. Because there is no cross reaction between BSA and bovine γ-globulin (BGG), the anti-BSA forms no precipitate with BGG and anti-BGG and anti-BSA form separate lines of precipitate.

(A)
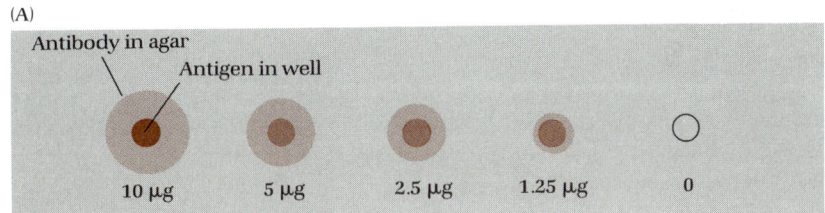

(B)
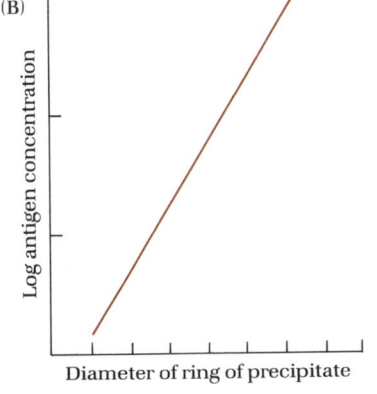

FIGURE 3 MANCINI TEST
(A) Antigen diffuses into antibody containing agar. The diameter of the ring of precipitate that forms is proportional to the log of the concentration of the antigen. (B) Standard curve. The concentration of antigen in an unknown sample is determined from a standard curve, which is prepared by using samples with known antigen concentrations.

assay is useful when we know the qualitative nature of the antigen but need an easy means of quantitation.

Immunoelectrophoresis (IEP)

A widely used variation of the precipitin reaction in a gel is IMMUNOELECTROPHORESIS (IEP). In this case one of the reactants, usually the antigen, is placed in a well cut in the agar. However, the antigen is not allowed to diffuse passively. Instead, the agar slab is subjected to electrophoresis, and the molecules in the antigen preparation each move in the

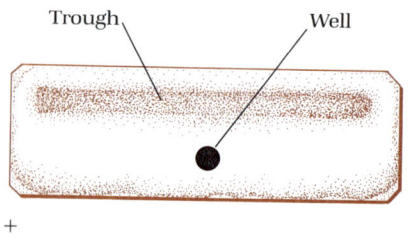

Antigen is placed in a small well cut into the agar.

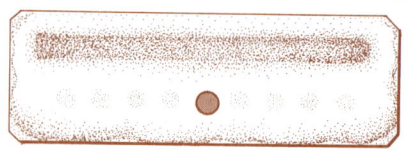

Antigen separates in an electrophoretic field.

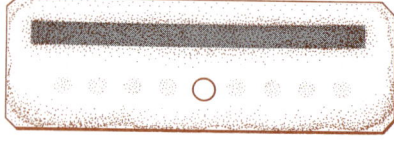

Antibody is added to the trough.

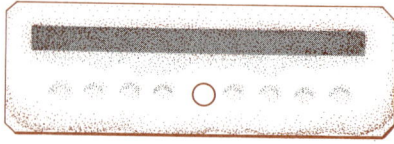

Antibody diffuses through the agar and reacts with separated antigen.

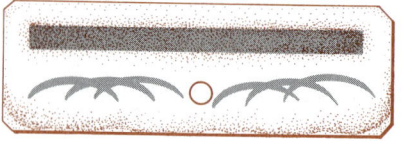

Precipitin lines form.

FIGURE 4 PRINCIPLE OF IMMUNOELECTROPHORESIS

The distance that the antigen in the well migrates in the electrical field is proportional to the antigen's charge. Antibody is added to the trough and diffuses through the agar. It reacts with the electrophoretically separated antigen, and a precipitate is formed.

MEASURING ANTIGEN–ANTIBODY REACTIONS

electric field according to their charge. In other words, the antigen is subjected to electrophoretic separation in the gel. To visualize the electrophoretically separated components, the investigator cuts a trough in the gel parallel to the direction in which the components have moved. Antiserum is placed in this trough and allowed to diffuse passively (*not* in an electrical field) into the gel. When the antibody reaches the electrophoretically separated antigen, AgAb complexes are formed. This test is illustrated in Figure 4.

This method allows the analysis of complex antigen–antibody systems such as serum (Figure 5). It can also be used as a means of identifying an unknown antigen, by determining whether the unknown has the same immunoelectrophoretic properties as a known antigen.

A variant of IEP, called ROCKET IMMUNOELECTROPHORESIS, is similar to the Mancini test and allows some quantitation of the reaction. Various concentrations of antigen are placed in wells that have been cut in the agar. In this test, the agar already contains antibody. The slab is subjected to an electric field, and as the antigen moves in the field it reacts with the antibody in the agar, resulting in the formation of characteristic "rockets." By compar-

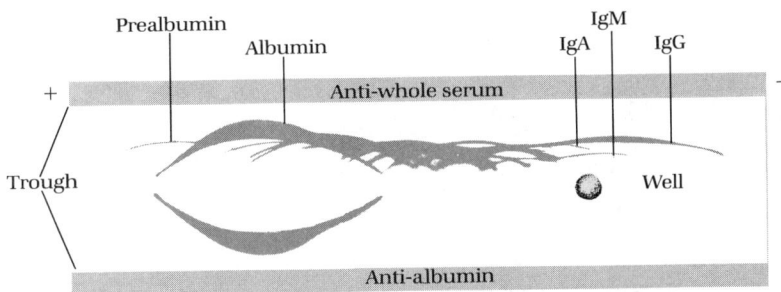

FIGURE 5 IMMUNOELECTROPHORETIC PATTERN OF HUMAN SERUM
Human serum was placed in the well and separated electrophoretically. The upper trough contains rabbit antiserum to whole human serum; hence the lines of precipitate form for all of the serum proteins. The lower trough contains rabbit anti-human albumin antiserum; hence the only precipitate that forms is with the human serum albumin. [Modified from Nisonoff (1984) *Molecular Immunology*, 2nd ed.]

CHAPTER EIGHT

ing the height of the "rocket" of an unknown with that of a standard, the concentration of antigen in the unknown can be determined (Figure 6).

Western Blotting

In recent years the separation of nucleic acids and proteins by gel electrophoresis has become a common analytical and preparative tool in cell and molecular biology. But characterization of the bands or spots that are resolved by the technique has been difficult in both one- and two-dimensional gels. One very potent method for achieving characterization is called WESTERN BLOTTING.

E. M. Southern introduced a method called Southern blotting in which electrophoretically fractionated DNA can be immobilized on nitrocellulose filters and used to analyze complementary sequences by hybridization in situ. An adaptation of this is to use RNA covalently attached to diazobenzyloxymethyl paper as a probe for complementary DNA. This method was amusingly called "Northern" blots by its inventors. The method of analyzing antigen–antibody complexes on nitrocellulose, which was invented by Burnette in Seattle, was called "Western" blotting.

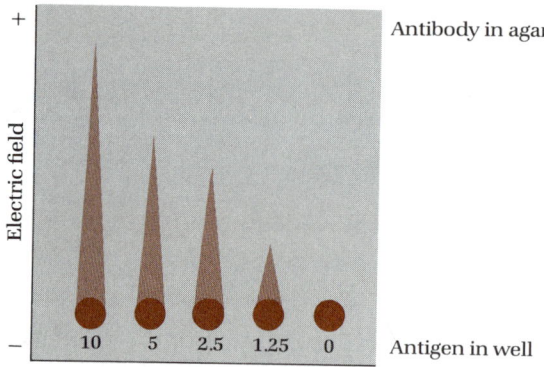

FIGURE 6 ROCKET ELECTROPHORESIS
Varying concentrations of antigen are separated by electrophoresis in agar containing antibody. By comparing the distance migrated by an unknown with data plotted on a standard curve, the concentration of antigen in the unknown sample can be determined.

MEASURING ANTIGEN–ANTIBODY REACTIONS

In Western blots the material that has been separated in the gel is transferred to a nitrocellulose membrane, usually by electroelution, and the nitrocellulose filter is reacted with antibody. If the antibody is directed against one of the components on the filter, an AgAb complex will form and be immobilized on the nitrocellulose filter. The AgAb complex can then be identified with a labeled reagent that reacts with the complex, usually radiolabeled anti-Ig (Figure 7). (Labeled antibody methods will be described later.)

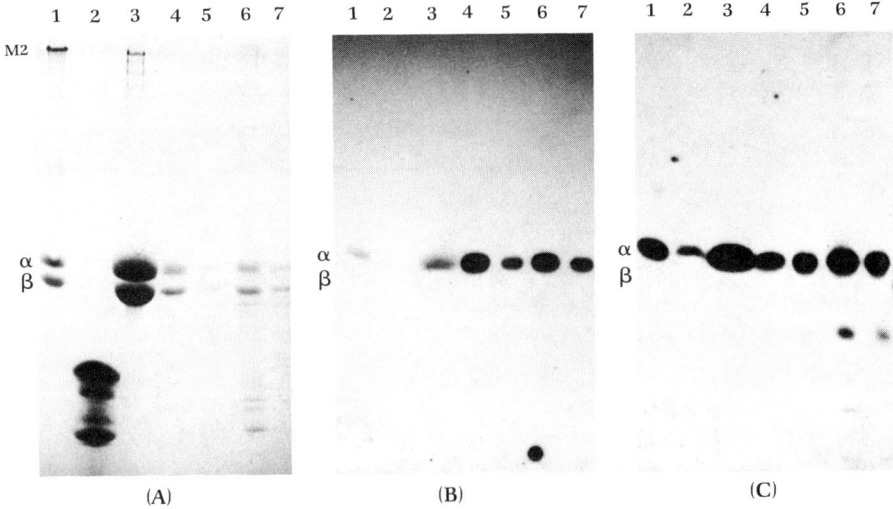

FIGURE 7 WESTERN IMMUNOBLOT

Microtubule proteins were prepared from various tissues and animals and separated by discontinuous SDS polyacrylamide gel electrophoresis, and probed with two different monoclonal anti-α-tubulin antibodies. (A) Gel stained with Coomassie Blue. (B, C) Autoradiograms of Western blots. Gels were probed with two different monoclonal anti-α-tubulin antibodies; antibody binding was detected by ^{125}I-labeled protein A. Samples: 1, cow brain microtubule protein; 2, bull spermatozoa; 3, chick brain microtubule protein; 4, sea urchin (*Strongylocentrotus purpuratus*) egg microtubule protein; 5, *S. purpuratus* sperm flagella; 6, *Lytechinus pictus* (another sea urchin) sperm flagella; 7, *Ciona intestinalis* (tunicate) sperm flagella. The tubulins split into their α and β subunits. Brain microtubule protein also contains high-molecular-weight associated proteins, marked M2 in (A). [Courtesy of David Asai]

CHAPTER EIGHT
Agglutination Reactions

When the antigen is particulate (for example, a cell), it settles to the bottom of the container and forms a visible pellet. If the cells have been reacted with antibody, however, the pattern of settling will be altered and the cells will *agglutinate*. This agglutination can produce various forms of AgAb complex, ranging from large clumps to fine material with the appearance of ground glass.

Unfortunately the agglutination reaction is useful only for qualitative work or for *relative* quantitation. Blood tests (Methods Box 2) are the most common qualitative use of the agglutination

---

METHODS BOX 2

RBC Typing

The most common agglutination test is that used for typing red blood cells. The major blood groups of humans are the ABO system. Donor and recipient must be compatible for successful blood transfusion; simple and accurate methods of red cell typing have been worked out.

To test for the presence of A or B antigens on the surface of red blood cells, the investigator takes two small drops of blood by fingerprick, places them on a slide, and adds a drop of anti-A to one and a drop of anti-B to the other. A positive reaction is seen by a rapid agglutination of the cells, as shown in the accompanying photograph. Agglutination in both drops indicates that the blood is type AB; no agglutination indicates that the individual is type O.

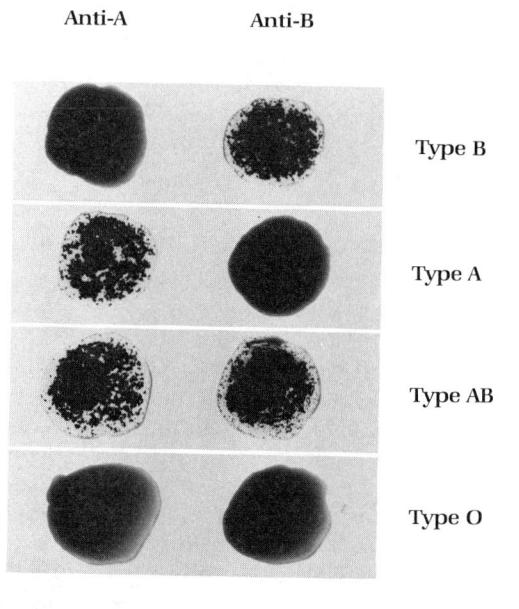

MEASURING ANTIGEN–ANTIBODY REACTIONS

reaction. In these tests the question being asked is usually "What is the blood type?" and not "What is the concentration of anti-red blood cell antibody?" The relative concentration of antibody in an antiserum can be determined by titrating the serum. For this titration, serial dilutions of the antiserum are prepared and reacted with a constant concentration of antigen. The last dilution to give a positive agglutination reaction is considered the end point, and the serum is said to have a TITER equivalent to the final dilution (for example, $1/20$ or $1/100$). In this way the amount of antibody in the serum can be compared to the amount in another antiserum measured in the same way. This can be used in the opposite direction, to determine the relative concentration of antigen, as well. In this case, a constant amount of a given antiserum is reacted with various concentrations of antigen.

Labeled Antibody Techniques

Because the essential problem of immunochemistry is to identify the AgAb complex, it is not surprising that there have been remarkable advances in the technology of labeling antibodies in order to identify them in the complex or to quantitate the complex. Radioactive, fluorescent, enzymatic, and electron-dense markers can be readily introduced onto an antibody molecule and are routinely used in both immunoassays and immunohistochemistry.

Primary and Secondary Antibody Methods

Two general methods are used to identify the AgAb complex using labeled antibody (Figure 8). In the PRIMARY METHOD we label all the Ig molecules in an antiserum, react the antiserum with antigen to form AgAb* complexes (in this case, with labeled antibody, Ab*), and then remove the unreacted molecules. This procedure leaves only those Ig molecules that are part of the AgAb* complex; and because these are labeled, the complex can be identified and studied.

A more sensitive, and thus more widely used, method is the SECONDARY METHOD. The first reaction is carried out with unlabeled reactants and unlabeled AgAb complexes are formed. A second antibody, labeled anti-Ig, is mixed with the AgAb complex formed

CHAPTER EIGHT

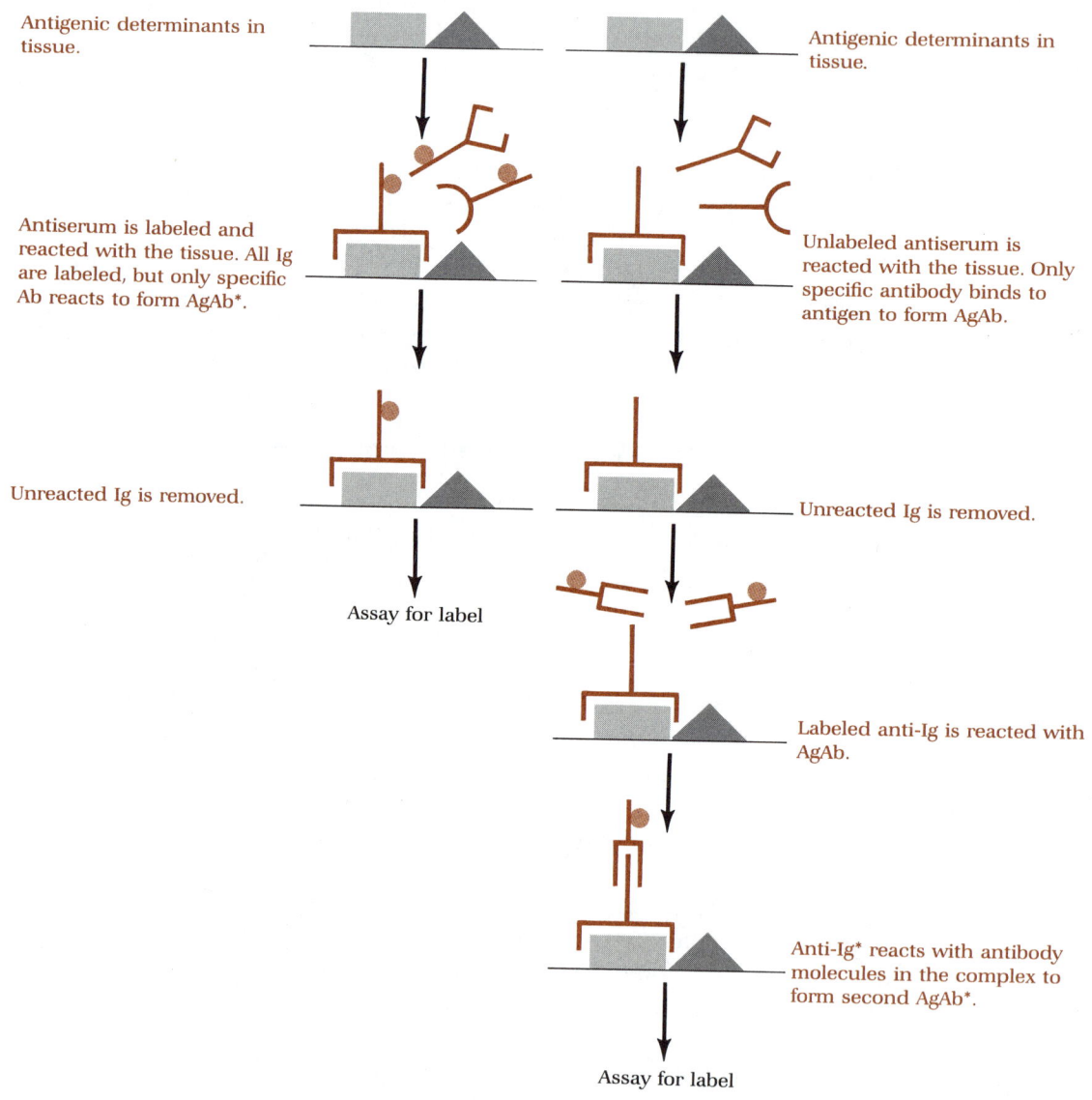

MEASURING ANTIGEN–ANTIBODY REACTIONS

FIGURE 8 IDENTIFICATION OF ANTIGEN:ANTIBODY COMPLEX WITH LABELED ANTIBODY

(A) Direct, or primary, method. The antibody is labeled directly and added to the sample. After the unreacted antibody is removed, the presence of the label is determined. (B) Indirect, or secondary, method. Unlabeled antibody is reacted with the sample. After unreacted Ig is removed, the second antibody, which is a labeled anti-Ig, is added and reacts with the AgAb complex. After unreacted second antibody is removed, the presence of the label is determined. Antibody can be labeled with radioisotope, enzyme, colloidal gold, or biotin.

in the first reaction. The labeled anti-Ig combines with all of the Ig molecules (i.e., antibody) in the AgAb complex and thereby labels them. This acts as an amplification step.

Radioactive Labels (RIA) Radioactive labels have been used in immunology and immunochemistry for a very long time. ^{125}I or ^{131}I can be attached to the tyrosine residues in a protein in such a manner that the immunological reactivity of the molecules is not altered. Because only a very small fraction of the immunoglobulin molecules in an antiserum are antibodies of the specificity being studied, it is not usually practical to label the primary antibody. Instead, a labeled second antibody is used (see preceding section). Radioactive labels are used for very sensitive assays called radioimmunoassays (RIA) which are described in Methods Box 3. They are also a very powerful tool for localizing antigens in tissue sections or on cell surfaces.

Enzyme Labels (ELISA) Antibodies to be used as second antibodies may also be conjugated to an enzyme. After the enzyme-labeled second antibody has reacted with the AgAb complex, the substrate for the enzyme is added. Enzyme–substrate combinations that can be identified by a color change are chosen; the presence of the color thus indicates the presence of the complex. The most commonly used enzyme is HORSERADISH PEROXIDASE (HRP). After the enzyme is conjugated to the anti-Ig,

METHODS BOX 3

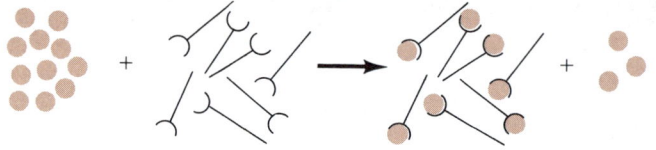

Control: A known amount of labeled antigen (●) is reacted with enough antibody (─⊂) to bind 70% of the antigen.

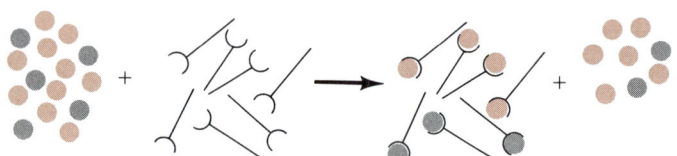

Experimental: An unknown antigen (●) is added and competes for binding of labeled antigen.

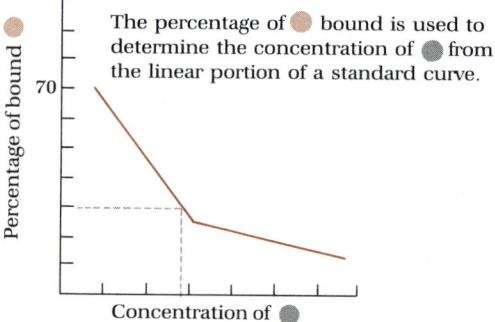

Standard curve

The percentage of ● bound is used to determine the concentration of ● from the linear portion of a standard curve.

Radioimmunoassays

RADIOIMMUNOASSAYS (RIA) have become the most commonly used and most powerful tools of immunochemistry. These assays are outgrowths of the assay developed in the 1960s by Solomon Berson (who died in 1973) and Rosalyn Yalow to immunologically quantify insulin. Rosalyn Yalow received the Nobel Prize for their work in 1977.

The principle of the RIA is that a very small amount of antigen in an unknown sample will *compete* with the binding of a known amount of radiolabeled antigen for a known amount of antibody. In this manner the concentration of *antigen* in an unknown sample can be determined by its ability to compete with labeled antigen. The principle is illustrated in the figure.

To carry out an RIA, a known concentration of labeled antigen X (Ag^*) is reacted with a known concentration of antibody (anti-X). The Ag^*Ab complex that forms can be quantitated by determining the amount of radioactive label. When unlabeled antigen (Ag) is added, it competes with the labeled antigen (Ag^*) for the constant number of combining sites on the antibody, thus *reducing* the amount of Ag^* in the complex. By setting up standard curves, we can quantify the amount of antigen (Ag) in the sample.

Radioimmunoassays are extremely sensitive (in the range of detection of nanograms per milliliter of antigen) and are widely used to quantify molecules present in very low concentration. They are especially useful for molecules in biological fluids, for example, insulin, steroid hormones, and neuropeptides. Commercial kits are available.

MEASURING ANTIGEN–ANTIBODY REACTIONS

the substrate, hydrogen peroxide, is added. The H_2O_2 is then converted to water in the presence of the electron donors diaminobenzidine or 4-chloronaphthol, whose oxidation products form a dark brown or purple color, respectively, and serve to localize the AgAb complex. The enzymes alkaline phosphotase, β-galactosidase, lactoperoxidase, and glucose oxidase can also be used in this technique.

In these enzyme-linked assays the amount of color is proportional to the amount of enzyme. We can thus use assays of this type to quantify the amount of AgAb complex. The enzyme-linked immunosorbent assay (ELISA) is described in Methods Box 4.

Fluorescent Labels

One of the great advances in the use of the immune system in diagnosis, histochemistry, and cell biology was made by the late Albert Coons at Harvard in 1944. Coons (who was a much-beloved figure in immunology) showed that a fluorescent label could be introduced into antibody molecules, so that when an AgAb complex is formed it can be visualized by virtue of the fluorescence.

Fluorescence is the property of a molecule that can absorb light of one wavelenth and emit light at another (Figure 9). The most commonly used fluorescent labels are fluorescein (which emits yellow–green light) and rhodamine (which emits red light). Figure 10 shows cells stained with fluorescein conjugated to anti-tubulin antibody.

The immunofluorescence technique takes advantage of the contrast between the emitted light and the nonemitting background. The method has a resolution limit of 200 nm. Higher resolution is achieved using electron-dense labels and electron microscopy.

Electron-Dense Labels

Electron-dense molecules such as ferritin or colloidal gold are markers used in electron microscopy. By attaching one of these labels to an antibody molecule, the specificity of the molecule can be used to localize antigens in tissue sections examined in the electron microscope. An example of "immunogold" is seen in Figure 11.

CHAPTER EIGHT

Because electron-dense labels absorb electrons, a tissue structure that has reacted with labeled antibody can be visualized. A powerful new method called IMMUNOPHOTOELECTRON MICROSCOPY has a resolution of 5 nm.

Immunophotoelectron microscopy is essentially the electron-optical analogue of immunofluorescence. In fluorescence microscopy the incident light stimulates the fluorescence emission

---

METHODS BOX 4

Enzyme-Linked Immunosorbant Assays (ELISA)

A variant of the enzyme-labeled localization technique used in histochemistry is the very popular ENZYME-LINKED IMMUNOSORBANT ASSAY, or ELISA. As the name suggests, the assay uses enzyme-linked methods. The test's uniqueness comes from the fact that one of the reactants, usually antigen, is immobilized (adsorbed) onto the surface of a test tube or microtiter well.

To determine the quantity of antibody in a sample, an aliquot of antiserum is reacted with the adsorbed antigen. The unreacted molecules are washed away, and an enzyme-linked anti-immunoglobulin is added. Finally, substrate is added and the amount of color that develops is determined. The amount of antibody present can be determined from standard curves, because the amount of color is proportional to the amount of enzyme-linked second antibody reacted.

An INHIBITION METHOD can also be used in ELISA assays. In these reactions, known amounts of unlabeled antigen are added to the unknown antiserum. This unlabeled antigen binds to the antigen-binding sites on the antibody and thus competes with the labeled antigen. A reduction in binding of the adsorbed labeled antigen is used to determine the quantity of antibody in the sample of serum.

ELISA assays can also be used to quantify the amount of antigen in a sample. This is done by adsorbing unlabeled antibody to a solid surface. The AgAb complex is quantified by adding enzyme-linked antibody directed against the antigen (i.e., labeled antibody of the same specificity as the unlabeled antibody already adsorbed to the surface, not an anti-Ig). This variation requires that the antigen have at least two accessible binding sites for antibody because two antibody molecules must be bound to the same antigen molecule.

ELISA kits for the detection of a very wide range of antigens are commercially available. The sensitivity of ELISA is in the range of nanograms per milliliter.

Direct method	Control	Inhibition method
Antiserum is added to the antigen, which has been absorbed onto a plate.	Known amount of antibody is added	Free antigen is added to antiserum.

Some Ig binds to Ag.

Unreacted Ig is washed away.

Enzyme-linked anti-Ig is added.

Substrate is added and enzyme activity is measured.

Standard curve is prepared

(Graph: Optical density (enzyme activity) vs. Antigen concentration)

The antibody concentration in an unknown serum is determined directly from the enzyme activity and the standard curve.

The antibody concentration in an unknown serum is determined by calculating the difference between the amount of enzyme bound in the control and the amount of enzyme bound in the test.

CHAPTER EIGHT

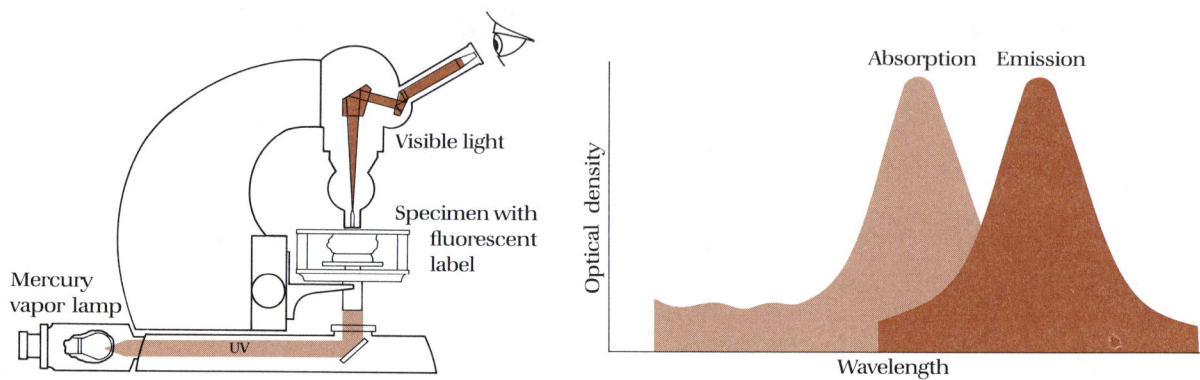

FIGURE 9 PRINCIPLE OF FLUORESCENCE MICROSCOPY

Excitation light at one wavelength (ultraviolet) is absorbed by the label and light of another wavelength (visible) is emitted and observed through the fluorescence microscope.

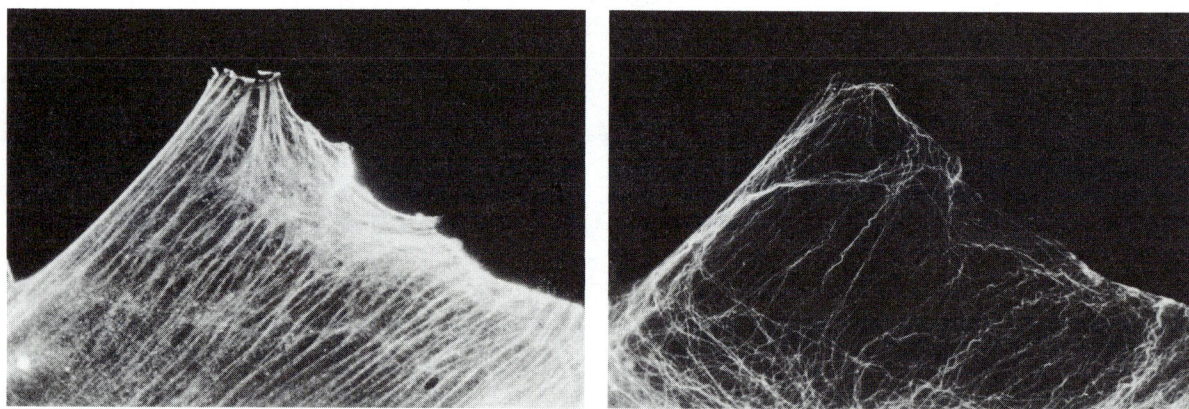

FIGURE 10 FLUORESCENCE MICROSCOPY

The same mouse fibroblast, double stained with one antibody that stains all microtubules (left) and another (right) that stains a subset of chemically distinct microtubules. Left, rabbit anti-tubulin rhodamine-labeled; right, mouse monoclonal fluorescein-labeled. [Courtesy of David Asai]

MEASURING ANTIGEN–ANTIBODY REACTIONS

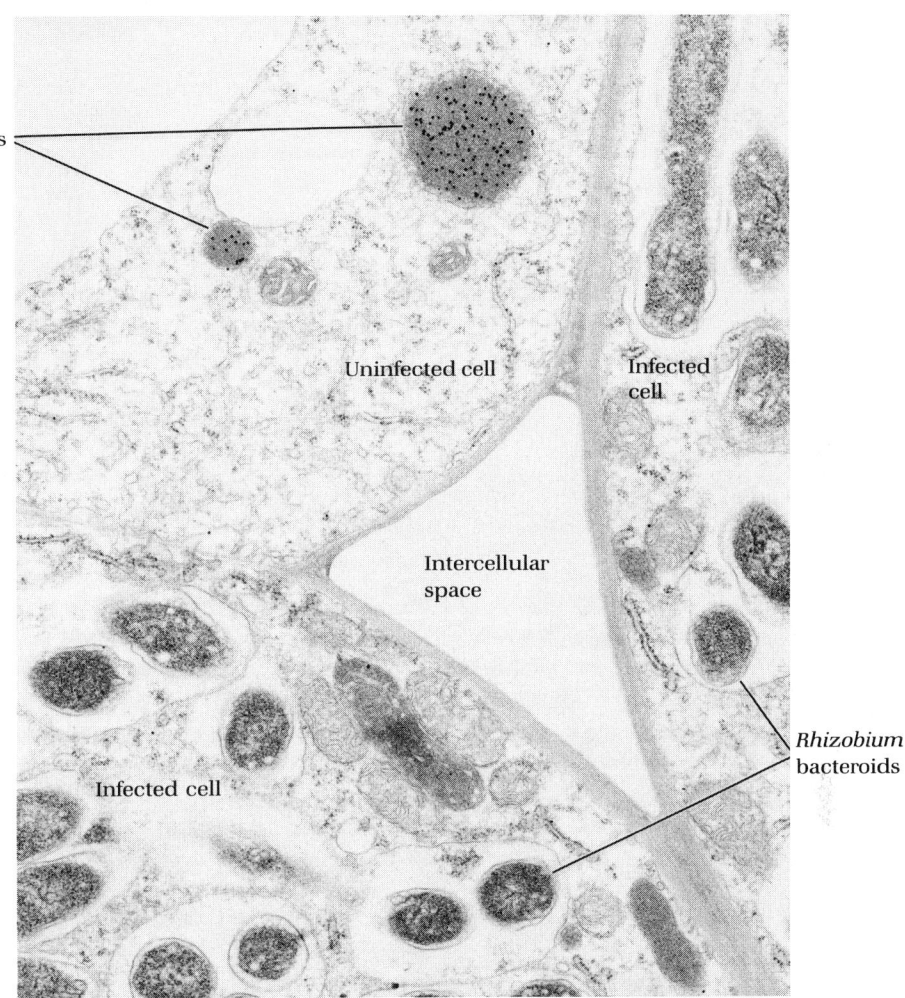

FIGURE 11   IMMUNOGOLD LABEL

Electron micrograph (17,280×) of a 3-week-old soybean nodule. The thin sections were incubated with rabbit antibody against a subunit of nodule-specific uricase. This was followed by 20-nm gold particles conjugated to protein A. The gold particles are found over the large peroxisomes in uninfected cells adjacent to cells infected by *Rhizobium*. It is thought that the *Rhizobium* fixes the nitrogen, which is then assimilated into the plant's uninfected cells using the uricase. [Courtesy of K. A. Vanden Bosch]

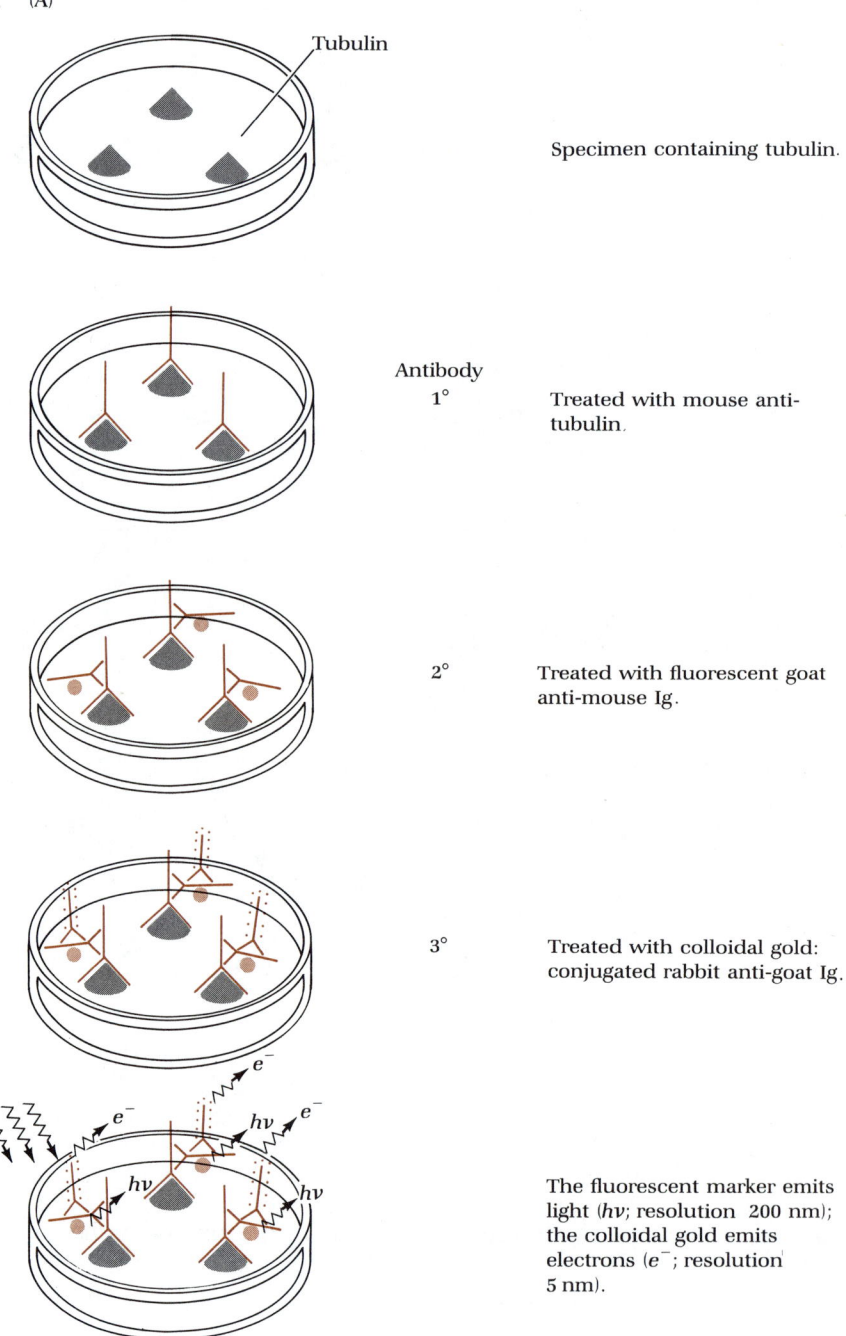

MEASURING ANTIGEN–ANTIBODY REACTIONS

from the dye, that is, light is emitted. In immunophotoelectron microscopy the incident light has a shorter wavelength and stimulates the emission of electrons from the label, which is colloidal gold. The electrons are then accelerated to high velocity and imaged.

In Figure 12 the specimens were simultaneously prepared for both fluorescence and immunophotoelectron microscopy. The *primary* antibody is a monoclonal anti-tubulin, which is reacted with the tissue specimen. The *secondary* antibody is a fluorescence-labeled goat anti-mouse Ig. The *tertiary* antibody is colloidal gold-labeled rabbit anti-goat Ig. The final AgAb complex can be visualized either in a fluorescence microscope or in the photoelectron microscope.

(B)

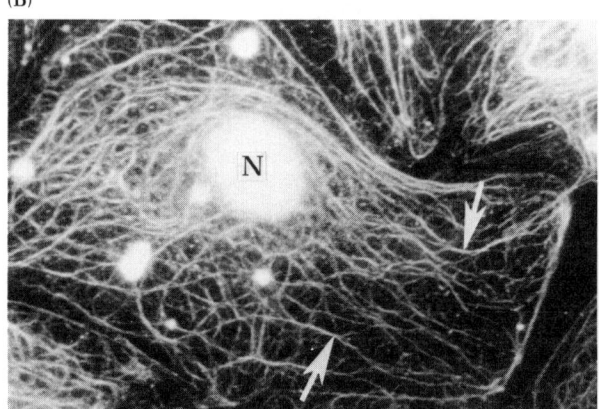 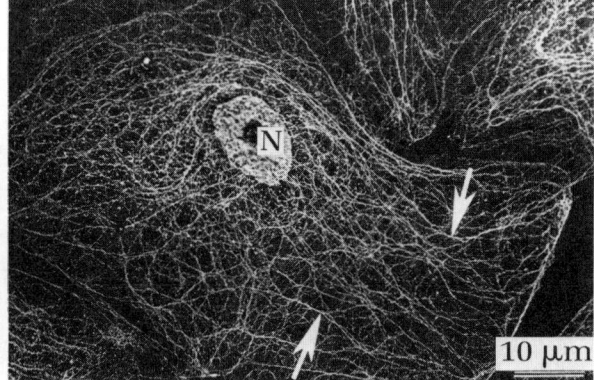

FIGURE 12 COMPARISON OF IMMUNOFLUORESCENCE AND IMMUNOPHOTOELECTRON MICROSCOPY

(A) Preparation of the samples. The sample is reacted with the primary antibody (monoclonal anti-tubulin), and antigen–antibody complexes form. A secondary antibody of fluorescence-conjugated goat anti-mouse Ig is reacted. The samples can now be used for fluorescence microscopy. A tertiary antibody of colloidal gold-conjugated rabbit anti-goat Ig is reacted. The samples can now be used for immunophotoelectron microscopy. (B) Immunofluorescence (*left*) and immunophotoelectron microscope pictures of tubulin:anti-tubulin specimen prepared in (A). Arrows identify some of the many microtubules that can be seen in both the fluorescence and photoelectron micrographs. [Courtesy of O. H. Griffith]

CHAPTER EIGHT

Nonspecific Binding to Immunoglobulin

There are some molecules that can bind nonspecifically to immunoglobulin molecules. We take advantage of this fact by labeling these special molecules with one of the labels discussed above.

PROTEIN A is a cell wall protein from *Staphylococcus aureus*; it has the property of binding nonspecifically to the Fc portion of immunoglobulin molecules. Heat-killed staph that express protein A can be used to precipitate Ig molecules from solution. Protein A can also be labeled and used as a probe for the AgAb complex.

Feeding large quantities of egg white to animals produces a biotin deficiency. This reduction in biotin was found to be due to a molecule in egg white that binds to biotin with extraordinary affinity. The molecule, a basic glycoprotein of 68,000 MW, is called AVIDIN. Many biotin molecules can be put on an antibody molecule without altering the antigen-binding properties of the antibody. Several molecules of avidin can bind to each biotin. When the avidin is labeled with an enzyme, this system can be used to examine the AgAb complex.

Flow Cytometry

A significant advance in technology has been the ability to either sort or analyze cells on the basis of their surface antigens using the technology of FLOW CYTOMETRY (Figure 13). Cells can be treated with an antibody conjugated to a fluorescent probe, so that when the cell passes through the laser beam fluorescent light is emitted. This light is collected and the intensity of the light from the individual cell is analyzed, and/or the light is used to put a charge on the droplet that forms around the cell as it leaves the nozzle assembly. The cells pass through charge deflection plates, and charged drops are deflected and collected.

Cells can also be sorted on the basis of the amount of light they scatter. Droplets that scatter predetermined amounts of light can have a charge placed on them and then be deflected.

MEASURING ANTIGEN–ANTIBODY REACTIONS

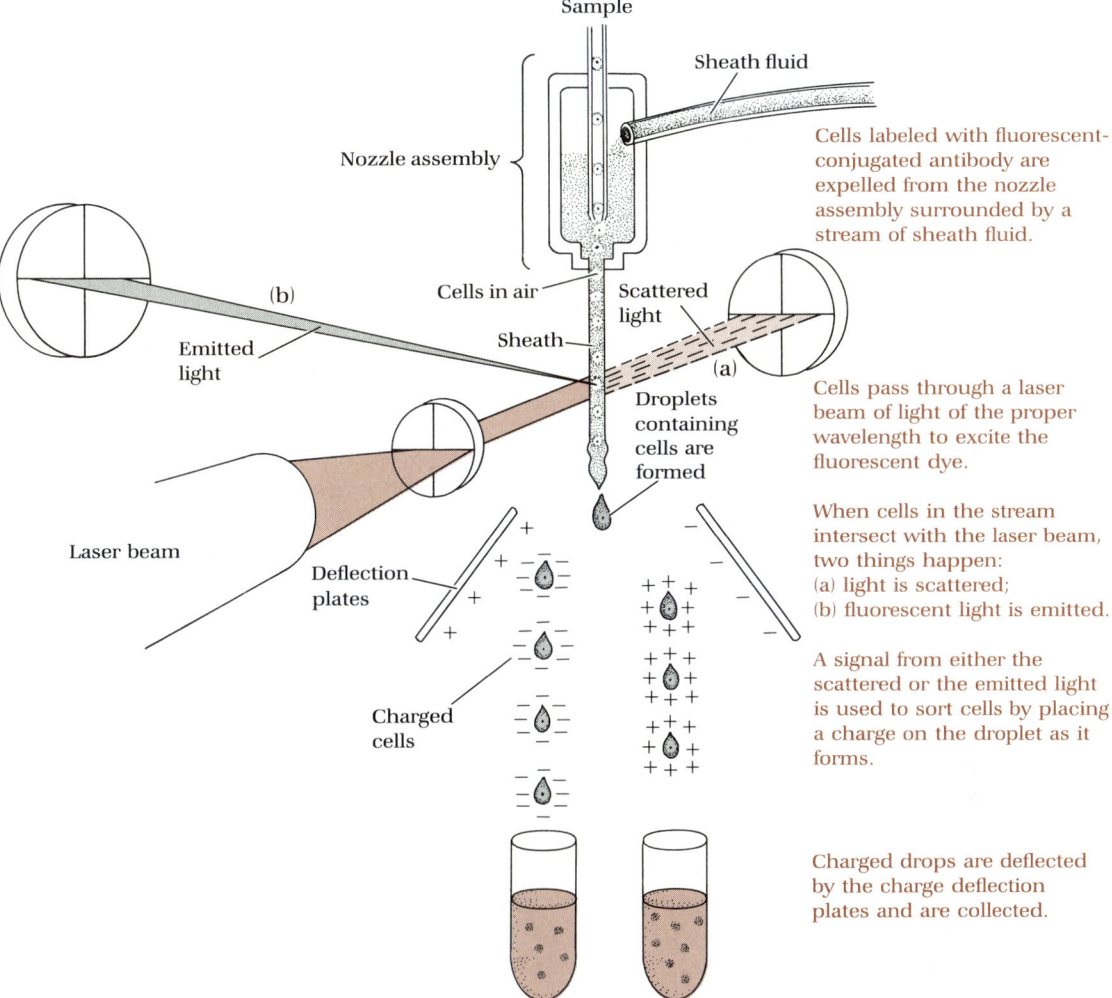

FIGURE 13 THE PRINCIPLE OF FLOW CYTOMETRY

Cells can be analyzed or sorted. The cells enclosed in a sheath of fluid pass through a laser beam. The amount of light scattered and the fluorescent light emitted are recorded. Either of these signals can be used to place a charge on the droplet so the cell can be deflected.

CHAPTER EIGHT

Summary

1. All methods of determining the presence, amount, or location of antigen or antibody depend on identifying or quantifying the AgAb complex.
2. Antigen–antibody reactions in which the antigen is soluble form precipitates. In quantitative precipitin reactions the amount of antibody is determined in the precipitate at the equivalence zone. Complexes formed in the presence of excess antigen do not form as much precipitate, and caution is needed in measuring the amount of precipitate. Precipitin reactions in gels allow the number of interacting antigen–antibody systems to be studied.
3. When the antigen is particulate (for example, a cell), formation of the AgAb complex results in an agglutination reaction. Agglutination reactions are usually qualitative only, the most common being the typing of red blood cells.
4. Modern methods of quantifying and localizing the antigen–antibody reaction rely very heavily on labeling one of the reactants. Radioactive and enzyme-linked labels are the most commonly used, but electron-dense labels are very useful in immunophotoelectron microscopy.
5. Radioimmunoassays (RIA) and enzyme linked immunosorbant assays (ELISA) are very sensitive (nanograms per milliliter) and very commonly used assays.

Additional Readings

Kabat, E. 1961. *Kabat and Mayer's Experimental Immunochemistry*, rev. ed. C. Thomas, Springfield, IL.

Lefkovits, I. and B. Pernis. 1979. *Immunological Methods*, vols. 1, 2, 3. Academic Press, New York.

Mishell, B. B. and S. M. Shiigi. 1980. *Selected Methods in Cellular Immunology*. W. H. Freeman, San Francisco.

Nowotny, A. 1979. *Basic Exercises in Immunochemistry*, 2nd ed. Springer-Verlag, New York.

Weir, D. M. et al. 1985. *Handbook of Experimental Immunology*, 4th ed. Mosby, St. Louis.

Williams, C. A. and M. W. Chase. 1967. *Methods in Immunology and Immunochemistry*, vols. 1, 2, 3. Academic Press, New York.

CHAPTER 9

COMPLEMENT

Overview The complement system, very much like the clotting and fibrinolysis systems, has evolved as a series of precursor molecules that are converted into active enzymes. Each enzyme uses the next molecule in the system as a substrate, converting it into its active form; hence the notion of a cascade. If this series of reactions occurs on the surface of a cell, the result is the formation of an attack complex that forms a transmembrane channel in the cell membrane. The presence of the channel leads to lysis of the cell.

The lytic pathway of the complement cascade can be described as a few discrete phases. In the classical pathway, the recognition phase occurs when one component of complement binds to the Fc portion of the antibody molecule in an AgAb complex. This phase leads, by several steps, to the activation phase, which is the crucial stage in the classical pathway. During the activation phase, the formation of the pivotal complement product, C3b, occurs. Component C3b is also formed without AgAb via the alternate pathway, which has a built-in amplification scheme for converting C3 to the active C3b. Finally, after generation of C3b, both pathways converge in the membrane attack phase to cause lysis of cells. Much of the confusion and fear about the study of complement comes about because of the nomenclature, and because there are several steps in each phase. This chapter is organized so that the discrete phases will be emphasized.

Discovery of the Complement System

The realization that in addition to antibodies there was some component in antiserum that was important in immune reactions came about at the end of the nineteenth century (which is known as the Golden Era of microbiology). The initial observation

---

METHODS BOX 1

The Complement Fixation Test

The binding of complement to the AgAb complex is stoichiometric, so by determining the amount of C bound (or *fixed*) to the complex we can determine the amount of complex. The principle of the complement fixation (CF) test is to determine how much lytic activity of complement has been removed from a sample of complement after an unknown amount of AgAb complex is added. This is an absolute value that gives the relative amount of complex present, although by using proper standard curves this number can be converted into the absolute amount of complex present.

Before carrying out the CF test, STANDARDS must be made: a sample of complement (usually normal guinea pig serum) is titrated by adding various amounts to a mixture of a known amount of red blood cells and a known amount of anti-red blood cell antibody. The red cell:anti-red cell mixture forms an AgAb complex, which lyses when C is bound. The titration is carried out to an end point, (expressed as percentage of lysis; in practice 60% is often used). We now have a set of reagents (namely, a known amount of complement and a test system of red cells and anti-red cells) that always gives the same amount of lysis when mixed together.

To carry out the CF test, the sample to be tested (for example, a sample of serum that may contain antibodies against molecule X) is mixed with X. If the sample contains anti-X, a small amount of X–anti-X complex will be formed. To determine how much X–anti-X has been formed, the amount of standard complement solution that results in 60% lysis of the standard red cell–anti-red cell complex is added. If any X–anti-X complex is present, some of the added complement will be "fixed" and the complement activity of the standard complement solution will be reduced by this amount.

To determine how much of the standard complement solution has been fixed to X–anti-X, the test red cell–anti-red cell mixture is added. Because the original amount of complement that was added was sufficient to lyse 60% of this test mixture, any *reduction* of lysis of the added red cells must be due to a reduction in the amount of complement available, that is, fixed to X–anti-X. The appropriate controls of standard complement plus X in the absence of the test serum must be done to rule out ANTI-COMPLEMENTARY EFFECTS in the serum (because the system is complex, the inactivation of one component in the cascade by some nonspecific factor could give a reduction in lysis that would be interpreted as a false positive).

METHODS BOX 1

(A) Standard

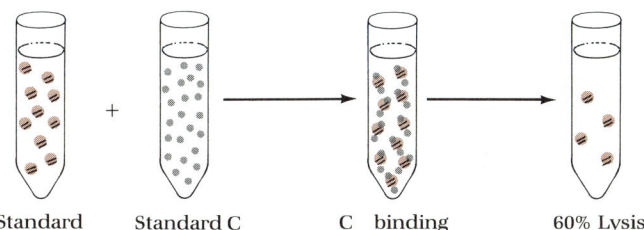

Standardized C is added to standardized RBC:anti-RBC (AgAb).

C binds to AgAb resulting in 60% lysis.

(B) Test for anti-X in unknown: reaction of unknown sample plus antigen to form AgAb

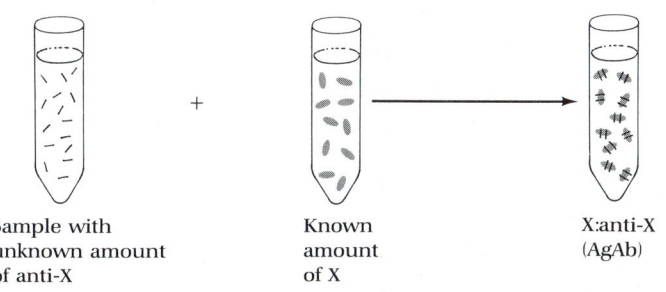

Unknown amount of anti-X in the sample is reacted with X. If sample contains anti-X, a complex of X:anti-X will form.

(C) Test for anti-X in unknown: addition of standard system to determine whether C is fixed

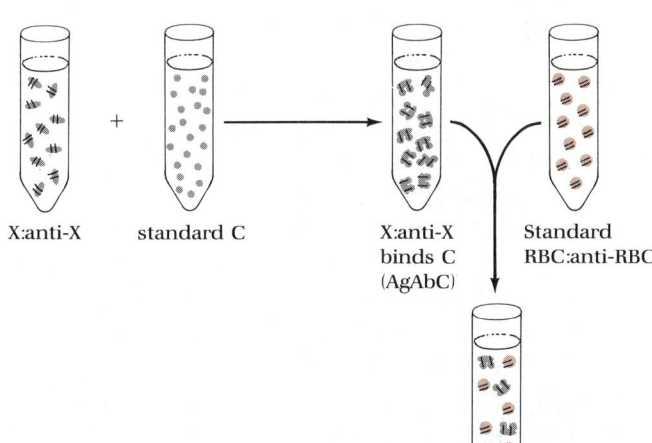

Standard C (as in A, above) is added to AgAb formed in (B); AgAbC forms.

The standard RBC:anti-RBC is not lysed because all of the C has been fixed by the unknown AgAb.

was made by Buchner in 1893, who noted that antisera that could kill bacteria lost their lytic activity when heated to 56°C. Jules Bordet followed this observation with the discovery in 1895 that the heat-labile substance was not antibody. He did this by showing that the lytic activity of a heat-inactivated anti-cholera antiserum could be restored by the addition of unheated *normal* serum. Bordet correctly concluded that antibodies were heat-stabile but that this other serum substance, which he called alexin, was heat-labile. (Ehrlich later renamed alexin *complement*.) Bordet also introduced the erythrocyte:anti-erythrocyte system as the experimental lytic system, a technical advance that significantly enhanced the study of complement. In 1919 Bordet received the Nobel prize for his work on complement.

The realization that complement was more than one substance came about over the next few decades. First it was found in 1907 that when fresh serum, which is used as a source of lytic complement, was dialyzed against water a precipitate formed. Neither the precipitate (after being redissolved in saline) nor the dialysis fluid had complement activity (that is, neither solution could restore lytic activity to a heat-inactivated serum). But when the two fractions were mixed together, activity was restored. This finding showed that complement had at least two components.

The two components then were shown to act sequentially. When erythrocytes were first reacted with heat-inactivated anti-erythrocyte antibody (so that the antibody would coat the red cells), the factor in the supernatant fluid was able to react only when the factor in the precipitate had reacted first. This finding showed that the reaction was sequential: antibody reacted with the antigen (forming what we now know to be an antigen–antibody complex), followed by the component in the precipitate, followed by the component in the supernatant fluid. Logically, the particulate factor (in the precipitate) was called "midpiece," and the soluble factor (in the supernatant fluid) was called "endpiece." Both midpiece and endpiece were heat-labile, so it seemed safe to conclude that—to use language that was appropriate at the time—"the heat-labile lytic factor in serum had two components, midpiece and endpiece." Midpiece was later re-

COMPLEMENT

named C1, and endpiece was renamed C2 (and we will now start using the modern terminology.)

The realization that things were more complicated than this came a few years later with the discovery that cobra venom destroyed the lytic activity of complement. The activity could be restored by addition of fresh normal serum (which was not surprising), but it could also be restored by addition of *heat-inactivated* normal serum. Because it was already known that C1 and C2 were heat-labile, this result meant that the cobra venom-labile but heat-stabile substance was another complement component; it was named C3. But now the easily visualized picture of midpiece–endpiece–lysis was replaced by a more complicated picture. Where did C3 fit into the reaction scheme? And, to paraphrase a song of the time, "Are there any more [components] at home like you?"

The answer to the question in the song was yes. It was noted that, believe it or not, when serum was mixed with yeast cells, the C3 was removed but *another* heat-stabile component remained. This component was named C4, and it was found to be inactivated by treatment with ammonia. It could be shown that the components reacted with the AgAb complex in the sequence C1, C4, C2, C3.

The situation remained like this until the late 1950s. At that time the modern era of complementology begins, as techniques of protein chemistry had advanced to the point where they could be applied to this obviously complex and important problem. The reader should once again be aware that although the advances in the modern era were possible because of advances in other areas, if the question had not been asked in terms of the immunology up to that point there would have been no problem on which to apply the new methodology.

As we progress in this chapter we will see that there are two pathways leading to lysis. One is called the classical pathway, and the second is called the alternate pathway. The pathways converge at the C3 step (Figure 1), and it would be wise for the reader to keep this point in mind while reading about the events in the complement cascade.

142
CHAPTER NINE

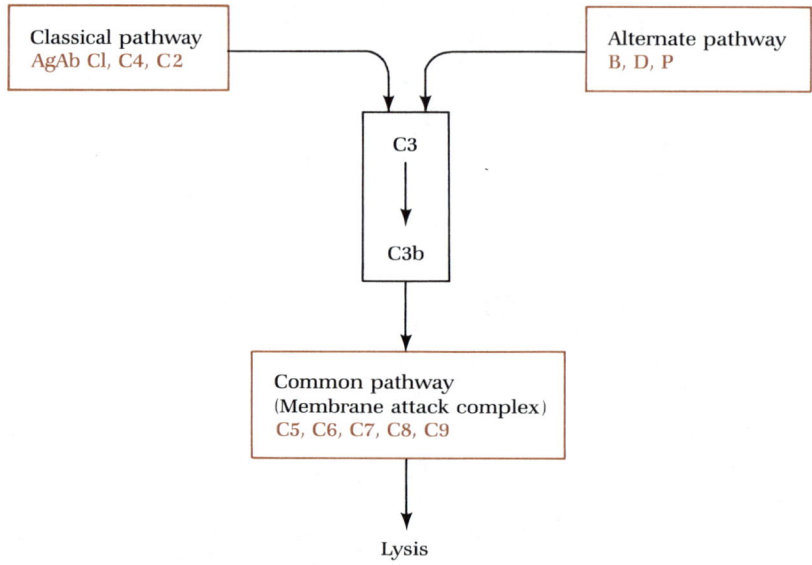

FIGURE 1 OVERVIEW OF THE COMPLEMENT EVENTS LEADING TO LYSIS

The classical and alternate pathways converge at the C3 ⟶ C3b step and lead into the common pathway, which ends with lysis.

The Classical Pathway

The Recognition Unit   The classical complement pathway begins when the first component of C (C1) binds to the AgAb complex. The result of this initial step is the formation of an activated C1.

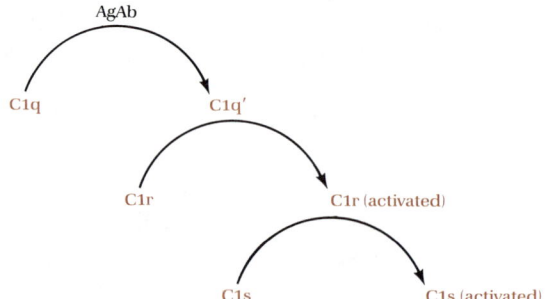

COMPLEMENT

C1 is a complex of three protein molecules called C1q, C1r, and C1s. Of these three proteins, C1q binds to the Fc portion of the antibody molecule. Only the C_H4 domain of IgM and the C_H2 domain of IgG have sites with which C1q reacts.

C1q is an unusual molecule that has the shape of a "bouquet of tulips" (Figure 2). It is composed of three sets of peptide chains, each set having six members, so the whole molecule is composed of 18 chains. The three sets of chains, called A, B, and C, associate to form the structure seen in Figure 2. The other two molecules of C1 (C1r and C1s) become altered after C1q combines with the Fc. It has been postulated that the reaction of C1q with Fc causes a configurational change that distorts one of the C1r

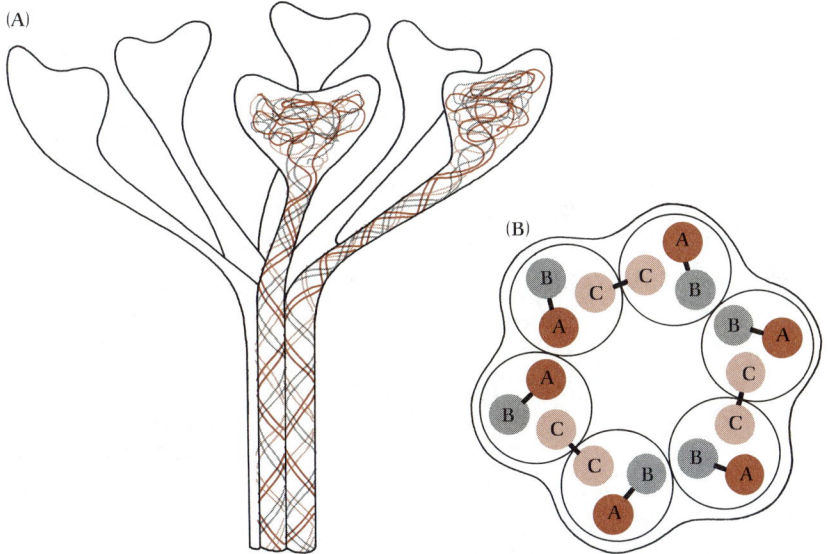

FIGURE 2 STRUCTURE OF THE C1q COMPONENT OF HUMAN COMPLEMENT

(A) The molecule consists of 18 chains and has a "bouquet of tulips" appearance. (B) Cross section through the "stalk" showing the six "stems" composed of A, B, and C peptides. The A and B chains in each stem are connected to each other by disulfide bonds. The C chain of one stem is connected to the C chain of another stem by disulfide bonds.

CHAPTER NINE

INFORMATION BOX 1

Synonyms for Products of the Complement Cascade

CLASSICAL PATHWAY		ALTERNATE PATHWAY	
C4C2a complex	C4C2 C3 convertase	Factor B	C3 proactivator Glycine-rich β-glycoprotein
C4bC2aC3b complex	C4C2C3b C5 convertase	Factor D	C3 proactivator convertase
		C3.B complex	Initiating C3 convertase
		C3Bb complex	Amplification C3 convertase
		C3bPBb complex	C5 convertase

---

molecules. This distortion exposes an enzymatic site on C1r, which in turn causes the cleavage of the second chain. The now activated C1r then cleaves the C1s chain, thereby generating two active fragments. This sequence is shown diagrammatically in Figure 3. As a result of this reaction the next components in the cascade, C4 and C2, can become activated.

The Activation Unit: C4 and C2

The first set of reactions generates activated C1s, which acts as the enzyme to catalyze the next reaction in the cascade:

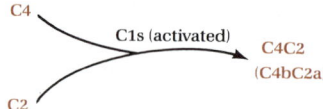

C1s cleaves low-molecular-weight peptides from C4 and C2 and exposes their active forms, C4a and C2a, which then fuse. These reactions are depicted in Figure 4A and 4B.

COMPLEMENT

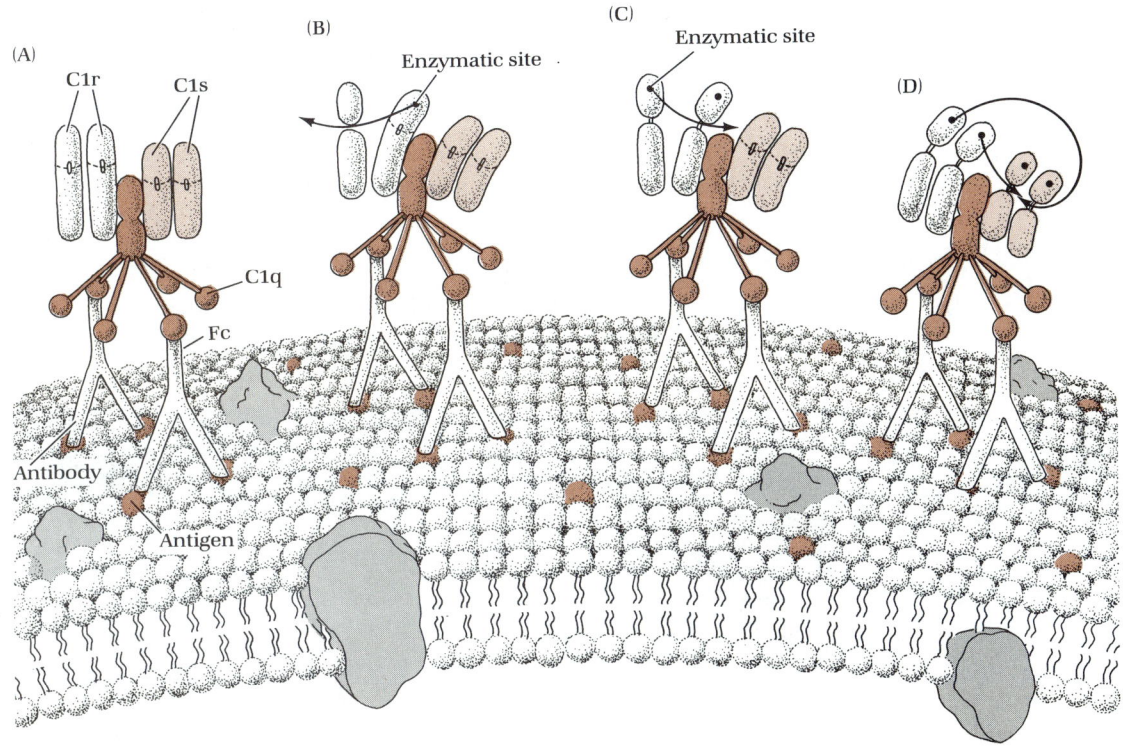

FIGURE 3 RECOGNITION UNIT OF THE COMPLEMENT SYSTEM

Two molecules of IgG are shown bound to the surface of a cell. (A) The C1q component of complement binds to the Fc portion of the immunoglobulins. This is the first step in the activation of the other C1 components. (B) Fc binding causes a change in the configuration of C1q, which then distorts one of the two polypeptide chains of C1r. This distortion exposes an enzymatic site on C1r and leads to cleavage of the chain. (C) The cleavage of the C1r chain opens an enzymatic site on the other C1r chain and cleavage of the second C1r chain occurs. (D) The activated C1r cleaves the C1s chains, thereby generating two activated fragments.

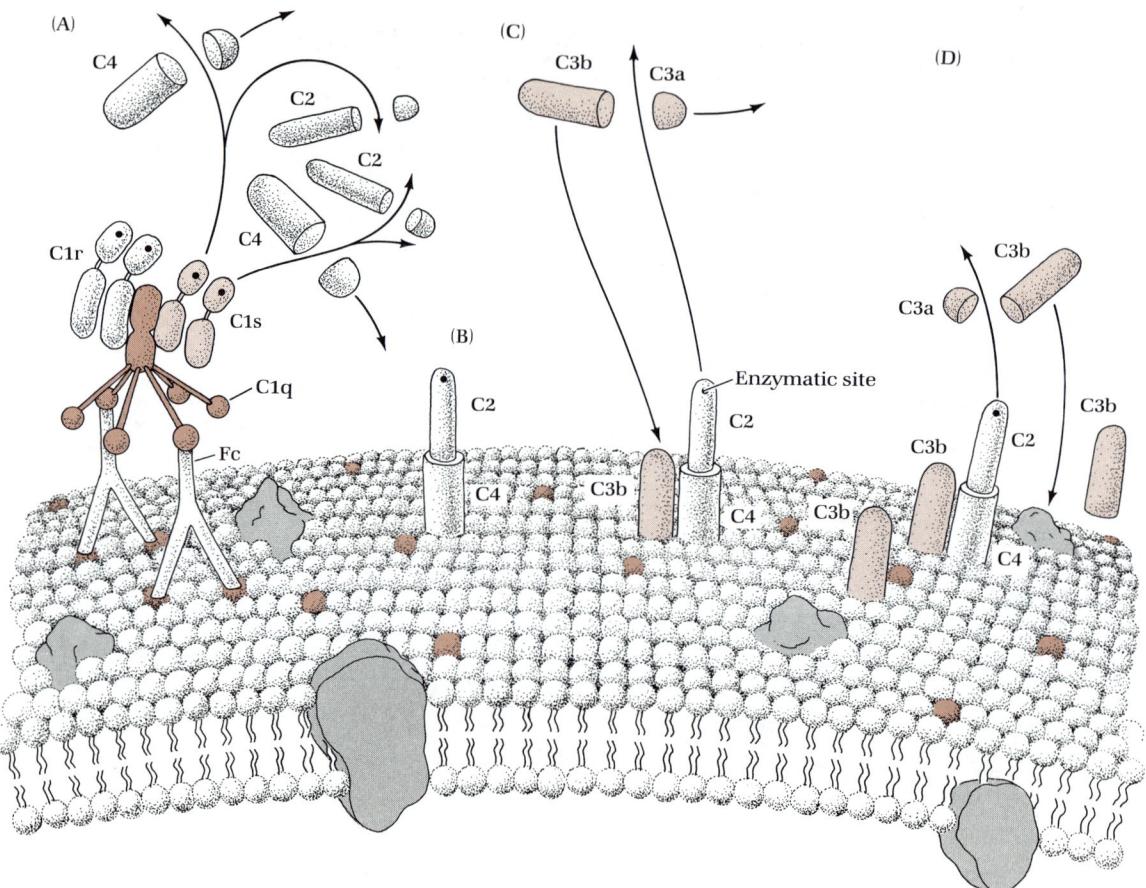

FIGURE 4   ASSEMBLY OF THE ACTIVATION UNIT
(A) Activated C1s attacks C4 and then C2, cleaving a small activation peptide from each. (B) Formation of a bimolecular C4C2 complex occurs, and the complex attaches itself to the cell surface. This complex is known as C3 convertase (see next panel). (C) The C4C2 complex acts on C3 in the serum, splitting off C3b, which forms a trimolecular complex C4C2C3b on the cell surface. (D) The C4C2 complex continues to act on serum C3 and many C3b molecules accumulate on the cell surface.

The C4bC2a complex (which we will abbreviate as the C4C2 COMPLEX) acts as an enzyme whose substrate is C3. For this reason it is also called C3 CONVERTASE. The enzyme C3 convertase splits C3 into two products, called C3a and C3b. The product C3b

COMPLEMENT

is the crucial component in the system and remains in the complement pathway by associating with the C4C2 complex.

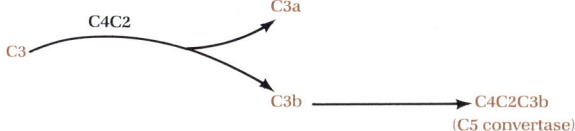

This is shown diagrammatically in Figure 4C and 4D. The C4C2C3b complex is an enzyme that reacts with the next component, C5, in the common pathway. For this reason, this complex is called a C5 CONVERTASE.

At this point the classical and alternate pathways converge to form the MEMBRANE ATTACK UNIT, which leads to the actual lysis of the cell. We shall pick up the narrative at the membrane attack unit after we examine those events in the alternate pathway that lead to the generation of C3b in a form that is also a C5 convertase.

The Alternate Pathway

The alternate pathway is associated with one of the tragic aspects of the scientific life. In the early 1950s Louis Pillemer, working at Western Reserve University in Cleveland, published papers in which he claimed to have discovered another complement pathway. This pathway did not need AgAb complexes to be activated; instead it was activated by sugar moieties in yeast and bacterial cell walls. Pillemer argued that a substance in serum, which he called PROPERDIN, or P, is able to activate C3. This idea met with criticism and acrimonious debate. Pillemer was an unusual man with a history of academic brilliance and emotional problems, and was apparently unable to withstand the pressures of this heated controversy. He took his own life a few years before his basic ideas were shown to be correct.[1]

The crucial points to be remembered about the alternate pathway are that the initiation can occur in the fluid phase

---

[1] The history of properdin and the controversy are covered in a brilliant essay by W. D. Ratnoff in *Perspectives in Biology and Medicine*, Summer 1980, p. 638. The essay was taken from Dr. Ratnoff's B.A. thesis at Harvard.

148
CHAPTER NINE

rather than on a cell surface, that it does not require the presence of the AgAb complex, and that it is an effective alternative method for producing C3b from C3.

Activation of the Alternate Pathway

The function of the activation unit in the classical pathway was to generate C3b. The C3b combined with the C4C2 complex to form the C4C2C3b complex, which connects to the membrane attack unit, a component common to both the classical and alternate pathways. The alternate pathway generates C3b in three ways, without the benefit of the AgAb complex or the C1 recognition unit.

The first way in which C3b is generated occurs when C3 reacts with a serum component called FACTOR B, a reaction that produces a C3.B complex.

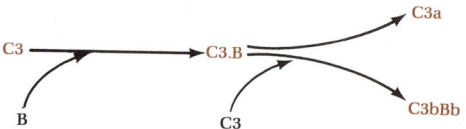

The Amplification Loop

The C3 part of the C3.B complex causes the B part to react with another C3 molecule, a reaction leading to the generation of C3b by cleaving the second C3 into C3a and C3b. Thus the complex, which contains C3, acts as an enzyme whose substrate is C3. (In the classical pathway it will be recalled that the C4C2 complex acts to convert C3 into C3a and C3b.) Because the C3.B complex is used in the generation of C3b from C3, this reaction is called the AMPLIFICATION LOOP.

The formation of the C3.B complex apparently occurs spontaneously in serum but the C3b product is inactivated as soon as it is formed by a C3B INACTIVATOR called C3bINA. In the presence of the inactivator the normal, very low serum level of C3b is maintained.

Another way that C3b is generated is by the interaction of C3.B with FACTOR D. This reaction results in the conversion of C3.B to C3bBb:

COMPLEMENT

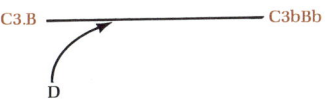

Thus we see that the interaction of C3 with either factor B, factor D, or the C3B complex results in the formation of the C3bBb complex.

Stabilization of the C3bBb Complex

The C3bBb complex is unstable unless it reacts with properdin to form a C3bPBb complex. Pillemer assumed that properdin was the *initiating* factor, but we now know that it is a *stabilizing* factor. (Most scientists would give a year's wages to be this close to being correct on a major discovery.)

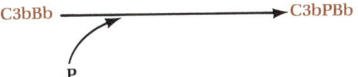

When a second C3b molecule is added to the C3bPBb complex, a conformational change occurs that makes the complex into a C5 convertase. At this step the alternate and classical pathways converge.

The Common Complement Pathway

The Membrane Attack Unit: C5b, C6, C7, C8, C9

We saw earlier how a C5 convertase is generated in both the classical and alternate pathways. Both of these C5 convertases can react with C5 to generate C5b. This C5b forms a tetramolecular complex with C6, C7, and C8; this complex attaches to the target cell membrane (Figure 5).

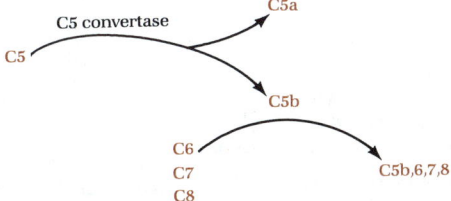

The C5b,6,7,8 complex catalyzes the polymerization of approximately 16 molecules of C9 to form a 160 Å × 100 Å tubule with a hydrophobic end that binds to lipids in the membrane. The poly-

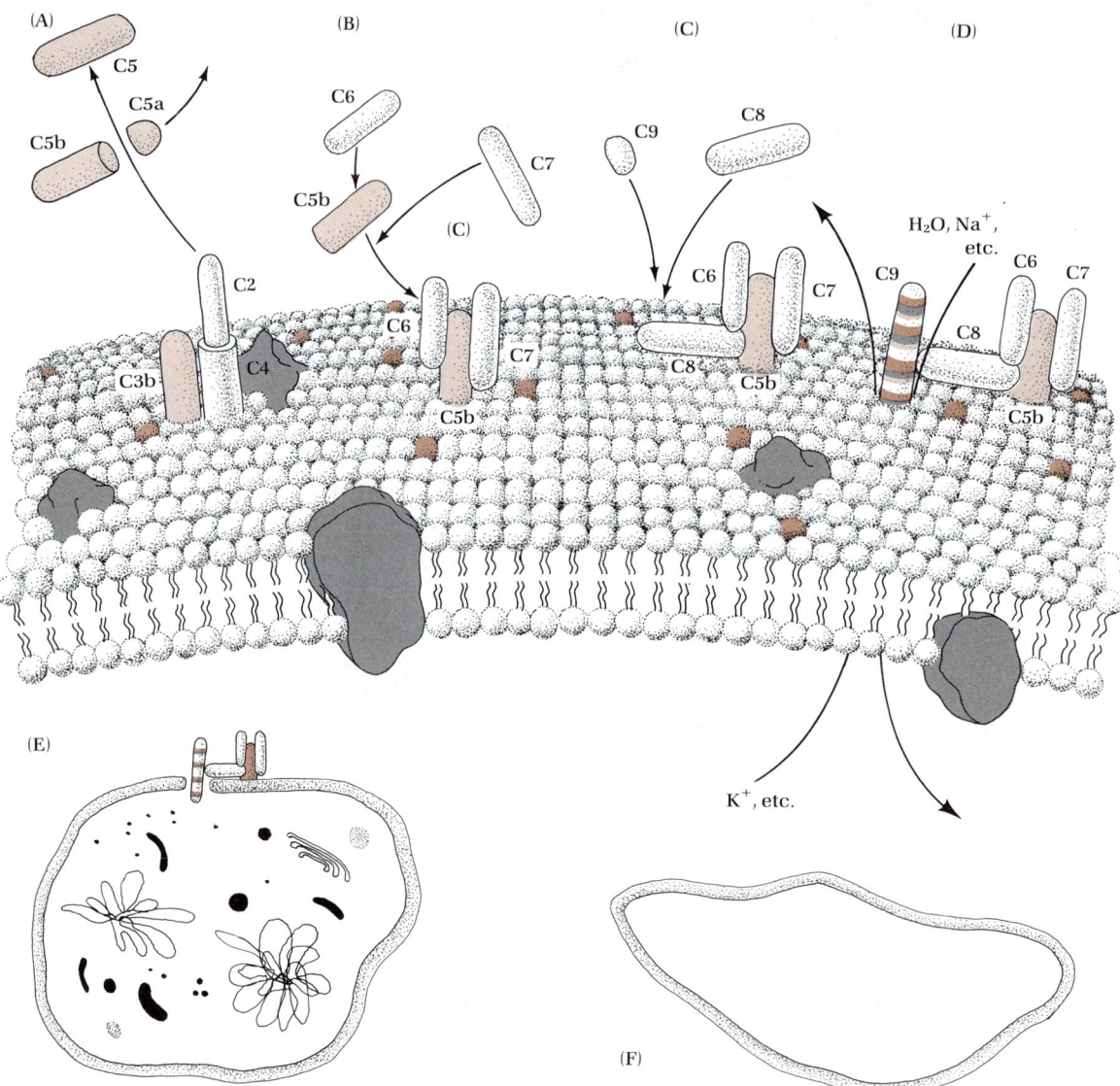

FIGURE 5   C4C3C3b COMPLEX AS C5 CONVERTASE

(A) The C4C2C3b complex cleaves C5 in serum to C5a and C5b. (B) C5b and C6 combine and form a complex on the cell surface. (C, D) C7, C8, and C9 are polymerized by the C5b-C8 complex, and the larger complex attaches to the membrane. (E, F) The polyC9 opens a transmembrane channel that allows potassium ions to leave the cell and water and sodium to enter. The cell swells, thereby allowing the intracellular contents to leave. Only an empty sac remains.

INFORMATION BOX 2

Complement Components

Component	MW	Concentration (µg/ml)	Component	MW	Concentration (µg/ml)
CLASSICAL PATHWAY			**ALTERNATE PATHWAY**		
C1q	410,000	180	B	93,000	200
C1r	170,000	50	Ba	30,000	
C1r (activated)	170,000		Bb	63,000	
C1s	85,000	100	D	25,000	1–5
C1s (activated)	85,000		P	184,000	25
C4	210,000	500	**COMMON PATHWAY**		
C4a	10,000				
C4b	200,000		C5	205,000	75
C2	115,000	30	C5a	11,000	
C2a	80,000		C5b	195,000	
C2b	35,000		C6	128,000	60
C3	195,000	1300	C7	121,000	55
C3a	9,000		C8	155,000	80
C3b	186,000		C9	75,000	200

merized C9 with the C5b,6,7,8 complex is called the MEMBRANE ATTACK COMPLEX (MAC). Manfred Mayer postulated a transmembrane channel that is active in lysis, and the MAC is probably the major component of this channel.

Figure 6 summarizes the classical, alternate, and common pathways.

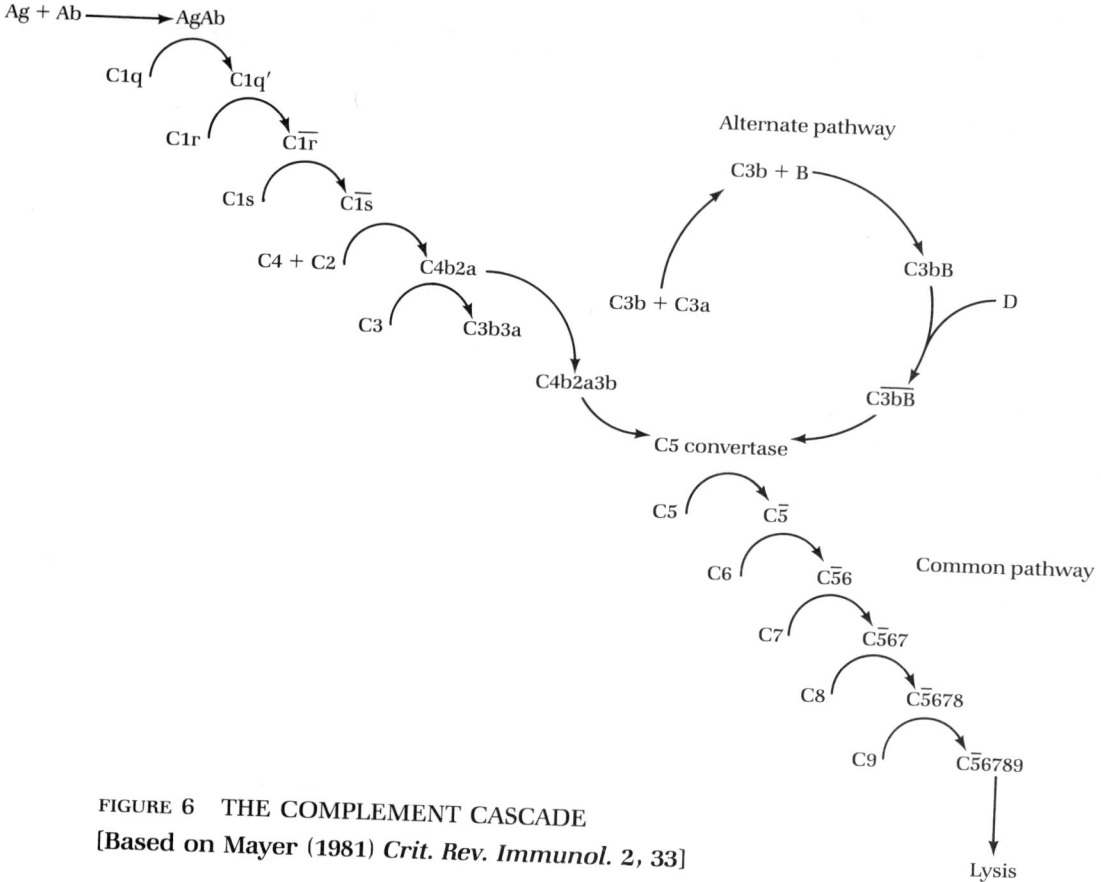

FIGURE 6   THE COMPLEMENT CASCADE
[Based on Mayer (1981) *Crit. Rev. Immunol.* 2, 33]

Summary

1. The complement system is a series of serum components that have the ability to combine with the AgAb complex. When the antigen is on the surface of a cell, reaction of the AgAb complex with the complement system results in lysis of the cell.
2. The complement components act as a cascade. The components react with each other, forming complexes that function as enzymes. These enzymes use the next component in the cascade pathway as substrate. There are three pathways: the classical pathway, the alternate pathway, and the central, or common, pathway. The classical and alter-

COMPLEMENT

nate pathways both form C5 convertase, which is the first component in the central pathway.

3. The classical pathway starts with a reaction in which C1 binds to the AgAb complex. C4 and C2 then bind to the activated C1, and this complex activates C3. The activated C4C2C3b complex is a C5 convertase.

4. The alternate pathway does not need AgAb complexes for initiation. C3 reacts with factor B or factor D to generate a C3bBb complex, which becomes stabilized by reacting with properdin (P). This results in a C3bPBb complex which is a C5 convertase.

5. The C5 convertase generated by either the classical or the alternate pathway leads to the activation of C5, which combines sequentially with C6 through C9. This complex is the membrane attack complex, which causes lysis of the cell.

Additional Readings

Mayer, M. M., D. W. Michaels, L. E. Ramm, M. B. Whitelow, J. B. Willoughby and M. L. Shin. 1981. CRC *Crit. Rev. Immunol.* 2:133.

Müller-Eberhard, H. J. 1983. Chemistry and function of the complement system. In F. J. Dixon and D. W. Fisher (eds.). *The Biology of Immunologic Disease*. Sinauer Associates, Sunderland, MA, p. 128.

Müller-Eberhard, H. J. and R. D. Schreiber. 1980. Molecular biology and chemistry of the alternate pathway of complement. *Adv. Immunol.* 29:1.

PART TWO
CELLULAR IMMUNOLOGY

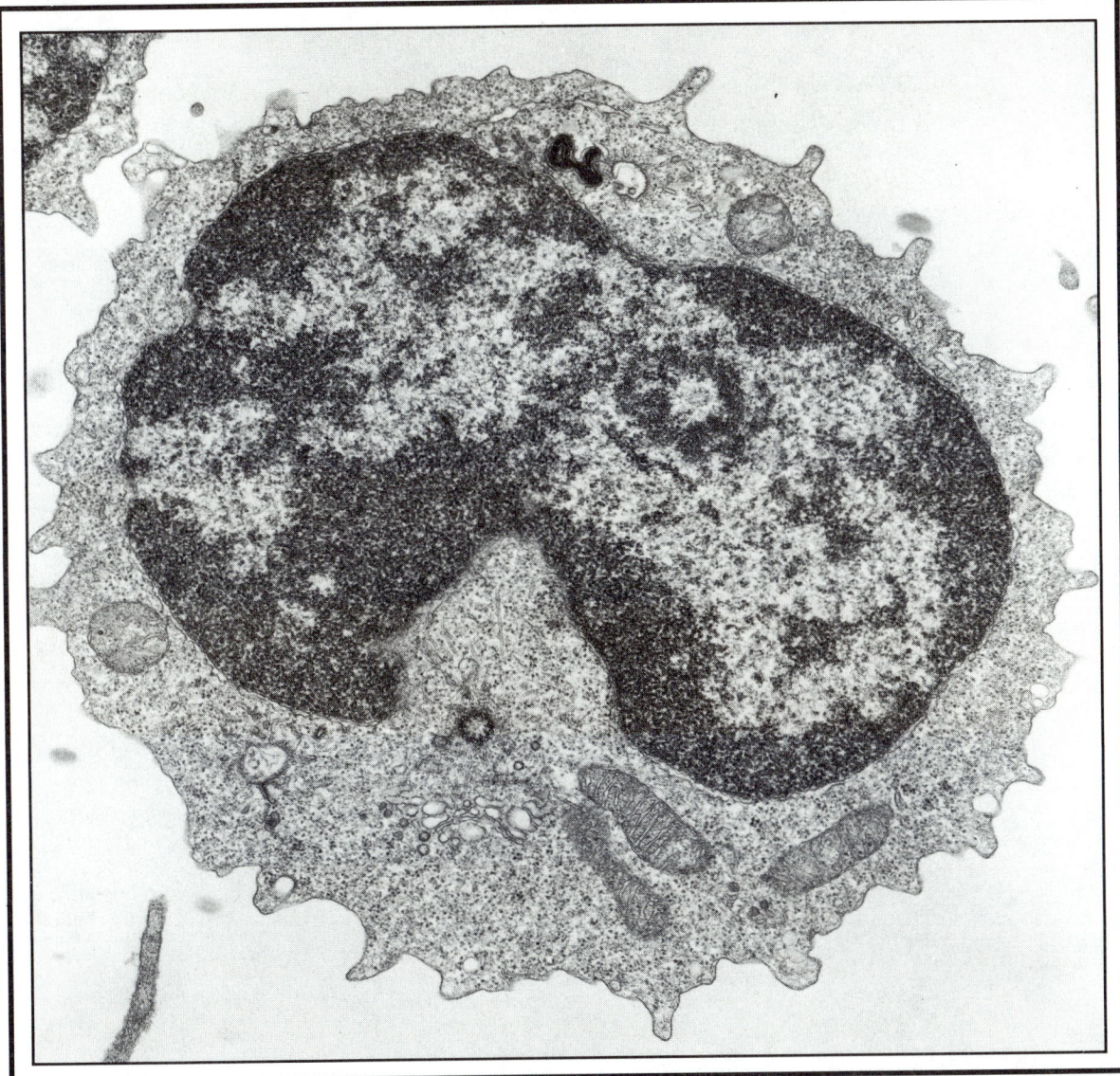

SECTION I
THE ORIGINS AND ORGANIZATION OF LYMPHOID TISSUE

> I must Create a System, or be enslav'd by another Man's.
> — WILLIAM BLAKE

The cells carrying out specific immune functions are in the blood system. In the four chapters of Section I we will examine the origin of these cells in the bone marrow; follow their differentiation in the bone marrow and thymus; describe their organization in the secondary lymphoid organs, the spleen and lymph nodes; and examine some of their surface properties.

The basic understanding of the properties of the immune system cells covered in this section is crucial to the understanding of the nature of cellular interactions in the immune response, which will be covered in Section II.

CHAPTER 10

HEMOPOIESIS

Overview The cells of the blood are constantly renewed during the life of an individual. The strategy that has evolved is one in which all of the blood cells are derived from a very small number of multipotent cells called stem cells. Differentiation can be viewed as a series of binary "decisions" that a cell must make. Each decision closes off a large series of differentiative options, thus limiting the number of options left to the cell's progeny. The first "decision" of the stem cell is really one of life or death, because its options are either self-renewal or commencement of differentiation into a terminal end cell. This chapter will discuss the nature of the decision process, the concept of determination, and the nature of commitment. The reader should keep in mind that the rules of hemopoietic differentiation are only now beginning to be worked out. Even though we are ultimately concerned with lymphocytes, we will often use evidence from erythrocyte and granulocyte differentiation to make the general points.

CHAPTER TEN

Hemopoiesis

The cells of the blood all have finite life spans and must be constantly renewed during the lifetime of the animal. When radiolabeled erythrocytes or granulocytes are injected into an animal, they disappear from the body. When the rate of disappearance is monitored, we see that the *proportion* of labeled cells gradually declines, but the *total* number of cells remains constant. This implies there is a state of homeostasis in which the rate of production of new cells is equal to the decline of old cells. The different mature cell types each have characteristic life spans. The half-life of red cells, for example, is months, whereas granulocytes have half-lives of hours. The process of blood cell formation, called HEMOPOIESIS, is a differentiation process that must occur throughout the life of the animal.[1] Red blood cells in humans are produced at the phenomenal rate of 2×10^6 cells per second.

Hemopoiesis is of interest to us not only because the blood-forming system is physiologically important, but also because it provides a very good system for studying some of the fundamental problems of differentiation. One of these problems concerns the ability of a cell to give rise to progeny, each of which is committed to differentiate into a different kind of cell. The fertilized egg is the ultimate example of this; but the blood-forming system is a good one in which to study cellular differentiation because blood cell formation occurs constantly in the adult animal.

The study of hemopoiesis has been facilitated by the fact that the blood-forming system is sensitive to X-irradiation. A mouse that has been subjected to lethal whole-body X-irradiation (approximately 800 r)[2] will die in about ten days because its blood-forming system has been destroyed. But irradiated animals can

---

[1] *Hemo* = blood, *poiein* = to make. It is interesting that the word *poiesis* is also the root of the word poetry. To the Greeks, the poet was the maker of words. This common root may strike the reader's fancy in a later section, when we discuss Niels Jerne's notion of the generative grammar of the immune system. I thank Professor Constance Jordan for, among other things, pointing out the common origins to me.

[2] The term r is rad, a unit of radiation; the unit of absorbed dose equal to 0.01 joule/kg in any medium.

HEMOPOIESIS

be rescued with an injection of bone marrow cells (that is, by performing a bone marrow transplant), because the procedure leads to a repopulation of the entire blood-forming system. Repopulated animals have normal numbers of all of the differentiated cells of the blood within a few days.

We have observed that injection of bone marrow cells results in the production of all of the mature cells of the blood. How does this come about? We can imagine two possibilities. Either the bone marrow contains *separate* cell types able to differentiate into each of the various mature blood cell types, or there is in bone marrow a *single* cell type that has the ability to give rise to all of the differential blood cells. This latter type of cell, one that can give rise to more than one type of cell, is called a STEM CELL. In fact, we now know that the irradiated mice are repopulated with the progeny of a multipotent hemopoietic stem cell.

Assay of Colony Forming Units

An assay that allowed the problem of the origin of the cells of the blood to be studied experimentally was devised by Till and McCulloch in Toronto. In this assay (Figure 1) mice are lethally irradiated and repopulated by intravenous injection of a small

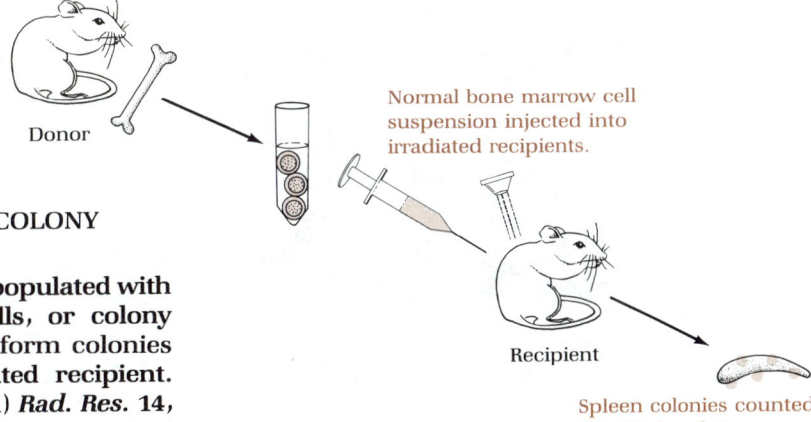

FIGURE 1 ASSAY FOR SPLEEN COLONY FORMING UNITS

Lethally irradiated mice are repopulated with bone marrow cells. Stem cells, or colony forming units-spleen (CFU-S), form colonies on the spleen of the irradiated recipient. [After Till and McCulloch (1961) *Rad. Res.* 14, 213]

CHAPTER TEN

number of bone marrow cells (ca. 10^5). When the spleens of these irradiated recipients are examined ten days later, discrete colonies can be seen on the spleen surface (Figure 2). The bone marrow cells that give rise to these colonies are called COLONY FORMING UNITS, or CFU. These are called colony forming units-spleen or CFU-S, to distinguish them from in vitro colonies, which will be discussed later.

One of the major problems in studying the nature of the CFU-S is their extremely low frequency. In the mouse bone marrow, for example, the frequency of the CFU-S is approximately 10^{-4} or one CFU-S per 10,000 bone marrow cells. The rarity of this cell makes direct study impossible, so experiments designed to determine whether the colony forming cell is a stem cell must be indirect.

Single-Cell Origin of Colonies

The number of spleen colonies is linearly related to the number of injected bone marrow cells (Figure 3). This is consistent with

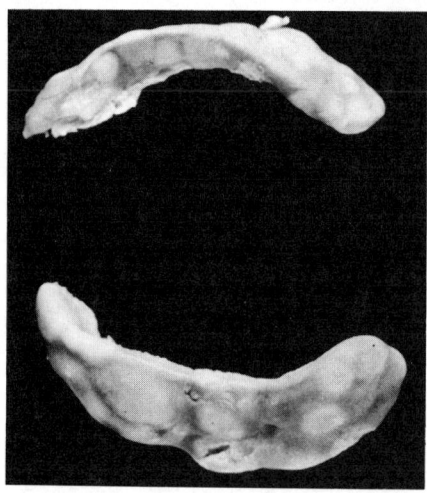
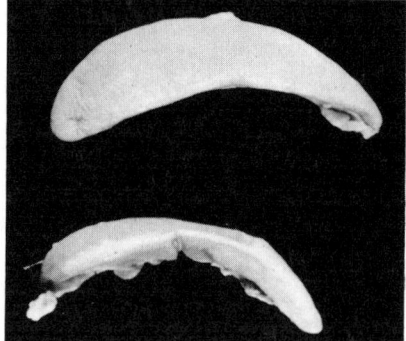

FIGURE 2 SPLEEN COLONIES IN THE CFU-S ASSAY

Left two spleens are from mice that received bone marrow and show colonies. Right two are from uninjected controls. Note the spontaneous colony on the upper control spleen.

HEMOPOIESIS

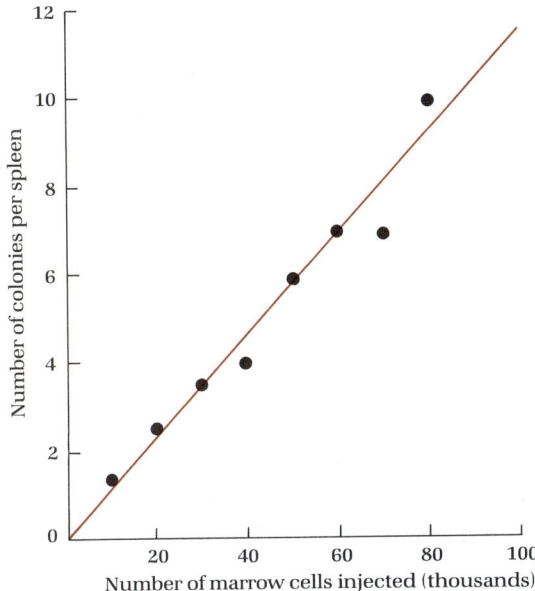

FIGURE 3 SPLEEN COLONIES FROM INJECTED CELLS

The relationship between the number of cells injected and the number of colonies. [After Till and McCulloch (1961) *Rad. Res.* **14**, 213]

the interpretation that the colony arises from a single cell. This conclusion is strengthened by experiments using chromosome markers. The CBA/T6 mouse carries a naturally occurring karyotypic alteration (an altered chromosome structure). When CBA/T6 bone marrow cells are injected into irradiated normal CBA mice (which do not have the altered karyotype and are designated +/+), over 90% of the cells in each colony examined contain the marker. This result strongly suggests that the cells in a colony are derived from the T6 cells. In another experiment, various ratios of marked and unmarked cells are injected. When this is done, it is found that the proportion of colonies with marked cells varies with the proportion of injected marked cells.

Multipotency of the CFU-S

Cytological examination of the spleen colonies shows that they are composed of several types of blood cells (erythrocytes, granulocytes, monocytes, and megakaryocytes). The fact that the colony is derived from a single cell and is composed of several cell types is the basis for the argument that a single cell type gives rise to different kinds of blood cells. In other words, the CFU-S is a *multipotent hemopoietic stem cell*. However, the direct test of this assertion is a difficult task.

The multipotency of the CFU-S has been tested in several ways but the most convincing of the experiments uses *unique* and rare chromosome markers. The T6 marker discussed above is carried by every cell in the CBA/T6 mouse, so the colonies in the experiments showing 90% marker-bearing cells could conceivably have been formed by more than one marked cell. The use of unique markers would allow this problem to be overcome. Unique markers can be introduced at random in the cells of a mouse by subjecting the animal to low levels of X-irradiation. This procedure causes breaks in chromosomes in some cells, resulting in rare and unique chromosome alterations. Most of these alterations are probably lethal to the cell, but an occasional cell will have a unique chromosome pattern and still retain normal function. If such a rare marker were to occur in a stem cell, then all of its progeny would have the same marker, and any cell in the colony that contained the marker almost certainly would be descended from the original marked cell. Therefore, the ideal test of the proposition that there is a multipotent hemopoietic stem cell would be to examine the cells in a colony to determine whether the cell types that are differentiating into erythroid and granuloid cells have the same characteristic chromosome marker.

The experiment (Figure 4), while easy to conceive, is very difficult to carry out for technical reasons. First of all, the number of marked cells is so low that they must first be enriched by growing them in a mutant mouse that is incapable of generating its own CFU-S. This mouse, the W/W^v mutant, serves as a biological test tube in which the numbers of marked cells can increase in the absence of normal stem cells.[3] Bone marrow cells from the irradiated mice are therefore grown in W/W^v mice for two months; during that time the number of marked cells increases.

---

[3] The mice must be repopulated with very low numbers of cells because the frequency of marked cells must be kept low. This means that irradiated recipients cannot be used because they would die before the small number of injected cells could effect a repopulation.

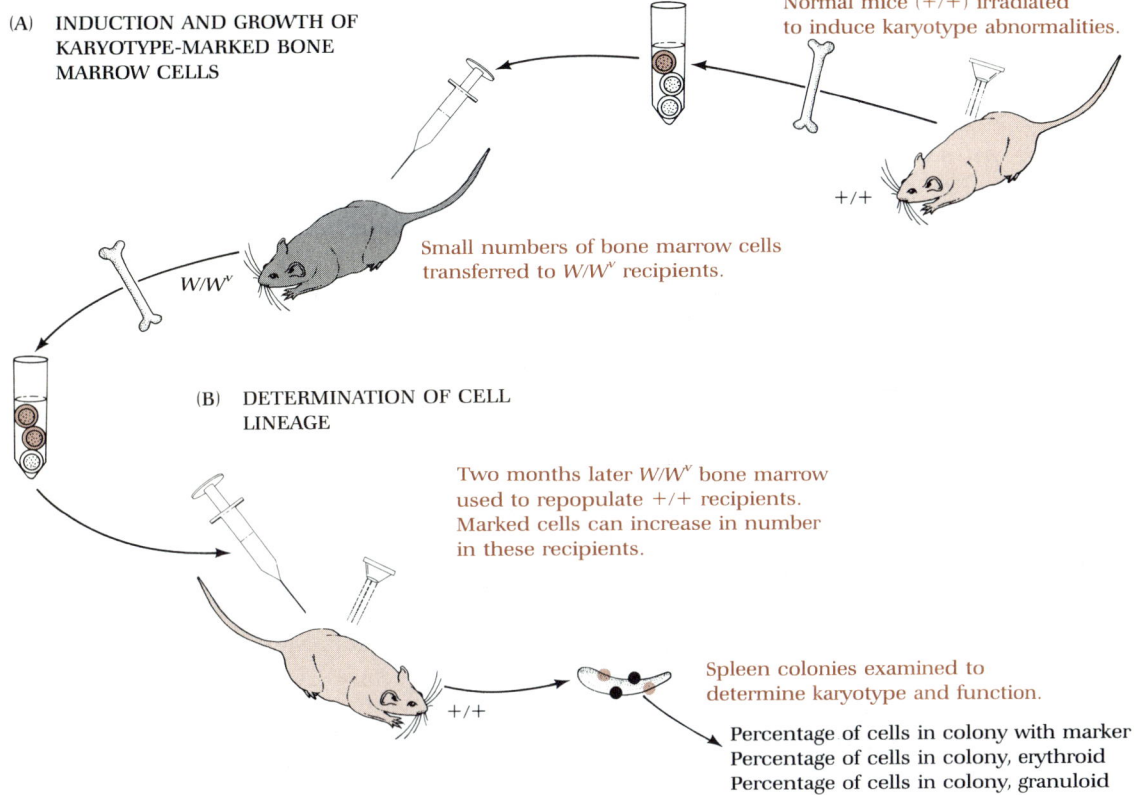

FIGURE 4 DETERMINATION OF ORIGIN OF DIFFERENTIATING CELLS

(A) Karyotypic markers are induced in normal bone marrow with X-rays. Bone marrow cells are expanded in W/W^v mice, and their bone marrow is used to repopulate +/+ mice. (B) Marked bone marrow is injected into +/+ mice; some cells from each colony are examined to determine whether the colony arose from a marked bone marrow cell (karyotype analysis). Cells from colonies with marked cells are tested for erythroid lineage (Fe incorporation) or granuloid lineage (presence of acid phosphatase). Because karyotype and function analyses cannot be carried out on the same cell, percentages of each are recorded from cells in the same colony. Typical results are shown in Table 1.

The W/W^v that can be shown to have been repopulated with marked cells are now used as a source of bone marrow cells for the experiment. They are injected into irradiated +/+ mice, and the spleen colonies of the recipients are examined ten days later. If the CFU-S is in fact a multipotent stem cell that can give rise to both erythroid and granuloid cells, then the cells differentiating into each of these types should have the marker. But now the second technical difficulty arises. It is not possible to do both a karyotype analysis to determine the presence of the marker and a histochemical analysis to determine cell function (erythroid or granuloid) on the *same* cell. Therefore, many cells in the colony must be examined and the conclusion drawn from a statistical analysis of the data.

Typical data from this experiment are shown in Table 1. Because the same cell cannot be examined for both marker and function, the first information needed is the percentage of cells that do *not* have the marker. It is possible that two cells, one marked and one unmarked, could have lodged in the same place in the spleen and produced a colony that is actually composed of cells derived from both of them. The value in column 1 of Table 1 tells us the maximum percentage of cells in the colony which could not have come from the marked cell. Columns 2 and 3 of Table 1 give the percentage of cells in each colony that are differentiating along erythroid and granuloid lines. Now, if the percentage of cells differentiating along both lines is higher than the percentage of cells without the marker, it must mean that at least some of the marked cells had to give rise to *both* erythrocytes

TABLE 1 Characteristics of spleen colonies examined in an experiment to determine the lineage of differentiating cells.

Colony	Percentage of cells without markers	Percentage of PMN	Percentage of RBC
I	10	52	32
II	1	14	28
III	0	12	16
IV	2	12	12
V	0	20	16

Source: After Wu et al. (1976), *J. Cell Physiol.* 69: 177.

HEMOPOIESIS

and granulocytes. Examination of the data in Table 1 shows that this is the result obtained. This experiment therefore shows that, because some of the cells in the colony came from a common cell, the CFU-S is in fact a multipotent stem cell.

Characteristics of the Hemopoietic Stem Cell

We will see that the cells derived from the stem cell are very sensitive to regulatory signals. The stem cells themselves, however, appear to be remarkably independent of these regulatory influences. The stem cell is a relatively quiescent cell with a very low rate of proliferation. This fact can be shown with "tritium suicide" experiments. In these experiments tritiated thymidine of extremely high specific activity is added to cultures of cells. The proliferating cells incorporate the highly labeled precursor into their DNA, and the radioactive disintegrations damage the DNA and prevent further replication of the cell. This procedure only works if the cell is synthesizing DNA and therefore using the labeled precursor. Suicide experiments have no effect on the stem cell, which shows that the cell is not an actively dividing cell. It replicates only often enough to maintain the normal physiological number (10^{-4}) of cells.[4]

Cells at different stages of differentiation express unique molecules on their surface. Antibodies raised against these molecules serve as very useful markers to identify cell types. The only known surface marker for the stem cell is an antigen shared with brain cells; but even though this fact has been known for a decade, it has not been possible to unequivocally use this antibody to isolate the stem cell. Some long-term bone marrow cultures allow the stem cell to be grown in vitro, but other cells are needed in these cultures. So far the stem cell cannot be maintained free of these other cells in culture. In short, this most interesting cell in the blood-forming system is still shrouded in mystery and offers an opportunity for a young investigator to make his or her reputation.

[4] The stem cells obtained from fetal liver, in contrast, are killed in the tritium suicide experiment and are thus actively proliferating cells.

CHAPTER TEN

Commitment and Differentiation

The stem cell carries out two functions, *self-renewal* and *differentiation*. Normal homeostatic levels of mature blood cells are maintained by regulation of both the number of stem cells and the rate at which they give rise to progeny (which differentiate into the various cell types of the blood). This regulation involves an obviously complex and delicate signal and feedback mechanism of which, except for the red blood cell, we know very little.

At some point, the stem cells become ready to initiate the events of differentiation into more mature cells. This act is called DETERMINATION. How a cell is determined to follow certain lineages and not others is one of the central questions in biology. Once a determined cell actually starts the changes down the lineage pathway leading to a terminally differentiated cell, it is called a COMMITTED CELL. The pathways of differentiation in the blood are shown in Figure 5.

Cellular differentiation can be considered as a process of *choices* by the cell.[5] It can be readily seen in Figure 5 that a cell can reach a certain point in its differentiation and still have several potential lineages to follow. By making a choice at such a branch point, the cell effectively closes off other potential lineages. Almost nothing is known about the decision making process; it is widely (but not universally) agreed that it is stochastic or random. But it is clear that in cellular differentiation, as in choosing a career or a lover, decisions made early in the process must be lived with for a long time. The cell's future is determined by its past.[6]

---

[5] The psychologist Steve Chorover has pointed out to me that by using the terms *choice* and *decision* we seem to be attributing to the cell a level of consciousness. This is, of course, not the intent. The words are used by differentiation biologists as a means of graphically describing the biochemical and molecular events that occur at a certain time.

[6] We should point out here that there is another problem in differentiation, called morphogenesis. MORPHOGENESIS is the establishment of form and pattern, as in an embryo or a limb bud. In this process it seems quite certain that positional effects (i.e., the cell's location) are important. These two problems—cellular differentiation and morphogenesis—are usually treated as separate phenomena, but they may be variations on the same theme of lineage establishment.

HEMOPOIESIS

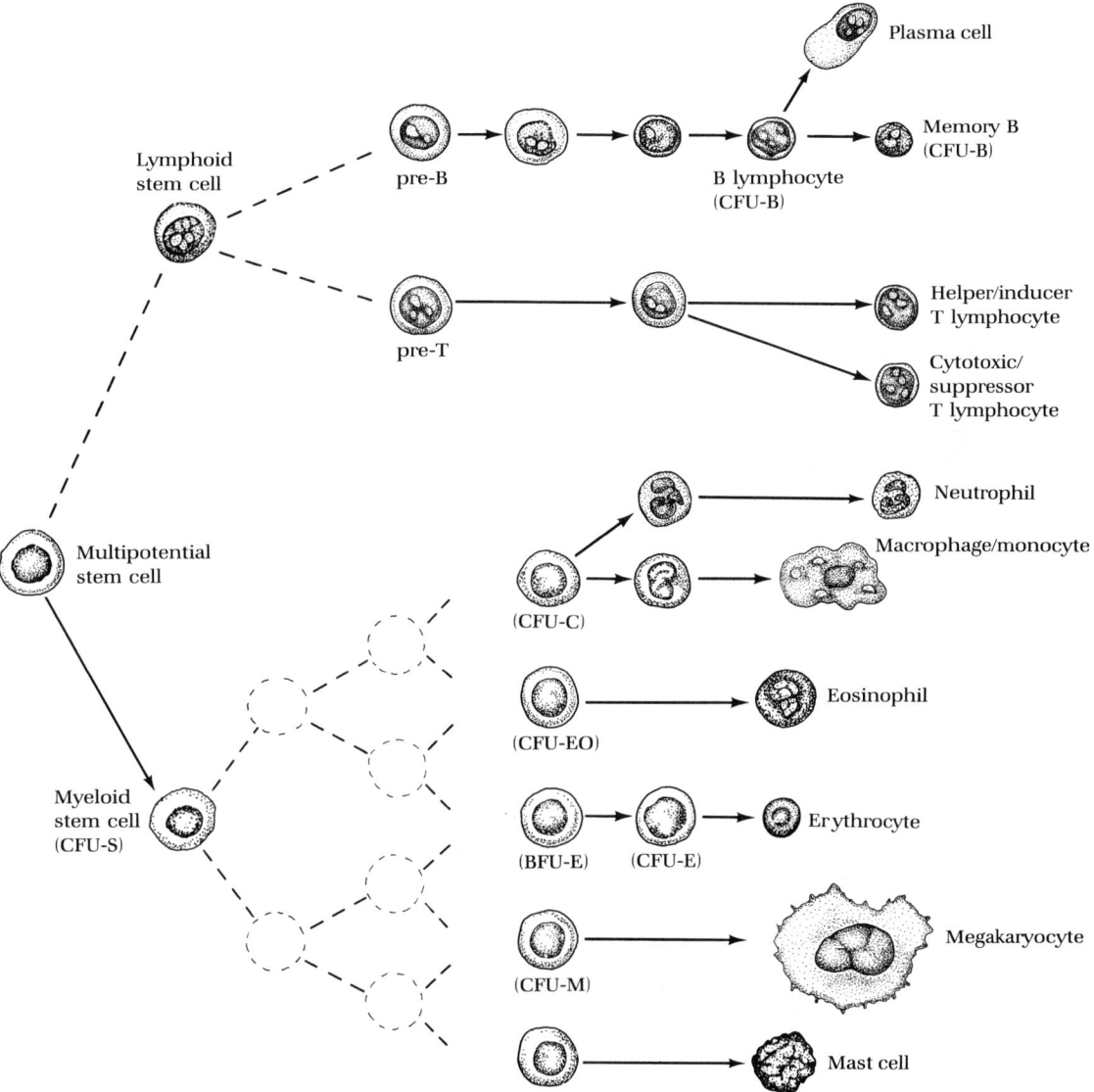

FIGURE 5   HEMOPOIETIC LINEAGES

The path of lineage establishment of the hemopoietic system starts with the multipotent stem cell. The first lineages that are established are lymphoid and myeloid. In this version, differentiation is seen as a string of "branch point decisions." The dotted outlines indicate proliferation and decision events which are not able to be studied.

CHAPTER TEN

Differentiation of Stem Cells into Progenitor Cells

The earliest committed hemopoietic cells are called PROGENITOR CELLS. The frequency of these cells, which are now in an established cell lineage, is about tenfold higher than that of stem cells (i.e., 10^{-3}). Progenitor cells are assayed in vitro in soft agar. These assays take advantage of the dependence of the progenitor cells on certain growth factors (discussed below). Cytological examination of the colonies formed in agar in the presence of a given growth factor shows that they contain cells that are differentiating along one or a limited number of pathways. It is important to realize that these growth factors probably do not cause the cell to become determined; rather they induce a determined cell to undergo the changes of the differentiative pathway—that is, to become committed.

We assume that the process of becoming determined must result in the expression of receptors for the inducing molecule. Reaction of the inducing factor with the receptor then results in the commitment and initiation of the differentiation process. The strategy of producing many cells from the stem cell requires that a small number of cells carry the potential to become a large number of cells of many different types; so along with differentiation, there must also be proliferation.

TABLE 2 Effect of growth factors on progenitor cells in vitro.

Growth factor	Response	Eryth.	Gran.	Mono.	Eosin.	Megakar.
GM-CSF	Proliferation	+	+	+	+	−
	Differentiation	−	+	+	+	−
G-CSF	Proliferation	+	+	+	+	?
	Differentiation	−	+	−	−	?
M-CSF	Proliferation	−	−	+	−	−
	Differentiation	−	−	+	−	—
IL-3	Proliferation	+	+	+	+	+
	Differentiation	+	+	+	+	—

Source: After Dexter (1984), *Nature* 309: 746. See also Walker et al. (1985), *Cell* 43: 269.

HEMOPOIESIS

Hemopoietic Inducing Factors

One of the most active areas of research involves the study of the factors that induce cells to differentiate and proliferate, since both normal function and cancerous growth are controlled by these factors. Table 2 lists a few of the known inducing factors in hemopoiesis. Most of the factors listed induce proliferation in many types of cells but induce differentiation in only a limited or specific subset of cells. The picture will become more complicated as these studies progress because in some differentiating systems there is an inverse correlation between proliferation and differentiation, whereas in others (granulocyte formation, for example) the two are directly correlated. Identification of physiologically significant inducing and proliferation factors is very difficult because many molecules, some of which cannot possibly be used in normal physiological conditions, are able to induce both proliferation and differentiation. Some of the properties of the "physiological" inducers are discussed in Information Box 1.[7]

The mechanisms by which the various inducing molecules affect the cells are unknown, but an in vitro experiment has shown that the progenitor is sensitive to the *concentration* of one of the inducing molecules, GM-CSF (see Information Box 1). As seen in Figure 6, which summarizes an experiment done by Metcalf, bone marrow cells were cultured on soft agar in the presence of high (2500 units) or low (50 units) concentrations of GM-CSF. After seven days, it was found that the low dose yielded almost exclusively monocyte colonies. In contrast, the high dose gave both granulocyte and monocyte colonies. To determine whether a single progenitor cell is sensitive to concentration or whether there are cells of two sensitivities in the progenitor cell population, the bone marrow cells were cultured in the presence of a high concentration of GM-CSF for 24 hours, after which the plates were examined and colonies containing two cells were identified and removed. The two daughter cells were placed in separate containers, one with a high and one with a low concentration of GM-CSF. Figure 6 shows that the daughter cells grown

---

[7] In my own research papers I have called these nonphysiological inducers "surrogate inducers," in contrast to "physiological inducers." How to distinguish them is the problem.

INFORMATION BOX 1

Myeloid Inducing Factors

ERYTHROPOIETIN

Erythropoietin is an inducer of erythroid differentiation. When bone marrow cells are cultured in vitro with erythropoietin, the colonies that form contain only cells of the erythroid series. In this case each colony is derived from a single progenitor cell, which is termed a BFU-E (burst-forming unit, erythroid). Erythropoietin is a glycoprotein of molecular weight 46,000 and is produced by the kidney. The production of erythropoietin is sensitive to the concentration of red blood cells in the circulation; a fall or rise in their numbers results in a compensating rise or fall in erythropoietin. (The concentration of oxygen is probably what is being sensed.)

Erythropoietin acts on erythrocyte progenitor cells in vitro at low concentration to stimulate the production of colonies of about 50 cells each in two days. These progenitor cells are called colony-forming unit, erythrocyte (CFU-E). At high concentrations, erythropoietin stimulates cells to produce colonies containing 5,000 cells in ten days. These progenitor cells are called BFU-E. BFU-E are cells at an earlier stage of differentiation along the erythrocyte pathway than are CFU-E (see Figure 5).

The gene for erythropoietin has recently been cloned.

COLONY STIMULATING FACTOR

Cells grown in the presence of factors called CSF, or COLONY STIMULATING FACTOR, give rise to colonies composed of cells differentiating along the myeloid (granulocyte–monocyte) line. (Goldwasser has coined the term MYELOPOIETIN for these molecules.) Three CSFs have been identified and studied extensively. The first of these, called GM-CSF induces progenitor cells to differentiate into both granulocytes and monocytes. GM-CSF has been purified to homogeneity, and the gene encoding it has been cloned. It is a glycoprotein of molecular weight 23,000 and is synthesized in small quantities in all tissues except in the lung, where it is synthesized in large quantity.

A factor called G-CSF induces progenitors only toward granulocytic differentiation. It is a protein of molecular weight 24,000. A glycoprotein called M-CSF, consisting of two chains, each with a molecular weight of 35,000, has also been identified. This molecule drives the cells along the monocyte lines. At the moment it is not known whether these three factors work at different points in the differentiative process.

INTERLEUKIN-3

Interleukin-3 (IL-3) is a glycoprotein of molecular weight 28,000 and stimulates in vitro growth of a wide variety of hemopoietic cells. Because of this it has been termed a "multi-specific" colony stimulating factor (a term that is scientific Newspeak for nonspecific). IL-3 has been shown to be identical to two other factors that stimulate the proliferation of stem cells (P-stimulating factor and stem cell-activating factor). The exact physiological role of IL-3 remains to be clarified, but it may act in concert with the specific inducing agents, perhaps to increase the proliferation rate of the differentiating cells.

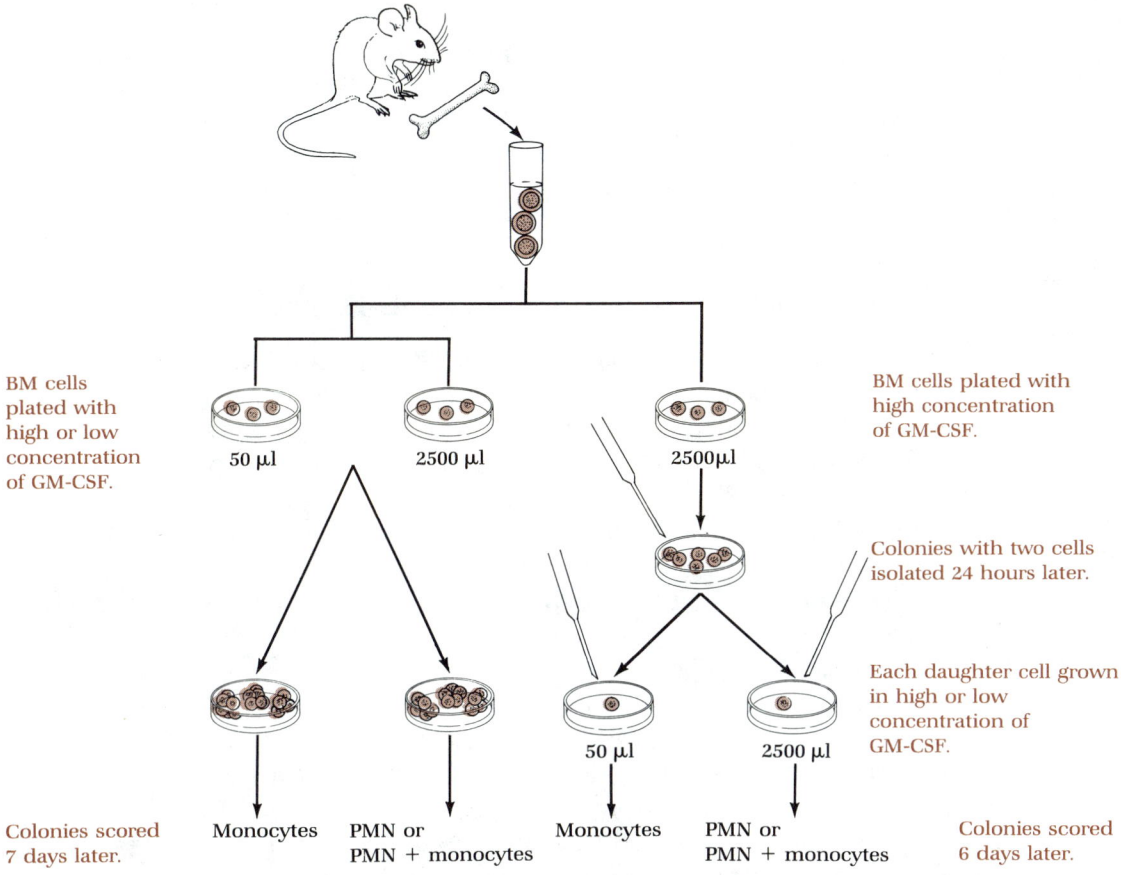

FIGURE 6 EFFECTS OF CONCENTRATION OF INDUCING FACTOR ON DIFFERENTIATION OF BONE MARROW

Bone marrow (BM) cells are plated with either high or low concentrations of GM-CSF. On the left, bone marrow populations are used. On the right, individual colonies are examined. Low concentrations of GM-CSF result in monocytes and high levels in granulocytes (PMN). [After Metcalf (1980) *Proc. Natl. Acad. Sci. USA* **77**, 5327]

in low concentrations gave rise to monocytes, and those grown in high concentrations gave rise to either mixed colonies of granulocytes and monocytes or to pure granulocyte colonies. This experiment indicates that the granulocyte–monocyte progenitor is indeed bipotential and that the choice of which differentiative pathway it will choose is a function of the concentration of the inducing agent.

CHAPTER TEN

We now know that all of the agents can act on small numbers of cells at very low concentrations (10^{-11} to $10^{-12}\,M$). The availability of inducible tumor lines (see below) at the moment offers one of the best means of studying their action.

Hemopoietic Inducing Microenvironments

Differentiation of myeloid cells such as erythrocytes and granulocytes from committed progenitors to mature end cells occurs primarily in the spleen and bone marrow. Because factors are needed to move the cells along the pathway of differentiation, we assume that these factors are found selectively in the sites of differentiation. With the exception of the thymus, as we will see in the next chapter, it has been very difficult to analyze the nature of the *hemopoietic inducing microenvironments*, or HIM. The bone marrow produces more active granulocytes than erythrocytes, whereas the spleen gives rise to more erythrocytes than granulocytes. In 1968 Wolf and Trentin grafted some bone marrow tissue into a discrete area of the spleen and found that the ratio of differentiating cell types was dependent upon the environment. The tissues could be shown to have the same number of progenitors but the environment allowed (or, perhaps more correctly, induced) the differentiation of one cell type.

Very recently the microenvironments supporting myeloid differentiation and those supporting lymphoid differentiation have been cultured in vitro. As a result of this advance it may be possible to determine the cells responsible and the nature of the regulation they exert upon the progenitor cells. Of course, we still have the problem of the small number of stem cells and progenitors, and until someone devises a method for growing these cells in pure cultures we must use indirect methods—mutant mice that have defects in their differentiation, or cloned tumor lines that mimic normal cells in some ways.

Mutant Mice and Cloned Tumor Lines

The low numbers of progenitor cells in the population of bone marrow cells makes their study almost as difficult as that of the

HEMOPOIESIS

stem cell. However, the use of mutant mice and cloned tumor cells are proving to be useful tools.

Mutant mice (Information Box 2) and certain disease states in humans have deficiencies in one or more of the progenitor cell types. By studying these blocks in differentiation, we can learn something about the normal process. The power of this type of analysis, using "experiments of nature," will be discussed later, in the section on human immunodeficiency diseases. The final proof of our understanding of the process of hemopoiesis will be our ability to cure the deficient state.

Work on the whole organism presents problems which in vitro studies do not have, and for the short term we will probably learn more about cellular differentiation by studying tumor cells in vitro. Many cultured tumor cells have been "trapped" at a certain state of differentiation but can still be induced to continue their differentiative pathway. Because tumor cells are able to grow clonally in the test tube, studies of homogeneous populations of cells is possible. However, experimenters must be aware of the possibility of merely exchanging artifacts because they are studying a regulatory process in a cell that, because it is a tumor, by definition has lost a significant part of its regulatory ability. Even with this caveat, however, to date a great deal has been learned about normal cell processes by studying cloned tumor cells.

Introduction of New Genes into Stem Cells

Because all the cells of the blood are derived from the multipotent stem cell, clinicians have long had the goal of treating inherited blood cell disorders in humans by introducing DNA into stem cells. Sickle cell anemia, for example, is a genetic disease caused by the substitution of a single incorrect amino acid in hemoglobin. If the gene for the nonsickle trait could be introduced into the stem cells of a person with the sickle cell trait, the introduced gene would be replicated during the self-renewal process of the stem cell and would be passed along to the progenitor cells during differentiation. This process would result in the production of normal terminally differentiated cells and the eventual

INFORMATION BOX 2

Some Mouse Mutants of Hemopoietic Development

Mutation	Chromosomal location	Phenotype
HEMOPOIETIC SYSTEM		
W series (*W*)	5	Anemia due to intrinsic hemopoietic stem cell defect
		Pleiotropic effect on germ and pigment cells
Steel series (*Sl*)	10	Anemia due to defect in hemopoietic microenvironment
		Pleiotropic effect on germ and pigment cells
Hertwig's anemia (*an*)	4	Anemia due to intrinsic hemopoietic stem cell defect
		Germ cell defect
ERYTHROID DEVELOPMENT		
Flexed-tail (*f*)	13	Hypochromic, microcytic anemia
Diminutive (*dm*)	2	Macrocytic anemia
Tail-short (*Ts*)	11	Prenatal anemia due to deficiency of blood islands in yolk sac
Sex-linked anemia (*sla*)	X	Hypochromic animals due to deficient intestinal iron transport
Jaundiced (*ja*)	—	Microcytic anemia
Hemolytic anemia (*ha*)	—	Neonatal hypochromic anemia, microcytosis; sterile

reduction of the sickle cell trait *in that individual*. The offspring, of course, would not be affected because the gene was not introduced into the germ line (the sperm and egg). The great advances in molecular genetics in the past few years have made gene transfer therapy a real possibility in the near future. One such TRANSFECTION EXPERIMENT in mice shows that the method is rapidly

INFORMATION BOX 2

Mutation	Chromosomal location	Phenotype
Spehocytosis (*sph*)	—	Hemolytic anemia
Microcytic anemia (*mk*)	15	Microcytic anemia due to defect in iron uptake from intestinal lumen to mucosa and plasma to erythroblasts
GRANULOCYTE DEVELOPMENT		
Beige (*bg*)	13	PMN granule defect; resembles Chediak-Higashi disease
Edematous (*oed*)	—	Increased granulocyte number
MACROPHAGE DEVELOPMENT		
Hepatitis virus susceptibility (*Hv*)	—	Resistance or susceptibility to hepatitis virus, associated with macrophage function
Myxovirus resistance (*mv*)	—	Resistance to infection with myxovirus, associated with macrophages
Tolerance to HGG (*Tol-1*)	—	Ease of immune tolerance induction, associated with macrophages
PLATELET DEVELOPMENT		
Beige (*bg*)	13	Serotonin granule defect
LYMPHOCYTE DEVELOPMENT		
Lipopolysaccharide response (*Lps*)	—	B cell defect in mitogen response to lipopolysaccharide
X-linked immunodeficiency (*xid*)	—	B cell response defect

approaching the point where we may soon be able to adapt it to some human conditions.

The principle of transfection experiments (Figure 7) is to introduce new genetic material into the genome of the mouse hemopoietic stem cell. The new genetic material in this case is a genome derived from Moloney sarcoma virus (MSV), which has

176
CHAPTER TEN

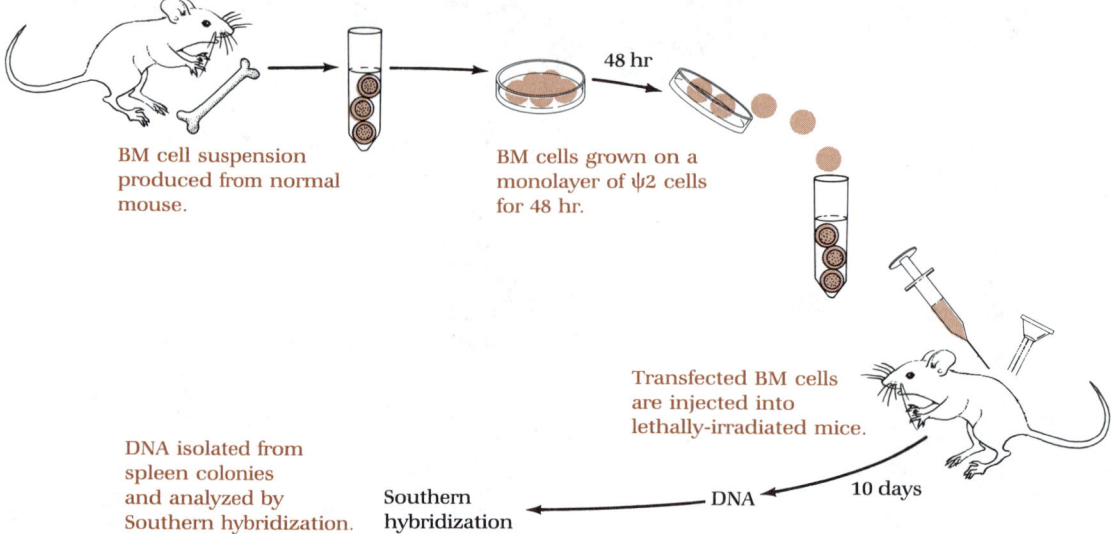

FIGURE 7 TRANSFER OF GENETIC MATERIAL INTO STEM CELLS

Moloney sarcoma virus (MSV) with dihydrofolate reductase (DHFR) and drug resistance genes is used to infect cells, which then serve as a monolayer for bone marrow cells. MSV genome is transfected into some bone marrow cells. The transfected cells are resistant to neomycin and are selected during growth in neomycin (not shown). The transfected cells are injected into lethally irradiated mice. DNA from spleen colonies is isolated and examined for DHFR gene by Southern blotting. [After Williams et al. (1984) *Nature* 310, 476]

been engineered to contain a segment of mouse cDNA encoding dihydrofolate reductase (DHFR) as well as a DNA segment that encodes resistance to the drug neomycin. These genes have no therapeutic value to the mouse. DHFR is a convenient gene to monitor, and the neomycin resistance gene is used in the selection process. Cells infected with this virus are grown as a monolayer, and normal mouse bone marrow cells are incubated on the monolayer for 48 hours. During this time virus infects the bone marrow cells and presumably integrates into the genome.

HEMOPOIESIS

The bone marrow cells are then removed from the monolayer and injected into irradiated recipient mice. After ten days the spleens of these mice are removed, and DNA is prepared from the spleen cells to determine whether the new gene is present. This DNA is treated with restriction enzymes which cleave it. The presence of the new genetic material in the mouse genome is then determined by Southern hybridization.

To show that the new gene was being carried by the stem cell population, investigators isolated colonies from the spleens of the mice inoculated with the transfected bone marrow cells and injected these colonies into another set of irradiated mice. The spleens of the second set of mice were examined for the presence of the new genetic material; it was present in two of the three recipients, a result indicating the new DNA had become associated with the stem cells and was present not only in the differentiating cells but also in the stem cell.

Had the recipient mouse had a genetic blood disease, and had the gene that was transfected been one with therapeutic value, the blood disease of the mouse would have been cured. But this process requires that the genes coding for normal traits be isolated and cloned. Research of this kind is going on at a very rapid rate, so there is good reason to believe that the power of the method can be applied to disease states in a short time.[8]

---

[8] Introducing genes into the germ line allows those genes to be passed on from generation to generation. This is now being done in mice. Mice that have had a new gene introduced into their germ line are called "transgenic mice." The reader should be aware of the fact that there are serious moral and ethical considerations involved with gene transfers. As biologists we must be cognizant of the fact that the gene pool of a species, including humans, can be altered, and we must not enter lightly into this new era of biotechnology. On the other hand, we must be aware that the era is here and that great potential value to humans can be derived by the rational use of the technology.

CHAPTER TEN

Summary

1. Hemopoiesis is the study of blood cell formation. All the cells of the blood are constantly being renewed in the adult animal and are derived from a multipotent hemopoietic stem cell.
2. Stem cells are assayed by an in vivo colony-forming assay and are called CFU-S (colony-forming units, spleen). Each colony is derived from a single cell.
3. Spleen colonies contain several kinds of blood cells. Because each colony is derived from a single cell but contains different kinds of cells, we conclude that a single cell can give rise to several cell types.
4. The process during which the stem cell establishes the lineage that it will follow during differentiation is called determination. Once a cell begins to differentiate along a pathway, it is called a committed cell. The earliest committed cells are called progenitor cells.
5. A variety of inducing molecules, some of which are specific for a given lineage, have been identified.

Additional Readings

Burgess, A., and N. Nicola. 1983. *Growth Factors and Stem Cells*. Academic Press, Sydney.

Goldwasser, E. (In press) Commitment in blood cell differentiation: does erythropoietin act as an instructive signal? In *Tenth Annual Frederick Stohlman Jr. Memorial Symposium*.

Golub, E. S. 1982. In vitro approaches to hemopoiesis. *Cell* 28, 687.

Hall, A. K. 1983. Stem cell is a stem cell is a stem cell. *Cell* 33, 11.

Metcalf, D. 1984. *Clonal Culture of Hemopoietic Cells: Techniques and Applications*. Elsevier, Amsterdam.

Ogawa, M., P. N. Pharr, and T. Suda. (In press) Stochastic nature of stem cell function in culture. In *Tenth Annual Frederick Stohlman Jr. Memorial Symposium*.

Schrader, J. W. 1984. Bone marrow differentiation in vitro. *C.R.C. Critical Rev. Immunol.* 4, 197.

CHAPTER 11

LYMPHOCYTES

Overview Cellular immunology is essentially the study of the biology of lymphocytes, their interactions, and their products. In the last chapter we discussed the evidence for the multipotency of the hemopoietic stem cell and noted that the spleen colonies contained cells of the myeloid series (erythrocytes, granulocytes, monocytes, and megakaryocytes) but not lymphocytes. In this chapter we will discuss the evidence that the lymphocytes also arise from the multipotent stem cell and show that the lymphocytes arise in two hemopoietic-inducing microenvironments (HIM), the thymus and the bone marrow. We will see that two kinds of lymphocytes, called B cells and T cells, differentiate in these two HIM. These cells, which cannot be distinguished on the basis of morphology, are profoundly different. They carry out very different functions, express different surface molecules and respond to different mitogens.

This chapter, in addition to developing the evidence for these two paths of differentiation of the lymphoid progenitor, will also describe and catalog many of the traits of the lymphocytes. This material will help us understand the experiments that show how the cells of the immune response interact (Section II).

CHAPTER ELEVEN

The Origins of Lymphocytes

Derivation of Lymphocytes from the Multipotent Stem Cell

Evidence that the lymphocytes are derived from multipotent stem cells comes from experiments very similar to those that showed that myeloid cells came from the CFU-S (Chapter 10). In the experiment diagrammed in Figure 1, unique chromosome markers were induced in +/+

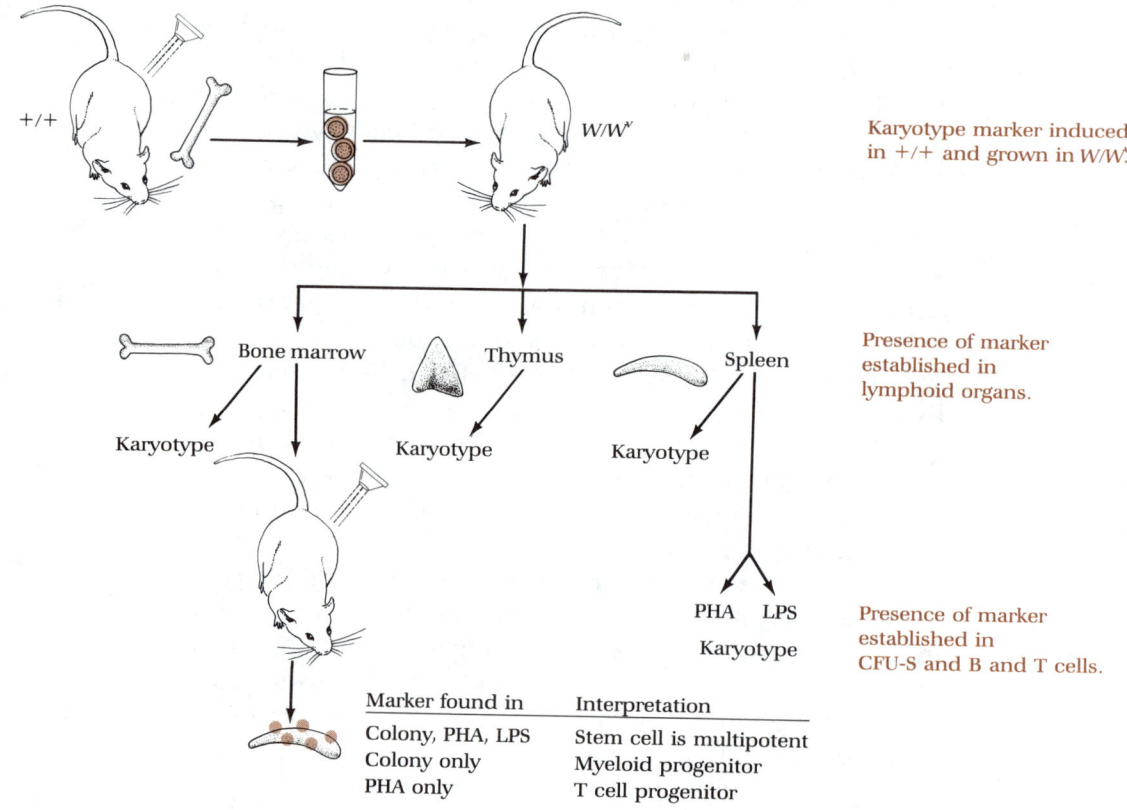

FIGURE 1 DETERMINING THE COMMON LYMPHOID PROGENITOR
Karyotypic markers are introduced by X-irradiation and marked cells are expanded in W/W^v hosts. Bone marrow cells are injected into irradiated +/+ mice and colonies are examined. Thymus cells and spleen cells are tested for karyotype, and spleen cells are tested for B cells and T cells by lipopolysaccharide (LPS) and phytohemagglutinin (PHA). [After Abramson et al. (1971) *J. Exp. Med.* 145, 1567]

LYMPHOCYTES

mice by X irradiation and the bone marrow cells passaged into W/W^v mutant mice so that the number of cells with karyotype alterations could be increased. After several months the bone marrow, two lymphoid organs, the thymus, and the spleen were removed from the W/W^v mice, and those mice with a high percentage of cells carrying a unique marker were analyzed further. The bone marrow cells from these animals were injected into irradiated +/+ mice to ascertain whether the CFU-S had the marked cells. The spleen cells were treated with reagents that stimulate lymphocytes to enter mitosis (these will be discussed in detail later in this chapter), and the cells of the thymus were examined for the marker. In this way the presence of the marker in the CFU-S as well as in lymphocytes from the spleen and thymus could be correlated.

Three marker patterns were obtained: some mice had the marker in both the CFU-S and the lymphocytes; some had the marker in the myeloid cells but not in the lymphocytes; and some had the marker only in the thymus-derived lymphocytes. These results show several things. First, even though lymphocytes are not found in the spleen colonies, the CFU-S gives rise to lymphocytes as well as to myeloid cells. The second important thing to be learned from this experiment is that at an early stage of differentiation there are progenitor cells that are determined to differentiate along myeloid or lymphoid lineages (recall Figure 5 of Chapter 10). This experiment argues that one of the first "decisions" made in hemopoietic differentiation is between the lymphoid and the myeloid pathways.

Primary and Secondary Lymphoid Organs

We saw in the last chapter that myeloid differentiation occurs in hemopoietic-inducing microenvironments, sites in which the myeloid progenitor cells are acted upon by specific inducing molecules. In an analogous manner, the differentiation of lymphocytes occurs in lymphoid-inducing microenvironments—the bone marrow and the thymus. The thymus is an organ whose sole function appears to be lymphoid differentiation. The bone marrow, in contrast, is also a site of erythroid and granuloid differentiation. In birds the BURSA OF FABRICIUS is a discrete site of lymphoid differentiation, and the

CHAPTER ELEVEN

mammalian bone marrow is thought of as the "bursal equivalent." These sites of differentiation of lymphoid progenitors to lymphocytes are called the PRIMARY LYMPHOID ORGANS.

After the lymphoid progenitor cells differentiate in the primary lymphoid organs, they migrate to the spleen and lymph nodes, which are called the SECONDARY LYMPHOID ORGANS. Figure 2 shows the locations of the primary and secondary lymphoid tissues. We will discuss the traffic of lymphocytes from the primary to the secondary organs and through the lymphatics, and the anatomy of the lymphoid organs in Chapter 12.

Lymphocytes are the cells that carry out the immune function. However, very few of the lymphocytes in the bone marrow

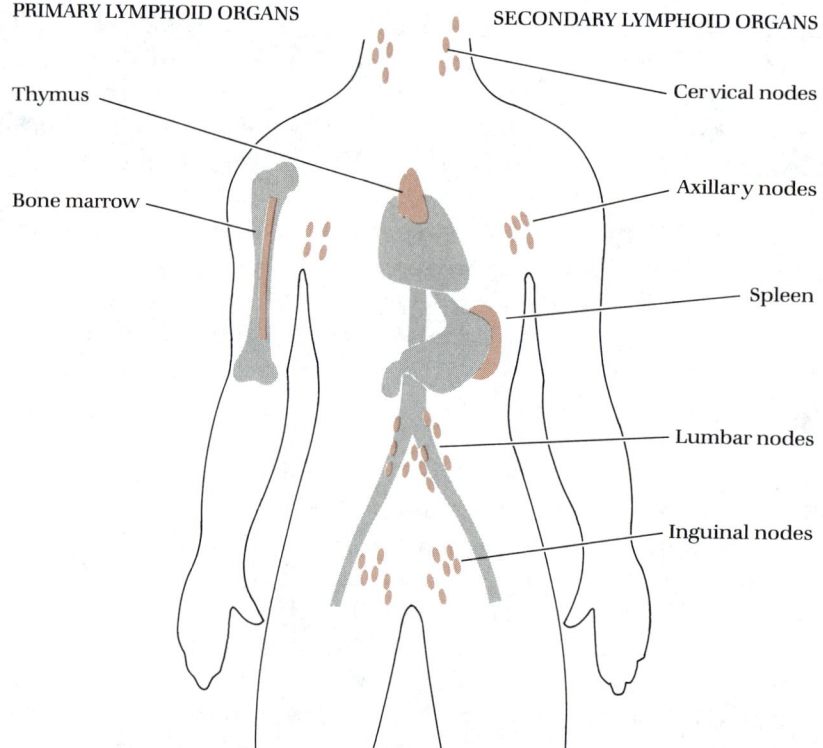

FIGURE 2   LOCATION OF HUMAN LYMPHOID TISSUE

LYMPHOCYTES

and thymus are functional. In contrast, the cells that are exported from these organs to the secondary lymphoid tissues are fully differentiated and functional. In addition, the ability of the thymus-derived lymphocytes to discriminate self from nonself—one of the most important functions of the immune system—is acquired during differentiation in the thymus.

B Cells and T Cells

The lymphocytes which differentiate in the bone marrow and the thymus are called B CELLS and T CELLS, respectively. B cells and T cells have similar morphology but differ in many fundamental ways. The most important difference between them is functional. B cells are antibody-forming cells, and the various subsets of T cells act as effector, helper, or suppressor cells. Thus the progeny of the cells that differentiate in each of the inducing microenvironments divide the labor of the immune response. Both B cells and the different functional subsets of T cells can also be distinguished by markers expressed on their surfaces and by their responses to certain substances, called mitogens, which induce cells to enter mitosis.[1]

The Concept of Differentiation Antigens

T cells and B cells can be distinguished by their totally different functions, but in the course of differentiation they acquire other sets of distinguishing characteristics, which in many cases seem to be independent of the cell's function. As we mentioned earlier, many of these characteristics are molecules expressed at the cell surface, called SURFACE ANTIGENS, and antibodies can be raised against them. Because antibodies are highly specific, they become potent, specific re-

---

[1] To illustrate the lack of morphological difference between the cells, the late Richard Gershon would often begin a talk about functional subsets of T cells by showing a slide of a lymphocyte, which he told the audience was a helper T cell. After describing it, he would flash up another slide of the *same* cell, which he would call a cytotoxic T cell. He would then give the same description he had given for the previous slide. Then he would call for the next slide, which was, of course, the same cell. He now called it a suppressor T cell and would begin the same morphological description. The audience quickly got the message: one cannot tell by sight alone what the function of the cell will be.

CHAPTER ELEVEN

agents that can be used to identify and detect the characteristic cell surface antigens. Used in conjunction with complement, they can also be used to eliminate the cells that express these antigens.

Furthermore, the expression of some of these surface antigens correlates with the stage of differentiation of the lymphocytes. Because of this correlation, they are called DIFFERENTIATION ANTIGENS. Differentiation antigens on T cells have proved to be exceptionally powerful tools for identification, characterization, and analysis. But B cells have few differentiation antigens, so other surface markers are used to identify them.

We do not know the function, if any, of differentiation antigens. It is conceivable that they are receptors for inducing agents. Some of them may play a role in the immune function of the cells. The concept of differentiation antigens was derived from studies on lymphocytes by Old and Boyse in New York, but the idea has much greater applicability. We know, for example, that the developing embryo has stage-specific antigens, and many other developing systems are being studied to determine whether the display of unique antigens at certain stages of differentiation is a general phenomenon in developing systems.

There are two methods of producing antibodies to differentiation antigens on lymphocytes. The original method involved the use of alloantigens and alloantibodies. The more modern method involves the use of monoclonal antibodies. These two methods of producing antibodies to cell surface markers are discussed in Information Box 1.

Differentiation Antigens on Murine T Cells

In the bone marrow, the common lymphoid progenitor cell gives rise to progeny, called PRE-T and PRE-B cells, which then undergo differentiation in the proper lymphoid HIM to become T cells or B cells. B cell differentiation, as we said, occurs in the bone marrow. The fact that the stem cells, lymphoid progenitors, pre-B cells, and pre-T cells all are found in the bone marrow makes the study of B cell differentiation rather difficult. In addition, myeloid progenitors are found in the bone marrow, and myeloid differentiation is going on in the same tissue. The study of T cell differentiation, while not a

INFORMATION BOX 1

Studying Differentiation Antigens with Alloantibodies and Monoclonal Antibodies

Alloantigens and Alloantibodies

ALLOANTIBODIES are antibodies made to antigens on the cells of members of the same species. The antigen expressed by one member of a species but not by another is called an ALLOANTIGEN. ISOANTIBODIES are antibodies made by an individual to its own antigens, and XENOANTIBODIES, or heteroantibodies, are antibodies made in another species.

Inbred mice are ideal for the production of alloantibodies, because they can be selected so that they differ in only one or a few antigens. Suppose cells of strain A express antigen a and strain B does not. When tissue from A is injected into B, it is recognized as foreign; and B produces antibody against a. This B anti-a antiserum is able to react with any cells that express a.

A good example of an alloantibody to a differentiation antigen is the Thy 1 antigen on T cells. Thy 1 is an antigen found on T cells of all strains of mice. The gene for Thy 1 has two allelic forms, Thy 1.1 and Thy 1.2. When thymus cells from a Thy 1.1 strain are injected into a Thy 1.2 strain, the Thy 1.2 strain will respond by producing antibodies to Thy 1.1. These anti-Thy 1.1 antibodies will react with the T cells of all strains that express the Thy 1.1 form of Thy 1. The use of alloantigens and alloantibodies therefore requires that there be at least two allelic forms of the antigen or that there be a strain that does not express the antigen at all. This is a limitation, but not one that is too severe.

The real limitation of the method is that we must rely on members of the same species to generate the antibodies. The problem is most evident when attempting to produce antibodies against surface antigens in humans. Even if there were no problem of allelic forms, a human alloantiserum would have to be raised in another human—a situation far from ideal. The advent of monoclonal antibodies has removed this problem, and we have reached the point where we now know more about the surface of human T cells than we do about those of the mouse.

Monoclonal Antibodies

Monoclonal antibodies were discussed in Chapter 6. The power of the technique is that we do not need allelic forms of an antigen and can raise the antibody in a different species. In the past the raising of xenoantisera (often called heteroantisera) was the only method of generating antibodies to human antigens. But because the species that was being immunized responded to so many antigens on the injected tissue, the resulting antiserum had antibodies to large numbers of antigens. The specificity of the antiserum could be increased by *adsorbing* out the antibodies of undesired specificities. This was done by adding tissue known to lack the antigen being studied but to express other antigens. Thus if we immunized a rabbit with human thymus cells, we would adsorb the antiserum with human liver cells to remove antibodies common to human cells. Liver would not, of course, have thymus-specific antigens, so these antibodies would not be removed or "adsorbed out" of the antiserum. Obviously this method was inefficient. The advent of monoclonal technology allows the investigator to immunize with tissue, fuse the lymphocytes, and, as long as he or she is clever enough, devise a selection method for the antibody desired and end up with a clone of cells producing antibody only to the antigen of interest.

CHAPTER ELEVEN

walk in the park, is easier because the thymus is a discrete inducing microenvironment.

Pre-T cells leave the bone marrow and enter the thymus via the blood. In the thymus they begin to undergo differentiation and express differentiation antigens that are characteristic of T cells. These antigens are molecules not expressed on stem cells or pre-T cells. Some of the more important murine T cell differentiation antigens are discussed in Information Box 2.

Lymphocytes in the thymus are found in the medulla and the cortex (Chapter 12). All thymic lymphocytes are Thy 1^+, but only medullary thymocytes express TL. The cells that are exported from the thymus to the secondary lymphoid tissues continue to express Thy 1 but are TL^-. The Lyt antigens become expressed in the thymus, where 85% of the cells are Lyt 1^+, 2^+. In the periphery only 30% of the cells express this phenotype. The percentage of Lyt 1^+ and Lyt 2^+ cells in the periphery varies according to tissue. These latter populations were originally associated with particular functions (Lyt 1^+ with helper and delayed-type hypersensitivity and Lyt 2^+ with cytotoxic and suppressor cells), but more recent analysis shows that the Lyt 1^+ and Lyt 2^+ cells are associated with different classes of MHC restriction (Section II).

It should be emphasized here that when cells are analyzed using very sensitive methods, most T cells express some level of Lyt 1. However, another molecule, called L3T4, is associated with the MHC restriction formerly associated with Lyt 1. For historical reasons we will continue to refer to Lyt 1 in some places, but the reader should be aware that most of the current literature will use L3T4 as the marker of choice.

Differentiation Antigens on Human T Cells

As in the mouse, the pre-T cell in humans enters the thymus and begins to undergo a series of differentiative changes which can be followed by the appearance of surface antigens. But in humans we obviously cannot take advantage of any potential allelic differences in the antigens by raising alloantisera. For many years this made the task of identifying differentiation antigens in humans very difficult. The advent of monoclonal antibodies, however, changed all that (see Information Box 1 and Chapter 6). In fact, we now know more about the surface antigens at different stages of differentiation in humans than we do in the mouse.

INFORMATION BOX 2

Properties of Murine T Cell Differentiation Antigens

Thy 1

One of the first differentiation antigens to be discovered was Thy 1 (originally called theta). Thy 1 is not expressed on the multipotent stem cell or on the pre-T cell, but *all* thymic lymphocytes are Thy 1^+. After the cells leave the thymus, they continue to express the Thy 1 antigen; so any lymphocyte in the periphery that is Thy 1^+ is, by definition, a thymus-derived lymphocyte. Thy 1 is thus the hallmark of a thymus-derived lymphocyte.

Thy 1 is a glycoprotein that has a molecular weight of 25,000 and is 50% carbohydrate. cDNA clones coding for Thy 1 show both DNA and protein sequence homology to two other surface proteins involved in the immune response—immunoglobulin and Class II MHC molecules.

Among lymphocytes, Thy 1 is unique to T cells. However, it is expressed on other types of cells, most notably brain cells and fibroblasts. It also can be induced in vitro on some other cells that are not lymphocytes. The distribution of Thy 1^+ cells in brain has allowed anti-brain antisera to be used as anti-T cell reagents. However, the presence of other hemopoietic antibodies in these antisera make them less useful than anti-Thy 1 raised as alloantibody or monoclonal antibody.

TL

The TL antigen, like Thy 1, is not expressed on the stem cell or pre-T cell but is expressed by lymphocytes in the thymus. Unlike Thy 1, however, TL ceases to be expressed on cortical thymus lymphocytes or on lymphocytes that are exported to the periphery, that is, functional T cells. This marker then is a useful one for functional cells within the thymus, but it cannot identify thymus-derived lymphocytes in the periphery.

Lyt

The Lyt antigens have been among the most useful in recent years because they have been used to define FUNCTIONAL SUBSETS of T cells. The Lyt antibodies were originally generated as alloantisera by taking advantage of the fact that there are multiallelic forms. Monoclonal antibodies are now available. The original antigen was identified on T cells, but more recently similar antigens on B cells have been named Lyb to distinguish them from those on T cells.

LYT 1 is a polypeptide that has a molecular weight of 67,000 and is coded on chromosome 9. Expression of this antigen was originally associated with helper T cells and cells that carry out delayed-type hypersensitivity reactions (Chapter 15). It is becoming clear, however, that Lyt 1 expression is really associated with Class II MHC restriction rather than with the function of the T cells. Using very sensitive flow cytometry technology, investigators have found that virtually all Thy 1^+ cells express some amount of Lyt 1, even though it may not be detectable by "ordinary" methods. Because of this, a molecule called L3T4 is now being used as a marker instead of Lyt 1.

LYT 2 and LYT 3 are genetically linked on chromosome 6. They have never been separated by recombination and are probably separate polypeptides on the same molecular complex. This complex is composed of two polypeptides of molecular weight 28,000–35,000. The Lyt 2 marker was originally associated with cytotoxic and suppressor cells, but now the association is thought to be with Class I MHC restriction.

CHAPTER ELEVEN

As monoclonal antibodies against human T cell antigens were generated, the antigens were quite naturally named by each investigator as he or she produced them. Because several workers independently produced monoclonal antibody against the same determinant, a plethora of designations sprang up before it was possible to compare the specificities of the antibodies to each other. Manufacturers of these antibodies were reluctant to change their designation even after it was known that two or three separately designated antibodies were identifying the same antigen. By common agreement the designation "T" followed by a number was adopted by most investigators. Thus, for example, we may see in the literature reference to T4 or T8 antigens on human T cells.

In 1982 the First International Workshop on Human Leukocyte Differentiation Antigens was held in Paris. At that meeting 139 monoclonal antibodies were tested by immunofluorescence, and the antibodies were grouped into "clusters" on the basis of the results. At the Fifth International Congress of Immunology held in Kyoto, Japan in 1983, the Nomenclature Subcommittee officially adopted this scheme of nomenclature. It was well known that certain human T cell differentiation antigens were found on certain subsets of T cells (T4 on helper cells, for example, and T8 on suppressor cells). The idea of the CLUSTER OF DIFFERENTIATION (CD) was to group all of the known antibodies that reacted with these identifiable subpopulations. In the future, any investigator who produces a new monoclonal antibody against a human T cell population can determine into which cluster group it falls. Information Box 3 describes the T antigen designation groups; and Information Box 4 gives the cluster of differentiation groupings of human T cell differentiation antigens.

Differentiation antigens by definition appear at certain stages of differentiation, and human T cell differentiation can be described as occurring in three stages. In STAGE I the T11 antigen is expressed. This antigen is associated with the binding of sheep erythrocytes to the surface of the human T cell, a phenomenon that was used in the past to identify human T cells. T11 remains expressed on the T cells throughout further differentiation. No other known antigens are expressed at this stage.

LYMPHOCYTES

INFORMATION BOX 3

Designation of Human T Cell Differentiation Antigens

Antigen	Distribution	Percentage of positive cells of peripheral blood	Other characteristics
T1, T3, T11, T12	Thymocytes, including functional subsets	70	—
T6	Thymocytes, but not functional subsets	0.5	—
T4	Helper cells	45	Class II MHC restriction
T8	Suppressor cells	30	Class I MHC restriction
T9	Activated T cells	—	Transferrin receptor
T10	Activated T cells	—	—
Tac	Activated T cells	—	IL-2 receptor

In STAGE II T6 is expressed. This antigen, like the murine TL, is expressed on cells only while they are in the cortex of the thymus. At about this same time two very important antigenic markers, T4 and T8, are *both* also expressed. Thus by the end of Stage II the developing T cells in the thymus are expressing T11, T6, T4, and T8. The cells of both Stage I and Stage II are located in the cortex of the thymus (Chapter 12). As further maturation occurs and the cells become medullary thymocytes, they no longer express T6 (hence the reason for referring to it as TL-like).

As the cells enter STAGE III they not only become T6$^-$, they also begin to express *either* T4 *or* T8. They also begin to express T3, which is associated with the T cell antigen-specific receptor. At the end of Stage III the cells are expressing either T11, T3, and

CHAPTER ELEVEN

> ### INFORMATION BOX 4
>
> ## Clusters of Differentiation
>
> The First International Workshop on Human Leukocyte Differentiation Antigens convened in Paris in 1982 and tested 139 monoclonal antibodies to human differentiation antigens. The results allow the antigens to be grouped into "clusters of differentiation." The table gives the clusters of differentiation for human T cell antigens.
>
> | Cluster designation | T designation | Population |
> |---|---|---|
> | CD1 [Thy,p45,12][a] | T6 | Cortical thymocytes |
> | CD2 [T,p50] | T1 | E rosette-forming cells |
> | CD3 [T,p19–29] | T3 | Mature T cells |
> | CD4 [T,p55] | T4 | Inducer T cells |
> | CD5 [T,p67] | T1 | Pan T + subpopulation of B cells |
> | CD6 [T,p120] | — | Mature T cells + subpopulation of B cells |
> | CD7 [T,p41] | — | Pan T |
> | CD8 [T,p32–33] | T8 | Cytotoxic/suppressor T cells |
>
> Source: Adapted from the Committee on Human Leukocyte Differentiation Antigens (1984), *Immunology Today* 5: 158.
>
> [a] In the nomenclature system devised by the Committee, each cluster of differentiation (CD) is given an arbitrary number, followed by an expression brackets indicating the typical cell, its chemical composition (e.g., p = protein; gp = glycoprotein), and molecular weight. Thus: CD# [cell, composition, MW]

T4 or T11, T3, and T8. The T4 cells are associated with helper phenomena and the T8 cells with suppression.[2]

T cells are not immunologically functional in Stages I and II, but acquire function in Stage III. The acquisition of specific im-

---

[2] The clinical significance of the cells bearing these markers will be seen in Chapter 29, where we will discuss the fact that the ratio of T4 to T8 cells changes drastically in acquired immune deficiency syndrome (AIDS). There is growing evidence that the T4 molecule acts as the receptor for HTLVIII, the virus that is the likely etiologic agent of the disease.

LYMPHOCYTES

munological function is no doubt due to the expression of the T3, which is a 20 to 25-kd glycoprotein associated noncovalently with the 90-kd heterodimer (sometimes called Ti) that is the T cell antigen-specific receptor.[3]

As we have said, the function of the T4 and T8 markers is not known, but the fact that they are expressed by functional subsets has naturally raised the possibility that they are in some manner involved in carrying out the function of the subset. Complementary DNA (cDNA) clones encoding T4 and T8 have been made by using gene transfer and subtractive hybridization (see Chapter 20 for details of this method). The deduced amino acid sequences indicate that T8 is a membrane-bound glycoprotein with an N-terminal domain that bears homology to the variable region of immunoglobulin light chains. The deduced sequence of T4 indicates that it bears homology to both variable and joining regions of immunoglobulin light chains. For this reason it has been suggested that they are members of the immunoglobulin superfamily (see Chapter 5).

Surface Markers on B Cells

Surface Immunoglobulin We have just seen that T cells have a wide variety of differentiation antigens which are used not only to define them as T cells but also serve as convenient indicators of their functional status. B cells, in contrast, have a more limited range of surface markers. Just as the hallmark of the T cell is Thy 1, the absolute criterion for a B cell is the presence of SURFACE IMMUNOGLOBULIN (sIg). When a population of lymph node cells, for example, is examined with fluorescence-labeled anti-Ig, only about 30% of them will be stained. When this exercise is carried out with a double stain—anti-Ig and anti-Thy 1—one population stains with anti-Ig and another with anti-Thy 1. So the hallmark of the B cell is to express surface sIg, whereas the hallmark of the T cell is to express a differentiation antigen.

---

[3] The complete discussion of the T cell receptor must await the discussion of the nature of cell interactions in the immune response. It will be covered in Chapters 20 and 21.

CHAPTER ELEVEN

Complement Receptor   B cells also express other surface markers that can be used to show that they are not T cells, but none of the markers, other than the surface immunoglobulins, are unique to B cells. One of these is a receptor for the third component of complement, C3. When C3 is activated on the surface of an erythrocyte, the red cells form rosettes with lymphocytes that bear the C3 receptor. These cells are called COMPLEMENT RECEPTOR-BEARING LYMPHOCYTES, or CRL. B cells are CRL, but there are also some non-Ig-bearing cells that have the C3 receptor.

Fc Receptor   Some, but not all, B cells express a receptor that binds to the Fc portion of the immunoglobulin molecule. This is not a very good marker because other cells, including some T cells, can express the Fc receptor and because not all B cells are Fc-receptor positive.

Surface Ig acts as the antigen-specific receptor. There has been speculation, but not agreement, about the possible functional role, if any, of the C and Fc receptors.

The Induction of Lymphocyte Differentiation

We have already discussed the fact that hemopoietic differentiation occurs in inducing microenvironments (HIM). Differentiation occurs in these areas through the action of specific inducing molecules, which act on the pre-T and pre-B cells. The two lymphoid HIM are the thymus and the bone marrow for T cells and B cells respectively. A great deal is known about the inducing molecules for T cell differentiation in the thymus but relatively little is known about B cell inducing mechanisms.

T Cell Inducing Factors   It is generally agreed that the inducing factors in the thymus are produced by the epithelial cells there. Several factors have been described, all of which are able to convert cells from the bone marrow into cells with surface markers associated with thymic lymphocytes. Some of the factors are also able to induce functional differentiation. As in myeloid differentiation, it is assumed that the determined cell (in this case the pre-T cell) is expressing receptors for the proper inducing molecule.

LYMPHOCYTES

THYMOSIN was the first of the factors to be described and was originally obtained from extracts of bovine thymus. Thymosin is actually a collection of molecules with different functions. One of these, thymosin Fraction 5, causes the expression of Thy 1 on treated pre-T cells. It is a protein of molecular weight 12,000.

Another factor, THYMOPOIETIN, is a protein of molecular weight 7,000 and induces the production of some differentiation antigens. Fractionation of thymopoietin has produced a 12-amino acid peptide that contains the inducing activity. This peptide has been synthesized in vitro, which led to the discovery that the N-terminal pentapeptide contains all of the inducing activity.

THYMIC HUMORAL FACTOR (Facteur Humoral Thymique) is a peptide that has both differentiation antigen-inducing activity and, under appropriate conditions, function-inducing activity.

It is not known whether one or all of these molecules is the physiological inducing molecule in the thymus.

Induction of B Cell Differentiation

As we stated earlier, there is no discrete anatomical HIM for B cells in mammals. In contrast, in the chicken B cells develop in the bursa of Fabricius. The mammalian "bursal equivalent" seems to be distributed in the bone marrow, and it is reasonable to assume that there are epithelial and reticular cells in the bone marrow secreting molecules that induce the differentiation of the pre-B cells into functional B cells. A molecule called BURSAPOIETIN was isolated from the bursa several years ago but has not been extensively studied. Studying B cell differentiation in mammals is difficult because of this lack of a discrete site.

Mitogen Responses of T Cells and B Cells

B cells and T cells also differ rather dramatically in their responses to agents that induce cell proliferation. These substances are called MITOGENS because they induce the cells to enter mitosis. Because mitosis involves the synthesis of new DNA, the ability of an agent to act as a mitogen can easily be determined by adding tritiated thymidine to cultures of cells and quantifying the amount of the isotope incorporated into the newly synthesized

CHAPTER ELEVEN

DNA. When this is done with a wide array of agents, we find that some agents preferentially induce B cells and some induce T cells.

Table 1 gives some of the more common B cell and T cell mitogens. This peculiar property allows us to identify a cell population, but as we will see in later chapters, mitogens are also of interest because they can act as surrogates for antigens. Surrogate antigens are needed because the frequency of any given antigen-specific cell is very low (about 10^{-6}). Because antigen will induce such a small number of cells, it is very often useful to study the events of lymphocyte proliferation by mitogens because they induce all the cells with which they react to proliferate.

TABLE 1 Some B and T cell mitogens.

Mitogen	Inhibitor	Cell
Phytohemagglutinin (PHA)	N-acetyl-D-galactosamine	T cells (human and mouse)
Concanavalin A (ConA)	αD-gluco and mannopyranosides	T cells (human and mouse); B cells if cross linked
Waxbean	—	T cells (human)
Pokeweed mitogen (PWM)	Di-N-acetylchitobiose	T and B (human and mouse but Pa-1 subunit acts only on B cells)
Lipopolysaccharide (LPS)	—	B cells (mouse, not human)
Aggregated tuberculin	—	B cells
Sodium periodate-reducing agents such as sodium borohydride (NaBH$_4$)	—	B cells
Dextran sulfate	—	Subset of B cells
Dextran polyvinylpyrrolidone	—	B cells
Trypsin, chymotrypsin	Leupeptin	B cells

LYMPHOCYTES

Summary

1. Lymphocytes are the cells that carry out the specific function of the immune response. They are derived from the multipotent hemopoietic stem cell, even though they do not appear in the spleen colonies.
2. Lymphocytes differentiate in two lymphocyte-inducing microenvironments, the thymus and the bone marrow (which is the mammalian equivalent of the avian bursa). Thymus-derived lymphocytes are called T cells and bursa-derived lymphocytes are called B cells. Functional T cells and B cells are morphologically similar but can be distinguished by several criteria.
3. Differentiation antigens are cell surface antigens expressed by cells when they reach a certain stage of differentiation. These antigens can be used to identify the origin of a cell and can themselves be identified by methods using either alloantibodies or monoclonal antibodies.
4. B cells and T cells respond to different mitogens (molecules that induce cells into mitosis).

Additional Readings

Ahmed, A., and A. H. Smith. Surface markers, antigens, and receptors on murine T and B cells. I. (1982) *CRC Critical Rev. Immunol.* 3, 331. II. (1983) *CRC Critical Rev. Immunol.* 4, 19. III. (1983) *CRC Critical Rev. Immunol.* 4, 95.

Boyse, E. A., and L. J. Old. 1969. Some aspects of normal and abnormal surface genetics. *Annu. Rev. Genet.* 3, 269.

Fitch, F. W. 1986. T-cell clones and T-cell receptors. *Microbial Rev.* 50, 50.

Littmann, D. R., Y. Thomas, P. J. Maddon, L. Chess, and R. Axel. 1985. The isolation of the gene encoding T8: a molecule defining functional classes of T lymphocytes. *Cell* 40, 237.

Maddon, P. J., D. R. Littman, M. Godfrey, D. E. Maddon, L. Chess, and R. Axel. 1985. The isolation and nucleotide sequence of cDNA encoding the T cell surface protein T4: A new family member of the immunoglobulin gene family. *Cell* 42, 93.

Scollay, R., and K. Shortman. 1983. Thymocyte subpopulations: an experimental review, including flow cytometry cross-correlations between the major murine thymocyte markers. *Thymus* 5, 245.

Seki, T., N. Spurr, F. Obata, S. Goyert, P. Goodfellow, and J. Silver. 1985. The human Thy 1 gene: structure and chromosomal location. *Proc. Natl. Acad. Sci. USA* 82, 6657.

CHAPTER 12

ORGANIZATION AND STRUCTURE OF LYMPHOID TISSUE

Overview We have learned that the cells of the immune system—lymphocytes and macrophages—arise from a common stem cell and undergo differentiation in specialized areas called hemopoietic inducing microenvironments. In addition, we have learned that the lymphocytes, both B cells and T cells, arise in primary lymphoid organs, the bone marrow and the thymus, and are then exported to the secondary lymphoid organs, the spleen and the lymph nodes.

In this chapter we will examine the structure of the primary and secondary lymphoid organs and the circulation pattern of the lymphocytes. We will see that the lymphocytes circulate throughout the body by passing between the blood and lymphatic vascular systems. The passage points are at the lymph nodes, which are accumulations of lymphoid cells with organized structure. At the point where a venule enters a lymph node there is a specialized endothelium, called the high endothelial venule; lymphocytes have receptors for this structure. As the B and T lymphocytes enter the nodes and the spleen they move to discrete areas of the organs.

ORGANIZATION AND STRUCTURE OF LYMPHOID TISSUE

Structure of Lymphoid Organs

The Thymus The thymus is a primary lymphatic organ. In humans it is located in the superior mediastinum, dorsal to the sternum. It is a bilaterally symmetrical organ divided into two LOBES. Each of the lobes is organized into broad, triangular LOBULES by connective tissue SEPTA which are continuous with the CAPSULE. The blood and lymphatic vessels run in the septa.

Lymphocytes and epithelial cells are the principal cells of the thymus. The lymphocytes are arranged in the lobules, forming a peripheral zone called the CORTEX and a central zone called the MEDULLA (Figure 1). Most proliferating lymphocytes in the thymus are found in the cortex. Although the medulla contains lymphocytes, it is relatively richer in epithelial cells than the cortex is. In addition, the medulla contains unique structures called HASSALL'S CORPUSCLES, which are concentric rings of tightly wound epithelial cells of unknown function.

The thymus has no afferent lymphatic supply. Blood reaches the organ through branches of the subclavian artery which enter at the medulla through the septa. The cortex is supplied by arterioles at the junction between the medulla and the cortex. The thymus connects to the lymphatic system by lymphatic vessels, which leave the medulla and drain into the mediastinal lymph nodes. Thus the traffic of pre-T cells to the thymus is via the blood, and the differentiated T cells leave through the efferent lymphatics or the venous drainage by the medullary vein. Lymphocytes can recirculate back into the thymus from the blood. Some factors involved in lymphocyte traffic will be discussed later in this chapter.

The thymus is large at birth and reaches its maximum size (ca. 40 gm in humans) at puberty, after which it begins to atrophy. As an animal ages, the parenchyma is replaced by fatty and fibrous tissue but the organ remains functional (Figure 2). We will see that this is true because only a small percentage of cells in the thymus are functional; as the organ atrophies, the percentage of functional cells increases.

Cortical and Medullary Thymocytes The lymphocytes in the thy-

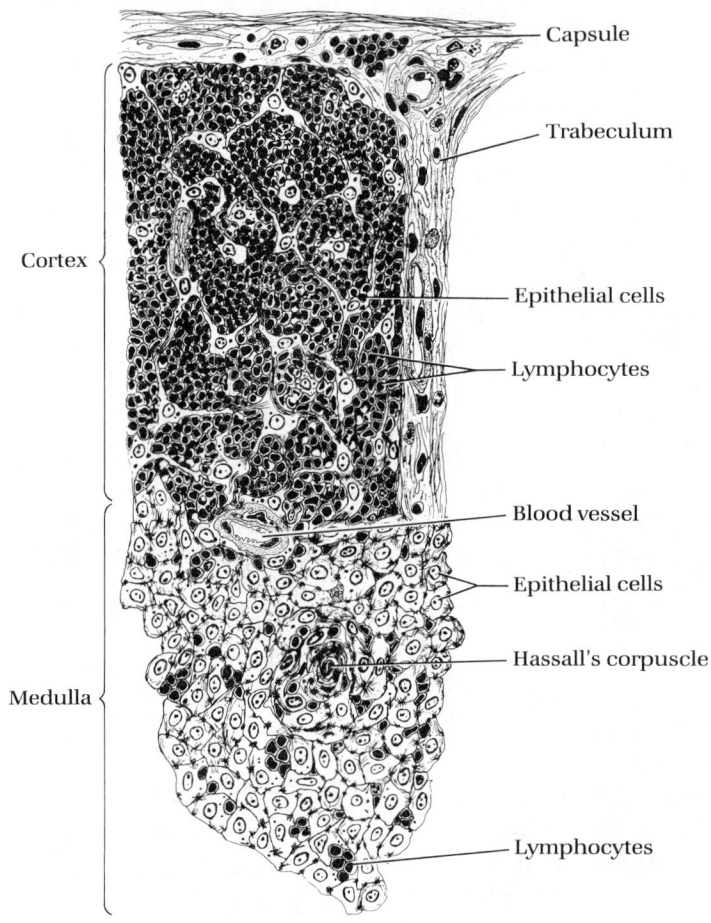

FIGURE 1 LOBULE OF THE THYMUS
A portion of a lobule in the human thymus. The cortex is rich in lymphocytes; the medulla is rich in epithelial cells; and the capsule and trabecula are rich in connective tissue and blood vessels. [From Weiss (1972), *The Cells and Tissues of the Immune System*]

mus are distributed in both the cortex and the medulla. One of the enduring mysteries about the thymus concerns the fact that the vast majority of thymocytes die in the thymus—only about 1% of the cells per day are exported to the periphery. The reason,

ORGANIZATION AND STRUCTURE OF LYMPHOID TISSUE

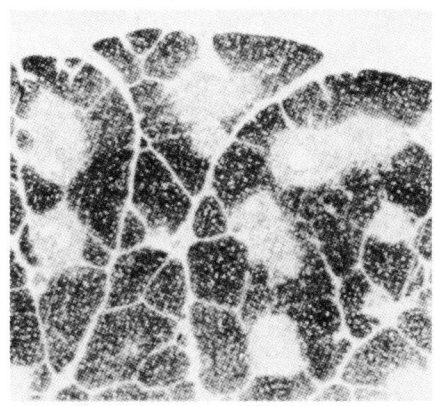
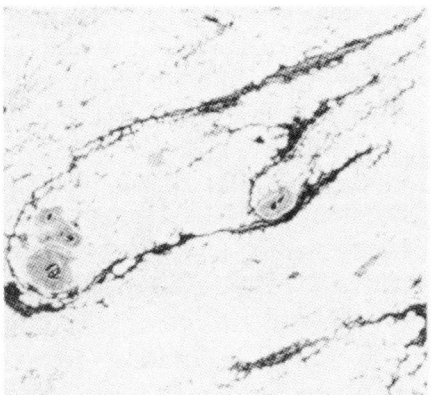

FIGURE 2 THYMUS BEFORE AND AFTER INVOLUTION

The tissue in the left micrograph is from a 3-month-old human infant; that on the right is from a 72-year-old adult. The lobular pattern in the young thymus is not seen in the involuted adult thymus, which is filled with fat and fibrous tissue (25×). [From Weiss (1983), *Histology: Cell and Tissue Biology*]

if any, for the large, apparently nonfunctional population is not known, but the bulk of the literature shows that it is the cells in the medulla that are the maturing population and the cells destined to be exported to the peripheral tissues. Cortical and medullary populations differ in levels of H-2 and Thy 1 as well as in their ability to be agglutinated by the lectin peanut agglutinin (PNA). The "immature" cortical thymocytes are predominantly Lyt $1^+,2^+$, whereas the "mature" medullary cells are Lyt 1^+ or Lyt 2^+, phenotypes consistent with function. One clue to the nature of the cells in the thymus comes from the following experiment. When a mouse is injected with cortisone, over 90% of its thymocytes die. The remaining cells, the CORTISONE-RESISTANT THYMOCYTES, or CRT, are medullary cells. So we have come to equate the maturing functional cells with CRT. In fact, when thymus cells are used in a variety of immunological reactions, they show very low reactivity. But after cortisone treatment all of the immunological activity of the thymus resides in the CRT.

The generally held view of maturation in the thymus can be

summarized as follows: cells enter as cortical cells, most of which die before maturing. A small number become medullary cells, acquire immunological function, and are exported to the peripheral lymphoid tissue. It must be noted, however, that there is some evidence that this may be an oversimplification, and that a small subpopulation of cortical thymocytes also become functional cells and are exported without ever entering the medulla.

The Spleen

The spleen is the secondary lymphoid tissue used most often in cellular immunology experiments. It is a fascinating organ that has many functions other than those of the immune response. A fine description of the functions of the spleen is given by Leon Weiss:

> The spleen may be best understood as a discriminatory filter, consisting of specialized vascular spaces through which blood flows. The foundation of its structure and its filtration capacities is a reticular meshwork fashioned of reticular fibers. There is no element of the blood, cellular or plasmal, which the spleen may not affect. It monitors the red blood cells in the circulation and destroys or modifies imperfect ones. It removes other blood cells when damaged or aged. It sequesters monocytes from the blood and facilitates their transformation into macrophages and holds them as splenic macrophages which act in antibody formation and other splenic functions. It traps T and B cells from the blood and sorts them into compartments, permitting them to interact with macrophages and antigen in immune responses. It stores as many as a third of the platelets of the body in a ready reserve. In certain species, it can also function as a reservoir for erythrocytes and granulocytes, capable of delivering them rapidly to the blood when needed. [Leon Weiss, 1977, *Histology: Cell and Tissue Biology*, 4th Edition, McGraw-Hill, New York.]

This wonderous organ is enclosed by a CAPSULE of dense connective tissue and is divided into communicating compartments by a network of TRABECULAE which come from the capsular surface (Figure 3). The tissue enclosed by the capsule is called the SPLENIC PULP (a term which conjures up visions of old, dreary, smelly dissection laboratories). The pulp is mostly red, but it contains clusters of gray-white zones. These areas quite naturally are called the RED PULP and the WHITE PULP. The junction between red and white pulps is called the MARGINAL ZONE.

ORGANIZATION AND STRUCTURE OF LYMPHOID TISSUE

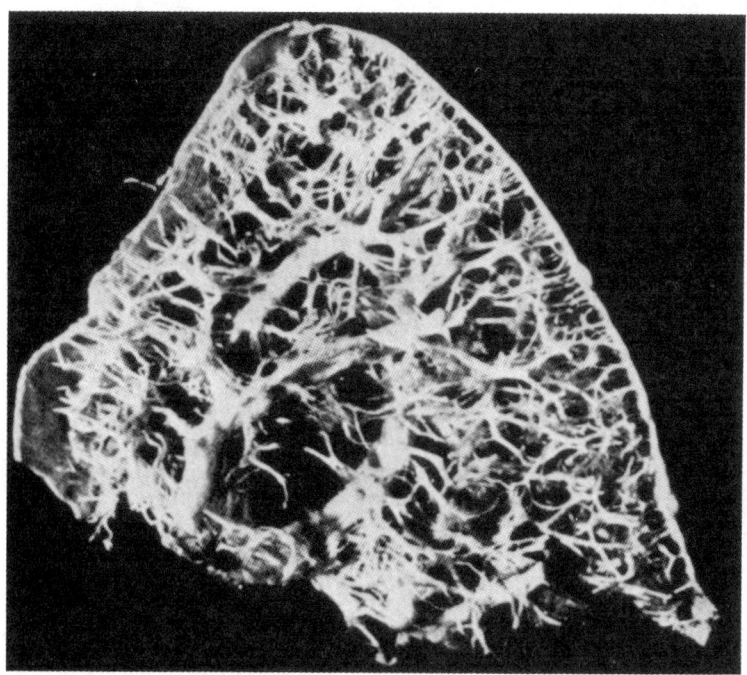

FIGURE 3 HUMAN SPLEEN
In this spleen specimen (magnification 4×) the trabecular framework and capsule remain after the pulp has been digested by a solution of sodium carbonate. [From Weiss (1983), *Histology: Cell and Tissue Biology*]

The red pulp is the site of storage of red blood cells (hence its color) and is composed of large, branching, thin-walled blood vessels called SPLENIC SINUSES. The tissue that lies between the sinuses is called the SPLENIC CORDS. The white pulp consists of cylinders surrounding the major arterial branches of the splenic pulp. These cylinders are called PERIARTERIAL LYMPHATIC SHEATHS, and within them are spherical clusters of lymphocytes called LYMPHATIC NODULES.

The white pulp, which contains the cells we will be most interested in, constitutes about 20% of the normal spleen and can be considered lymphoid tissue. It contains lymphocytes, macrophages, and other cells lying free in a reticular meshwork surrounding the arterial vessels. B cells and T cells are localized in the white pulp in what are known as T-dependent and B-dependent areas. The T-DEPENDENT AREAS of the spleen are primarily the lymphatic sheaths; the B-DEPENDENT AREAS are primarily the nodules.

CHAPTER TWELVE

Blood enters at the SPLENIC ARTERY through the hilus and branches into the trabeculae as TRABECULAR ARTERIES. These turn out of the trabeculae and enter the periarterial lymphatic sheaths; at this point they become CENTRAL ARTERIES. Lymphatic vessels are found within the trabeculae and in the white pulp closely associated with the central artery. The lymphatics drain into the lymph nodes near the hilus.

Lymphatic Vessels and Lymph Nodes

The lymphatic vessels, like the blood vessels, are a system of endothelium-lined tubes that transport cells and fluid. Unlike the blood vessels, the lymph vessels do not form a continuous, closed system. The lymphatic vessels carry their contents, called LYMPH, in only one direction—from connective tissue spaces toward the major lymphatic vessel (the THORACIC DUCT) and then into the venous system. The major function of the lymphatic vessels is to recover fluids that have escaped into the connective tissue spaces from the blood capillaries and venules and return them to the blood.

LYMPH NODES are structures along the path of the collecting lymphatic vessels. Because the cells of the lymph percolate through them, they are a major site of lymphocyte accumulation; it is in the lymph nodes that the exchange of material between blood and lymph occurs. Lymph nodes are surrounded by a CAPSULE (Figure 4). The afferent lymphatic vessels enter the node through the capsule at several sites and leave through a single site at the HILUS, an indentation on one surface. The blood vessels both enter and leave the node at the hilus. Figure 5 shows the organization of the lymph node in diagrammatic form.

Lymphocytes are the major cell type of the lymph node and lie in a fine meshwork called the RETICULUM. In the peripheral CORTEX the lymph nodes are rather tightly packed; toward the hilus they are less dense and form the MEDULLA. At the periphery of the cortex are NODULES, or FOLLICLES, which are clearly discernible concentrations of lymphocytes. PRIMARY NODULES are tightly packed and uniform and may contain a central zone of larger lymphocytes and macrophages. The central zone is called a GERMINAL CENTER. The deep part of the cortex between the nodules and the medulla is called the TERTIARY CORTEX. B cells are found in the primary nodules, and T cells are found in the tertiary cortex.

ORGANIZATION AND STRUCTURE OF LYMPHOID TISSUE

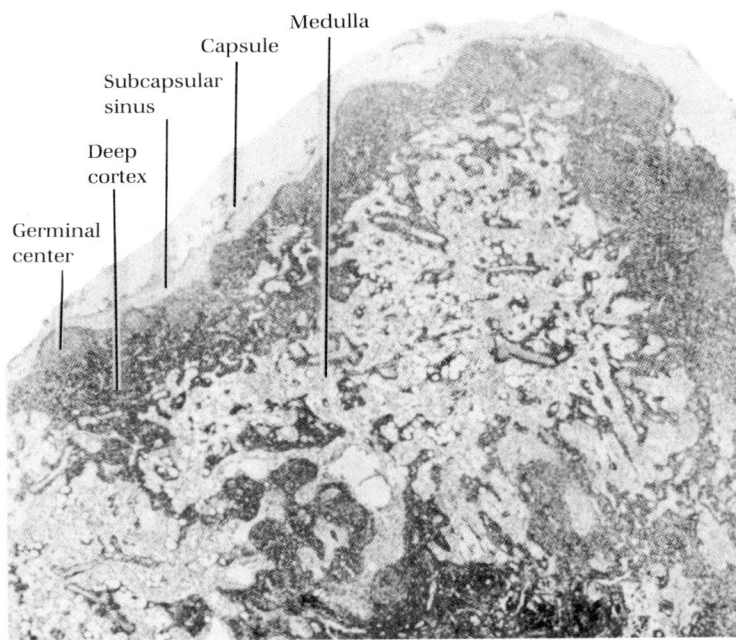

FIGURE 4 HUMAN LYMPH NODE

A portion of a lymph node, showing the capsule, medulla, and cortex. (Giemsa stain, 30×.) [From Weiss (1983), *Histology: Cell and Tissue Biology*]

Circulation of Lymphocytes

As noted earlier, the lymphocytes circulate through the body, passing between the blood and lymphatic vascular systems at the lymph nodes. In the 1960s J. L. Gowans and his co-workers carried out what are now considered classic studies on lymphocyte traffic. In these studies lymphocytes collected from the thoracic duct were labeled with tritiated adenosine and then transfused into normal animals. The fate of the transfused cells was determined by autoradiography at various time periods.

These studies revealed the remarkable fact that recirculating cells enter the lymph nodes from the venous circulation by adhering to and then migrating through a specialized set of postcapillary venules (Figure 6). These specialized vessels are called HIGH ENDOTHELIAL VENULES (HEV), a name that describes the tall, plump shape of their lining cells (Figure 7). Because the emigration from blood into lymph nodes occurs only at HEV and at no other endothelia, it was assumed that lymphocytes have receptors that

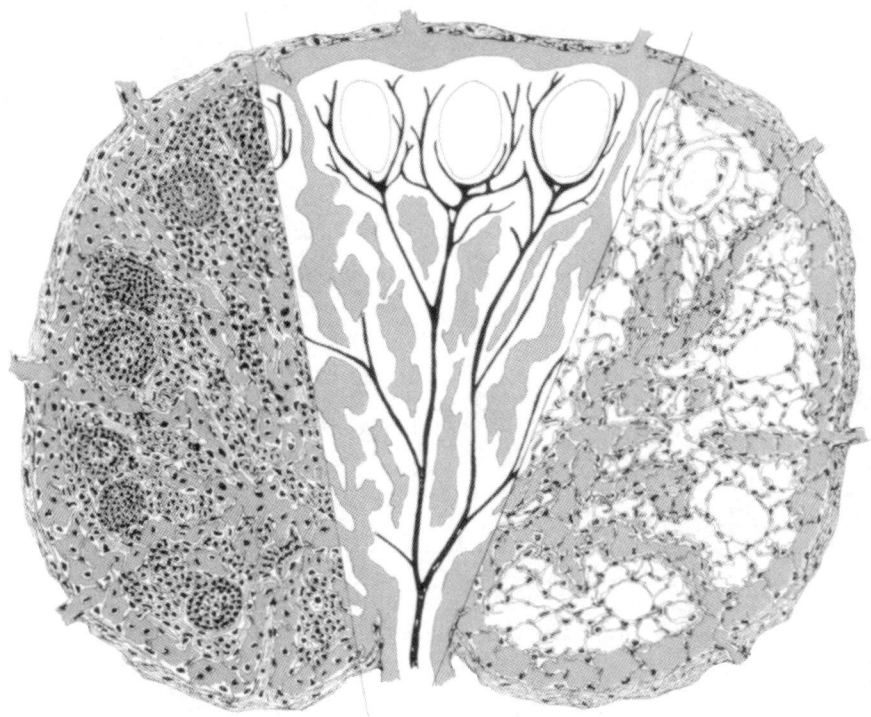

FIGURE 5 LYMPH NODE

Three diagrammatic views of a lymph node. Right: reticular cells; center, distribution of veins; left, distribution of lymphocytes. [From Weiss (1972), *The Cells and Tissues of the Immune System***]**

recognize these structures. Recently a molecule on the surface of virtually all peripheral B and T cells has been identified by Weissman and his colleagues at Stanford; this molecule seems to be the one involved in recogniton of the HEV. It is defined by a monoclonal antibody called MEL-14. The HEV-recognizing molecule is a glycoprotein with a molecular weight of ca. 80,000.

Preincubation of lymphocytes with anti-MEL-14 in the absence of complement inhibits their binding to HEV in the in vitro test system. However, the ability of anti-MEL-14 to block binding to HEV is seen only for cells in the peripheral lymph nodes and not for those in Peyer's patches. Cells that bind to Peyer's patch

ORGANIZATION AND STRUCTURE OF LYMPHOID TISSUE

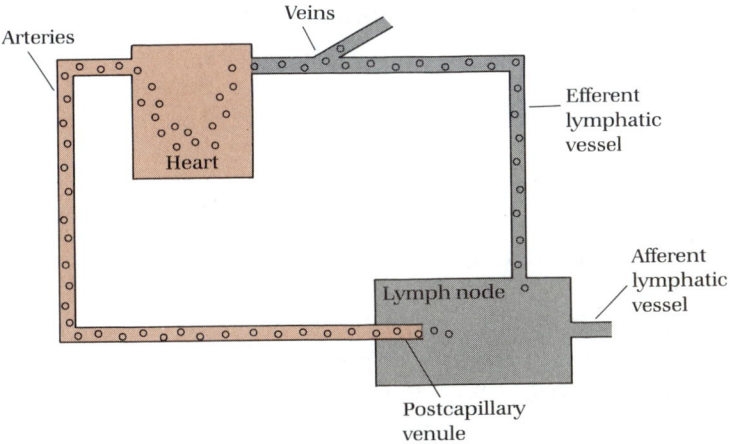

FIGURE 6 PATHWAY OF LYMPHOCYTE RECIRCULATION

Small lymphocytes leave the lymph node via an efferent lymphatic vessel and enter the lymphatic circulation. They enter the blood through the veins, then enter the arterial circulation, to be carried back to the lymphoid tissue. The thymus is the only lymphoid organ not in this route of recirculation.

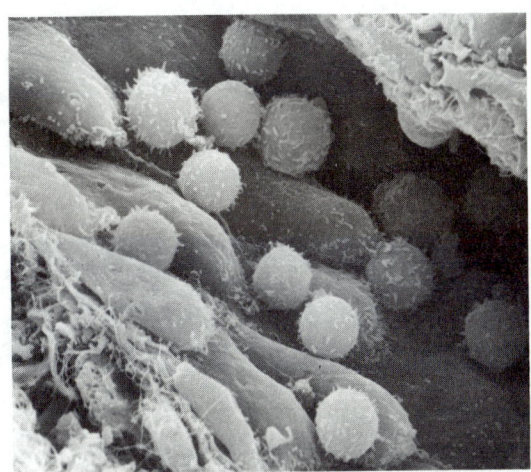

FIGURE 7 HEV IN A MOUSE LYMPH NODE

Scanning electron micrograph showing luminal surface of HEV in a mouse lymph node. Numerous lymphocytes are tightly bound to the plump endothelial cells. [Courtesy of E. C. Butcher and I. L. Weissman]

CHAPTER TWELVE

HEV can be shown to have reacted with the anti-MEL-14 antibody even though they can still bind to the HEV. This argues for the existence of two means of recognition of endothelial surfaces: one in the peripheral nodes and one in the Peyer's patches.

B and T Cell Regions of Lymphoid Organs

After the lymphocytes cross the HEV and enter the lymph node or enter the white pulp of the spleen from the marginal zone, they become segregated into discrete areas. The B cells move to primary follicles in the lymph nodes, while T cells remain diffused throughout the paracortex of the lymph node (Figure 8) and the periarteriole cuff in the spleen.

The reason for this segregation by cell type is not known, but one reason currently being considered is based on the reticular cells found in the two areas. A cell called the INTERDIGITATING CELL (IDC) is found in the T-dependent areas. In contrast, the B cell-rich areas have a reticular cell called the FOLLICULAR DENDRITIC CELL (FDC). It is not known, but has been predicted, that B cells and

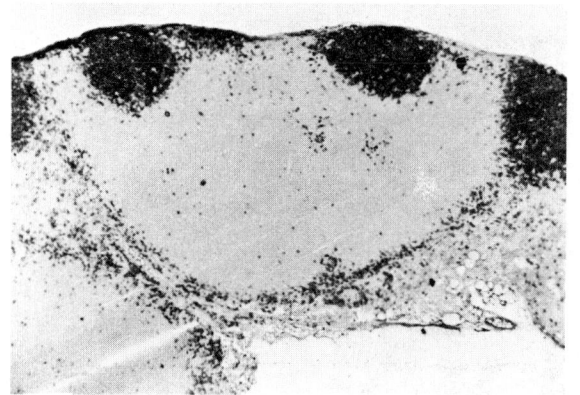 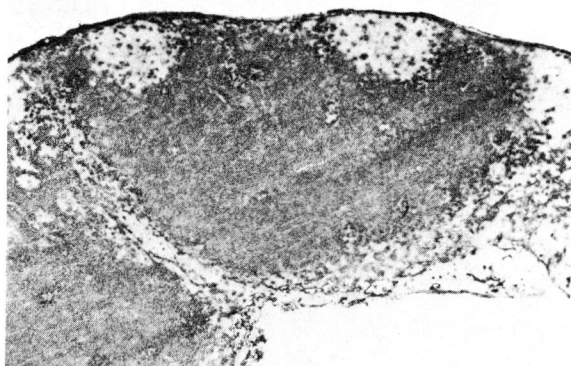

FIGURE 8 SEGREGATION OF B AND T CELLS
Immunoperoxidase staining of frozen sections of an unstimulated mouse lymph node, demonstrating the segregation of B and T lymphocytes into discreet domains. (Left) Anti-IgD reveals the localization of B cells to discrete follicles in the outer cortex. (Right) Anti-Thy 1 staining defines the paracortical T cell region. [Courtesy of R. Reichert]

ORGANIZATION AND STRUCTURE OF LYMPHOID TISSUE

T cells interact preferentially with one or the other of these reticular cells. As we progress through the next chapters, we will be discussing B cell and T cell interactions and will see that many of the advances in cellular immunology have been made using dispersed cultures in vitro. The reader is urged to keep in mind at the end of those chapters that the time may now be right to go back to the animal, or at least to the lymphoid tissue in its actual in situ organization, to determine what happens in the animal.

Summary

1. The thymus is a primary lymphoid organ composed of lymphocytes and epithelial cells. Pre-T cells enter the thymus via the blood and differentiate into thymic lymphocytes (or thymocytes). The thymocytes are found in both the cortex and the medulla.
2. The medullary thymocytes are the "mature" cells and differ from the cortical thymocytes in surface markers and cortisone sensitivity. The medullary cells are the cortisone-resistant thymocytes (CRT), which are the functional cells of the thymus.
3. Lymphocytes circulate between the blood and the lymphatic vascular systems. They leave the venous circulation to enter the lymph nodes through vessels lined with specialized endothelia, called high endothelial venules (HEV). Virtually all circulating B and T cells have a receptor for the HEV; this receptor is defined by a monoclonal antibody called MEL-14.
4. Lymphocytes are distributed in T- and B-dependent areas of the spleen and lymph nodes.

Additional Readings

Gallatin, M., T. P. St. John, M. Siegelman, R. Reichert, E. C. Butcher, and T. L. Weissman. 1986. Lymphocyte homing receptors. *Cell* 44, 673.

Gowans, J. L., and E. J. Knight. 1964. The route of re-circulation of lymphocytes in the rate. *Proc. R. Soc. London B.* 159, 257.

Siegelman, M., M. W. Bond, W. M. Gallatin, T. St. John, H. T. Smith, V. A. Fried, and T. L. Weissman. 1986. Cell surface molecule associated with lymphocyte homing is a ubiquitinated branched-chain glycoprotein. *Science* 231, 823.

Weiss, L. 1972. *The Cells and Tissues of the Immune System.* Prentice Hall, Englewood Cliffs, NJ.

CHAPTER 13
THE MAJOR HISTOCOMPATIBILITY COMPLEX

Overview We will see in the next few chapters that the products of a gene complex called the major histocompatibility complex (MHC) are involved in antigen recognition and cell interactions in the immune response. The MHC was studied for many years by a small group of enthusiasts, but only recently has the significance of the complex to the immune response been recognized. The MHC, which is called H-2 in the mouse and HLA in man, is a multiallelic locus of genes that encode surface molecules; these molecules are involved in virtually every aspect of the immune response.

The genes of the MHC and their products are grouped into three classes. Class I genes encode surface molecules which are found on all cells of the body. Class II encode molecules—the so-called Ia antigens—which are found primarily on cells of the immune system. The class III genes encode a serum protein called the Ss protein and a complement component. The genes for the MHC products have been cloned.

In the mouse there is a gene complex called the T locus, which is on the same chromosome as the MHC. The products of the T locus are thought to be candidates for molecules involved in cell interactions during embryogenesis.

THE MAJOR HISTOCOMPATIBILITY COMPLEX

The Discovery of the Major Histocompatibility Complex

The development of our understanding of the major histocompatibility complex (MHC) is an instructive example of the merging of ideas and discoveries in many areas to produce the view we have at the present time. It is occasionally necessary, when we begin to feel very modern, to look at how we got to where we are today. By this exercise we are reminded that, even though we work at the very edge of the known, we are really part of a continuum of development of scientific thought; today's discoveries are important not only for the solution of the problem as it is formulated today, but also as discoveries that will be used in a very different light further along the continuum.

The study of the MHC grew out of early work in cancer research. When it was realized that the only way to propagate experimental tumors in mice was by using genetically homogeneous inbred strains, geneticists began to develop such strains. Because an inbred strain was either "susceptible" or "resistant" to a given tumor, a genetic theory of tumor susceptibility developed. All of this was happening at the turn of the century when the germ theory of disease was being proved and the role of the immune system in defense against disease was the driving impetus of research. It was natural to link the two by predicting that the genes for resistance encoded structures that were important in immunity. But no immune theory of defense could explain why the tumors grew in the inbred strain in which they arose, because these mice should be able to respond to the tumor.

The great geneticist J. B. S. Haldane in 1933 introduced the contrary notion that the "immunity" was not directed against something unique to the tumor, but instead that normal tissue antigens on the surface of the tumors similar to the blood group antigens Landsteiner had discovered a few years earlier were what determined whether a tumor that arose in one strain would grow in another. In other words, he suggested that the immune response leading to rejection of the tumor would be directed against normal cellular antigens unique to that *strain* rather than against tumor-specific antigens unique to the *tumor*.

CHAPTER THIRTEEN

The testing of this hypothesis led to the search for tissue specific antigens in mice. In the late 1930s Peter Gorer discovered four blood-group antigens using the few inbred strains available at the time. He named these I, II, III and IV. The growth or rejection of a tumor correlated with the expression of antigen II, and he found that C57BL mice that rejected a tumor from A-strain mice developed antibodies that reacted against antigen II on normal cells from strain A. The importance of this work cannot be overstated.

> Gorer's early work established two important facts. First, it demonstrated that the genes for susceptibility to tumor transplants were identical with the genes coding for alloantigens. Second, it provided firm evidence for the immunological nature of resistance to tumor transplants by showing that rejection of a tumor is accompanied by production of alloantibodies. These two discoveries led Gorer to formulate the concept of tissue transplantation. According to Gorer, "normal and neoplastic tissues contain iso-antigenic factors which are genetically determined. Iso-antigenic factors present in the grafted tissue and absent in the host are capable of eliciting a response which results in the destruction of the graft." This immunological theory of transplantation represented one of the major advances in biological sciences of the twentieth century and marked the beginning of the era of transplantation immunology. Curiously, this fact was never formally recognized by prize-awarding committees, which often hailed discoveries of far less significance.
> [J. Klein, *Biology of the Mouse Histocompatibility-2 Complex*, p. 7]

While Gorer was carrying out his work in England, an equally remarkable investigator was examining the relationship between genetics and tumor susceptibility in the United States. George Snell joined the recently organized Jackson Laboratory in Bar Harbor, Maine, in 1935. The director of the laboratory was the great geneticist C. C. Little (called "Prexy" because he had been president of both the University of Michigan and the University of Maine). Snell took advantage of the inbred strains of mice available at Jackson to initiate a study of the formal genetics of the antigens responsible for tissue rejection. In 1948 he coined the term HISTOCOMPATIBILITY ANTIGENS, or H antigens, for these antigens. The genes that coded for the H antigens he termed HISTOCOMPATIBILITY GENES.

THE MAJOR HISTOCOMPATIBILITY COMPLEX

The work Snell had done for his doctorate at Harvard was on linkage analysis in the mouse, and he applied that approach to the transplantation problem. One of his more important contributions was the production of congenic mice (which will be discussed later). Using these mice, which differed only at the H locus, he found that the H genes were linked to a gene called *fused tail* (*Fu*) and that the gene coding for Gorer's antigen II was also linked to *Fu*.

Gorer and Snell began a lifelong friendship and collaboration in which Gorer spent his summers at the Jackson Lab (a tradition that many scientists have continued over the years). When they realized that the two systems were the same they combined the names, calling the antigens which were responsible for graft rejection H-2. This work was awarded the Nobel prize in 1980. Unfortunately, Peter Gorer died in 1961 and could not share the prize, but his contributions are known and appreciated by all biologists interested in this area of work.[1]

Traits Controlled by the Major Histocompatibility Complex

We noted earlier that the original reason for studying the major histocompatibility complex (MHC) of both mouse and human was its clinical application to tumor growth and then graft rejection. But graft rejection is just one aspect of the response of the host to MHC antigens on foreign tissues. Graft rejection is a cell-mediated response brought about by effector T cells (Section II). Because, as we will see later, graft rejection is the archetypical cell-mediated response, the MHC antigens have been extensively studied as a means of understanding the mechanisms of cell-mediated responses.

As might be expected, the introduction of foreign tissue into a host also results in the production of antibodies against the MHC antigens. Of the two responses, the cell-mediated response is much more significant. The antigens that induce antibody forma-

---

[1] A fairly detailed and highly readable history of the MHC can be found in J. Klein (1975), *Biology of the Mouse Histocompatibility-2 Complex: Principles of Immunogenetics Applied to a Single System*, pp. 3–15.

CHAPTER THIRTEEN

tion are called SEROLOGICAL ANTIGENS, and the antigens involved in cell-mediated responses are called TRANSPLANTATION ANTIGENS.

During the course of research on the MHC, it gradually became clear that many other aspects of the immune response were also controlled by genes within the MHC. The traits controlled by the genes of the MHC are given in Table 1. What will become clear in Section II is that the traits with which the MHC is involved affect the entire range of the immune response.

The MHC is a large gene complex, consisting of 1.5 recombination units in the mouse and 2 recombination units in humans. On the basis of the genetic data, the MHC region should be several million base pairs long, but we are not certain of this fact because in the mouse suppression of recombination occurs between H-2 and another multigene locus called the T locus, which is also located on chromosome 17.

TABLE 1 Traits controlled by the MHC in the mouse.

	Region					
		I				
Trait	K	A	E	J	S	D
Serological antigens	++	++	++	+	++	++
Transplantation antigens	++	+	+	−	−	++
Cell-mediated lympholysis	++	+	+	?	−	++
Mixed lymphocyte reaction	±	++	±±	+	−	±
Control of immune response	±	++	++	?	−	±
T–B interaction	−	++	++	?	−	−
MHC restriction, T_C	+	−	−	−	−	+
MHC restriction, T_H	−	+	+	?	−	−
Suppressor cells	−	−	−	+	−	−
Complement activity	−	−	−	−	+	−

Key: ▢ Class I   ▨ Class II   ▨ Class III

THE MAJOR HISTOCOMPATIBILITY COMPLEX

Mapping the MHC Genes by Function and Gene Product

There is an appropriate assay for each of the traits in Table 1; thus the genetics of each of the functions can be worked out. When the genes controlling these traits are mapped by standard genetic methods, it is found that they are all located as a gene complex on chromosome 17 in the mouse and on chromosome 6 in humans. The order of the genes as mapped by their *function* is seen in Figure 1. The various traits can be mapped to *regions* which were originally called K, I, S, and D. Later it was found that the I region had several *subregions* called A, B, J, E, and C, and that there was a region called L adjacent to the D region. The Tla region for many years had been considered not to be a part of the MHC proper, but it is of increasing importance in the immune response and now is always considered along with the MHC.

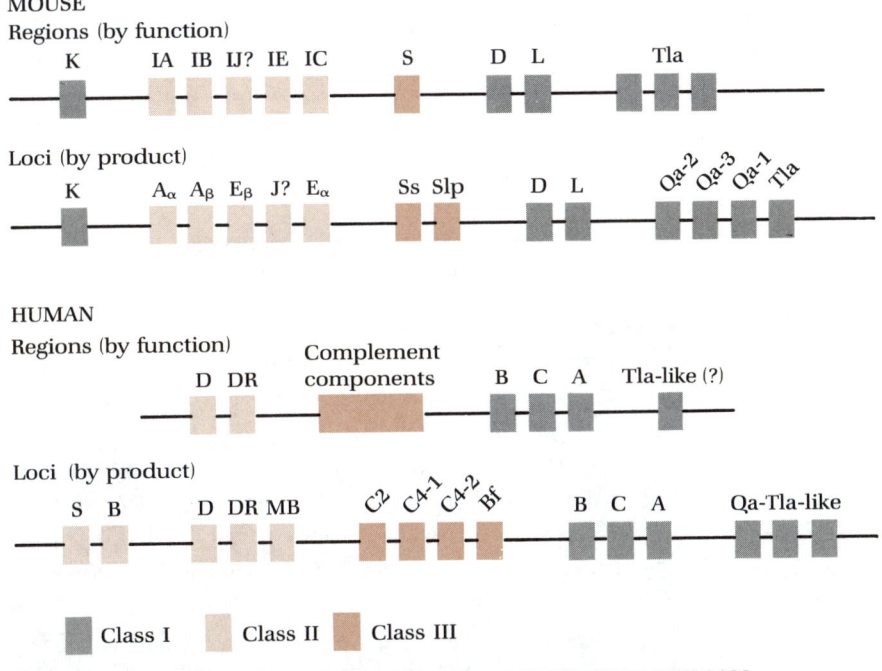

FIGURE 1   MHC REGIONS AND LOCI OF MOUSE AND HUMAN

CHAPTER THIRTEEN

The MHC genes are divided into three classes. CLASS I GENES encode cell surface transplantation antigens and serological antigens. CLASS II GENES encode a series of antigens, called Ia antigens, that are expressed primarily on lymphocytes. Class II genes also control the level of the response to some antigens. For this reason they are also called *Ir* (immune response) genes. CLASS III GENES control the expression of some components of the complement system.[2]

Figure 1 also shows the gene map of the MHC, as determined by an analysis of the gene products. The differences between the genetic map by *function* and by *product* is most striking in the I region. Recall that the only way to map a gene by function is to isolate a mutant with an altered function so that mating studies can be carried out. Map distances in these cases are really a reflection of the frequency of recombination of genes. By this method it was found that there are five subregions of I. When another approach was used—isolation and analysis of molecules from cells—it was found that only products for the IA and IE subregions could be found. There is still some controversy about IJ (note the question mark in the figure), which we will discuss later in this chapter.

Polymorphism of the Major Histocompatibility Complex

MHC, Multigenic and Multiallelic

As work progressed on the MHC and as details of its organization and wide-ranging functions became known, some investigators argued that this may be the major system by which individuals distinguish *self* from *nonself*—one of the more profound problems in biology. Any system allowing an individual of the species to distinguish its tissues from the tissues of other members must be highly polymorphic; that is, there must be many forms of the antigens dis-

---

[2] The MHC is being introduced at this point in the book, in part because an understanding of the Class I and Class II molecules are needed to understand the cellular events in the immune response, which will be discussed in Section II. For that reason we will focus on these structures and not discuss the Class III genes or products.

THE MAJOR HISTOCOMPATIBILITY COMPLEX

tributed among the various individual members of the population. The MHC is, in fact, one of the most highly polymorphic gene complexes known. Indeed, it is both *multiallelic* and *multigenic*.

Each of the genes in Figure 1 has several allelic forms (i.e., every member of the species has the gene, but different members have different forms of the gene), and a brief glance at the Information Boxes shows that polymorphism in the MHC is extremely high. Some genes exhibit greater polymorphism than others; for example, in the mouse there are more than 50 alleles of the Class I antigens K and D, whereas Qa-2, also a Class I antigen in the Tla region, has only a few alleles.

It has been argued that the polymorphism of the I region (Class II molecules) and of the K, D, and L molecules (Class I molecules) must reflect selective pressure for those molecules. It will be seen as we go along that K, D, and L molecules function as recognition molecules in cytotoxic lymphocyte responses and

---

INFORMATION BOX 1

Class I Determinants of Some Commonly Used Mouse Strains

Each haplotype has public and private K and D determinants. Several strains may share a public determinant, but private determinants are unique to each strain.

H-2 haplotype	Public K determinants[a]																Private K determinant	Public D determinants												Private D determinant
	1	3	5	8	11	25	34	35	36	37	38	39	42	45	46	47		1	3	5	6	13	35	36	41	42	43	44	49	
b	−	−	+	−	−	−	+	+	−	−	+	−	−	+	−	−	33	−	−	−	+	−	−	−	−	−	−	−	−	2
d	−	+	−	+	−	+	−	−	−	−	−	−	−	−	+	+	31	−	+	−	+	+	+	+	+	+	+	+	−	4
k	+	+	+	+	+	−	−	−	−	−	−	−	−	+	−	+	23	+	+	+	−	−	−	−	−	−	−	−	+	32
q	+	+	+	−	+	−	+	−	−	−	−	−	−	+	−	−	17	−	+	−	+	+	+	+	−	−	−	−	+	30
s	+	−	+	−	−	−	−	−	−	−	−	+	+	−	−	−	19	−	+	−	+	−	+	+	−	+	−	−	+	12

[a] +, presence of determinant; −, absence of determinant.

that the I region molecules act in the regulation of lymphocyte function. Polymorphism in these genes serves to increase the range of responses that the individual can mount. The absence of polymorphism in the Class I molecules of the Tla region and in the complement components (Class III molecules) must, by similar reasoning, reflect a need for conservation of these products.

The Notion of the Haplotype

The combination of all of the alleles and loci within the complex is called the HAPLOTYPE. In the mouse the H-2 haplotype is denoted by a superscript, for example, $H-2^d$. This shorthand indicates the allelic form of each of the several genes in the MHC of that strain. In this case, all of the alleles are called d. There are several mouse strains that have been termed TYPE STRAINS and serve as the arbitrarily chosen prototype for the haplotype. Some H-2 haplotypes of common strains are given in Table 2. Note that several strains can have the same H-2 haplotype. In other words, the allelic forms of all the H-2 genes in those strains are the same. But A and B10.A, for example, are different strains because their alleles for other genes are different.[3] Table 2 also shows that some strains are recombinants of two haplotypes; for example, strain A is a recombinant of the $H-2^k$ and the $H-2^d$ haplotypes.

Public and Private Specificities

A given haplotype has unique, serologically defined antigens, called PRIVATE SPECIFICITIES. Each haplotype has a private specificity, or determinant, that is unique to the haplotype. For example, all $H-2^k$ mice have the same serologically defined antigens (numbers 23 and 32). There are many strains of mice with the $H-2^k$ haplotype, and they all contain these private specificity determinants.

In addition to the private specificities, there is a set of serologically defined antigens called PUBLIC SPECIFICITIES, or public determinants. These antigens are not restricted to a given haplotype; one strain may have several of them, whereas another strain may have some of these as well as an array of other specificities.

---

[3] As we go along it will seem to the reader that there are, in fact, no other genes than those that encode immunoglobulins and MHC. The reader should rest assured that there are many other genes known in both mouse and human, and some of them are even of some importance.

THE MAJOR HISTOCOMPATIBILITY COMPLEX

TABLE 2   H-2 haplotypes of commonly used mouse strains and congenics.

H-2 haplotype	Alleles present in MHC regions					Strains with haplotype
	K	IA	IE	S	D	
$H\text{-}2^a$	k	k	d	d	d	A B10.A
$H\text{-}2^b$	b	b	b	b	b	B10 C57BL/6
$H\text{-}2^d$	d	d	d	d	d	DBA/2 BALB/c B10.D2
$H\text{-}2^k$	k	k	k	k	k	C3H CBA B10.BR

For example, some strains with the $H\text{-}2^k$ haplotype have antigen specificity 3, but this antigen is shared by virtually all haplotypes; it is therefore a public specificity antigen.

Selected H-2 and HLA determinants are given in Information Boxes 1, 2, and 3.

INFORMATION BOX 2

Class II Determinants of Some Commonly Used Mouse Strains

H-2 haplotype	A molecule determinants[a]																				E molecule determinants			
	1	2	3	4	5	6	8	9	10	11	12	13	14	15	16	17	18	19	20	24	7	21	22	23
b	−	−	+	−	−	+	+	−	−	−	−	−	+	−	−	−	+	−	−	−	−	−	−	−
d	−	−	−	−	+	+	−	−	+	−	−	+	−	−	−	−	+	−	+	−	+	−	−	+
k	+	−	+	−	−	−	−	−	−	−	−	−	−	+	−	+	+	+	−	−	+	−	+	−
q	−	−	+	−	+	−	−	+	+	−	−	+	−	−	+	−	−	−	−	−	−	−	−	−
s	−	−	−	+	+	−	−	+	−	−	+	−	−	−	−	+	+	−	−	+	−	−	−	−

[a]+, presence of determinant; −, absence of determinant.

INFORMATION BOX 3

New and Old Nomenclature for Human Lymphocyte Antigens

	New	Old		New	Old
HLA-A	A1	A1	HLA-B	B5	A5
	A2	A2		B7	A7
	A3	A3		B8	A8
	A9	A9		B12	A12
	A10	A10		B13	A13
	A11	A11		B14	W14
	Aw19			B15	W15
	Aw23	W23		Bw16	W16
	Aw24	W24		B17	W17
	A25	W25		B18	W18
	A26	W26		Bw21	W21
	A28	W28		Bw22	W22
	A29	W29		27	W27
	Aw30	W30		Bw35	W5
	Aw31	W31		B37	Bw37, TY
	Aw32	W32		Bw38	W16.1
	Aw33	W19.6		Bw39	W16.2
	Aw34	MALAY 2		B40	Bw40, W10
	Aw36	MO		Bw41	SABELL
	Aw43	BK		Bw42	MWA
				Bw44	B12 non-TT
				Bw45	TT$^+$
				Bw46	HS, SIN 2
				Bw47	407$^+$, MO66, CAS, Bw40C
				Bw48	KSO, JA, Bw40.3
				Bw49	Bw21.1, SL-ET

THE MAJOR HISTOCOMPATIBILITY COMPLEX

INFORMATION BOX 3

	New	Old		New	Old
	Bw50	Bw21.2, ET	HLA-D	Dw1	LD 101
	Bw51	B5.1		Dw2	LD 102
	Bw52	B5.2		Dw3	LD 103
	Bw53	HR		Cw4	LD 104
	Bw54	Bw22J, SAP 1, J1		Dw5	LD 105
	Bw55	W55, 21.1		Dw6	LD 106
	Bw56	W56, 22.2, Te92, Da30		Dw7	LD 107
	Bw57	W67, 17.1, 17A, 17 long		Dw8	LD 108
	Bw58	W68, 17.2, 17B, 17 short		Dw9	TB9, OH
	Bw59	W69, HOK-1, 8.2		Dw10	LD 16
	Bw60	W60, 40.1		Dw11	LD 17
	Bw61	W61, 40.2		Dw12	DB4, DHO
	Bw62	W64, 15.1-TO53, 15B, Te72		DRw1	LB1
	Bw63	W65, 15.2-TO52, 15A, Te71		DRw2	LB2
	Bw4	W4, 4a		DRw3	LB3
	Bw6	W6, 4b		DRw4	LB4
				DRw5	LB5
				DRw6	LB6
HLA-C	Cw1	T1		DRw7	LB7
	Cw2	T2		DRw8	WIAS
	Cw3	T3		DRw9	WIA4x7
	Cw4	T4		DRw10	ST-1, LTM
	Cw5	T5			
	Cw6	T7			
	Cw7	CVE, TOK			
	Cw8	T8, T9			

Source: Compiled at the Eighth International Histocompatibility Workshop (1980).

CHAPTER THIRTEEN

Congenic Mice

For experimental purposes, it is essential to have mice that differ in only one allele of the MHC. When mice differ at one locus but are the same at all other genetic loci, they are called CONGENIC. An example of congenic mice would be B10 mice that have different H-2 haplotypes or even different alleles of one of the genes but are identical at all other loci.

For example, suppose we wanted to test the role of the H-2 complex on some aspect of the immune response. We would need mice that differ *only* at H-2 and not at any background genes—that is, mice with identical background genes but different H-2 genes.[4] This arrangement would allow us to compare the response of B10 mice, which are H-2^b, with the response of mice with some other haplotype, say H-2^a. If there were a difference in the response being tested it could be attributed to a difference in H-2 genes and not to a difference in background genes. The mice that have B10 background genes and H-2^a genes would be congenic for H-2.

Congenic strains are designated by the background strain, a dot and then the donor of the differing gene. In the example used above, the background strain is B10. If the donor of the H-2^a genes is strain A, then the congenic is designated B10.A (the term is spoken "B10 dot A"). It is essential not to confuse this notation with the designation of an F_1, which shows both strains within parentheses. An F_1 of B10 and A would be $(B10 \times A)F_1$.

Production of Congenic Mice

The production of mice that differ at only one specified gene requires some fancy genetic footwork. The genetic method of constructing congenic mice was worked out by George Snell. Suppose we have two strains, X and Y. A certain tumor is accepted (will grow) when injected into strain X but will be rejected (will not grow) by strain Y. The object is to introduce the genes of strain Y (the ability to reject this tumor) onto the genetic background of strain X so that we end up with an X.Y mouse in which the only Y trait present is the ability to reject the tumor.

---

[4] In the chauvinistic jargon of the MHC crowd, all genes in the mouse that are not MHC genes are referred to as "background."

THE MAJOR HISTOCOMPATIBILITY COMPLEX

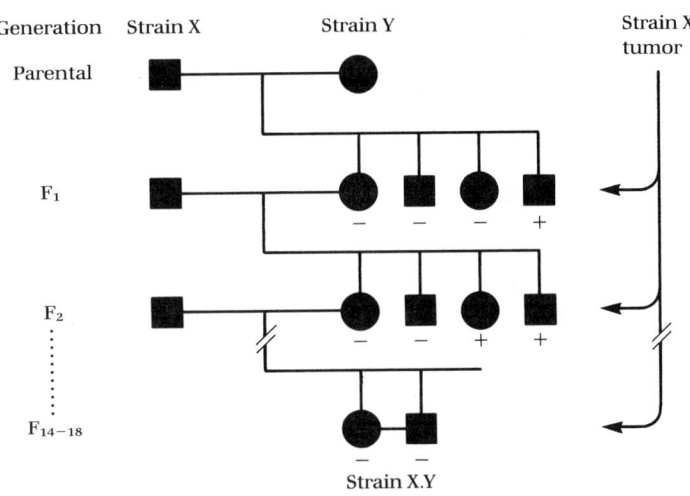

FIGURE 2 PRODUCTION OF CONGENIC MICE

Strains X and Y are mated and some F1 progeny are backcrossed to X. At each generation only the Y animals that express the desired trait are backcrossed to X.

The genetics involved are diagrammed in Figure 2. The procedure involves crossing an animal with the ability to reject the tumor (in this case, strain Y) with a member of the strain that does not (strain X). The offspring will have genes from both X and Y, so they must be screened to determine which animals have the ability to reject the tumor (i.e., are expressing the trait of Y). These animals are then backcrossed to X, and the offspring of this F_2 generation are screened for the ability to reject the tumor. It is clear that in the backcross to X the Y genes have been diluted, but the mice are screened for only a single trait of Y. So even though the general gene contribution of Y is reduced, the gene for tumor rejection has been enriched. Those animals that are able to reject the tumor are once again backcrossed to strain X and the offspring again screened for the Y trait. With each backcross there is further dilution of the Y genes, except for the genes determining the trait being selected. In contrast, there is a progressive enrichment of the X background genes. Somewhere around the fifteenth backcross generation the dilution is almost complete, and the result is a strain that has background genes of strain X and graft rejection genes of strain Y; the new strain is now an X.Y congenic.

The example above is a scientific one, but an intuitive example may be of some use. Suppose you decide to systematically determine the amount of vermouth you want in your martini. You could start by adding to a chilled glass one jigger of vermouth, one jigger of gin, and an olive. After sipping it, you decide it should be drier, so you discard half the martini (retaining the olive) and add an equal volume of gin. Another sip tells you that this is still not dry enough, so you discard half the martini, retain the olive, and add an equal volume of gin. Another sip, another discard (not the olive, though) and another addition of equal volume follow. If you do this ten times you will have a chilled glass that contains over 99 percent gin and the olive. Consider the gin to be the background and the olive to be the desired gene, and you have the notion of a congenic mouse.[5]

Structure of MHC Molecules

Class I Molecules — The antigens encoded by the Class I genes are the classic transplantation antigens involved in graft rejection and the serological antigens that induce antibody formation. Class I antigens are found on all cells of the body in various concentrations.

The Class I antigens are composed of two chains, a variable chain called the α CHAIN and an invariant chain called β_2-MICROGLOBULIN (Figure 3). The α chain has a molecular weight of 45,000 and β_2-microglobulin has a molecular weight of 12,000. The β_2-microglobulin is noncovalently linked to the α chain. The antigenic specificity of the Class I molecules is in the α chain, so it is responsible for the allelic variation. All individuals of the species have the same β_2-microglobulin, no matter what their MHC haplotype.

The α chain of the Class I molecules is composed of five distinct domains. There are three EXTERNAL DOMAINS (termed α1, α2, and α3, each of approximately 90 residues); a TRANSMEMBRANE

---

[5] I thank Jan Klein for this instructive illustration.

THE MAJOR HISTOCOMPATIBILITY COMPLEX

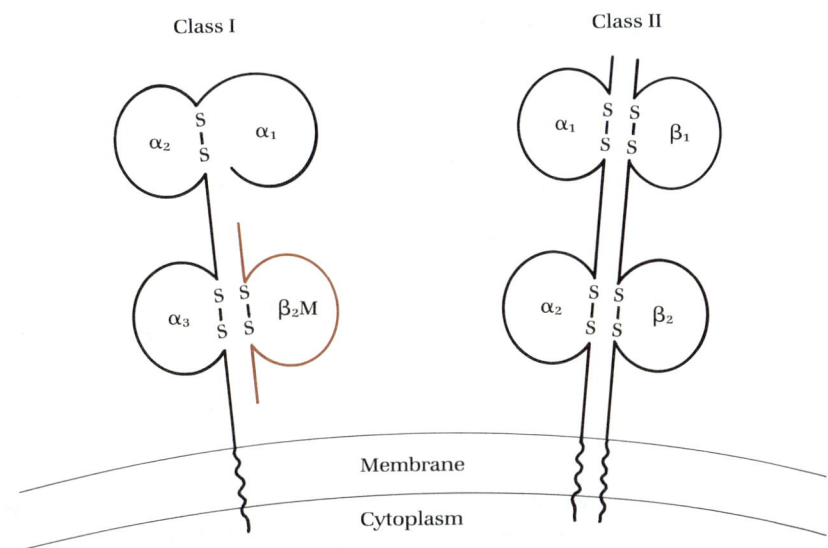

FIGURE 3 STRUCTURE OF CLASS I AND CLASS II MHC MOLECULES
In Class I the α chain is variable but β_2-microglobulin is invariant. In Class II both α and β chains are variable.

DOMAIN of 43 residues; and a CYTOPLASMIC DOMAIN. β_2-microglobulin associates with the α chain at the α3 domain.

Class II Molecules The Class II molecules of the mouse have proved very interesting. By genetic analysis there are five subregions of the I region (Figure 1), but the gene products of only three of them—A, E, and J—can be identified. The IB and IC genes regulate the level of immune responses toward certain antigens but do not code for cell surface antigens. IJ, on the other hand, is associated with suppressor function and codes for a serologically identifiable molecule; but, as we will see below, there is some controversy about the location of the gene. The structure of Class II molecules is shown in Figure 3.

Class II molecules are found on a limited array of cells, all of which are associated with the hemopoietic system (Chapter 10). This distribution is of very great importance in cell–cell interactions in the immune response (Chapters 14–18).

CHAPTER THIRTEEN

Class II molecules are composed of two chains, called α and β. Unlike Class I molecules, in which the β_2-microglobulin chain is invariant, Class II molecules have two variant chains. The α chain has a molecular weight of 33,000–35,000 and the β chain has a molecular weight of 28,000–30,000.

Organization of the MHC Genes

Several Class I and Class II genes have been cloned and sequenced. The exon–intron relationship of MHC genes is shown in Figure 4. Note the precise correlation between the exons and the domains of the molecules discussed above.

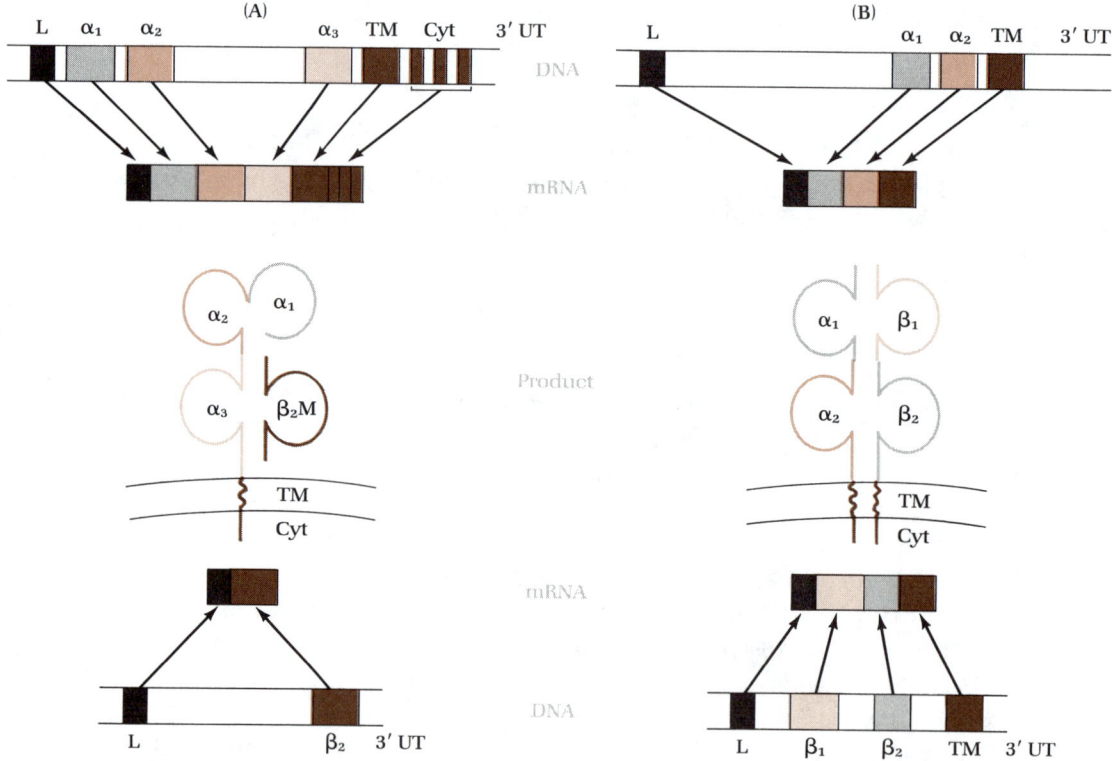

FIGURE 4   ORGANIZATION OF MHC GENES
The exons encoding the domains are shown. TM = Transmembrane; Cyt = cytoplasmic. (A) Class I molecules and β_2-microglobulin. (B) Class II molecules.

THE MAJOR HISTOCOMPATIBILITY COMPLEX

The features of Class I genes resemble those of other eukaryotic genes. For example, the upstream and downstream intron boundaries have GT/AG nucleotides that are important in RNA signal splicing. Sequences characteristic of promoter regions are also present. The sequenced Class IIE$_\alpha$ genes have a single exon for the transmembrane and cytoplasmic exons. The sequenced human DR$_\alpha$ gene has the same exon–intron relationship as the mouse E$_\alpha$ gene.

Probes from various regions of a 230-kb clone of I region DNA have been prepared and used to do a "chromosome walk" of the I region. The A$_\alpha$, A$_\beta$, and E$_\beta$ genes were found to be encoded in the IA region of the genetic map. E$_\alpha$ was in the IE subregion. The IA and IE subregions, however, are separated by only 3.4 kb of DNA, leaving no room for IB and IJ genes. Part of this paradox can be explained by the suggestion that the IB subregion is due to complementation between the IA and IE subregions. IB, it will be recalled, does not code for a known peptide.

There are, however, known peptide products of IJ. These peptides are associated with soluble suppressor factors (Chapter 23) and require much more than 3.4 kb of DNA. A possible explanation for this "IJ paradox" may be that the IJ product is due to complementation between two genes. One of the genes is on chromosome 17 in the H-2 region (probably IE) and the other, termed Jt, is on chromosome 4.

Recombinant Class I–Class II Molecules

It has been possible, using the methods of gene splicing and cloning, to construct a gene that is a recombinant of a Class I and a Class II gene (Figure 5). A portion of the gene for the β chain of IA^k (A$_\beta^k$) and a portion of the gene for H-2D^d starting at DC2 were joined and transfected into an L cell. The gene consists of the leader and β1 domains of IA covalently linked to exons encoding the C2, transmembrane, and cytoplasmic domains of D^d. The chimeric molecule expressed has a molecular weight of 30,000–40,000 and two external domains (Figure 5). The outermost domain is Class II (A$_\beta^k$), and the domain closest to the membrane is Class I (D^d). The hybrid molecule is precipitated with monoclonal antibodies to either IA^k or H-2D^d.

The cell lines that express these hybrid MHC molecules are

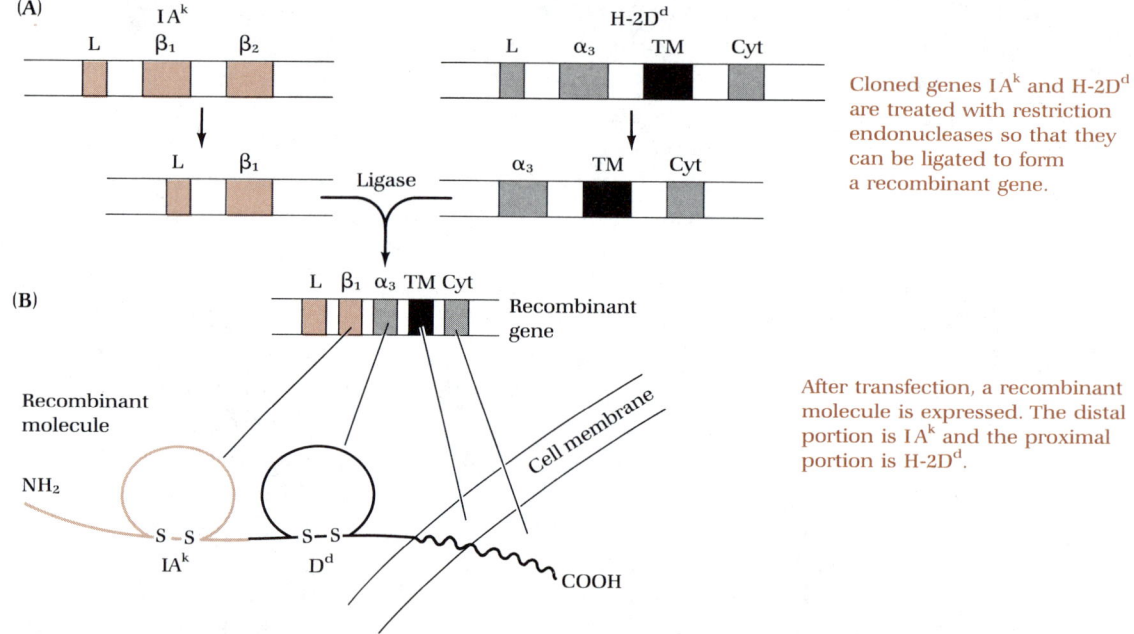

FIGURE 5 CONSTRUCTION OF A RECOMBINANT CLASS I/CLASS II GENE AND MOLECULE

(A) The cloned Class I and Class II genes are clipped in a manner that will allow them to be joined by a ligase. (B) The recombined gene encodes a hybrid molecule that is a Class I protein at the NH terminus but has a C terminus containing the cytoplasmic, transmembrane, and a proximal half of a Class II molecule. [After McClusky, Germain, and Margulies (1985) *Cell* **40**, 247]

now being used to determine the role of the various portions of the molecule in cell-mediated responses (Section II).

Expression of MHC Molecules

The expression of Class I molecules is coordinately controlled with β_2-microglobulin, which is on chromosome 2. A human Burkitt lymphoma cell line called Daudi, for example, does not express HLA-A, HLA-B, or HLA-C, even though there are normal amounts of mRNA for the α chains from these regions in the cytoplasm. There is, however, no β_2-microglobulin protein or its

THE MAJOR HISTOCOMPATIBILITY COMPLEX

mRNA. Similarly, the embryonic tumor ECC lines do not express Class I antigens and also have no β_2-microglobulin. Thus, in some manner the expression of H-2 molecules depends upon the expression of β_2-microglobulin.

The expression of the two chains of Class II molecules is also coordinately controlled. Some haplotypes, such as H-2^b, do not express IE because they have defective promoter regions for E_β, even though they have normal cytoplasmic levels of E_α. In normal cells the α and β chains are noncovalently associated with a 31,000-dalton invariant chain called Ii, which plays some role (though not a crucial one) in transporting the complex to the cell surface. Ii is present in these mice, which do not express IE, suggesting that the major coordinate control is at the α–β chain complex level rather than at Ii.

The Immunoglobulin Superfamily

Sequence Homology between MHC, Immunoglobulin, and Thy 1

Figure 6 is a diagrammatic representation of four molecular structures involved in the immune response: Class I and II MHC molecules; the immunoglobulin molecule; and Thy 1, a T cell differentiation antigen that was

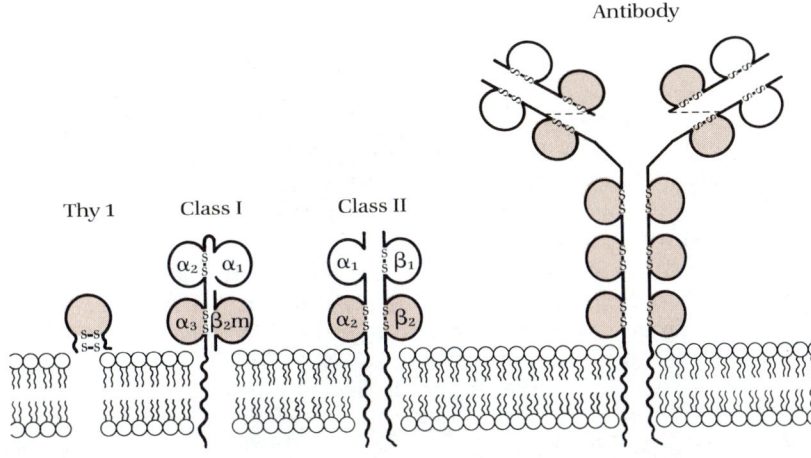

FIGURE 6 IMMUNOGLOBULIN SUPERFAMILY

The colored areas display sequence homology and are thought to have a common evolutionary ancestry. [From Hood, Steinmetz, and Malissen (1983) *Annu. Rev. Immunol.* **1, 529]**

CHAPTER THIRTEEN

discussed in Chapter 11. The similarity in the chain structures of the four molecules is rather striking. Furthermore, the DNA sequences of the exons of Class I$_{\alpha 3}$, Class II$_{\alpha 2}$, Class II$_{\beta 2}$, and β_2-microglobulin are homologous to the exon sequences encoding antibody-molecule constant regions. There is also homology in protein sequences with Thy 1. The homology between the structures is seen in the shaded areas of Figure 6. We saw in Chapter 11 that T cell differentiation antigens T4 and T8 also fall into this family.

All of this homology among molecules functioning in the immune system has led to the speculation that the structures may have arisen from a common molecule which has undergone divergent evolution. These homologous molecules constitute the IMMUNOGLOBULIN SUPERFAMILY.[6]

The T Locus

The T LOCUS is a cluster of genes located, like H-2, on chromosome 17 of the mouse. It is an interesting locus because it may play a role in cell recognition in the embryo and thus may be an embryonic counterpart of H-2. The locus has a fascinating history, described here by Dorothea Bennett, one of the leaders in T locus research.

> The study of mutant genes at the T locus in the mouse had an inauspicious beginning more than 50 years ago, when Nelly Dobrovolskaia-Zavadskaia, a Russian cancer researcher interested in radiation biology, made an unwanted discovery. A mouse she had treated with X-rays produced some progeny with short tails, and although she looked on this as a diversion from more important things, Dobrovolskaia-Zavadskaia nevertheless felt obligated to define the abnormality she had produced. First she demonstrated by breeding tests that the short-tailed animals carried a dominant mutation that she named Brachyury but was later symbolized by T, for tail, in English. In further experiments she found it impossible to obtain a true-

---

[6] Because the Thy 1 antigen is also found in brain—even brain of animals that have not yet evolved an immune system—Av Michison has suggested that the family be called the "Thy 1 superfamily." This name would suggest that the gene conserved and used in many facets of the immune response developed first as a brain antigen.

THE MAJOR HISTOCOMPATIBILITY COMPLEX

INFORMATION BOX 4

Control of Immune Responses by Ir Genes

The responses that mice make to some antigens is under the control of Class II genes, which are called Ir genes for this reason. The figure shows the responses of various haplotypes to a variety of antigens.

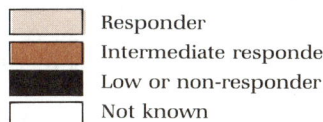

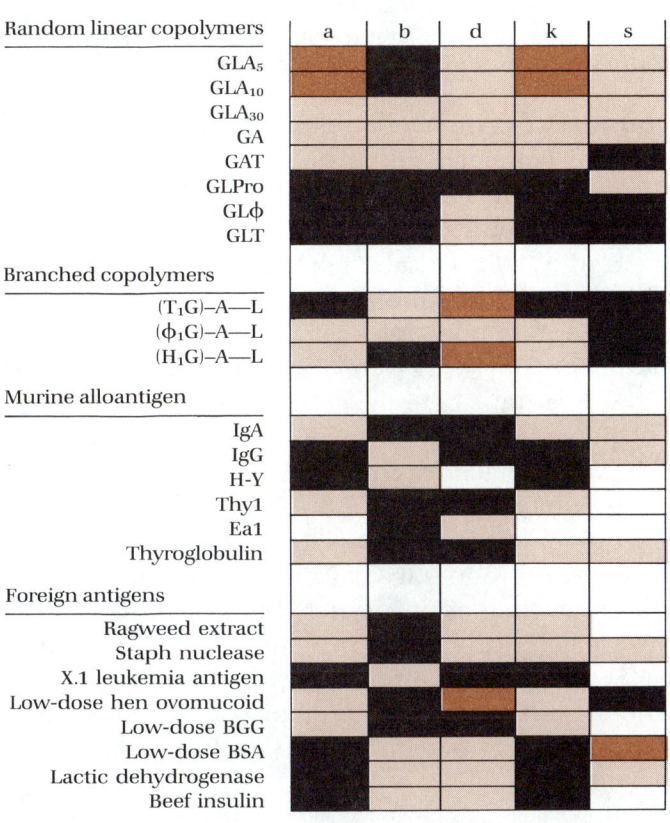

CHAPTER THIRTEEN

> breeding line of short-tailed mice, and so she came to the correct conclusion that homozygotes for the new mutation died before birth. Eventually, she made the mistake of outcrossing short-tailed animals to two unrelated lines of apparently normal mice; one was a French strain of uncertain origin, and one was derived from a wild mouse trapped by Dobrovolskaia (who was by this time apparently a dedicated mouse fancier) while she was on vacation near the Spanish border. To her surprise, some offspring of both these crosses had a sharply different abnormality: they had no tails at all. The logical next step was to inbreed the tailless offspring from each cross; this was done, and the results were completely perplexing to the cancer researcher because this time the abnormal phenotype clearly bred true, and two tailless parents produced only tailless offspring. At this point, Dobrovolskaia threw in the sponge. She visited the laboratory of L. C. Dunn at Columbia University and apparently pleaded with him to take over her animals.
> [D. Bennett (1980), *Harvey Lectures* 74, 1.]

Dunn and his students were able to show that the tailless mice constituted a "balanced lethal" system in which both homozygous classes die and heterozygotes breed true. Mutations at t are lethal in homozygotes because they result in pathology and embryonic death. The lethals fall into eight complementation groups, each with a unique pathology at a different time in embryonic development (Figure 7).

Bennett and Boyse in New York were able to show that the sperm from t mutant heterozygotes had antigens which defined several of the complementation groups. The t antigens, like H-2, have multiple specificities, some of which are common and some of which are unique (similar to public and private specificities in H-2). The unique antigens seem to be associated with the lethal factor and the common ones with the tail abnormality.

Research on the t antigens and their role as cell surface differentiation antigens (Chapter 11), which are important in embryogenesis, is a very active and important area of work at the moment. The introduction of gene cloning and molecular probes is proving to be a very powerful tool in understanding this fascinating gene complex.

THE MAJOR HISTOCOMPATIBILITY COMPLEX

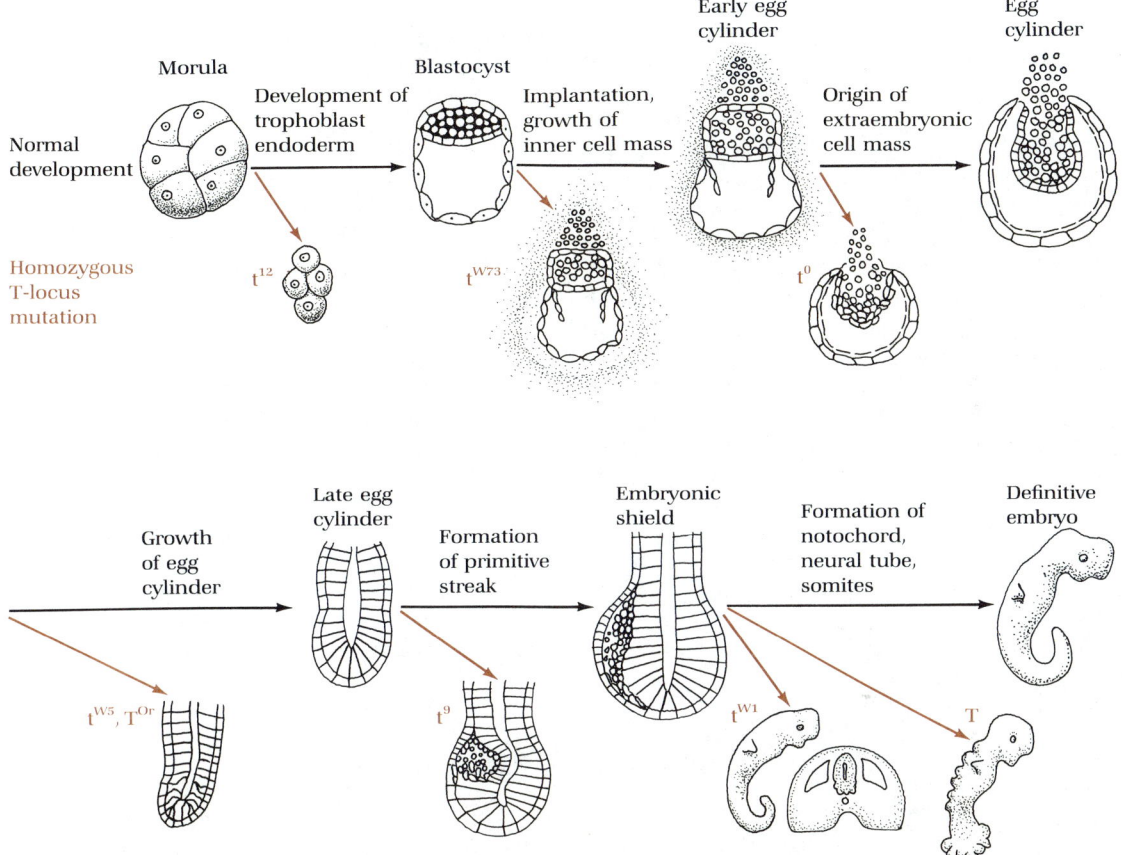

FIGURE 7   PATHOLOGY OF T-COMPLEX MUTATIONS IN THE MOUSE

Along with the H-2 gene complex, chromosome 17 in the mouse carries the T locus, whose products are thought to control numerous cell–cell recognition events in the developing embryo. In the homozygous state, various T locus mutations are lethal at the stage of development indicated in the lower diagrams. For example, in an embryo homozygous for the earliest acting mutation, t^{12}, the cells of the morula fail to undergo compaction into a blastocyst. [After Bennett (1975) *Cell* 6, 441]

CHAPTER THIRTEEN

Summary

1. The major histocompatibility complex (MHC) is a complex of genes that encodes molecules involved in various aspects of the immune response.

2. The MHC gene products can be grouped into three classes, called I, II, and III. Class I products are found on all cells, Class II products are found on cells of the immune system (Ia antigens), and Class III products are serum products, some of which are associated with the complement system.

3. The MHC is one of the most highly polymorphic systems in biology. Each of the genes of the system has many alleles. The collection of all of the alleles is called the haplotype.

4. Some of the antigens encoded by the MHC are expressed by members of more than one haplotype and are called public specificities. Other MHC antigens are expressed only by the members of a given haplotype and are called private specificities.

5. By selective backcrosses, mice can be bred to have the MHC genes of one haplotype and the background genes of another. These are called congenic mice.

6. Class I antigens have a variant chain called α and an invariant chain called β_2-microglobulin. Class II antigens have two variable chains, α and β.

7. The T locus in the mouse may function as the embryonic counterpart of the MHC.

Additional Readings

Bennett, D. 1978. The T complex in the mouse: An assesment after 50 years of study. *Harvey Lectures* 74, 1.

Hood, L., M. Steinmetz, and B. Malissen. 1983. Genes of the major histocompatibility complex of the mouse. *Annu. Rev. Immunol* 1, 529.

Klein, J. 1975. *Biology of the Mouse Histocompatibility-2 Complex: Principles of Immunogenetics Applied to a Single System.* Springer-Verlag, New York.

Klein, J., F. Figueroa, and Z. A. Nagy. 1983. Genetics of the major histocompatibility complex: The final act. *Annu. Rev. Immunol.* 1, 119.

Klein, J., A. Juretič, C. N. Baxevanis, and Z. A. Nagy. 1981. The traditional and a new version of the mouse H-2 complex. *Nature* 291, 455.

Mengle-Gaw, L., and H. O. McDevitt. 1985. Genetics and expression of murine Ia antigens. *Annu. Rev. Immunol.* 3, 367.

THE MAJOR HISTOCOMPATIBILITY COMPLEX

Mitchison, N. A. 1981. The case for functional nomenclature. *Immunol. Today* September, 167.

Möller, G. (ed.). 1985. *Immunological Reviews*, Vols. 84, 85, and 86. Volume 84, Molecular genetics of Class I and II MHC antigens 1. Volume 85, Molecular genetics of Class I and II MHC antigens 2. Volume 86, Molecular genetics of Class III MHC antigens.

Snell, G. D., J. Dausset, and S. Nathenson. 1976. *Histocompatibility*. Academic Press, New York.

SECTION II

CELL COOPERATION

If it aint complicated it dont matter whether it works or not because if it aint complicated up enough it aint right. So even if it works, dont believe it.

WILLIAM FAULKNER, *The Town*

In these five chapters we will discuss the cellular events that lead to an immune response, revealing the various layers of complexity of the cellular events in that response. The solution to the problem of cellular events in the immune response is a fascinating one that has taken many unexpected twists and turns. To understand that story and the current status of the problem, which involves B cells, various functional subsets of T cells, Lyt phenotypes, and the role of the MHC (all of which were introduced in the previous section), it is necessary to follow the flow of discoveries which elucidated the role of each of these components. Furthermore, it will be necessary to understand the material in this section before the reader can fully comprehend the material in the next section, on receptors.

CHAPTER 14

THE DIVISION OF LABOR

Overview There are two kinds of immune responses: humoral and cell-mediated. A division of labor is apparent among the cells that carry out the two kinds of responses; indeed, the responses are carried out by different sets of cells. The first clue that this division of labor existed came from experiments in which the thymus was removed from mice at birth; these neonatally thymectomized animals had impaired immune responses. A similar discovery was made with the avian bursa; it was found that neonatally bursectomized birds also had impaired responses to antigen. To complicate matters further, it was then found that removal of macrophages from in vitro cultures of spleen cells prevented the lymphocytes in these cultures from making immune responses. Together all of these studies showed that there is a need for two kinds of lymphocytes—B cells and T cells—and macrophages in the immune response.

This chapter will develop the evidence for the division of labor. It will also introduce the reader to some of the methodology that will be needed to understand all cellular immunology experiments.

CHAPTER FOURTEEN

Humoral and Cell-Mediated Immune Responses

The Immunocompetent Cell

The introduction of antigen into an animal causes a complex series of events that result in a variety of responses. Because we almost always are interested in only one or a very few of these responses, we call the response to antigen *the immune response*, even though *the immune responses* is probably more appropriate.

It has been known since long before the modern era that the cells that carry out the immune response are LYMPHOCYTES. In 1958 Peter Medawar coined the term *immunologically competent cell* to define a cell that is "fully qualified to undertake an immunological response." Medawar later noted (1963) that he meant the term to indicate that the cells had the *potential* to carry out a response, and that to "describe an immunologically activated cell, a cell actually doing something, as immunologically competent strikes me as supererogatory (*sic*), like describing an aircraft already overhead as competent to engage in flight."[1]

The important point is that at the start of the Modern Era, circa 1960, the best immunological thinkers viewed the immune response as the domain of one kind of cell, the lymphocyte. It was known that there were large and small lymphocytes and that antibody was produced by a specialized lymphocyte called a PLASMA CELL, but there was little reason to think that there was a profound difference between lymphocytes.

Traditionally the immune response has been divided into the HUMORAL, or ANTIBODY RESPONSE, and the CELL-MEDIATED RESPONSES. The humoral response results in the production of antibody, so all of the effects that are observed or measured are the result of this *product* of lymphocytes. Cell-mediated responses, on the other hand, are reactions that are carried out *directly* by the lymphocytes themselves. We now know that all lymphocytes are not the same and that different sets of lymphocytes are responsible for carrying out the humoral and cell-mediated responses.

---

[1] Although we may see some examples of immunologists who think as well as Sir Peter, we certainly will not see many in these pages who write as well as he does.

THE DIVISION OF LABOR

Cell-Mediated Responses Defined

In Chapter 8 we discussed the methods used to describe and quantify the antibody response. Before we examine some of the evidence concerning the mechanisms of cell-mediated responses, it will be necessary to understand the nature of these reactions. The reader should consult Methods Boxes 1–5 to read about the various cell-mediated responses.

The designation "cell-mediated response" is used to distinguish these reactions from immune reactions in which antibody is not involved. Although many cell-mediated responses involve tissue destruction, other tissue-destroying reactions are caused by antibody. The reactions involving antibody are called immediate hypersensitivity reactions and will be discussed in Chapter 26.

METHODS BOX 1

Delayed-Type Hypersensitivity

Delayed-type hypersensitivity (DTH) is the traditional form of cell-mediated response and is best exemplified by the TUBERCULIN TEST. If an individual has come in contact with *Mycobacterium tuberculosis* (the organism that causes tuberculosis), that individual becomes *sensitized* to antigens of the organism—that is, that individual has made an immune response to some of these antigens. Most individuals tend to make a stronger cell-mediated response than antibody response to this organism (which is why it was chosen as an example). To test for the presence of sensitized cells (i.e., to test for a cell-mediated response), a small amount of antigen (usually supernatant fluid from the medium in which the organisms were grown) is injected into the skin. If the individual has sensitized cells, these cells will accumulate and cause other cells to be attracted to the site of the injected antigen. The result is a lump, visible and palpable by 48 hours after injection. If the response were due to antibody (immediate hypersensitivity), the reaction would reach a maximum in 24 hours. In experimental animals, DTH reactions can be quantified by measuring the size of the lump that forms, or by injecting the antigen into the footpad of a mouse and measuring the amount of swelling after 48 hours. The footpad that received antigen is then compared with the other, which received a control injection of diluent without antigen.

METHODS BOX 2

Allograft Rejection

An ALLOGRAFT is a graft of tissue from one member of a species to a different member of the same species. For example, grafts from one human to another are allografts. A graft between members of two different strains of mice is also an allograft. If tissues from one strain of mouse are grafted onto animals of another strain, the tissues will begin to grow; but after several days the immune system will cause the grafts to stop growing and die. This reaction is called GRAFT REJECTION. In humans, organ transplants (such as skin, kidney, and heart transplants) are allografts, and when rejection occurs the immunological mechanisms are the same as those seen in experimental animals. Graft rejection is a cell-mediated phenomenon because it can be transferred to normal animals only with lymphocytes and not with serum.

Immediate hypersensitivity reactivity can be transferred to a normal animal with serum from an immune animal. Cell-mediated responses, however, can be transferred only to a normal animal by injecting the lymphoid cells of a sensitized animal. This result implies that the product of the B cell (antibody) is responsible for immediate hypersensitivity reactions but lymphocytes themselves are responsible for cell-mediated responses.

Division of Labor among Cells in the Immune Response

One of the most important realizations in the development of our understanding of the nature of the immune response was that the notion of the immunocompetent cell was correct, but incomplete. In fact, as mentioned earlier, antibody and cell-mediated responses are carried out by different sets of cells; and even among these different populations there can be subpopulations of cells. Furthermore, in addition to the lymphocytes (which are responsible for the specificity of the immune response), accessory cells (macrophages) are also involved.

THE DIVISION OF LABOR

We will now begin to analyze the various levels of complexity of the cellular basis of the immune response. As you begin to see the beauty at any of these levels, remember that there is still another level to come. The whole process will be very much like peeling an onion, during which you uncover layer after layer and are often moved to tears during the process. If you like onions the whole thing is worthwhile.

Effect of Neonatal Thymectomy

Lymphocytes arise from the multipotent hemopoietic stem cell through the action of inducing factors in the lymphocyte-inducing microenvironments—the bone marrow and the thymus (Chapter 10). The Modern Era of the study of the cellular basis of the immune response can be looked upon as beginning with the simultaneous but independent observations on the role of the thymus by Robert A. Good in Minneapolis, J.F.A.P. Miller in London, and Byron Waksman in New Haven. Good, an immunologist and clinician, noted that in patients with thymomas (tumors of the thymus) there are often accompanying disorders of the immune system, especially acquired hypogammaglobulinemia (a severe reduction in the concentration of serum immunoglobulins). He and his colleagues carried out a very large series of experiments in which the thymus was removed from experimental animals, and the effect of this THYMECTOMY on the immune response was studied. Miller, an Australian working in England, was studying lymphocytic leukemia in mice. Because the thymus was known to be the target organ of the disease, he asked what the effect of removal of the thymus would be. He showed that in the absence of the thymus the mice did not develop leukemia; but, perhaps of more importance, he also saw that the removal of the thymus had far-reaching effects on the immune response. Waksman was interested in the mechanism of cell-mediated tissue destruction, and he also found that the removal of the thymus at birth impaired the immune function of the adult.

These three investigators all found that removal of the thymus of mice within the first few days after birth (neonatal thymectomy) resulted in a severe *reduction* in immune potential. When the neonatally thymectomized mice reached several weeks

METHODS BOX 3

Graft-versus-Host Reaction

In the allograft reaction the host is immunologically competent, and the graft, usually skin, does not contain immunologically competent cells. Therefore, the host recognizes the antigens of the graft as foreign and responds against them. In such a case, the host rejects the graft. In the graft-versus-host (GVH) reaction, the roles are reversed. As the name implies, it is the graft that recognizes the antigens of the host and responds against them. Therefore, the graft in a GVH reaction must contain immunocompetent cells.

The GVH reaction is widely used in the laboratory; but, like delayed sensitivity and allograft rejection, it also has clinical implications, especially in bone marrow transplantation. If any immunocompetent lymphocytes have recirculated into the bone marrow, these cells will be transferred with the transplanted bone marrow cells (the graft); they can then react against the recipient (the host). In experimental situations the host is usually rendered immunologically incompetent either by treatment with X ray or by experimental design—that is, by the use of very young mice that have not yet acquired full immune competence. These immunologically incompetent hosts are injected with lymphocytes that can react against antigens of the host. As in all cell-mediated responses, the ability to carry out a GVH reaction is limited to cells; antibody does not play a role.

In the mouse, one of the consequences of a GVH reaction is the enlargement of the host's spleen. Interestingly, it is primarily the host's own cells that infiltrate and enlarge the spleen, although they do this because of the presence of the graft cells, which are carrying out a reaction against the host. The amount of spleen enlargement, or SPLENOMEGALY, is taken as a measure of the severity of the GVH reaction. Splenomegaly is expressed as the SPLEEN INDEX:

$$\text{Spleen index} = \frac{\frac{\text{weight of experimental spleen}}{\text{total body weight}}}{\frac{\text{weight of control spleen}}{\text{total body weight}}}$$

Control animals in a GVH reaction are recipients that are the same age and sex as the recipients of the experimental group but are injected with cells of the same type of host, that is, syngeneic cells. Injecting syngeneic cells into a recipient should cause no effect, because the control cells will not recognize the host as foreign. If there is no splenomegaly in the experimental animal, it will have the same ratio of spleen to body weight as the control, and the spleen index will be 1.0. By convention, a spleen index of 1.3 is considered indicative of a positive GVH reaction.

In experimental situations, the recipients in the GVH reaction are usually F_1 mice and the donors one of the parental strains. In this manner the host does not recognize the transferred cells as foreign. This procedure is diagrammed in Figure A. Spleen cells of strain A are injected into $(A \times B)F_1$ hybrids. The A cells (the graft) induce a GVH reaction in $(A \times B)F_1$ hosts but not in the A host, because the immunocompetent cells of the A graft recognize the antigens of B on the $(A \times B)F_1$ host cells. The cells of the $(A \times B)F_1$, however, do not recognize anything as foreign on the A cells. To be sure, the A cells are different be-

METHODS BOX 3

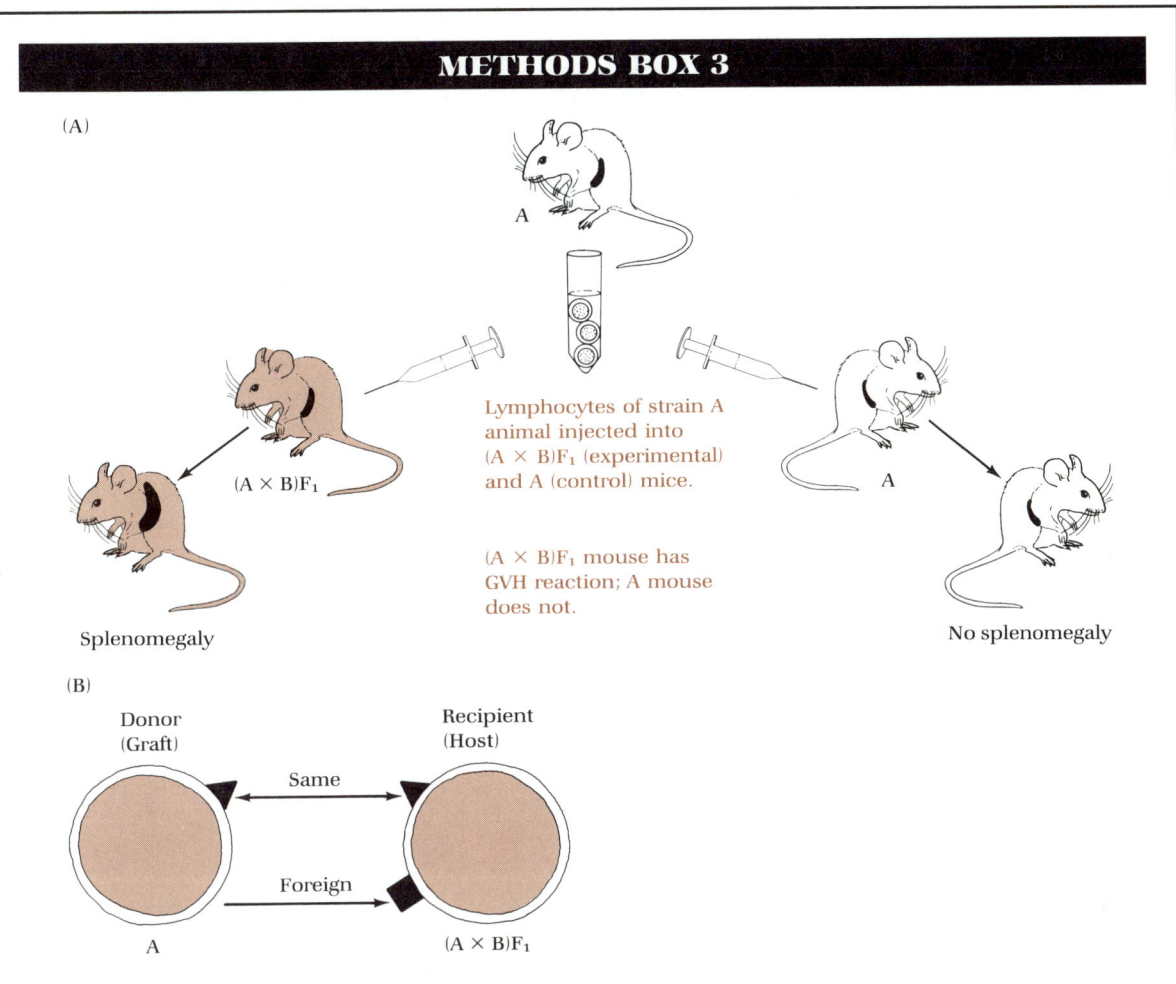

cause they do not have the B antigens, but it is important to remember that the immune response is directed only to the presence of different antigen, not to differences resulting from the absence of antigen. This experiment is diagrammed in Figure B.

of age, they either were given skin from mice of other strains to test their ability to reject grafts (a test of their cell-mediated response), or were inoculated with antigen to test their ability to produce antibody (the humoral response). The neonatally thymectomized mice failed to reject skin grafts, produce antibody, or give delayed skin reactions, whereas sham-thymectomized con-

METHODS BOX 4

Cytotoxic Lymphocyte Reaction

The two commonly used in vitro models for cell-mediated responses are diagrammed in the figure. The model in which test cells are lysed in vitro is called the CYTOTOXIC LYMPHOCYTE REACTION. Cytotoxic lymphocytes (CTL) are also called KILLER CELLS. The reaction that generates these cells is also called the CELL-MEDIATED LYMPHOLYSIS (CML) response. In this reaction cells of one strain of mouse react against antigens on the cells of another strain. (Or in humans, one individual's cells react with those of another individual.) Cells of strain A can be injected into animals of strain B, so that the strain B animals are sensitized to A cells; or the cells can be sensitized in vitro. In the assay to measure the degree of sensitization, the responding cells (in this case, the cells of strain B) are mixed with TARGET CELLS bearing the relevant antigens of A in vitro. Target cells can be cells from strain A or from a closely related strain that has some of the same antigens as cells of strain A on their surface. These target cells are labeled with radioactive chromium (^{51}Cr). Chromium has the fortunate property of entering cells rapidly but leaving them very slowly, as long as the cell membrane is intact. When the membrane is damaged, the chromium is rapidly released. Thus by quantifying the amount of chromium released from the cells, we can determine how much membrane damage (i.e., killing) has been done by the sensitized cells. CTL data is reported as the percentage of kill of a population of target cells at a defined "effector:target" ratio (E/T). The results are often expressed as the slope of the straight line that is generated when percentage of killing is plotted against a range of E/T.

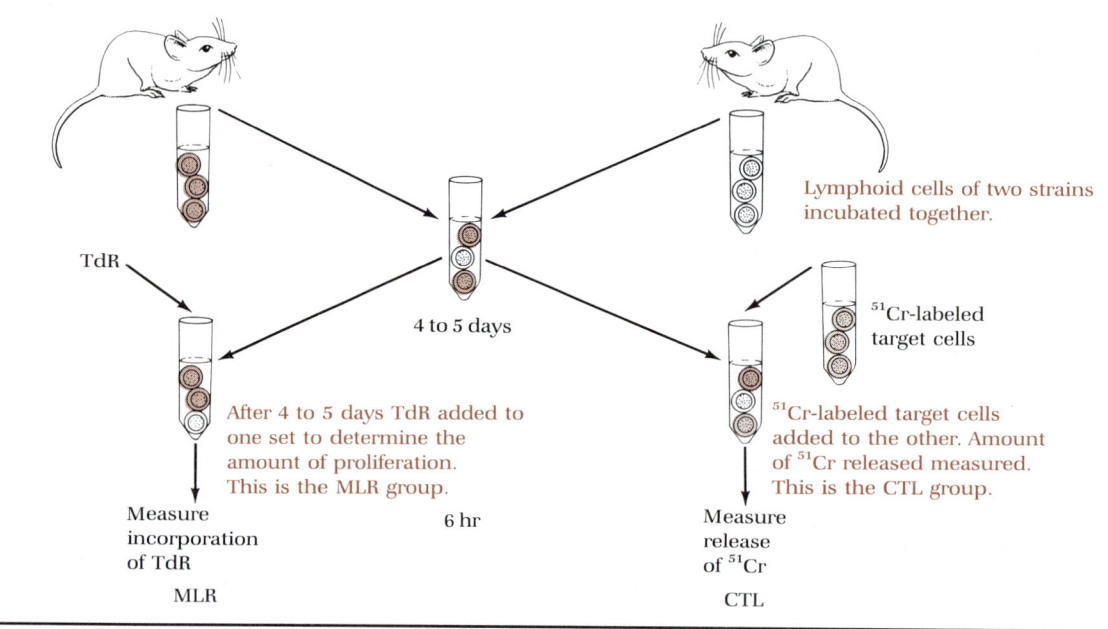

> ## METHODS BOX 5
>
> ### Mixed Lymphocyte Reactions
>
> Another in vitro cell-mediated response is called the MIXED LYMPHOCYTE REACTION (MLR). This reaction measures the amount of cell proliferation that sensitization causes. In this reaction, cells from two individuals or strains that have different surface antigens are mixed together in vitro. If one cell population recognizes the other as foreign, it will begin to proliferate. This proliferation can be quantified by determining the amount of incorporation of radiolabeled precursors into DNA (tritiated thymidine, for example). In practice the cells are allowed to react for 4 or 5 days, then the tritiated thymidine is added to the culture. If proliferation is taking place, the tritiated thymidine will be incorporated into newly synthesized DNA. By extracting the DNA and determining the amount of radiolabel incorporated, a measure of the degree of proliferation is obtained. Because both populations will recognize each other and respond by proliferation, one population can be treated with agents such as mitomycin C that prevent proliferation. After this treatment the cells can still stimulate but cannot respond. This response is called a ONE-WAY MLR.

trols made normal responses.[2] If these neonatally thymectomized mice were repopulated with thymocytes when they reached several weeks of age, their ability to generate responses was restored. These results are shown in Figure 1.

These studies showed that the thymus plays a crucial role in the immune response. Furthermore, the data could be interpreted as showing that the thymus is both necessary and sufficient to allow an animal to carry out both kinds of immune responses. The thymus then seemed to be the source of the immunocompetent cell. Unfortunately, this reasonable assumption is wrong. Nevertheless, this pioneering work can be looked upon as the foundation of modern cellular immunology.

Effect of Bursectomy

The bursa of Fabricius is a lymphoid organ in the cloacal region of the chicken. Removal of this organ also leads to impaired immune function. This remarkable and important discovery was made in 1954 by Bruce Glick, then a graduate student at Ohio State University. He relates

---

[2] In sham thymectomy, the animal is subjected to all aspects of the surgical procedure except the physical removal of the thymus. This control tests the effect of the stress of the thymectomy on the immune response.

CHAPTER FOURTEEN

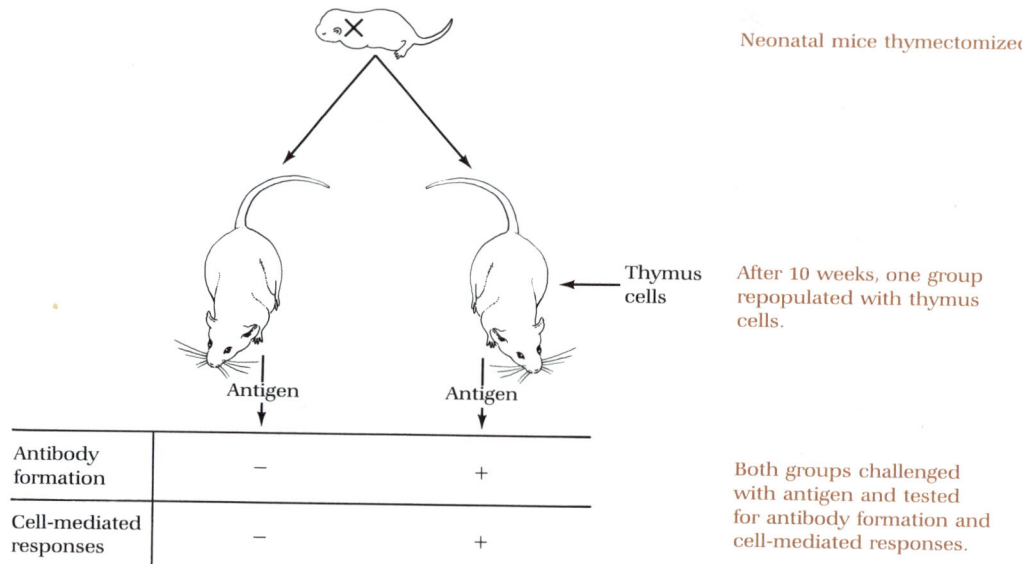

FIGURE 1 EFFECT OF NEONATAL THYMECTOMY

Neonatal mice are thymectomized and one group repopulated with thymus cells. After both groups are challenged with antigen, antibody formation and cell-mediated responses are tested.

how he discovered the fact that the bursa plays a role in the immune response:

> Up to the summer of 1954, bursectomy experiments had failed to reveal a specific function for the bursa. At this time nine of my 6-month-old experimental birds were used by Timothy S. Chang, a fellow graduate student, in a class demonstration which consisted of injecting chickens with *Salmonella typhimurium* O antigen and then determining the antibody titer of the serum. Six of the birds died immediately after the injection. Three survived, but to our surprise, their sera produced no agglutination when mixed with the homologous antigen. The wing-band numbers were checked with the record book, which revealed that all nine birds had previously been bursectomized. It appeared that the bursa was responsible for the result since the normal pen mates reacted to the injections by producing normal antibody titers.
> [Bruce Glick (1964) *The Thymus in Immunobiology*, p. 348.]

THE DIVISION OF LABOR

This rather startling result meant that both thymectomy and bursectomy could cause a severe depression of immune potential. It was soon found, however, that removal of the bursa did not impair the immune response in the same manner as did thymectomy. After neonatal thymectomy both the graft rejection and the antibody responses (cellular and humoral responses) were depressed. After neonatal bursectomy, however, antibody responses were depressed but skin graft rejection was normal. Indeed, bursectomized chickens rejected grafts as well as sham-operated controls.

These facts were a major piece of evidence leading to the insight that there is division of labor among lymphocyte populations. Other evidence indicated there is even further division of labor, because the lymphocytes must interact with accessory cells (macrophages) to generate an immune response.

The Role of the Macrophage

The importance of a nonlymphoid cell—the MACROPHAGE—in the generation of immune responses in vivo had long been suspected, but it was not until the invention of in vitro methods for generating immune responses that more precise experiments could be carried out. Mishell and Dutton in La Jolla and Marbrooke in Melbourne devised tissue culture methods for generating primary in vitro antibody responses in 1966. These methods were very quickly modified so that in vitro cell-mediated responses could also be carried out. One of the first problems to be explored using these new techniques was the role of the macrophage in generating immune responses.

Antibody Responses In Vitro: The Mosier Experiment

Cells from the mouse spleen can be separated into two functional populations by their differential ability to adhere to the surface of glass or plastic petri dishes. A few hours after introduction of cells to the containers, those cells not firmly attached to the surface are removed. The nonadherent cells are lymphocytes. The adherent cells are predominantly macrophages. When antigen is added to the unfractionated spleen cell population in vitro, antibody is produced. But when antigen is added to either the adherent or nonadher-

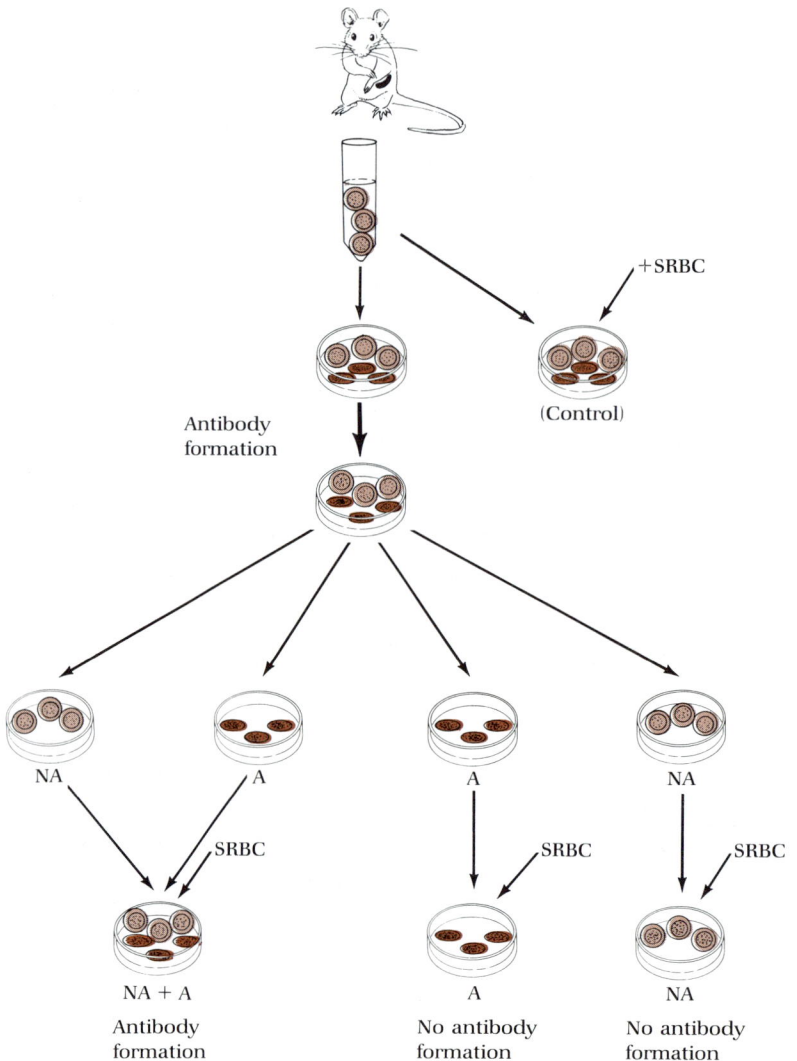

FIGURE 2 NONADHERENT AND ADHERENT CELLS IN ANTIBODY PRODUCTION

Adherent (A) cells (macrophages) and nonadherent (NA) cells (lymphocytes) are prepared from normal spleens. Neither population can respond to antigen by producing antibody, but the combined preparations do respond. [After Mosier (1967) *Science* 158, 1573]

ent population, no antibody is produced. When these two populations are recombined, however, there is antibody production (Figure 2). This classic experiment was the first to show unequivocally that lymphocytes must interact with a nonlymphoid cell to be able to generate an antibody response.

Cytotoxic T Cells

Macrophages were soon found also to be required for the generation of cytotoxic lymphocytes (CTL), as shown in Figure 3. In this experiment, spleen cells from CBA ($H-2^k$) mice were immunized in vitro against cells from

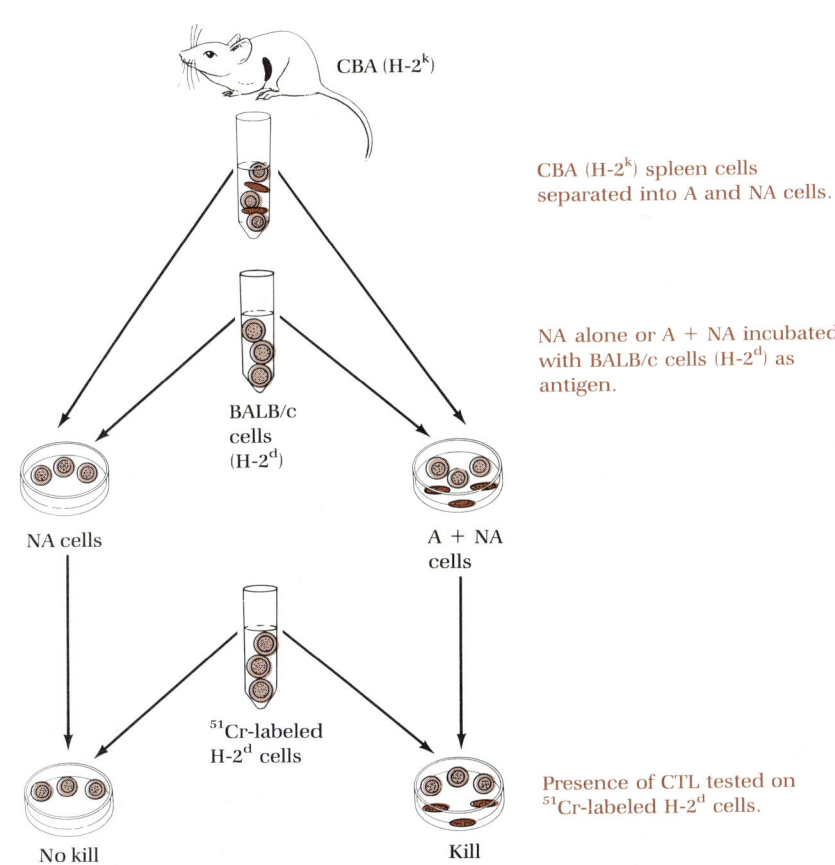

FIGURE 3   GENERATION OF CTL EFFECTOR CELLS
Nonadherent (NA) cells (lymphocytes) cannot generate cytotoxic T cells in the absence of macrophages (A cells). [After Wagner et al. (1972) *J. Exp. Med.* **136**, 331]

BALB/c (H-2^d) mice in the presence or absence of macrophages. Cytotoxic cell activity was determined by the release of ^{51}Cr from DBA/2 target cells. (DBA/2 mice are also H-2^d.) It can be seen that in the absence of macrophages the numbers of cytotoxic cells generated were greatly reduced, showing the need for these cells in the generation of a CTL response.

Proliferative Responses to Mitogens

The data in Table 1 show that a proliferative response to mitogens (PHA and ConA) requires macrophages. In the absence of macrophages, there is a poor proliferative response to either mitogen. The addition of macrophages to the cultures, however, results in the generation of the responses to control levels.

All of these experiments show that there are various forms of the immune response and that lymphocytes and macrophages must interact to generate them. This is another way of stating that there is a division of labor among the cells of the immune response.

TABLE 1 Need for macrophages in proliferative responses to mitogens.

Cells in culture	^{3}H incorporation (cpm)		
	No mitogen	ConA	PHA
T lymphocytes alone	94	233	412
T lymphocytes + macrophages	279	5900	55,200

Source: From Rosenstreich et al. (1976), *J. Immunol.* 116: 131.

Summary

1. The immune response consists of the humoral, or antibody, response and cell-mediated responses. Lymphocytes are responsible for both.

THE DIVISION OF LABOR

2. In the antibody response lymphocytes produce a product—antibody—which has immune function. In cell-mediated responses the lymphocytes themselves carry out the immune function.

3. Delayed-type hypersensitivity (DTH), allograft rejection, and the graft-versus-host reaction (GVH) are examples of in vivo cell-mediated responses. Cytotoxic lymphocyte responses (CTL) and the mixed lymphocyte reaction (MLR) are examples of in vitro cell-mediated responses.

4. Removal of the thymus at birth abolishes antibody and cell-mediated responses. Restoration of thymus cells restores the responses. Removal of the bursa of Fabricius from chickens at birth abolishes antibody but not cell-mediated responses.

5. Macrophages are required for the generation of antibody and for cytotoxic and proliferation responses.

CHAPTER 15

HELPER AND EFFECTOR CELLS

Overview In the last chapter we saw that there is a division of labor among the cells of the immune response. In this chapter we will begin to see *how* the labor is divided. We will develop the evidence for the remarkable fact that there are cell interactions in both humoral and cell-mediated responses. These interactions take the form of cell cooperation in which some cells carry out the immune functions (these are called effector cells) and some cells act as helpers.

Cell-mediated responses are carried out by effector T cells. B cells also are effector cells because they produce antibody; but they also require helper cells. Helper cells participate in the generation of the effector cells and in both humoral and cell-mediated responses are T cells. The *principle* of cooperation between helper and effector cells is the same for both humoral and cell-mediated responses. In this chapter we will first examine evidence for cooperation and then examine other evidence for helpers and effectors. Examples from both humoral and cell-mediated responses will be considered together for each point.

HELPER AND EFFECTOR CELLS

Evidence of Cooperating Cell Populations

In the early 1960s the picture that was emerging from the neonatal thymectomy and bursectomy studies showed that there was division of labor within the lymphocyte population. The bursa (or its equivalent in mammals) appeared to control some aspects of antibody formation, while the thymus appeared to be involved in both antibody formation and graft rejection. The almost universal view of the thymectomy studies was that the thymus, a primary lymphoid organ, was both necessary and sufficient for the immune response and was seeding the secondary tissues with functional cells. This arrangement had been predicted at the turn of the century, as shown in the following quote, which was made at a time when people could be more certain about both science and nationalism.

> It has fallen to my lot to show that the first leucocytes arise in the thymus, from its epithelial cells, and that the thymus must be regarded as the parent source of all the lymphoid structures of the body. It does not cease to exist in later life no more than would the Anglo-Saxon race disappear, were the British Isles to sink beneath the waves. For just as the Anglo-Saxon stock has made its way from its original home into all parts of the world, and has there set up colonies for itself and for its increase, so the original leucocytes, starting from their birthplace and home in the thymus, have penetrated into almost every part of the body, and have there created new centres for growth, for increase and useful work for themselves and for the body.
> [J. Beard (1899) The true function of the thymus. *Lancet* i, 144. Quoted by Defendi (1964) in *The Thymus in Immunobiology*]

This comforting notion—that all immunocompetent cells come from the thymus—was shaken by experiments from at least two sources, which showed that the situation might not be this simple. Two groups, one in America and one in England, did experiments having different designs but addressing the same question and coming to the same conclusion. This kind of situation occurs over and over in science and should make us all aware that there are times when a question can be posed in such a manner that it can be answered and the likelihood is that more than one creative person will realize this.

CHAPTER FIFTEEN

Bone Marrow–Thymus Reconstitution: The Claman Experiment

One set of experiments was carried out by Claman and his co-workers in Denver, who X-irradiated mice to abolish their immune systems and then attempted to restore immune function with thymus cells. Given the view of the day, thymus cells should have restored the ability of the mice to produce antibody. In this experiment (Figure 1), the thymus and bone marrow of normal mice are removed and made into

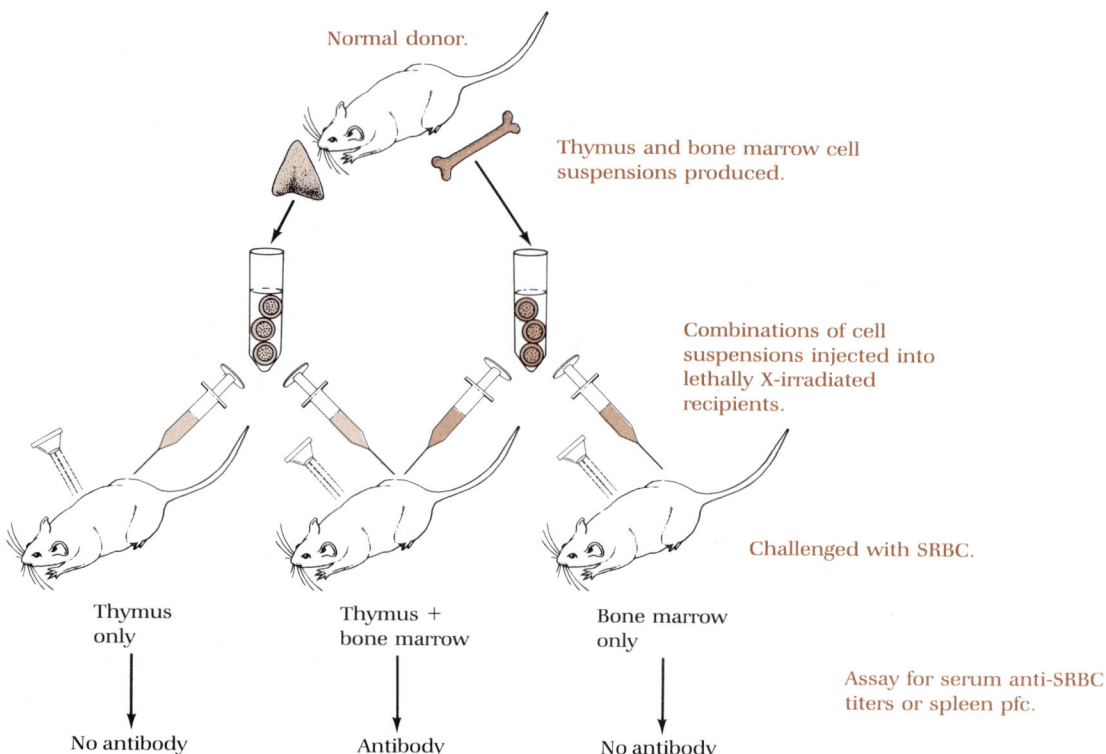

FIGURE 1 THE CLAMAN EXPERIMENT

Bone marrow–thymus reconstitution. Irradiated mice do not have their immune function restored if they are repopulated with either bone marrow or thymus cells alone. The ability to produce antibody in response to antigen is restored by repopulating the irradiated mice with both bone marrow and thymus cells. [After Claman et al. (1969) *J. Immunol.* 97, 828]

HELPER AND EFFECTOR CELLS

single-cell suspensions. An aliquot of each of the two cell populations is then injected into groups of lethally X-irradiated, syngeneic recipients. Marrow and thymus are injected into one group, only thymus into another group, and only marrow into a third group. In this way the experiment has the necessary experimental and control groups to determine whether either population alone produces antibody or whether the two populations must both be injected. The mice are challenged with antigen (sheep red blood cells, SRBC), and after an appropriate interval the amount of antibody produced is determined.

The results of the experiment in Figure 1 showed that repopulating irradiated mice with either marrow alone or thymus alone was *not* sufficient to generate a significant titer of antibody. However, injection of cells from *both* of the primary lymphoid organs resulted in restoration of the antibody response. This finding showed clearly that thymus cells alone were not able to reconstitute the antibody response and immediately opened to question the view that the thymus exports all of the functional cells in the immune responses.

The second kind of experiment raising doubt that all immune function was due to the cells of the thymus was done by Davies and his co-workers in London using cells with the T6 chromosomal marker. In these experiments, mice were lethally irradiated and repopulated with either bone marrow or thymus cells. By use of this marker it was possible to show that thymus cells proliferated in response to antigen but did not make antibody. Bone marrow cells injected into irradiated recipients who then received antigen but no thymus cells neither proliferated nor produced antibody. But when bone marrow and thymus cells were injected together and the animals challenged with antigen, antibody was produced. So this experiment, like the one discussed previously, shows that thymus cells alone do not restore irradiated animals, but a combination of cells from the thymus and the bone marrow does.

These two experiments showed that there were at least two lymphocyte populations involved in antibody formation and that some form of *cellular cooperation* was occurring between them. The inescapable conclusion from these experiments is that there was cellular cooperation between bone marrow and thymus cell populations and one or both of them were then able to produce antibody. The question then became, Which cell population was producing the antibody—the cells from the thymus or the cells derived from the bone marrow, or both?

Cell Cooperation in Graft-versus-Host Reaction

Cell cooperation in cell-mediated responses was first shown in 1970 by Asofsky and his colleagues at the NIH, using the graft-versus-host reaction (GVH; Figure 2). The recipients were newborn (BALB/c × C57BL/6)F_1 mice. Various numbers of parental thymus *or* peripheral blood cells were injected into the F_1 and the spleen index for each concentration of injected cells was noted. A third group of F_1 recipients was inoculated with both thymus cells *and* peripheral blood cells. The resulting spleen index was greater than the sum of the two reactions to each of the cell types alone. The important point in the presentation of the data (Figure 2) is that by varying the number of cells injected, a titration curve relating the spleen index to the number of cells injected can be obtained. From this titration curve the number of thymus or peripheral blood cells required to give a positive spleen index of 1.3 can easily be deter-

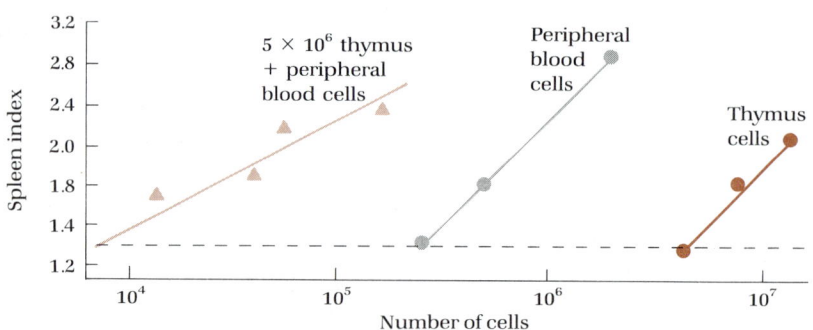

FIGURE 2 GVH REACTION

Titration curves of cell populations alone or in combination in generating a GVH reaction. The mixture of thymus cells and peripheral blood cells is more effective than either population alone. [After Asofsky et al. (1971) *Prog. Immunol.* 1, 369]

HELPER AND EFFECTOR CELLS

mined. In the experiment in Figure 2 an index of 1.3 was achieved with 5×10^6 thymus cells or with 2×10^5 peripheral blood cells. When thymus and peripheral blood cells are injected together, a synergistic reaction occurs, because mixing 5×10^6 thymus with as few as 3×10^4 peripheral blood cells gives an index *greater* than 1.3. Because it requires 2×10^5 peripheral blood lymphocytes alone to give an index of 1.3, this result shows that the thymus cells and peripheral blood cells together are over *10 times* more effective than they would be if the response was additive. This experiment also shows that in cell-mediated responses, as in antibody formation, there is some sort of cell cooperation going on.

Evidence for Effector and Helper Cells

Reconstitution after Neonatal Thymectomy: The Mitchell-Miller Experiment

Because repopulation of neonatally thymectomized mice with thymus cells reconstituted the ability of these mice to produce antibody, it was logical to assume that the thymus lymphocytes were the eventual antibody-forming cells. The bone marrow–thymus reconstitution experiments, however, suggested that cooperation was occurring between the thymus and bone marrow cells; and the experiments with chromosomally marked cells suggested that the thymus-derived cells were not the ones producing antibody. So it was crucial to definitively determine which cell was producing the antibody and what the other cell type was doing.

The experiment that gave the first clear answer to this question was performed by G.F. Mitchell and J.F.A.P. Miller and is one of exceptional elegance. This experiment requires readily identifiable markers for the cells of the thymus-derived population and another set of markers for the cells of the bone marrow-derived population. H-2 antigens serve as perfect markers for this purpose. (At this point the reader should review Chapter 13 on the MHC, if needed.)

The idea of the Mitchell-Miller experiment (Figure 3) was to repopulate at eight weeks of age a neonatally thymectomized mouse of one H-2 haplotype with thymus cells from a mouse of another H-2 haplotype. We already know that injecting thymus

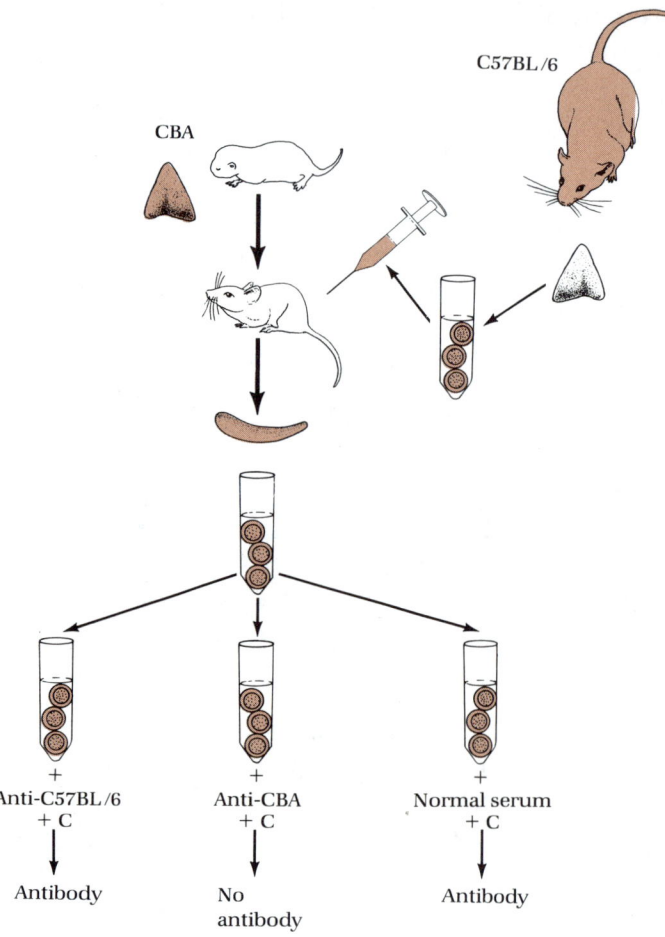

FIGURE 3 THE MITCHELL-MILLER EXPERIMENT

Experiment determining whether thymus cells become antibody-forming cells. Neonatally thymectomized CBA mice are repopulated with C57BL/6 thymus cells and challenged with antigen. Before the assay to determine the number of antibody-forming cells is carried out, aliquots of spleen cells are treated with anti-C57BL/6, anti-CBA, or normal serum, plus complement. Absence of antibody-forming cells after treatment with anti-CBA indicates that the cells producing antibody are from the thymectomized host and not from the injected thymus cells. [After Mitchell and Miller (1968) *Proc. Natl. Acad. Sci. USA* **59**, 296]

HELPER AND EFFECTOR CELLS

cells will restore the ability of the thymectomized animal to produce antibody-forming cells. The crucial part is to then determine which H-2 antigens are on the surface of the antibody-producing cells. If they are the same as those of the injected thymus cells, then the thymus-derived cells are the cells that produce antibody. If they are not the same as those of the injected thymus cells but belong to the haplotype of the thymectomized host, then a cell already present in the host is producing the antibody but is unable to do so until the thymus cells are present.[1]

Anti-H-2 antiserum is used to determine the H-2 type of the antibody-forming cells in the following manner. Anti-H-2 antibody reacts with cells with the appropriate H-2 antigen on their surfaces and then allows complement to bind to the Ag–Ab complex. Thus these cells will be lysed in the presence of complement and will no longer be able to carry out any function. If these cells are antibody-forming cells, then the number of antibody-producing cells in the population will be drastically reduced. The appropriate controls for this experiment are to react the cells with an antiserum that contains antibodies against some H-2 antigens other than those on the cell surface and also with normal serum, which contains no anti-H-2 antibodies.

This experiment led to one of the great surprises in modern immunology and clearly showed the nature of the division of labor among lymphocytes. Figure 3 shows that there was no reduction in antibody-producing cells after treatment of the cells of the repopulated animals with antibodies directed against the H-2 of the injected thymus cells. However, there was almost complete abolition of the antibody-forming cells after treatment with an antiserum directed against the cells of the neonatally thymectomized host. This experiment shows that the thymus cells do not become antibody-producing cells but do allow some cell type already present in the neonatally thymectomized mouse to be-

---

[1] Virtually all of the experiments discussed from now on describe the quantification of the antibody-forming cells rather than the determination of the titer of antibody. The invention of a plaque-forming assay by Niels Jerne made this possible. The Jerne plaque assay is described in Methods Box 1.

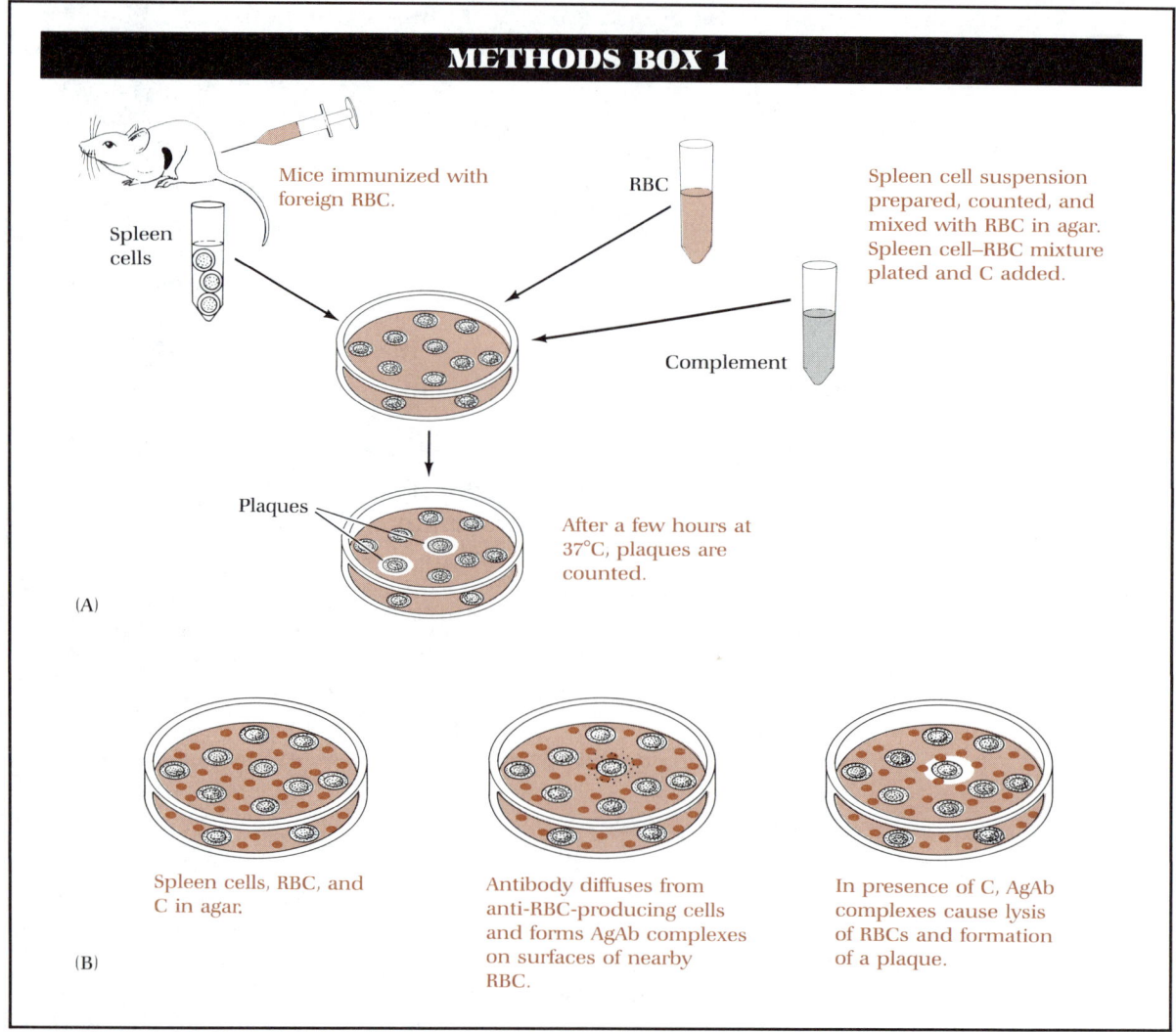

come an antibody-forming cell. In other words, the presence of the thymus cell is required for the conversion of some host cell to an antibody-forming cell. The thymus cell thus acts as a "helper" cell for some other cell, which becomes an "effector" cell (i.e., an antibody-forming cell).

HELPER AND EFFECTOR CELLS

METHODS BOX 1

The Jerne Plaque Assay

In 1963 Niels Jerne devised an assay to determine the number of antibody-forming cells in a cell suspension. This assay, called the HEMOLYTIC PLAQUE ASSAY or the JERNE PLAQUE ASSAY, made possible the quantitative study of the cellular events in antibody formation and was as important to the development of cellular immunology as the quantitative precipitin reaction was to immunochemistry.

When a cell that is producing antibody is immobilized in agar, the antibody molecules it produces will accumulate in the vicinity of the cell. If antigen is suspended uniformly in the agar, then an AgAb complex will form in an area surrounding the antibody-producing cell. When the antigen is an erythrocyte or a molecule that has been conjugated to an erythrocyte, lysis of the erythrocytes surrounding the antibody-producing cell occurs, producing a clear space, or "plaque" (Figures A and B).

The number of antibody-forming cells in the starting suspension of cells can be determined because the experimenter knows the total number of cells per milliliter in the suspension and the volume plated into the antigen-containing agar. By counting the number of plaques in the agar, the number of PLAQUE-FORMING CELLS (pfc) can easily be calculated. This is usually expressed as either pfc/spleen or pfc/10^6 cells.

REFERENCES

Jerne, N. K., and A. A. Nordin. 1963. Plaque formation in agar by single antibody-producing cells. *Science* 140: 405.

Golub, E. S., R. I. Mishell, W. O. Weigle, and R. W. Dutton. 1968. A modification of the hemolytic plaque assay for use with protein antigens. *J. Immunol.* 100: 133.

Mishell, B. B., and S. M. Shiigi. 1980. *Selected Methods in Cellular Immunology*, Chapter 3. Freeman, San Francisco.

The Failure of Allogeneic Bone Marrow–Thymus Reconstitution

Having shown that the thymus-derived cells act as helper cells but do not become antibody-producing cells, the next logical step is to determine whether the effector cells—the antibody-producing cells—are cells from the other primary lymphoid organ, the bone marrow. The experiment seemed simple to do: merely carry out the marrow–thymus reconstitution experiment with bone marrow of one H-2 donor and thymus of another type and treat the antibody-forming cells with anti-H-2 antiserum—that is, carry out a combined Claman and Mitchell-Miller experiment. Surprisingly, when the first part of this experiment was attempted (the allogeneic reconstitution), researchers found that no antibody-forming cells could be generated when bone marrow and thymus cells were of different H-2 haplotypes. In other words, attempts at allogeneic marrow–thymus interactions were unsuccessful. This is an important fact, and will be further emphasized later, but at the time the problem remained to determine whether the bone marrow cells were in fact the cells producing antibody.

Experimenters once again took advantage of markers, but this time of chromosomal markers, not cell surface markers. And, once again, the T6 marker was used. T6 bone marrow and +/+ thymus were injected into irradiated +/+ mice. The antibody-forming cells were then examined and did indeed contain the T6 marker. This result showed that the bone marrow-derived cells produced the antibody. When the experiment was carried out in the other direction—i.e., with thymus cells which had the marker and bone marrow cells which did not—none of the antibody-forming cells contained the T6 marker.

The results of this experiment show that the bone marrow-derived cells produce antibody and thus are the *effector cells* in antibody formation, and that the cells of the thymus act as *helper cells*, because the bone marrow cells alone cannot produce antibody. Thus we see that there is B cell–T cell cooperation in the generation of an antibody response. It is also safe to conclude that in the thymectomy experiments the cells of the thymectomized animal that were producing antibody were the bone marrow-derived lymphocytes.

However, the reader should keep in mind that allogeneic thymus cells can reconstitute a neonatally thymectomized mouse, but allogeneic bone marrow and thymus cells cannot cooperate in reconstituting an irradiated host. We will return to this point later and show that when this apparent contradiction was later studied in greater detail it led to an understanding of a whole new level of complexity in cell cooperation.

HELPER AND EFFECTOR CELLS

Varied Nature of Cell-Mediated Responses

The experiments described above show the flow of discoveries leading to the idea that there are helper cells and effector cells in antibody formation. We will now look at some of the experiments showing that there are also helper cells and effector cells in cell-mediated responses.

Delayed hypersensitivity reactions had been studied for many years. When allograft rejection came to be investigated as a means of studying skin and organ transplantation, it was soon realized that allograft and delayed hypersensitivity reactions were similar because both were cell-mediated responses. With the discovery that the GVH reaction was a form of rejection phenomenon, it made sense to unify all the cell-mediated reactions and to think of them as being roughly equivalent. When in vitro reactions such as CTL and MLR were found to be cell-mediated reactions, there was initial jubilation because it appeared more precise and quantitative means of measuring cell-mediated reactions would be available. But, as with most initial unifying notions in science, more and more exceptions were found, until it became clear that all cell-mediated responses were not merely manifestations of the same phenomenon measured in different ways. In fact, the various cell-mediated reactions each measure a separate effector and helper function.

Just as the rapid advances in helper and effector cell cooperation in antibody formation came to dominate so much of immunological thought in the 1960s, helper and effector cell cooperation in cell-mediated responses came to dominate much thought in the 1970s. We will see in later chapters that the role of the major histocompatibility complex in these reactions has come to dominate cellular immunological thought in the 1980s.

T cells are the Effector Cells in Cell-Mediated Responses

In antibody formation the T cell acts as a helper cell and the B cell is the effector cell. Figure 4 shows the result of an experiment designed to determine whether the effector cell in cell-mediated responses is a B cell or a T cell. This experiment is especially easy to carry out because it merely involves generating a response and pretreating the cells with anti-Thy 1 and complement before carrying out the reaction.

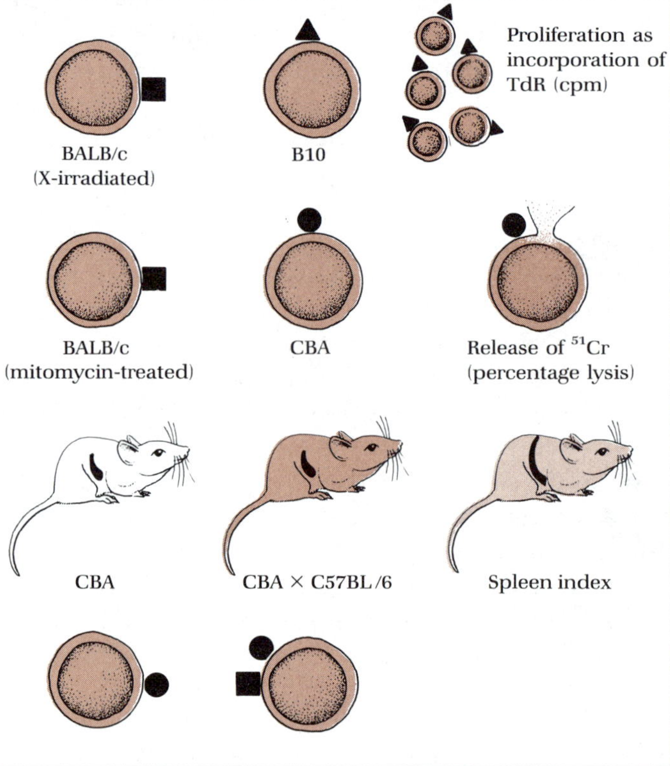

Reaction	Stimulator cell	Responder cell	Reaction	Effect of anti-Thy 1 treatment of responder cell		
				Normal serum	Anti-Thy 1	Percentage reduction
MLR (cpm)	BALB/c (X-irradiated)	B10	Proliferation as incorporation of TdR (cpm)	8249	331	94
CTL (percentage lysis)	BALB/c (mitomycin-treated)	CBA	Release of ^{51}Cr (percentage lysis)	100	4	96
GVH (S.I.)	CBA	CBA × C57BL/6	Spleen index	1.32	0.91	

FIGURE 4 ABOLITION OF CELL-MEDIATED RESPONSES
Treatment of cells with anti-Thy 1 and complement abolishes cell-mediated responses.

The MLR, CTL, and GVH reactions are all abolished by pretreatment with anti-Thy 1 and complement, which shows that the effector cell in cell-mediated responses is a T cell.

Evidence for Cell Cooperation in the Generation of CTL

In this section we will present evidence that the helper cell in the MLR, CTL, and GVH reactions is also a T cell, indicating T cell:T cell cooperation in cell-mediated responses. In these reactions, one T cell is the helper and another the effector. We will also see that there are

HELPER AND EFFECTOR CELLS

distinct subpopulations of T cells, which can be identified by surface antigens.

The experiments described in the preceding section show that the cells involved in cell-mediated reactions are T cells; these experiments require a marker (Thy 1) that distinguishes T cells from B cells. The experiments described in this section show T cell:T cell interaction in the generation of a CTL response, and require a marker that distinguishes different subpopulations of T cells. Such antigenic markers exist as a series of surface antigens, called Lyt antigens (see Chapter 11). There are three well-studied Lyt antigens: Lyt 1, Lyt 2, and Lyt 3.

In the experiment diagrammed in Figure 5, lymph node T cells were used to generate an in vitro CTL response. These lymphocytes were pretreated with various antisera *before* the addition of antigen, in the following manner: treatment of cells with anti-Lyt 1 and complement eliminated all cells that expressed Lyt 1 on their surfaces but left cells expressing Lyt 2 and Lyt 3. Similarly, treating another cell population with anti-Lyt 2 and anti-Lyt 3 eliminated Lyt 2^+, 3^+ cells and left Lyt 1^+ cells. When the Lyt 1^+ cells were used to generate the CTL, they were incapable of generating a response. When Lyt 2^+, 3^+ cells were used, they were able to carry out CTL at only 30 percent of the control value. This result shows the situation is rather complicated, and signals that cell cooperation is probably occurring. When Lyt 1^+ and Lyt 2^+, 3^+ populations were combined, however, control levels of CTL were generated. This result shows that there are two populations of T lymphocytes that interact synergistically in CTL responses. One of these is the effector cell, but it needs the helper cell to fully generate its cytotoxic capacity.

Helper and Effector Cells To determine which cells were the helpers and which the effectors, another experiment was done (Figure 6). CTL were generated with lymph node T cells that were *not* treated with any antiserum. After the response had developed, however, and before the cells were assayed for their ability to cause ^{51}Cr release, they were treated with either anti-Lyt 1 or anti-Lyt 2,3 antiserum and complement. The cells remaining after this treatment were then tested for their ability to

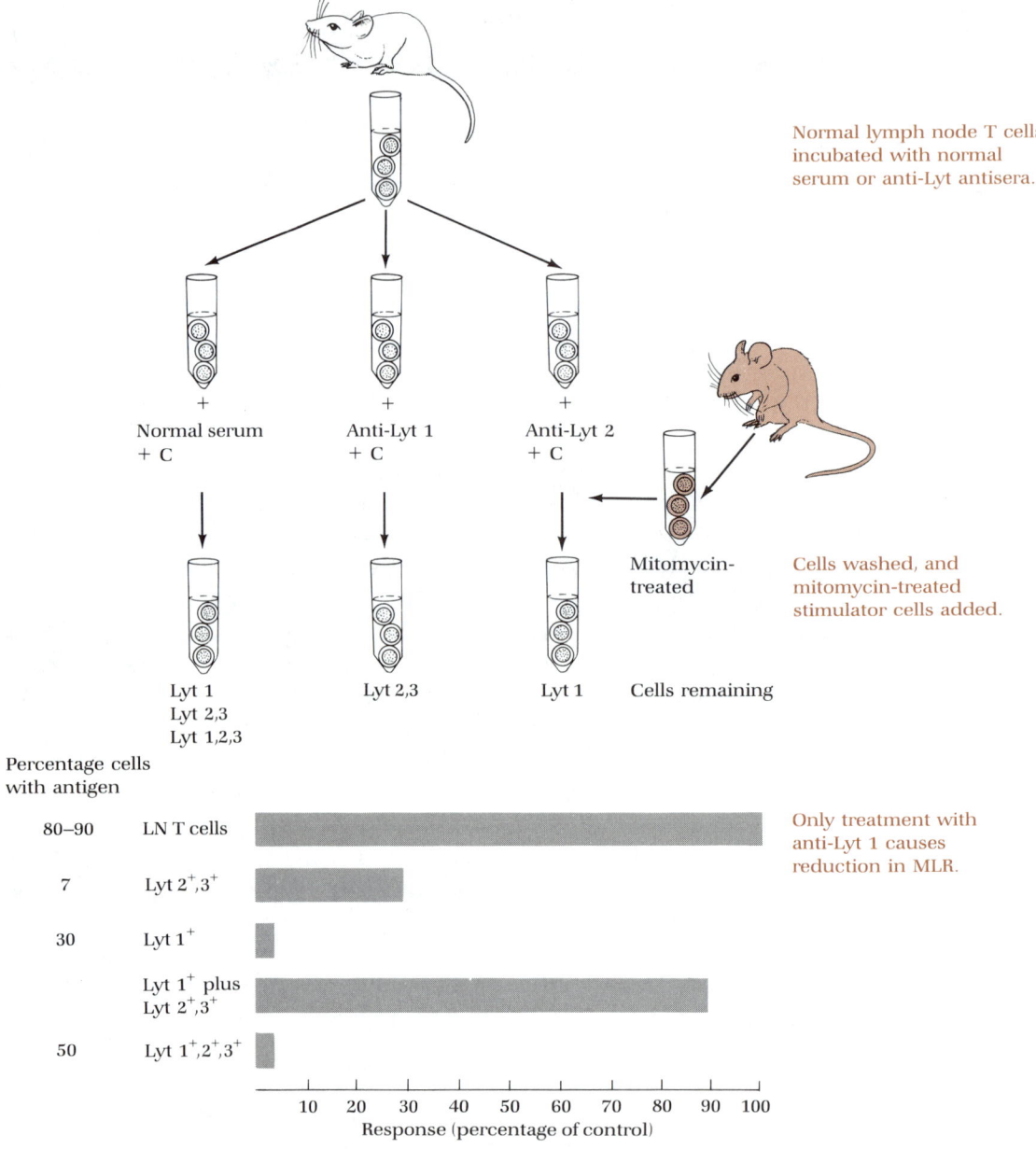

FIGURE 5 CELL COOPERATION IN CTL

(A) Normal spleen cells are treated with either normal serum plus C (as control), anti-Lyt 1 plus C (leaving Lyt 2,3 cells), or anti-Lyt 2 plus C (leaving Lyt 1 cells). Mitomycin-treated stimulator cells are added to each population. (B) Response of the cell population in A. Control cells (LN T cells) give 100%, Lyt 2,3 cells give 30%, and Lyt 1 cells give 5% of control. Combining Lyt 1 and Lyt 2,3 populations gives 100% of control, showing that there is cell cooperation. [After Cantor and Boyse (1975) *J. Exp. Med.* 141, 1376 and 1390]

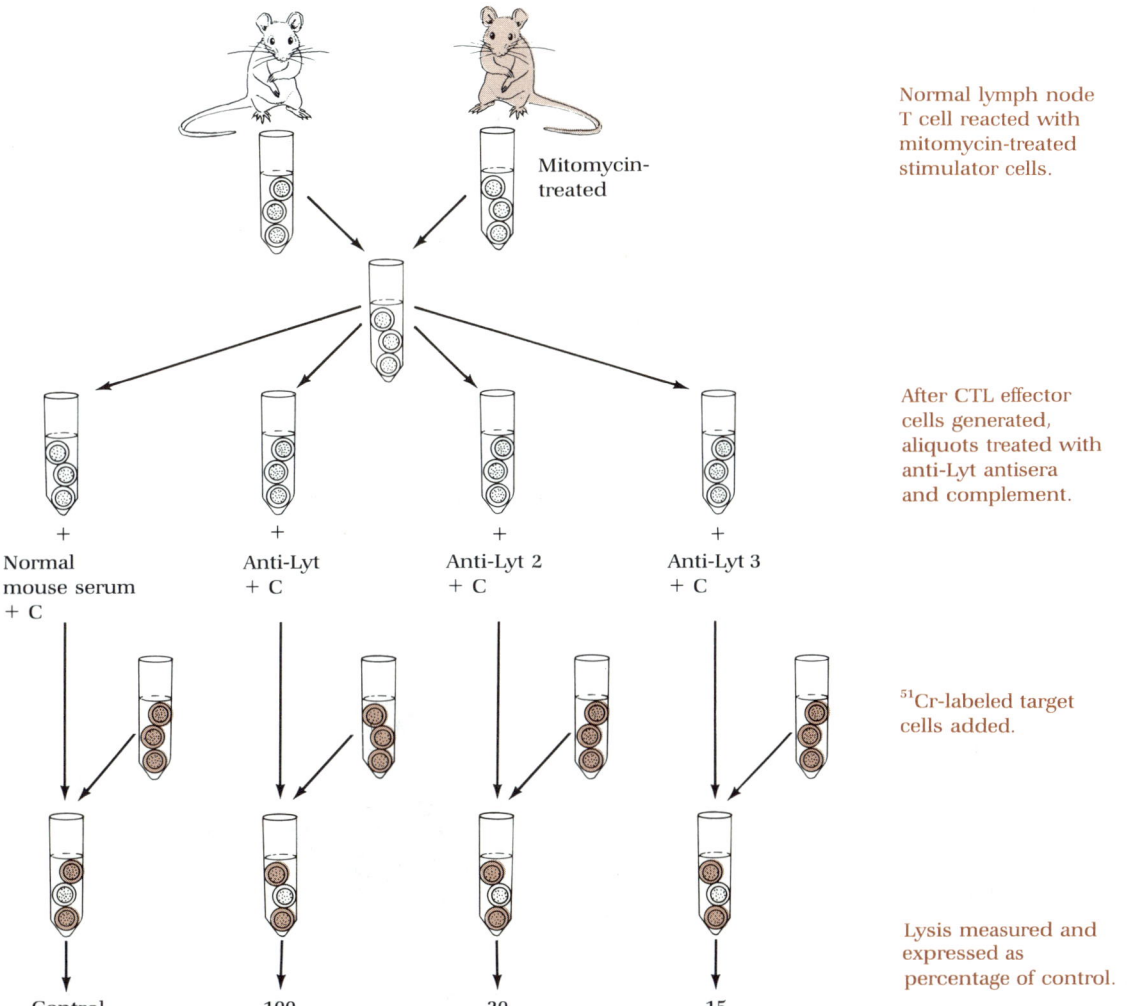

FIGURE 6 LYT PROFILE OF CTL EFFECTOR CELLS

CTL are generated by reacting mitomycin-treated stimulator cells with normal lymph node T cells. After several hours, the cells are treated with anti-Lyt antiserum and complement and subsequently reacted with the ^{51}Cr-labeled targets. Treatment with anti-Lyt 1 (Lyt 2,3 cells remaining) does not reduce the percentage of lysis, but treatment with anti-Lyt 2, 3 does. Thus, the CTL effector is Lyt 2, 3. [After Cantor and Boyse (1975) *J. Exp. Med.* 141, 1376]

CHAPTER FIFTEEN

act as effector cells in CTL. In this way it was possible to determine the Lyt phenotype of the *effector* population. It was found that only treatment with anti-Lyt 2 or anti-Lyt 3 abolished the ability of the cells to carry out lysis of the target cells. This result shows that the Lyt 2^+, 3^+ cells are the *effector* cells and that the Lyt 1^+ cells act as *helper* cells.

Summary

1. Repopulating an irradiated mouse with either bone marrow *or* thymus cells does not reconstitute its antibody response. Repopulating with bone marrow *and* thymus cells does. This shows there is cell cooperation in generating antibody responses.
2. Experiments in which T cell populations are treated with anti-Lyt antiserum and complement show that Lyt 1^+ and Lyt 2^+, 3^+ T cells cooperate in the generation of cytotoxic T cells.
3. In antibody formation, B cells are the effector cells and T cells are the helper cells. In the cytotoxic T cell responses, Lyt 2^+, 3^+ cells are the effector cells and Lyt 1^+ cells are the helper cells.

CHAPTER 16

HELPER AND EFFECTOR DETERMINANTS

Overview In the last chapter we saw that in both antibody formation and cell-mediated responses, one set of cells acts as effector cells and the other acts as helper cells. The next layer of complexity involves the means by which helper and effector cells interact with antigen. As we examine both humoral and cell-mediated responses, we will once again see the same basic pattern. There are helper and effector determinants in each of the types of responses.

The reaction of helper T cells and effector B cells with different antigenic determinants (or epitopes) was discovered through the use of haptens and carriers. The explanation of what had been a rather mysterious phenomenon called the carrier effect allowed us to see that the helper cell (the T cell) reacts with the carrier portion of the antigen and the effector cell (the B cell) reacts with the haptenic determinant. This means that for a molecule to initiate an immune response (that is, to be an immunogen), it must have at least two kinds of determinants, helper and effector. In cell-mediated responses, the same pattern of reaction by the helper and effector cells is seen. The reader should keep in mind the symmetry that is beginning to emerge in humoral and cell-mediated responses. Both use the strategy of helper cell and effector cell, each of which reacts with helper determinant and effector determinant respectively on the antigen.

CHAPTER SIXTEEN

Antibody Formation

We already know that the B cell is the effector cell and the T cell is the helper cell in antibody formation. Our understanding of helper and effector cell interactions in antibody formation came about through our understanding of the roles of *haptens* and *carriers*.

In Chapter 2 we saw that haptens were classically defined by Landsteiner as molecules that can react with antibody but cannot induce antibody formation (i.e., are antigenic but not immunogenic). However, a hapten can be made immunogenic by conjugating it to an immunogenic molecule, such as a foreign protein. In this way, hapten–carrier conjugates (H-C) elicit anti-hapten and anti-carrier responses when injected into an animal. When a hapten such as DNP is conjugated to any of a variety of immunogenic proteins, the animal responds by producing anti-DNP antibodies as well as antibodies to the carrier. This finding naturally led to the idea that the carrier was only a passive vehicle, whose only function was to transport the hapten. The experiments below describe the *carrier effect* and show this idea to be an oversimplification.

The Carrier Effect

The carrier portion of the hapten–carrier conjugate has more than the mere transport role it was originally thought to play. An example of what came to be called the CARRIER EFFECT is shown in Figure 1. Dinitrophenyl (DNP) is a hapten. When it is injected alone, it does not stimulate antibody formation. Bovine γ-globulin (BGG) is a carrier. When it is injected alone, it stimulates anti-BGG antibody production. In the experiment shown in Figure 1, animals were immunized with DNP conjugated to BGG (DNP-BGG). After suitable intervals, the serum of the animals was assayed for anti-DNP antibody. The animals were then re-injected with either DNP-BGG (the homologous hapten–carrier conjugate), DNP-egg albumin (DNP-EA) (the same hapten on a different carrier protein), or BGG (the original carrier without hapten). Only the animals that received a second injection of DNP-BGG made a good secondary response to DNP. Thus, even though all the animals had received a first injection of

HELPER AND EFFECTOR DETERMINANTS

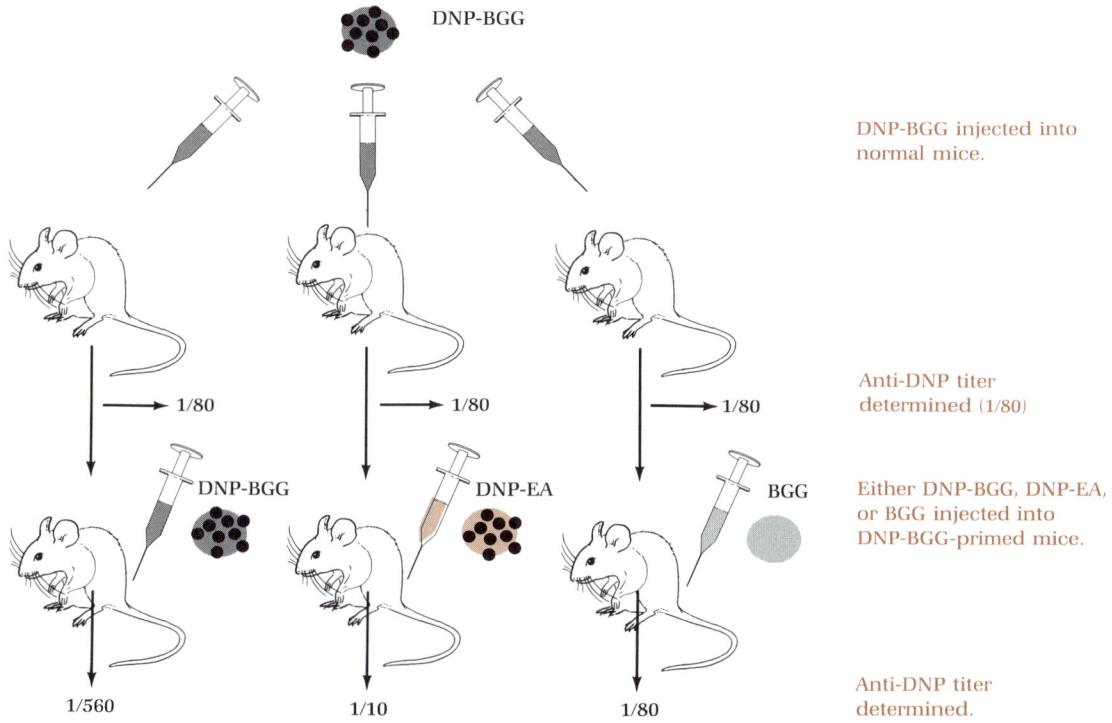

FIGURE 1   THE CARRIER EFFECT

A secondary anti-hapten response is obtained only when the hapten is on the same carrier in both the primary and secondary injections. This is true even though the mice have made comparable primary anti-hapten responses. [After Ovary and Benacerraf (1963) *Proc. Soc. Exp. Biol. Med.* 114, 72]

DNP (were primed to DNP), they made a secondary response to the second confrontation of DNP only when it was conjugated to the *same* carrier used in the initial injection. This experiment shows that even though an animal is injected with the same hapten for both the primary and secondary responses, it will make a secondary or augmented response to the second injection of hapten only when the hapten is on the same carrier for both injections. In other words, the carrier molecule plays more than a passive role.

CHAPTER SIXTEEN

Adoptive Transfer of the Carrier Effect

To analyze the cellular events responsible for this surprising result (the carrier effect), Mitchison and his co-workers in London carried out a series of experiments using *adoptive transfer* of the carrier effect. The idea of these experiments is to use an irradiated mouse as a biological test tube. Various spleen cell populations are injected into the irradiated mouse; in this manner the experimenter can determine the role played by a particular cell population in the cellular interactions leading to antibody formation. The beauty of this system is that a variety of experimental manipulations can be made on the spleen cells before transfer. By use of this experimental design the carrier effect can be transferred adoptively, as shown diagrammatically in Figure 2.

In these adoptive transfer experiments mice are lethally irradiated and injected with spleen cells from syngenic mice. The donor mice have usually been primed to either of two hapten–carrier complexes that we will call hapten–carrier I (HC-I) and hapten–carrier II (HC-II). (In this case, the second carrier is designated C-II.) Unprimed donor mice are used as a source of control cells. After repopulation with the primed cells, the recipients are challenged with HC-I. Figure 2 shows that only recipients that were primed with HC-I make a secondary anti-hapten response.

Overcoming the Carrier Effect by Carrier Priming

We saw in the experiment in Figure 2 that the carrier effect could be transferred adoptively with spleen cells. The carrier effect can be overcome (that is, a secondary response to HC-II can be obtained) if the recipient mice in the adoptive transfer are repopulated with HC-I-primed cells *plus* cells from mice *primed to the heterologous carrier alone* (C-II). This experiment is diagrammed in Figure 3.

Part A of this experiment is a repeat of the adoptive transfer of the carrier effect. In part B there are two groups of donors, one primed to HC-I and one primed only to the heterologous carrier, C-II. The irradiated recipients receive primed cells from each set of donors and are then challenged with hapten conjugated with the heterologous carrier, HC-II. The amount of anti-hapten antibody produced by these recipients is comparable to that in the mice in Figure 2 that received homologous hapten–carrier conju-

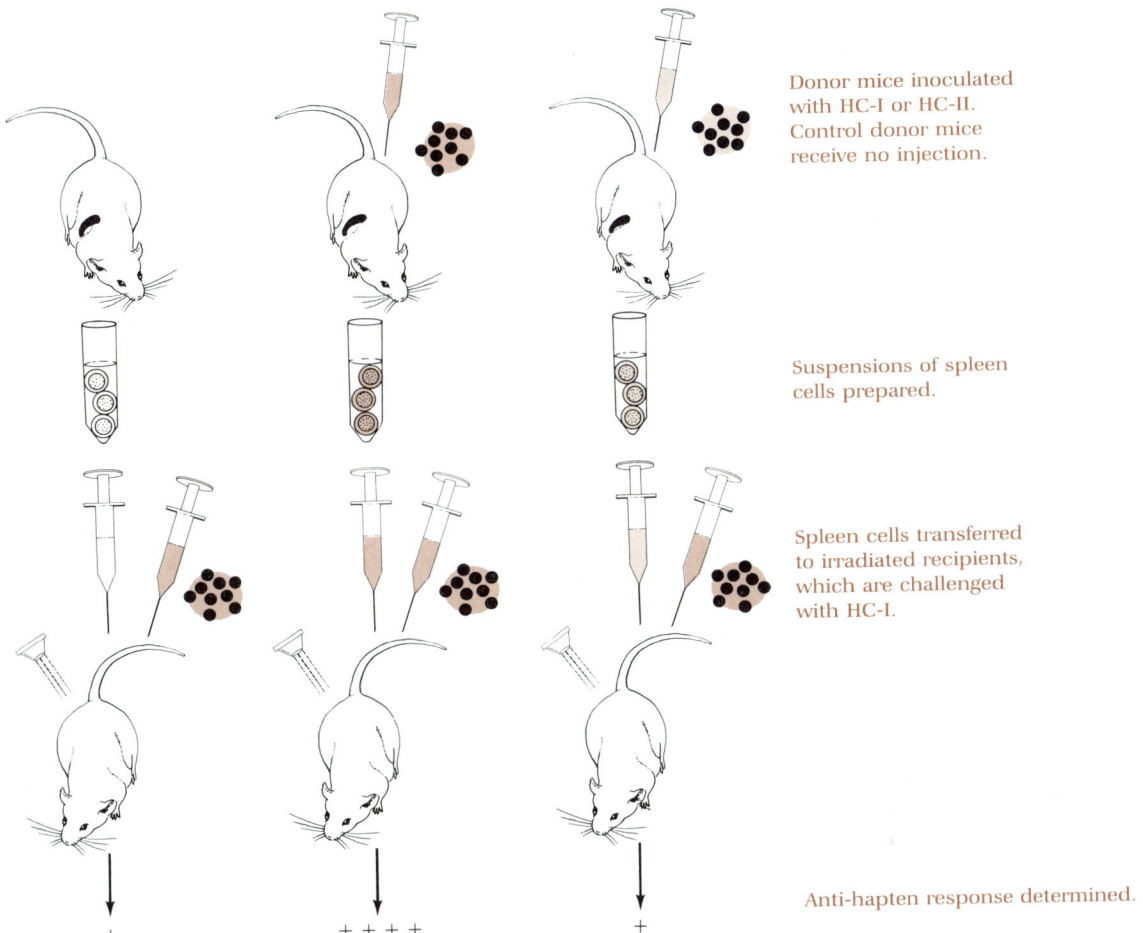

FIGURE 2 ADOPTIVE TRANSFER OF THE CARRIER EFFECT

Mice are immunized with either HC-I or HC-II and their spleen cells transferred to syngeneic, irradiated recipients. The recipients are challenged with HC-I. The carrier effect is seen in the new hosts that received spleen cells from HC-I-treated donors.

gate. This result means that the presence of the C-II-primed cells overcame the carrier effect. The C-II-primed spleen cells could not be contributing the extra anti-hapten antibody because they were not primed to the hapten, but it is clear that they were necessary for the production of a response by the anti-hapten-producing cells.

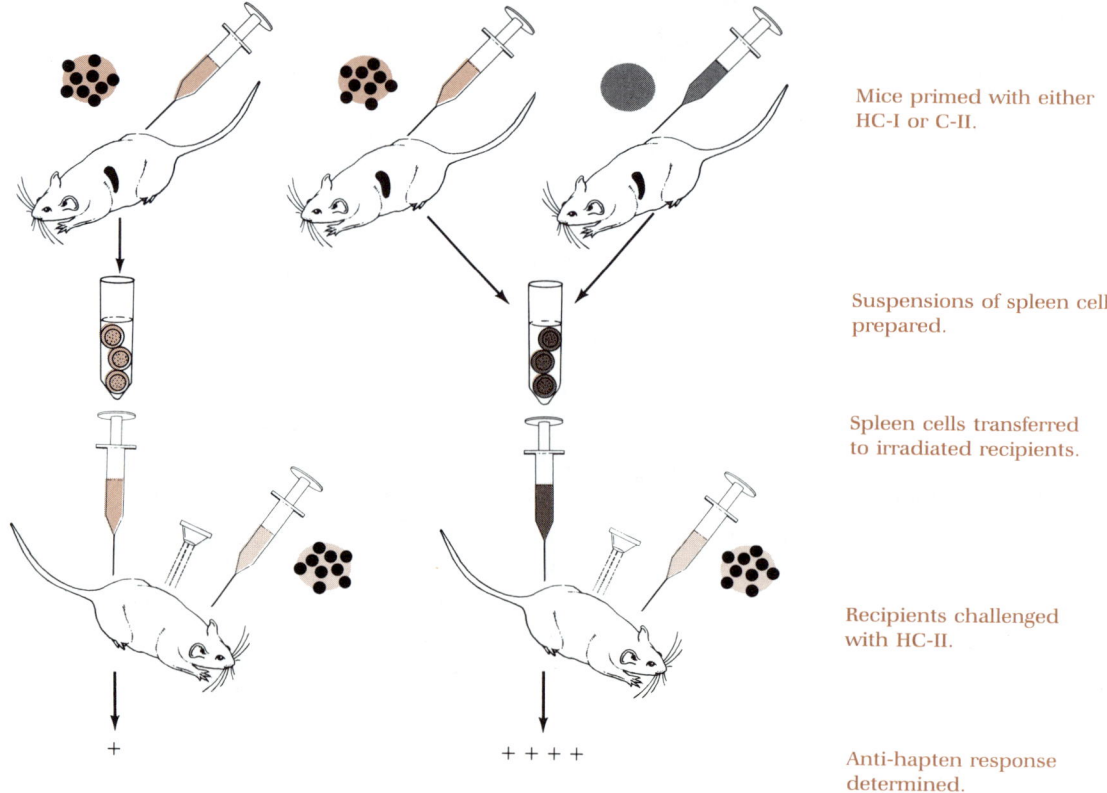

FIGURE 3   CARRIER PRIMING

Carrier priming overcomes the carrier effect in an adoptive transfer experiment. Irradiated recipients that receive a mixture of spleen cells from mice primed with HC-I and mice primed with C-II (with no hapten conjugated) produce a secondary response to HC-II.

This experiment shows some form of *cooperation* between the hapten-primed and the carrier-primed populations. It appears that when one set of cells is primed to hapten (HC-I) and one to carrier (C-II), they interact to produce a secondary response to the hapten even though it is conjugated to the heterologous carrier. Thus if we can understand the cellular basis of the carrier effect, we will be on the path to understanding the nature of the cell cooperation in the generation of an antibody response.

HELPER AND EFFECTOR DETERMINANTS

Hapten-Reactive and Carrier-Reactive Lymphocytes: The Raff Experiment

The experiment that explained the cellular basis of the carrier effect and gave the first indication of the nature of the division of labor among B cells and T cells was carried out by Martin Raff in London in 1970.

The plan of the experiment is elegantly simple. It is essentially the carrier-priming experiment described in Figure 3, with the additional step of treating the primed cells with either anti-Thy 1 or normal serum before transferring them to irradiated recipients. Treatment with anti-Thy 1 antiserum and complement will lyse T cells; in this way it can be determined whether the T cells in the primed mice have responded to hapten or to carrier.

The experiment and results are shown in Figure 4. In part A, one group of mice is primed with HC-I and another with C-II. After a suitable interval (approximately one week) the adoptive transfer is carried out. However, the carrier-primed cells are treated with anti-Thy 1 antiserum plus complement before transfer. In other words, the T cells in the carrier-primed suspension are lysed. The hapten-primed cells are treated with normal serum plus complement, so the T cells in this group are unaffected. The two populations are mixed and injected into irradiated hosts, which are then challenged with hapten conjugated to carrier II (HC-II). (Figure 3 serves as the control for this experiment—that is, no anti-Thy 1 treatment. The result is a secondary anti-hapten response.) We see in Figure 4 that treating the carrier-primed population with anti-Thy 1 results in a poor anti-hapten response; that is, the carrier effect is *not* overcome. This means anti-Thy 1 treatment of the carrier-primed population abolished the ability to overcome the carrier effect. This experiment demonstrates that the T cells have reacted with the carrier.

In contrast, in part B, when the hapten-primed spleen cells are treated with anti-Thy 1 antiserum plus complement and the carrier-primed cells are treated with normal serum, the carrier effect *is* overcome. This result shows that killing the T cells has no effect on the hapten-primed population. We know that antibody-producing cells are B cells and that antibody is being produced against the hapten. Therefore this experiment dramatically shows that helper T cells respond to carrier.

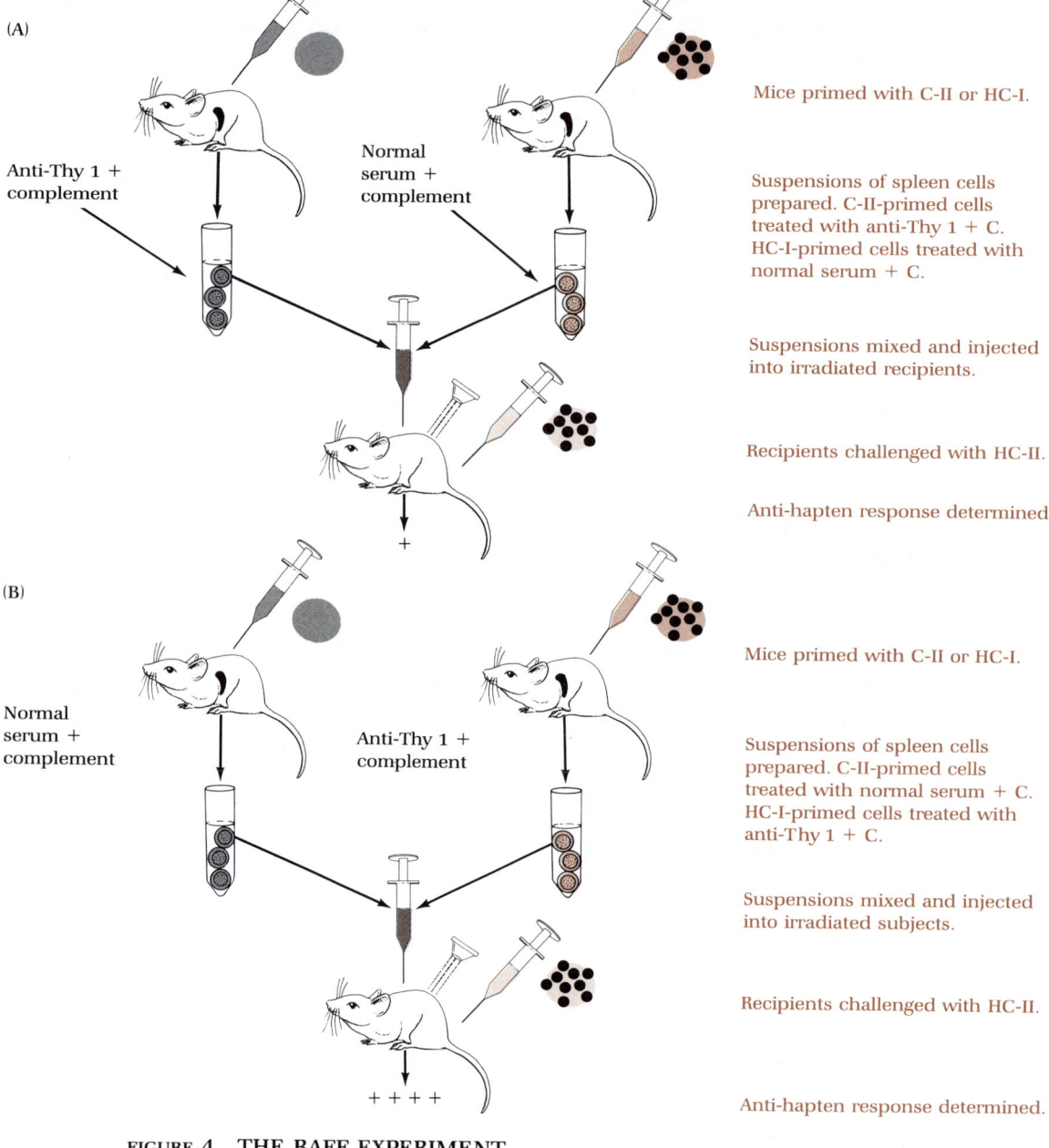

FIGURE 4 THE RAFF EXPERIMENT
This experiment shows carrier-primed cells are T cells, because when they are treated with anti-Thy 1 and complement the carrier effect is not overcome. In contrast, there is no effect when hapten-primed cells are treated with anti-Thy 1 and complement. [After Raff (1970) *Nature* 226, 1257]

HELPER AND EFFECTOR DETERMINANTS

The result of this experiment shows that the effector cells and the helper cells in antibody formation each react with a different part of the immunogen. It also shows that we must think of an immunogen as being composed of helper determinants and effector determinants.

Overcoming the Carrier Effect with Allogeneic Cells: The Allogeneic Effect

The experiment in Figure 3 showed it is possible to overcome the carrier effect with carrier priming and that this second effect is the result of a reaction between helper T cells and carrier determinants on the antigen. David Katz and his co-workers, first at the NIH and then in Boston, found that it is possible to overcome the carrier effect in another, quite different way. They observed that the injection of *allogeneic cells* could also allow the animals to respond to HC-II with a secondary anti-hapten response.

As shown in Figure 5, an HC-I primed animal makes a secondary anti-hapten response to HC-II when allogeneic cells are injected. The allogeneic cells must be viable, so they probably carry out some form of GVH reaction. During the course of the allogeneic response that results from the injection of these cells, a soluble factor is produced; it can substitute for the allogeneic cells. Thus if one generates an allogeneic response in vitro (i.e., an MLR) and uses the supernatant fraction from this reaction in place of the cells, one gets a comparable result—the overcoming of the carrier effect.

We will see later that this phenomenon, which probably is not of physiological importance, time and again plays an important part in experiments designed to analyze the cellular events in immune responses. It is also one of the first indications that the MHC can play a crucial role in the cellular interactions leading to an immune response.

Cell-Mediated Responses

T cell:T cell cooperation in the generation of cytotoxic lymphocytes (CTL) was elegantly shown through the use of anti-Lyt antiserum (Chapter 15). In those experiments, neither the Lyt 1^+ nor the Lyt 2^+ T cells alone were able to generate large numbers of CTL effector cells. Combining the Lyt 1^+ and the Lyt 2^+ popula-

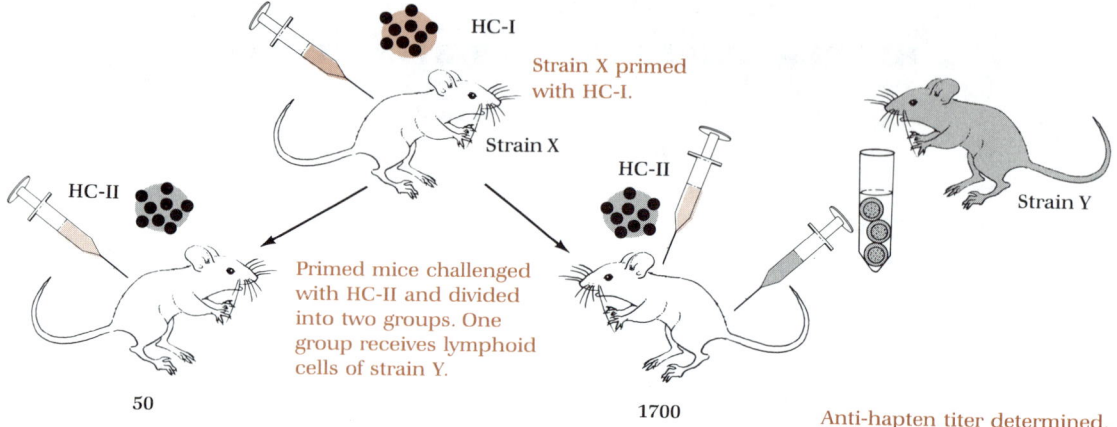

FIGURE 5 THE ALLOGENEIC EFFECT
The carrier effect can be overcome by injecting allogeneic spleen cells that have not been carrier primed. [After Katz et al. (1971) *J. Exp. Med.* 133, 169]

tions, however, restored CTL activity to levels comparable to those of the untreated cells. By treating cells with anti-Lyt antiserum *after* a CTL had been generated, it was shown that the effector cell was the Lyt 2^+ cell and the helper cell the Lyt 1^+ cell.

MLR and CTL Responses and MHC Antigens

An important series of experiments by Bach and his co-workers in Madison showed that there are separate *subpopulations* of T cells, which react with different antigens of the MHC complex.[1] The general plan of these experiments was to test the ability of cells to stimulate an MLR using cells from strains of mice with known differences in the H-2 complex. By choosing the proper congenic strains, it is possible to test the contribution to the MLR of an antigenic difference in only one region of H-2. To test the role of the antigens of the D region, for example, one could choose as responder a strain that

---

[1] In the rest of this chapter we will be discussing the generation of cytotoxic lymphocytes (CTL), the mixed lymphocyte reaction (MLR), and the major histocompatibility complex (MHC). It will be necessary to lapse into "immunologese" at times. The reader is urged to review CTL and MLR in Chapter 14 and MHC in Chapter 13 before proceeding.

HELPER AND EFFECTOR DETERMINANTS

is bbbb ($K^b I^b S^b D^b$). The stimulator cell (which is treated with mitomycin C so that it cannot proliferate) could then be bbbk. In this case the only difference is in the D region of the H-2 complex: b in one case, k in the other. Similar combinations can be set up for the K region or the I region. Recall that the results of MLR stimulation studies are expressed as a stimulation index (SI), which is calculated as

$$SI = \frac{\text{cpm of experimental}}{\text{cpm of control}}$$

If the incorporation in the experimental group is the same as that in the control group, the SI is 1.0. If the experimental is six times the control, the SI is 6.0, and so on.

When a large number of combinations were examined, a pattern emerged (Table 1). The greatest stimulation of the MLR came from differences at the I region of H-2 (Class II MHC molecules). Similar kinds of experiments were also carried out in the generation of CTL, the idea being to vary only one region of H-2 and examine the effect on CTL. These results showed that differences at the I region gave little or no CTL but differences at K and D regions gave good stimulation (Table 1). Thus we see that the MLR is associated with Class II molecules and the CTL with Class I molecules.

TABLE 1 Effect of various regions of the H-2 complex on the generation of MLR and CTL.

Difference between responder and stimulator cells	MLR	CTL
K	Poor	Good
I	Very good	Poor
S	Poor	Poor
D	Poor	Good
K or D plus I	—	Very good

CHAPTER SIXTEEN

The "Three-Cell Experiment"

The most dramatic results of this series of experiments came from Bach's "Three-Cell Experiment." Now we know that cells that differ in Class II give the best MLR and cells that differ in Class I give good CTL. If the MLR and CTL are manifestations of helper and effector cell stimula-

MLR (proliferation, as cpm [^{3}H]thymidine)	Stimulator cell	Responder cell	CTL (cytotoxicity, as percentage of ^{51}Cr release)
10,000	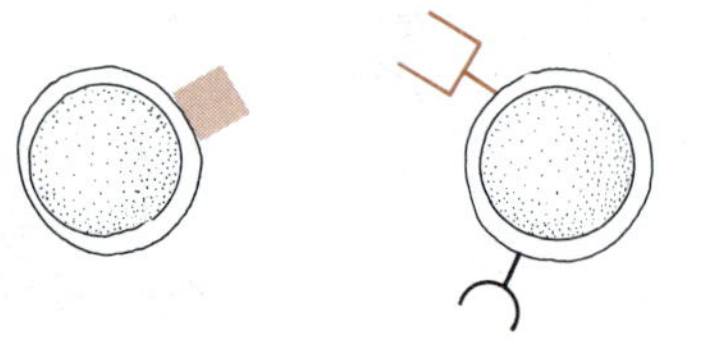	Stimulator and responder cells differ at Class II	0
3000	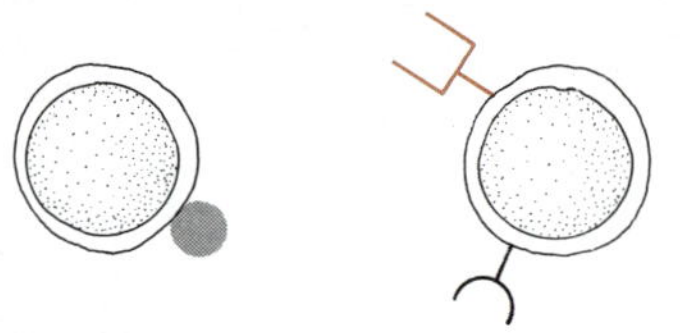	Stimulator and responder differ at Class I	15
10,000	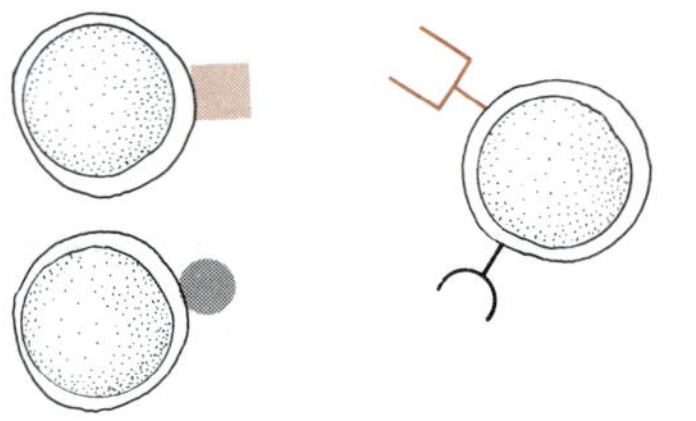	Stimulator and responder differ at both Class I and Class II	50

FIGURE 6   THE THREE-CELL EXPERIMENT

There is collaboration between Class I and Class II MHC antigens in the generation of CTL. [After Schendel et al. (1976) *Nature* 259, 273]

HELPER AND EFFECTOR DETERMINANTS

tion, then combining the cells with the differences seen in Table 1 should give strong MLR and even stronger CTL responses. Figure 6 shows that this is exactly the result obtained. Although differences at Class I antigens give good responses and differences at Class II antigens give poor responses, the combination of differences at Class I and Class II gives a very good response.

Other experiments using anti-Lyt antiserum carried out at about this time showed that the MLR reactive cell was an Lyt 1^+ cell. This finding leads to the conclusion that the cells reactive with Class II MHC antigens (I region determinants) are the *helper* cells and cells reactive with Class I determinants are the *effector* cells in cell-mediated reactions. Thus in cell-mediated responses, just as in antibody responses, there are helper cells and effector cells, each of which react with unique determinants on the antigen. This association of help with Class II and effector cells with Class I will be a recurring theme in the following chapters.

Summary

1. The nature of the cell interactions between helper cells and effector cells in antibody formation can be studied using haptens and carriers. Haptens are molecules that do not induce the production of antibody by themselves but do when conjugated to an immunogenic molecule called a carrier.
2. The carrier effect is the requirement for the hapten to be conjugated to the same carrier in both the primary and secondary challenge. Hapten conjugated to a second carrier for the second challenge does not lead to a secondary anti-hapten response. The carrier effect can be adoptively transferred.
3. Priming with heterologous carrier overcomes the carrier effect. When carrier-primed cells are pretreated with anti-Thy 1 and complement and transferred with cells primed to hapten on heterologous carrier, the carrier effect is not overcome. This shows that T helper cells are primed to carrier.
4. Antigen can be thought of as having two determinants: haptenic determinants that react with B cells and carrier determinants that react with T cells.
5. In cell-mediated responses, MLR cells react with Class II (I region) MHC determinants and CTL react with Class I (K/D) MHC determinants.

CHAPTER 17

MHC RESTRICTION

Overview We have been dropping tantalizing hints that the MHC plays a central role in generating immune responses. In this chapter we will present some of the evidence showing that this is the case. The first inkling of the importance of the MHC in the generation of immune responses came when we saw that the responder–nonresponder trait mapped to the MHC. The next important realization came when it was found that cell cooperation apparently could occur only between syngeneic cells. This finding led to the notion that there was like:like interaction between helper and effector cells. However, the use of animals repopulated with allogeneic hemopoietic stem cells (called bone marrow chimeras) and thus having allogeneic hemopoietic cells showed that like:like interactions could not be the case. In fact, the best explanation is that the T helper cell must recognize MHC antigen, which means it must have a receptor for "self" as well as for foreign antigen.

One of the more surprising results we will see is the phenomenon of "adaptive differentiation," in which self-reactivity can be acquired or learned.

Thus, in this chapter we will see revealed yet another level of complexity of cell interactions. The picture that will emerge is one of joint recognition. The activation of helper T cells requires the recognition of antigen in association with MHC on the surface of an antigen-presenting cell.

MHC RESTRICTION

MHC Restriction in Antibody Formation

Mitchell-Miller Revisited: The Need for Syngeneic Cells

The Mitchell-Miller experiment (Chapter 15) was one of the crucial experiments in the development of the idea of cell cooperation in the immune response. In that experiment, neonatally thymectomized mice of one H-2 haplotype were repopulated with thymus cells from mice of another haplotype (allogeneic thymus cells) to determine whether the thymus-derived lymphocytes were the antibody-producing cells. The haplotype of the antibody-forming cells was shown to be that of the host rather than that of the donor of the thymus cells, proving that the thymus cells did not produce antibody, but only acted as helper cells for a cell already present in the thymectomized mouse. However, a difficulty developed when the approach of using different H-2 haplotypes as markers could not be used in a Claman-type experiment of bone marrow–thymus reconstitution of irradiated mice. In that experiment allogeneic bone marrow and thymus cells failed to cooperate in an irradiated host. This inability to cooperate across an H-2 barrier was thought to be merely a technical nuisance. As we will now see, the "nuisance" became a profound observation. There is probably some great lesson of social significance to be learned from this.

Repopulation Failure in Nude Mice

The inability of allogeneic bone marrow and thymus cells to cooperate was seen again in some very important experiments carried out by Bernice Kindred and Don Shreffler. They found that nude mice (which are congenitally athymic) could have their immune response restored only transiently with allogeneic thymus cells. In these studies, BALB/c nudes were repopulated with thymus cells from syngeneic BALB/c mice ($H-2^d$) or with allogeneic thymus cells of CBA ($H-2^k$) or C57BL/6 ($H-2^b$) mice. If the animals were challenged with antigen and assayed for antibody within a few days after reconstitution, they produced a good antibody response, whether reconstituted with either syngeneic or allogeneic thymus cells. But if there was an interval of several days between repopulating with thymus cells and challenge with antigen, only the animals reconstituted with the syngeneic thymus cells responded. The lack of response by the animals repopulated with allogeneic thymus

CHAPTER SEVENTEEN

cells was not due to the disappearance of the allogeneic cells or to reaction by the host against them, but was, rather, a reflection of an inability to cooperate.

Kindred went on to do a large series of experiments with thymus grafts and was able to show clearly that the responses of nude mice were restored much more efficiently with syngeneic than with allogeneic grafts. It seems safe to assume that the transient restoration seen using allogeneic cells is caused by the allogeneic effect. The irony is that this probably means the Mitchell-Miller experiment—the crucial experiment showing helper and effector cells, upon which so much followed—gave "correct" results for the wrong reason. The B cells that were activated in that experiment were almost certainly activated not by the T helper cells, but by an allogeneic effect.

Claman Revisited: The Need For I Region (Class II) MHC Identity

The examples of the inability of bone marrow and thymus-derived cells to cooperate across H-2 barriers were studied extensively by Katz and his co-workers, who showed that a fundamental principle in the immune response was involved. Using a reconstitution system that was designed to *rule out the allogeneic effect*, they primed T cells to carrier (C-I) in one strain (B10.A) of mice and primed B cells to hapten (HC-II) in mice of homologous (B10.A) and heterologous (A) strains. The system, which is a variation of the original Claman experiment, is diagrammed in Figure 1. These primed populations were then allowed to cooperate in an irradiated F_1 of the two parental strains. The recipient was then challenged with hapten (HC-I), and the anti-hapten response was tested.[1] In this

---

[1] Many experiments in this and the next chapter will use congenic mice; the reader may want to review Chapter 13. A thorough understanding of the carrier effect (Chapter 16) is also needed at this point.

FIGURE 1 MHC RESTRICTION IN ANTIBODY FORMATION
Cells with the same MHC but different backgrounds cooperate in antibody formation. (A) Mice of different strains are carrier primed or hapten primed and injected into unirradiated F_1 mice, which are challenged with hapten and carrier. (B) When the MHC is the same, there is cooperation leading to antibody formation. [After Katz et al. (1973) *Proc. Natl. Acad. Sci. USA* 70, 2624]

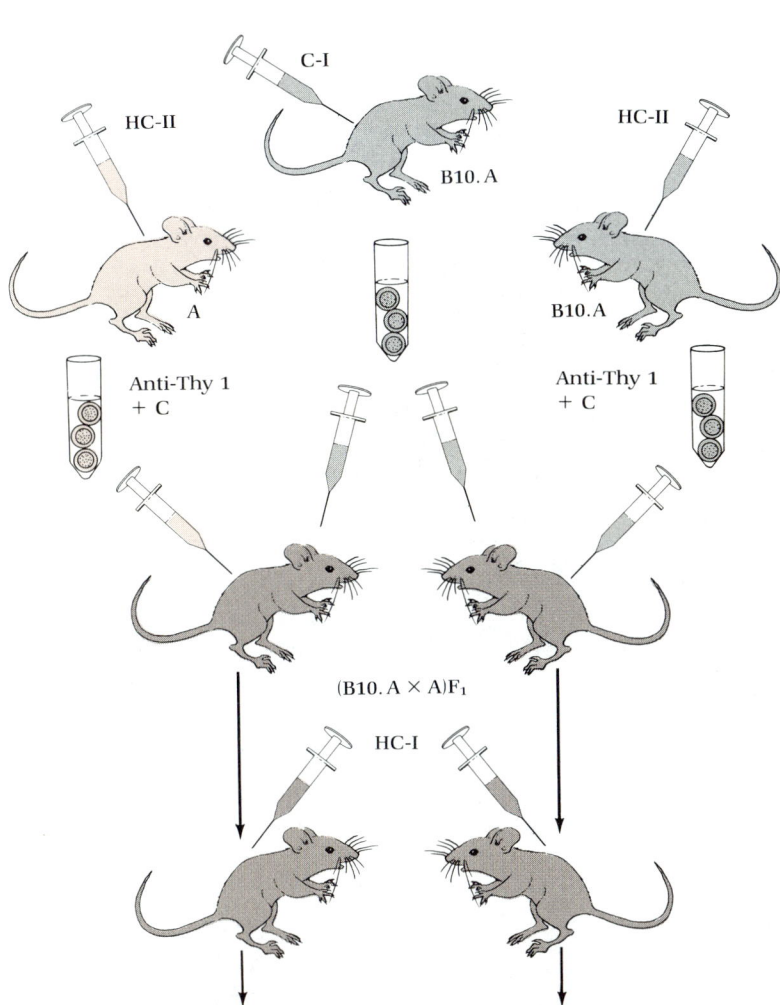

way, they were able to determine whether carrier-primed T cells could cooperate with B cells of any H-2 haplotype or whether there was genetic restriction in the interaction of T cells and B cells. Figure 1 shows that when both cell populations were from the same strain (B10.A), there was good cooperation—as expected. When the cells were from strains that were allogeneic at both background and H-2 (for example, B10 and A.By), there was poor cooperation. The crucial groups here are Groups III and IV. In Group III, the H-2 regions are identical ($H-2^a$), but the backgrounds are different (B10 and A). Nevertheless, there is good cooperation, indicating that any barrier to cooperation is not found in the background but in H-2. In Group IV, the backgrounds are identical (B10 and B10.A), but the H-2 is different. This arrangement results in poor cooperation. From this experiment Katz concluded that identity at H-2 is required for B cell:T cell cooperation.

The results in Figure 1 show that there can be cooperation of populations when background genes are different, but no cooperation unless the H-2 genes are identical. But these results do not show *which* region of H-2 must be shared. Experiments of similar design using other recombinant strains showed that the crucial differences in the H-2 complex were localized in the I region (Class II genes). It is a generally accepted conclusion, based on many years of experimental results, that the MHC restricted cooperation is the physiologically important one and the non-MHC restricted cooperation seen in the allogeneic effect is not of physiological significance. The most important experiments in cellular immunology in the last several years are based upon this conclusion.

MHC Restriction in Cell-Mediated Responses

Shortly after Katz showed that there was MHC restriction in the generation of an antibody response, two groups working independently showed that there is also MHC restriction in the generation of cell-mediated responses.

MHC RESTRICTION

The Zinkernagel-Doherty-Shearer Phenomenon

The generation of cytotoxic T cells for antigens other than allogeneic H-2 is also MHC restricted. This phenomenon was demonstrated for virus by Zinkernagel and Doherty in Australia and Shearer at the NIH. It was soon extended to minor histocompatibility antigens (non-H-2) and the male H-Y antigen. It is now seen as one of the basic rules of the immune response.

The basis of the phenomenon is shown in Figure 2. Mice of

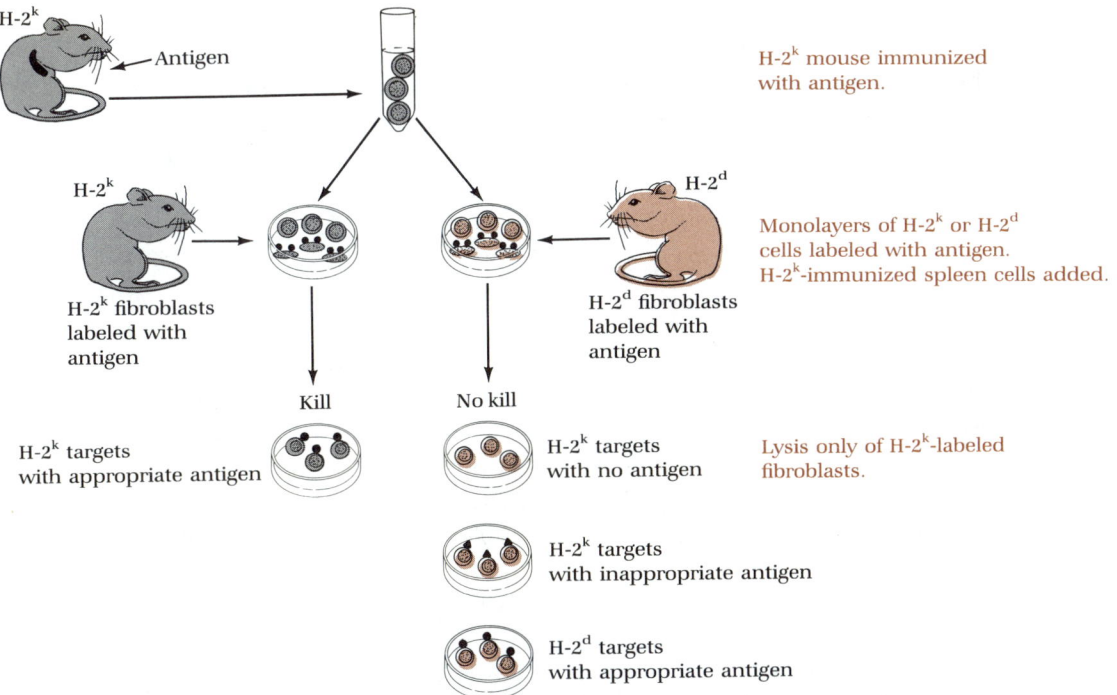

FIGURE 2 MHC RESTRICTION IN CELL-MEDIATED RESPONSES

Mice are challenged with antigen, which can be virus [Zinkernagel and Doherty (1974) *Nature* 248, 701]; TNP-modified self cells [Shearer (1974) *Eur. J. Immunol.* 4, 527); minor H antigens [Bevan (1975) *J. Exp. Med.* 142, 1349]; or H-Y antigens [Gordon et al. (1975) *J. Exp. Med.* 142, 1108]. Antigen-specific lysis of appropriate target cells is seen only when target and effector cells share MHC antigens.

one strain are immunized with antigen to generate CTL. After an appropriate interval their spleen cells are added to ^{51}Cr-labeled antigen-coated target cells of the same or a different strain. When the antigen (virus, TNP, minor H, or H-Y) is on a target cell of the same H-2 haplotype as the immunized mouse, killing of the target cells occurs (Group A). The following controls show that the spleen cells are cytotoxic cells specific for the antigen on the target cells. When the sensitized spleen cells are added to cells of the same H-2 haplotype that have no antigen (Group B) or an inappropriate antigen (Group C), no killing occurs. This result shows that the injection of antigen has resulted in antigen-specific cytotoxic cells. The important group is Group D, in which the specific antigen is on target cells of another H-2 haplotype. In this group, no killing occurs. This means that even though antigen-specific cytotoxic cells were generated, they could only kill target cells displaying the appropriate antigen when the target cells were also of the same H-2 haplotype. Thus, there is MHC restriction in cytotoxic cells, just as there is in antibody formation.

Site of Restriction

The MHC restriction in antibody formation was localized to the I region, that is, the region coding for Class II MHC antigens. When similar analysis was done in the cytotoxic cell system, it was found, using congenic mice, that the restriction is exerted not in the I region, but in the K and D regions (Class I). This is shown in Table 1. We thus have a situation in which the generation of helper cells is restricted at the I region (Class II) and the generation of cytotoxic effector cells is restricted in the K/D regions (Class I).

Compatibility between Responder and Stimulator

The data in Figure 2 could be interpreted to mean that there is MHC restriction between the cytotoxic cell and target (that is, in the effector or killing phase of the CTL reaction), or it could indicate MHC restriction in the generation of the cytotoxic cells. To distinguish between these possibilities, several groups did the following experiment (Figure 3) in each of the model systems described above. $(A \times B)F_1$ ani-

MHC RESTRICTION

TABLE 1 MHC restriction (K/D regions) in generation of cytotoxic effector cells.[a]

Virus system	Immune spleen							Percentage ^{51}Cr release from macrophages		
	Strain	Haplotype						SJL sssss	BALB/C ddddd	CBA/H kkkkkk
		K	A	E	J	S	D			
LCM	A.TL	s	k	k	k	k	d	25	64	1
	CBA/H	k	k	k	k	k	k	2	1	34
	A/J	k	k	k	d	d	d	0	64	30
Ectromelia	A.TL	s	k	k	k	k	d	32	47	0
	CBA/H	k	k	k	k	k	k	0	15	43
Sendai	A.TL	s	k	k	k	k	d	63	24	5
	A.TH	s	s	s	s	s	d	63	59	3
	A/J	k	k	k	d	d	d	3	65	49

Source: From Doherty et al. (1976), *Transplant. Rev.* 29: 89.
[a] Areas in brown show significant differences.

mals were challenged with antigen that was associated with cells of either parent A or parent B. The spleen cells were then tested for killing on antigen-coated targets from parent A and parent B. If the MHC restriction is only between effector and target, then the (A × B)F_1 cells should kill both A and B targets, because the F_1 effector has both. If, however, the MHC restriction is between the responding precursor cell and the stimulating cell in the generation of the cytotoxic cell, an (A × B)F_1 challenged with antigen on the cells of parent A should lyse only A targets because only A MHC was present at the initiation of the response. Conversely, challenge of the F_1 with antigen-coated cells of B would lead to killing of B but not A targets. As shown in Figure 3, the killing was restricted to the parental haplotype used for immunization, indicating that the restriction occurs during the generation of the cytotoxic cells and not during the effector phase.

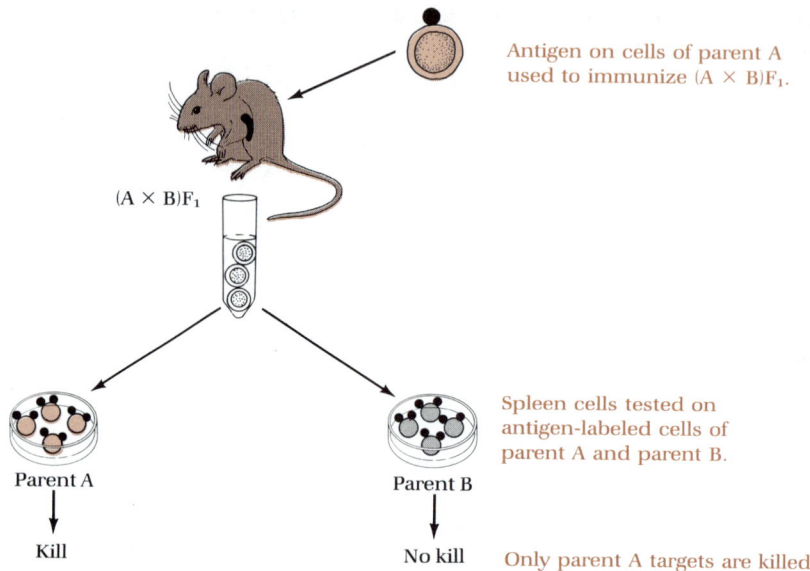

FIGURE 3 MHC RESTRICTION OCCURS DURING THE GENERATION OF CYTOTOXIC CELLS

F_1 mice are challenged with antigen on one parental-type cell. Killing is seen only when the effector cell is reacted with antigen-conjugated cells of that parental type. This result shows that the restriction occurs not during the effector phase of the reaction but during the generation of the effector cytotoxic cells.

Lyt Phenotype and Recognition of MHC Class

So far we have seen that Lyt 1^+ cells are helper cells in both cell-mediated responses and antibody formation (Chapter 15), and that helper cells are restricted to Class II antigens whereas cytotoxic cells are restricted to Class I (this chapter). These facts led originally to the conclusion that the Lyt phenotype of a T cell correlates with the functional subclass of the cell. It seemed logical to assume that the Lyt antigens were obligate markers for the subclasses, but we know now that this is not the case. Rather, the Lyt phenotype correlates with the class of MHC antigen that the cell recognizes. In other words, T cells that are restricted to Class I molecules are Lyt 2^+ and those that are restricted to Class II molecules are Lyt 1^+. This very

MHC RESTRICTION

important fact comes from experiments in which cells that are the exception to what was thought to be the rule were studied. For example, Susan Swain and her co-workers in La Jolla found that under the appropriate conditions they could generate helper T cells against Class I antigens, and that the cells that carry out this helper function express Lyt 2. Conversely, under conditions in which cytotoxic cells are generated against Class II antigens, the effector cells express Lyt 1. In addition, if these cells are treated with anti-Lyt 2 antibody in the absence of complement so that the Lyt 2 antigens are blocked, their cytotoxic activity is blocked. Treating with the antibody before challenge with antigen blocks the induction of functional cells.

Many other groups have produced results similar to this, and there is now general agreement that the class of MHC antigen to which the cell exhibits restriction is correlated with the Lyt phenotype. The functional significance and mechanism are not known, but the fact that anti-Lyt 2 blocks function and that the human counterparts, T4 and T8, have regions of homology with immunoglobulin variable regions will probably be crucial clues.

Cell Interaction Molecules   At the time, the most popular and intellectually satisfying explanation for the MHC restriction data was that T cells and B cells coooperated through the interaction of identical I region molecules. Katz called these CELL INTERACTION molecules (CI). This explanation means that the lymphocytes use their I region molecules (the CI molecules) to identify each other from among the myriad of cell types in the body, because Class II molecules are expressed only on lymphocytes and macrophages. It also means that the nature of the interaction is like:like. Because so many of the interactions in biology and biochemistry are the exact opposite of this—that is, like:unlike interactions (e.g., receptor–ligand, antigen–antibody, enzyme–substrate)—there was some hesitancy in accepting the idea of like:like interactions in the immune response. In fact, at the time that the idea was proposed, Katz also proposed an alternative theory that said there was an acceptor on the surface of one cell for a molecule on the other. The problem would become to define the nature of the "acceptor."

CHAPTER SEVENTEEN

It might be mentioned in passing that a former immunologist, G. M. Edelman, who received the Nobel prize for his work on antibody structure, has developed the theory that nerve cells interact with each other through like:like interactions between nerve cell adhesion molecules (NCAM). It remains to be seen whether like:like interactions are used by the nervous system. We will see in the following sections that they are *not* used by the immune system. Something akin to the acceptor alternative, but with much more surprising ramifications, is involved in cell interactions in the immune system.

Studies Using Chimeras

As so often happens in science, further advances required the introduction of another experimental model to open new ways of examining the means by which cells interact in an MHC-restricted manner. This system was the use of the CHIMERIC MOUSE. The original chimera in Greek mythology was a fire-breathing monster, usually represented as a composite of a lion, a goat, and a serpent. Chimeric mice are more gentle creatures. They are animals containing tissues that are from two genetically distinct parents; the tissues exist side by side in the same animal. This is in contrast to an F_1 animal, in which the characteristics of each of the parents are expressed in each cell. Chimeras provide the opportunity, if they can be constructed, of having cells of two different genotypes functioning in the same animal.

Allophenic Chimeras The most exotic chimeric mouse is the TETRAPARENTAL, or ALLOPHENIC, chimera used so elegantly by Beatrice Mintz and her co-workers in Philadelphia to study questions of differentiation. Allophenic mice are produced by combining the eight-cell stage embryos of two different animals and allowing them to develop in the uterus of a pseudopregnant mouse (Figure 4). Because each embryo has two parents, the combined embryo of each of the two parents has four parents (hence the term *tetraparental*). The animals that come out of this strange union have cells from both sets of donor parents, so that if one starts with embryo A and embryo B, the chimeric animal will have cells of A and B living side by side. By

MHC RESTRICTION

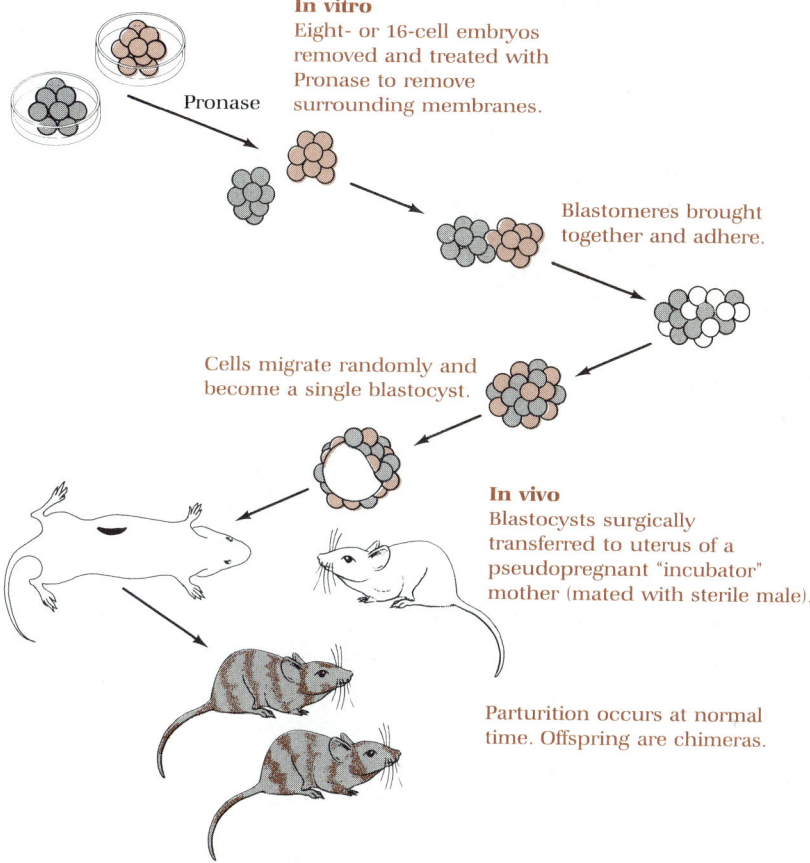

FIGURE 4   PRODUCTION OF ALLOPHENIC MICE

Eight- or sixteen-cell embryos are fused, and the single blastocyst that forms is implanted into a pseudopregnant mother. The offspring are chimeras that have cells of both parents existing side by side. [After Mintz (1967) *Proc. Natl. Acad. Sci. USA* **58,** 344]

combining embryos of different H-2 haplotypes, it is possible to develop chimeras that contain cells of both parental haplotypes. These different cell types have grown up in the same environment and have become tolerant of each other.[2]

[2] See Chapter 24 for a discussion of immunological tolerance. For the present it is sufficient to know that tolerance is the inability to make an immune response to a specific antigen—in this case, the cells of the other haplotype.

CHAPTER SEVENTEEN

It was thought that perhaps the allogeneic cells were not cooperating in the experiments described earlier because they were reactive to each other—a problem that would be overcome in allophenic mice. The original report of experiments designed to determine whether B cells and T cells with different H-2 antigens from the same allophenic mouse could cooperate showed that they were indeed able to cooperate. However, other experiments using allophenics came to the opposite conclusion. It soon became obvious that the technical difficulties involved in producing these mice make the number of experiments that can be done and the number of investigators who can do them a limiting factor. This problem was overcome by using bone marrow chimeras.

Bone Marrow Chimeras

BONE MARROW CHIMERAS are adult animals that are lethally irradiated and then repopulated with bone marrow cells from other strains. Because lymphocytes differentiate from stem cells in the bone marrow, the animals eventually contain lymphocytes derived from the donor strain, but all other tissues are from the irradiated recipient. This point will become important later.

The chimeras can be made by injecting parental bone marrow cells (P) into an F_1, F_1 into a parent, or one strain into another. The nomenclature for chimeras is as follows:

$P_1 \rightarrow F_1$ indicates injection of bone marrow from one parent into an F_1 of that parent and another parental strain.

$P_1 + P_2 \rightarrow F_1$ indicates injection of bone marrow from each parent into an F_1.

Any recirculated T cells in the bone marrow are killed before injection so that the chance of graft-versus-host reaction is lessened. The method used by von Boehmer and Sprent for making bone marrow chimeras is illustrated in Figure 5.

Experiments Using $P_1 + P_2 \rightarrow F_1$: Evidence for Histoincompatible Cooperation

The first experiments that used chimeras to determine whether B cells of one parental H-2 could cooperate with T cells of another are diagrammed in Figure 6. In this experiment, the bone marrow of two parental

MHC RESTRICTION

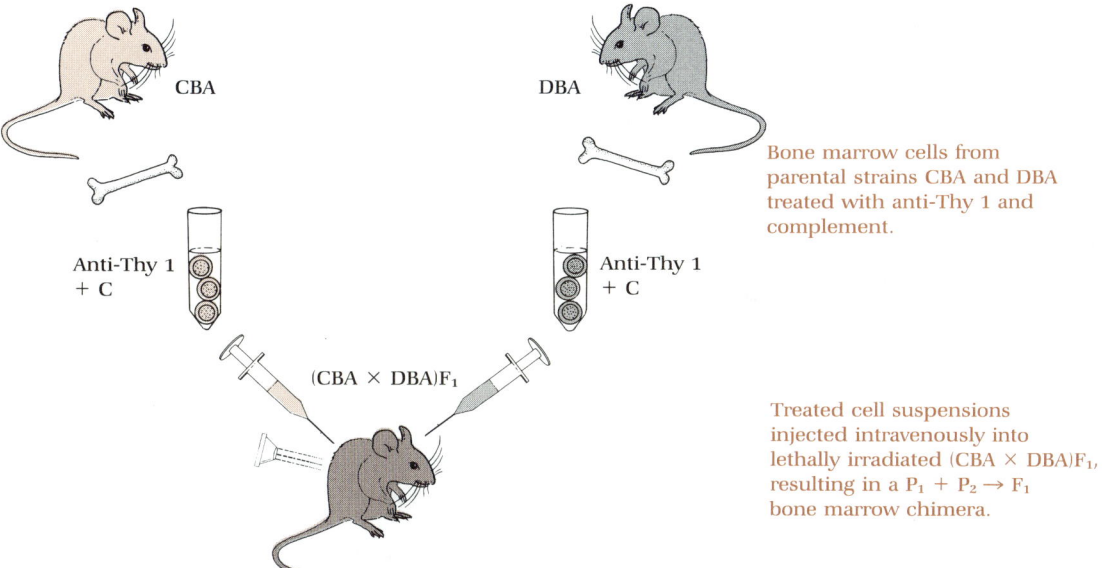

FIGURE 5   PRODUCTION OF BONE MARROW CHIMERAS
Bone marrow is treated with anti-Thy 1 and complement to remove any recirculated T cells and injected into an irradiated recipient. The production of $P_1 + P_2 \rightarrow F_1$ chimera is illustrated [After von Boehmer et al. (1975) *J. Exp. Med.* 141, 322]

types (CBA and DBA) were injected into irradiated (CBA × DBA)F_1 mice; that is, $P_1 + P_2 \rightarrow F_1$ chimeras were produced. Several months later, cells from the lymph nodes of these chimeras were obtained and passed over an anti-Ig column to remove B cells. These cells were a mixture of cells of the two parental haplotypes; half the cells expressed H-2^d (from the DBA parent) and half the cells expressed H-2^k (from the CBA parent). The DBA cells were then eliminated by treating the population with anti-H-2^d antiserum plus complement, and the dead cells were removed, thus leaving a population of CBA (H-2^k) T cells. These CBA T cells from the chimera were then injected into irradiated F_1 mice along with B cells of the same or different haplotype, and the recipients were challenged with antigen. The number of antibody-forming cells was then determined. It can be seen from the

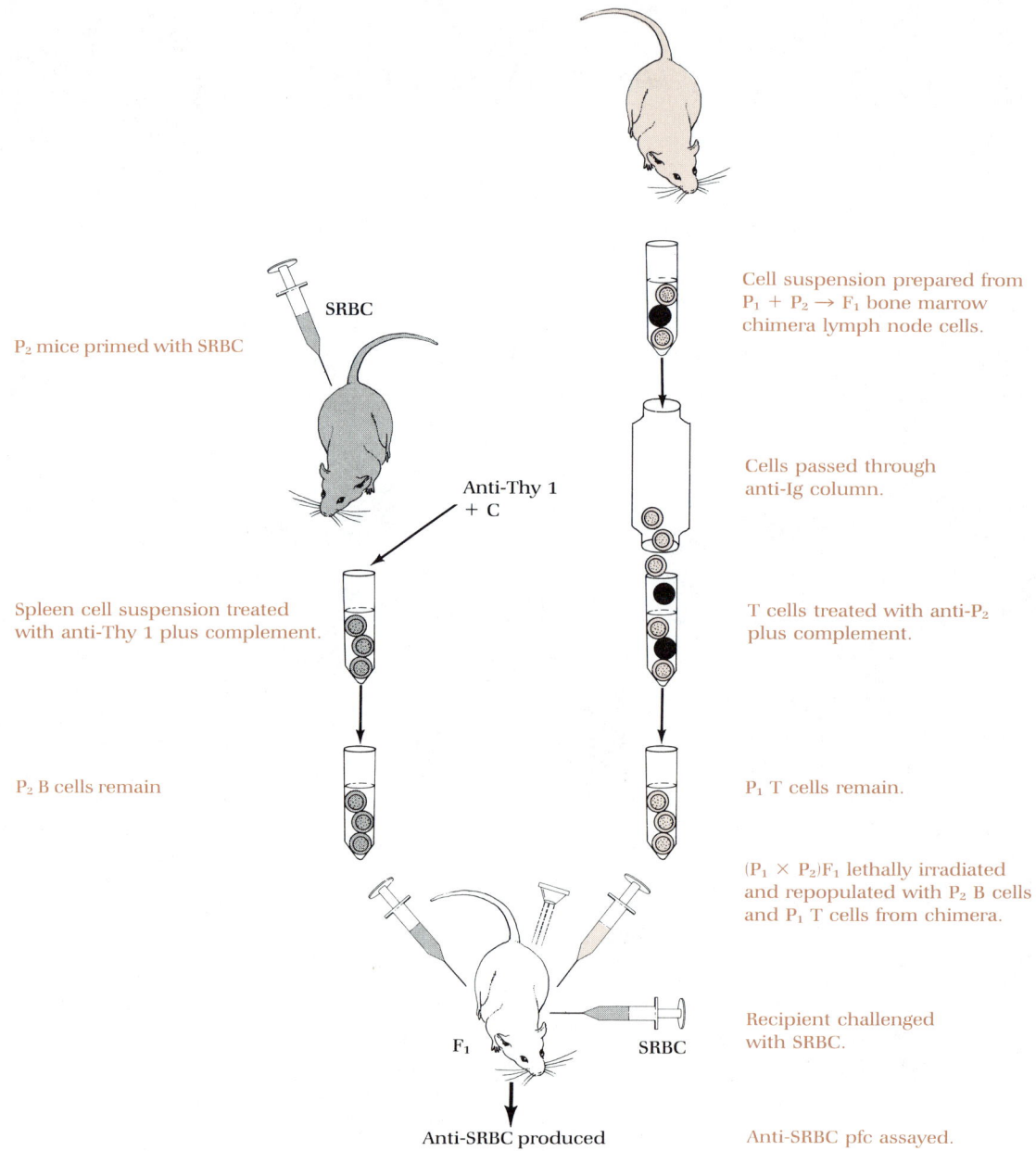

FIGURE 6 COOPERATION OF ALLOGENEIC T AND B CELLS

Lymph nodes from a $P_1 + P_2 \rightarrow F_1$ chimera are passed through an anti-Ig column to remove B cells. The remaining T cells are treated with anti-P_2 and complement, a treatment leaving only chimeric P_1 T cells. These cells are injected into an irradiated F_1 along with B cells from a normal P_2 mouse, and the recipient is challenged. Antibody production shows that under these conditions the allogeneic B and T cells are able to cooperate. [After von Boehmer et al. (1975) *J. Exp. Med.* 142, 989]

MHC RESTRICTION

data in Table 2 that there was cooperation between chimera-derived T cells of the $H-2^k$ haplotype and normal B cells of the $H-2^d$ haplotype. In other words, there was allogeneic cell cooperation, but in this case it was in the absence of an allogeneic effect.

This result presented a real dilemma. The data in several experimental systems had shown clearly that there was MHC restriction in cell interaction in the generation of immune responses, yet in this system it appeared that there was no such restriction. The resolution of this dilemma revealed another previously unthought of layer of complexity in the cell interactions leading to immune responses: the idea that there is enough plasticity in the immune system so that MHC restriction can be changed or "learned."

Experiments Using $F_1 \rightarrow P_1$: Adaptive Differentiation

To explain the difference between the results obtained in the allogeneic experiments and the results in the chimera experiments, David Katz once again came to the rescue. He developed a theory called ADAPTIVE DIFFERENTIATION. According to this theory, cells can in some manner "adaptively" acquire the ability to cooperate by differentiation in the environment of the allogeneic haplotype. Thus, if thymus-derived cells of the $H-2^k$ haplotype can differentiate in the environment of the $H-2^d$ haplotype, the $H-2^k$ cells will be able to cooperate with the $H-2^d$ cells. They will have "adaptively" differentiated the ability to interact.

Experiments using $F_1 \rightarrow P_1$ chimeras were carried out by Katz and his co-workers in an antibody-forming system and by Mi-

TABLE 2 T cells from bone marrow chimeras act as helper cells for syngeneic and allogeneic B cells.

Cells transferred	Plaque-forming cells
CBA chimeric T cells alone	964
CBA chimeric T cells + CBA B cells	35,107
CBA chimeric T cells + DBA B cells	17,763

Source: From von Boehmer et al. (1975), *J. Exp. Med.* 142: 989.

chael Bevan in a cell-mediated system. In the antibody experiment, shown in Figure 7, the $F_1 \rightarrow P_1$ chimeras were produced and after a suitable interval were primed with carrier. Their spleen or lymph node cells were then used as a source of carrier-primed T cells. These carrier-primed T cells from the chimera were then injected into lethally irradiated F_1 recipient mice along with hapten-primed B cells from conventional mice of either parental strain or the F_1. The recipient was then challenged with hapten and carrier. In this manner adaptive differentiation was being tested by asking if the F_1 T cells from the chimera (which should be able to cooperate with either parental type of B cell) will "adapt" to being able to react preferentially with only one parental haplotype.

As an example, parental strains A and C serve as irradiated recipients for bone marrow from $(C \times A)F_1$ donors in forming $F_1 \rightarrow P_1$ or $F_1 \rightarrow P_2$ chimeras. The T cells from the F_1 will differentiate in the environment of either one or the other parental H-2 haplotypes. If the idea of adaptive differentiation is correct, these F_1 cells should show a preference (or a restriction) in their interaction by cooperating with B cells of the haplotype of the strain of the parent in which they differentiated. Figure 7 shows that this is the result obtained.

In these experiments, the top group in the figure are controls, showing that F_1 bone marrow cells differentiating in an F_1 environment ($F_1 \rightarrow F_1$) are able to cooperate well with B cells of the F_1 and of each of the parental strains. The bottom part of the figure shows the experimental group. Here we see that T cells from an $F_1 \rightarrow P_1$ cooperate preferentially with B cells of the parental type in which they differentiated but not with the other parental type. This result indicates that F_1 cells that have undergone differentiation in an F_1 environment can cooperate with either parental type (the controls); but when differentiation occurs in one of the parental types, there is cooperation only with that parental type of cells (the experimental groups). Thus, even though the primed T cells should have the genetic potential to cooperate with B cells of both parental types because they are of F_1 origin, they are restricted in their cooperation to the B cells of the parental type in which they differentiated.

MHC RESTRICTION

(A)

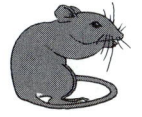

Conventional parental strain (P_2) mouse primed with HC-II.

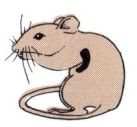

$F_1 \to$ parent (P_1) bone marrow chimera primed with C-I.

Primed B cells prepared from spleen cells treated with anti-Thy 1 plus complement.

Primed T cells prepared from spleen cells.

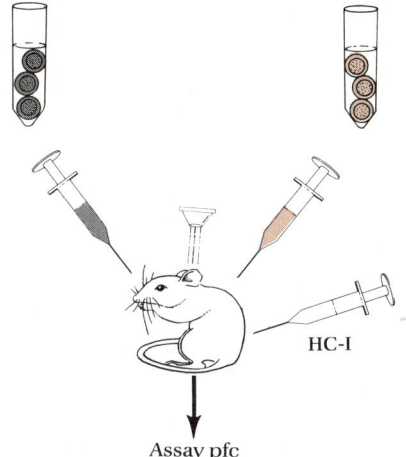

T cells (P_1) from carrier-primed chimera ($F_1 \to P_1$) and B cells (P_2) from hapten-primed conventional (P_2) mouse injected into irradiated, conventional F_1 recipient.

Recipient challenged with HC-I.

Assay pfc

Anti-hapten pfc assayed.

(B)

Source of chimeric T cells	Source of conventional B cells	Response	Interpretation
$F_1 \to F_1$	P_1	▬▬▬	Chimeric $F_1 \to F_1$ T cells cooperate with F_1 and both parental B cells.
	P_2	▬▬▬	
	($P_1 \times P_2$)F_1	▬▬▬	
$F_1 \to P_1$	P_1	▬▬▬	Chimeric $F_1 \to A$ T cells cooperate with F_1 T cells and T cells of the strain in which they differentiated.
	P_2	▬	
	($P_1 \times P_2$)F_1	▬▬▬	

FIGURE 7 ADAPTIVE DIFFERENTIATION
(A) T cells from an $F_1 \to P_1$ bone marrow chimera primed with C-I are injected into an irradiated recipient along with HC-II-primed conventional B cells. If there is adaptive differentiation, then the F_1 T cells should cooperate preferentially with P_1 B cells. (B) $F_1 \to A$ T cells cooperate with A cells but not C cells. [After Katz et al. (1978) *J. Exp. Med.* **148,** 727]

CHAPTER SEVENTEEN

Similar results were obtained in cell-mediated responses. When F_1 cells were allowed to differentiate in the environment of only one parental type, they preferentially lysed targets of that H-2 rather than those of the other haplotype. We see then that in both antibody and cell-mediated responses there is MHC restriction, but it is more complicated than just the sharing of the same MHC genes. Somehow MHC restriction can be "learned."

Summary

1. The immune response of nude mice can be restored with syngeneic but not allogeneic thymus cells, and the immune response of irradiated mice can be restored only with bone marrow and thymus cells that are syngeneic at the I region of MHC (Class II).
2. Cytotoxic T cells can lyse only targets that have the appropriate antigen and express the same Class I MHC antigens.
3. Lyt phenotype correlates with MHC class restriction but not with function. Lyt 1^+ cells are reactive with Class II and Lyt 2^+ cells are reactive with Class I MHC antigens.
4. Studies using bone marrow chimeras have shown that the T helper cell must recognize the self MHC on the antigen-presenting cell. By a phenomenon called "adaptive differentiation," the self-MHC can be learned.

Additional Readings

Golub, E. S. 1980. Know thyself: autoreactivity in the immune response. *Cell* 21, 603.

Katz, D. H. 1980. Adaptive differentiation of lymphocytes: theoretical implications for mechanisms of cell–cell recognition and regulation of immune responses. *Adv. Immunol.* 29, 138.

Swain, S. L. 1981. Significance of Lyt phenotypes: Lyt 2 antibodies block activities of T cells that recognize Class I major histocompatibility complex antigens regardless of their function. *Proc. Natl. Acad. Sci. USA* 78, 7101.

CHAPTER 18

ACQUISITION OF THE RESTRICTION REPERTOIRE

Overview So far in this section we have developed the ideas that the cells that cooperate to generate both antibody and cell-mediated responses react with different portions of the antigen and require the presence of accessory cells. Two surprising facts emerged: that these responses are MHC restricted, and that the MHC restriction can be "learned." We will see that the restriction is not learned in the usual sense of the word; rather, it involves selection.

In this chapter we will develop evidence to support two unexpected conclusions. The first is that MHC restriction is between the T cell and the antigen-presenting cell. The second conclusion is that the interaction is not between macrophage MHC and T cell MHC, but between macrophage MHC and a receptor for self-MHC on the T cell.

Finally, we will make the very important point that an F_1 animal has T cells able to cooperate in an MHC restricted manner with one or the other of the parental-type macrophages. In this respect, the T cells of an F_1 are similar to those of a chimera. This curious fact will be used to explain experiments in both bone marrow and thymus chimeras. These experiments show that the MHC of the thymus in which the T cell differentiates becomes the "self" with which the T cell cooperates. In the thymus, those lymphocytes that express receptors for the thymic MHC are selected whereas those expressing receptors for other MHC haplotypes are not. It is in this manner that the self-recognition in MHC restriction is acquired.

CHAPTER EIGHTEEN

MHC-Restriction and Accessory Cells

We saw in Chapter 14 that macrophages are necessary for many immune functions. We will now develop this idea in detail for T cell activation; that is, we will examine the evidence that shows MHC restriction is between antigen-presenting cells (macrophages) and T cells.

Macrophage Activation of T Cells

A population of resting T cells exhibits the capacity to carry out functions only after antigenic stimulation. This response is termed ANTIGENIC ACTIVATION. One of the most dramatic aspects of activation is the induction of proliferation of the antigen-specific cells (this process is one of the basic tenets of clonal selection).

The experiment of Rosenthal and Shevach (Figure 1) shows that macrophages are required for the activation of T cells. In this experiment peritoneal exudate cells (PEC), which are 75%–85% macrophages, are harvested from guinea pigs and allowed to adhere to glass for several hours. The nonadherent cells are then removed and discarded. This procedure produces a population of cells that contain over 98% macrophages. The adherent cells are then incubated with antigen (a process called "antigen pulsing"). T cells obtained from lymph nodes are then added to the antigen-pulsed macrophages, and after a suitable interval the amount of T cell proliferation is determined by adding tritiated thymidine. Figure 1 shows that proliferation of the T cells occurs only when both antigen and macrophages are present. This result indicates that one of the crucial initial steps in the generation of the immune response—the activation of T cell proliferation by antigen—is a step that requires the presence of an accessory cell.

Role of MHC Haplotype of Macrophages and T Cells

The experimental system in Figure 1 was used to test the role of the MHC in the activation of T cells by antigen and macrophages. Guinea pig macrophages of one MHC haplotype were pulsed with antigen, then T cells from animals of another MHC haplotype were added. The amount of T cell proliferation was determined (Table 1). When

ACQUISITION OF THE RESTRICTION REPERTOIRE

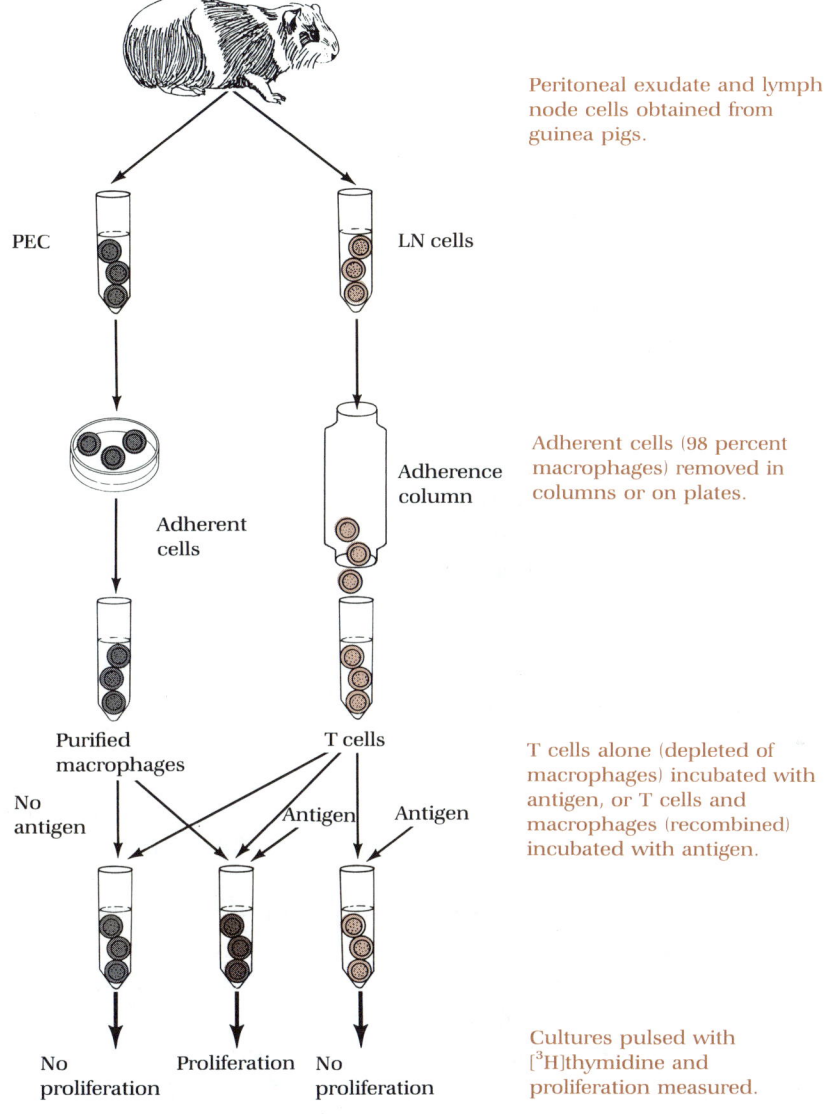

FIGURE 1 ANTIGEN-INDUCED T CELL PROLIFERATION
Removal of macrophages from a lymph node cell preparation removes the ability of the cells to proliferate in response to antigen. The addition of peritoneal exudate macrophages restores the ability of the cell to proliferate. [After Rosenthal and Shevach (1974) *J. Exp. Med.* 138, 1194]

TABLE 1   MHC restriction of T cell activation.

	Source of T cells		
Macrophage	Strain 2	Strain 13	$(2 \times 13)F_1$
2	25.4	2.9	5.3
13	0	18.2	6.0
$(2 \times 13)F_1$	10.5	7.6	11.00

Source: Data from Rosenthal and Shevach (1974), *J. Exp. Med.* 138: 1194.

macrophages from Strain 2 guinea pigs were pulsed with antigen and added to T cells of Strain 2, Strain 13, or a $(2 \times 13)F_1$, there was proliferation only with Strain 2 or the $(2 \times 13)F_1$ macrophages. Similarly, the antigen-pulsed macrophages from strain 13 were able to activate only Strain 13 or the F_1 T cells. This experiment shows clearly that even though macrophages are required for the induction of antigen-specific T cell proliferation, the macrophages and T cells must have the same MHC haplotype. In other words, T cell activation by antigen and macrophage is MHC restricted.

Two Populations of T Cells in the F_1

When T cells were incubated with antigen-pulsed macrophages of one strain for four days and then *restimulated* with the same or different antigen-pulsed macrophages, there was an enhanced or secondary stimulatory response. As one would expect, this secondary stimulation is also MHC restricted. But the picture is very complex (Table 2). When both the primary and secondary stimulation of the $(A \times B)F_1$ T cells was with antigen-pulsed macrophages from parent A, there was good secondary proliferation. But when the second stimulation was with antigen-pulsed B macrophages, the secondary response was poor. This is surprising, because the responding T cells are F_1 and therefore have both A and B MHC molecules on their surfaces (we know that MHC molecules are codominantly expressed on F_1 cells). Therefore the result cannot be because A or B molecules are not present on the F_1 T cells;

ACQUISITION OF THE RESTRICTION REPERTOIRE

TABLE 2 Response of F_1 T cells to parental macrophages.

Primary stimulation	Secondary stimulation	Proliferation of F_1 cells
A	A	Yes
	B	No
	(A × B)F_1	Yes
B	A	No
	B	Yes
	(A × B)F_1	Yes
(A × B)F_1	A	Yes
	B	Yes
	(A × B)F_1	Yes

Source: After Paul et al. (1977), *J. Exp. Med.* 145: 618.

some other explanation is needed for this preference for one parental haplotype. The similarity between these results and the adaptive differentiation experiments in which T cells preferentially cooperated with one parental type of cells after residence in a $F_1 \rightarrow P_1$ chimera is evident. In fact, this experiment is one of the first of the chain of experiments leading to our current explanation of adaptive differentiation, and it reveals an important aspect of MHC restriction.

The best explanation for the MHC restriction of the secondary stimulation seen in the above experiment is that there are *two subpopulations of T cells in the F_1*. The reaction of one population is restricted to one parental haplotype and the other is restricted to the other. This idea, if correct, would be very unusual indeed, because it would mean that in this respect a normal F_1 animal behaves like a chimera.

To test the possibility that there are two separate sets of restricted T cells in an F_1 animal, a system was used in which any cell that responds to the first stimulation is killed. If there are two subpopulations of T cells, then the one that responds during the first stimulation will be killed and not be able to respond to that antigen in the second stimulation. There should, however, be a normal response to the second parental haplotype macrophages, because the cells responding in the presence of these MHC determinants will not be stimulated and killed during the primary stimulation. To carry out this experiment, F_1 T cells are incubated with antigen-pulsed macrophages of one parental type, and after a few hours the drug bromodeoxyuridine (BUdR) is added. This drug is incorporated into newly synthesized DNA in such a manner that when the cells are exposed to light any cell that has incorporated BUdR is killed. This is a clever and generally useful way of selectively killing proliferating cells.

When this method was used on F_1 T cells that had been stimulated with macrophages of one parental type, it was found that there was no proliferation to that parental type upon secondary stimulation. This is what would be expected of cells responding to the first antigen, because cells that respond are killed. In contrast, there was a normal response to antigen on macrophages of the other parental haplotype. This result means that the F_1 cells that were able to respond to the antigen-pulsed macrophages of the second parental haplotype had not proliferated during the first stimulation. Because the responding cells are from the F_1, this experiment confirms the notion that there are two subpopulations of T cells in the F_1, each displaying MHC restriction to one of the parental antigens.

MHC Restriction Is for an Accessory Cell

Two of the observations we have discussed now come together as we try to make sense out of the flow of discoveries. The $F_1 \to P_1$ chimera experiments show that the T cells of an F_1 react preferentially with P_1 cells over P_2 cells. The experiments showing two sets of T cells in the F_1 suggest a mechanism for this preference. An elegant and important series of experiments by Al Singer and his co-workers at the NIH seem to offer the start of the possible explanation.

First, these investigators constructed bone marrow chimeras in all possible combinations (Table 3). The spleen cells of these chimeras were challenged with antigen in vitro and the number of antibody-forming cells determined. This experiment becomes a test for the ability of the cells of one MHC that have developed

ACQUISITION OF THE RESTRICTION REPERTOIRE

TABLE 3 Antibody responses of intact spleen cells from bone marrow chimeras and reconstituted controls.

Reconstitution type	Strains used	Antibody response (pfc/culture)
CONTROLS		
$P_1 \to P_1$	B10	184
$P_2 \to P_2$	B10.A	118
$F_1 \to F_1$	(B10 × B10.A)	175
CHIMERAS		
$P \to F_1$	B10 → (B10 × B10.A)	102
	B10.A → (B10 × B10.A)	126
$F_1 \to P$	(B10 × B10.A) → B10	252
	(B10 × B10.A) → B10.A	143
$P_1 \to P_2$	B10 → B10.A	1
$P_2 \to P_1$	B10.A → B10	1
MIXING EXPERIMENT		
—	B10 + B10.A → B10	90
—	B10 → B10.A + B10.A → B10	327

Source: Data from Singer et al. (1981), *J. Exp. Med.* 153: 1286.

in different MHC environments to cooperate. The controls are homologous reconstitutions—for example, $P_1 \to P_1$.

It was found that all of the combinations except the completely allogeneic $P_1 \to P_2$ and $P_2 \to P_1$ spleen cells were able to give responses equivalent to the controls. One of the conclusions from this experiment is something that we already know—that under appropriate circumstances allogeneic cells can cooperate. The intriguing group is the $P_1 \to P_2$ that were not able to respond. Because the macrophage is needed in these responses and must be of the same MHC as the T cell, it was hypothesized that the MHC restriction might be for an accessory cell in the host (the X-rayed recipient of the bone marrow).

CHAPTER EIGHTEEN

To test this idea, the spleen cells were fractionated into lymphocytes and macrophages (nonadherent and adherent cells; Figure 2). We know from the Mosier experiment done in the Dark Ages of cellular immunology that the lymphocytes will not react unless macrophages are present. When P_1 or P_2 macrophages were added to the chimeric lymphocytes, the results in Table 4 were obtained. The lymphocytes from $P_1 \rightarrow F_1$ chimeras were able to cooperate with both P_1 and P_2 macrophages. This means that the P_1 T cells maturing in an F_1 environment had acquired the ability to react with macrophages of both parental types. The lymphocytes from $F_1 \rightarrow P_1$ chimeras, in contrast, can cooperate only with P_1 and not with P_2 cells. This result shows that even though there are two populations of T cells in the F_1, the environment in which the cells mature determines their MHC restriction.

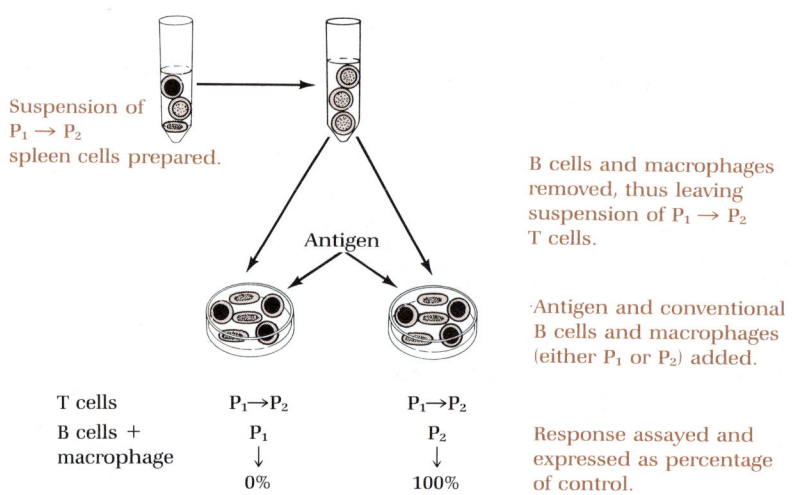

FIGURE 2 HOST OR T CELL DETERMINATION OF MHC RESTRICTION

T cells are prepared from bone marrow chimeras and incubated with B cells and macrophages from conventional mice. Antigen is added and the number of pfc determined. In this way it is possible to determine whether the restriction is for the host MHC (P_2 in this diagram) or the T cell (P_1 in this diagram) [After Singer et al. (1981) *J. Exp. Med.* **153**, 1286]

ACQUISITION OF THE RESTRICTION REPERTOIRE

The $P_1 \rightarrow P_2$ cells that do not respond when unfractionated (Table 3) cooperate fully with macrophages from the P_2 host but not with those from the P_1 donor. This shows that the P_1 T cells can react *only* with macrophages having the same MHC haplotype as that of the cells among which they matured. Similarly, $P_2 \rightarrow P_1$ T cells can cooperate only with P_1 macrophages.

Clearly, then, the MHC haplotype of the cells in the environment in which the T cell differentiates determines the MHC haplotype of the accessory cell with which it can react.

Synthesis: MHC Restriction is Self:Anti-Self

Because we have been drawing evidence together from several lines of experiments, this midpoint summary may be of value to the reader.

The original explanation for what appeared to be the requirement for MHC identity in cell cooperation was that identical molecules on the surfaces of cells had to interact with each other (the CI molecules; Chapter 17). This explanation was called into

TABLE 4 Antibody responses of chimeric T cells.

Chimera T cells	Accessory cells	Antibody response (percentage of control)
$P_1 \rightarrow F_1$	P_1	100
	P_2	100
$F_1 \rightarrow P_1$	P_1	100
	P_2	0
$F_1 \rightarrow P_2$	P_1	0
	P_2	100
$P_1 \rightarrow P_2$	P_1	0
	P_2	100
$P_2 \rightarrow P_1$	P_1	100
	P_2	0

Source: After Singer et al. (1981), *J. Exp. Med.* 153: 1286.

CHAPTER EIGHTEEN

question by the results of the chimera experiments, which showed that under appropriate circumstances cells with different MHC haplotypes could interact and give an immune response. The notion of adaptive differentiation was introduced to accommodate this fact. But if the idea of adaptive differentiation is correct, then the idea of like:like interaction of CI molecules cannot be correct, because we know that the cells that are productively cooperating have different MHC molecules on their surfaces. The F_1 cell that can cooperate only with a P_1 cell still expresses both P_1 and P_2 MHC molecules. The subtle but important point here is that the adaptation takes place not in the ability to *express* MHC molecules of a different haplotype but in the ability to *interact* with MHC molecules of a different haplotype.

All of this data must be explained, and probably the most logical synthesis which has emerged is the idea that the interaction between T cells and accessory cells is a *self:anti-self* interaction. This means that the T cell interacts with the accessory cell of the appropriate MHC haplotype through some form of receptor for those MHC molecules—an idea that runs counter to 85 years of immunological thought. Until now, every theory that was meant to explain any part of the immune response had to have some proviso for preventing the reaction to self.[1] But this very complex recognition system seems to have evolved so that the T cell becomes activated by recognizing foreign antigen in the context of self. Psychologists have known for years that the mind can only discern differences between two objects when it has a point of reference; so an individual learns to identify self as separate from mother, and then learns to identify others as nonself. The immune system appears to need to identify self so that it does not carry out destructive reactions against self. In the chapters on the T cell receptor we will discuss the nature of the molecules at the cell surface that carry out this reaction, and in the chapter on immune tolerance we will discuss some possible strategies that have evolved.

[1] It has been argued by some that the self:anti-self interactions described above are not *reactions* but only *recognitions*. This is not a good argument, however, because recognition without reaction is like virtue without temptation, and has no evolutionary significance.

ACQUISITION OF THE RESTRICTION REPERTOIRE

The Thymus as a Site of Acquistion of MHC Restriction

The experiments showing that the MHC restriction of the T cell is for MHC antigens on an accessory cell are clear evidence that the MHC products for which the restriction occurs are determined not by the T cell but by the host.[2] The question now becomes, How does the restriction of the host MHC become imposed, and where is the site of the acquisition of this restriction in the host?

Studies with Thymus Chimeras

One site that immediately comes to mind as a possible candidate for an event that is associated with T cell maturation is the thymus. One approach to determining whether the thymus is indeed the site is to produce bone marrow chimeras which have no thymus and then implant into them a thymus of any desired MHC haplotype. In this way the pre-T cell from the donor bone marrow of one haplotype can mature in a thymus from a mouse of another haplotype. This is accomplished by thymectomizing mice shortly before irradiation and bone marrow repopulation (Figure 3). After a suitable interval, the mice are implanted with several intact lobes of thymus so that these animals become both bone marrow and thymus chimeras. The MHC restriction they display after immunization can thus be used to determine the role that the thymus plays in the acquisition of the restriction repertoire.

Zinkernagel and his co-workers did the first series of experiments using thymus chimeras. Table 5 shows the results of an experiment in which F_1 bone marrow develops in F_1 recipients with transplanted thymuses from one or the other of the parental types: the restriction is for the haplotype of the *thymus*. It will strike the reader that this experiment gives the same result as the $F_1 \rightarrow P_1$ experiment, which was used as the test of the adaptive differentiation hypothesis. The conclusion seems to be that the thymus is the site of adaptive differentiation, which is really another way of saying that the thymus is the site of acquisition of MHC restriction.

[2] We have said before that this acquisition of the repertoire of restriction has been termed "learning," but we consider this to be an unfortunate choice of terms.

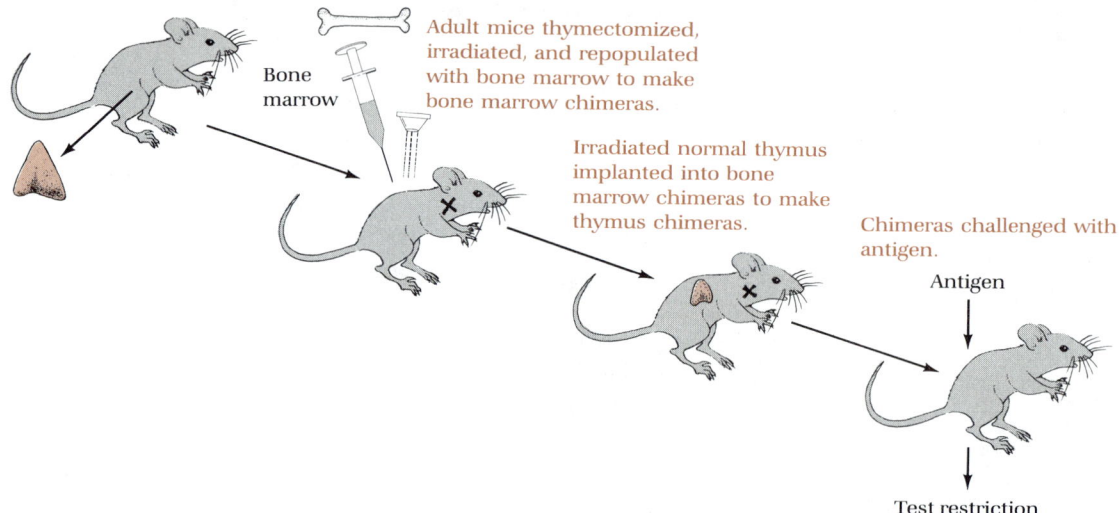

FIGURE 3   ROLE OF THE THYMUS IN THE GENERATION OF MHC RESTRICTION
[After Zinkernagel et al. (1978) *J. Exp. Med.* **147**, 882]

Studies with Nude Mice

Another experimental approach to test the possible role of the thymus in conferring MHC restriction involves the use of nude mice. Because these mice are congenitally athymic, they have no environment in which T cells can differentiate into functional, immunocompetent cells. However, they do have normal pre-T cells; so if they are provided with a thymus, these pre-T cells can differentiate into functional T cells. Therefore, if the thymus from a mouse with an MHC haplotype that differs from that of the nude mouse is implanted into these animals, the pre-T cells will mature in this thymus. But because the T cells are derived from host stem cells, they will be of host origin, even though they matured in a thymus with a different haplotype. The question now is, Will these host T cells show restriction for the host MHC or for the MHC of the donor thymus?

ACQUISITION OF THE RESTRICTION REPERTOIRE

TABLE 5 Influence of transplanted irradiated thymus on MHC restriction.

Bone marrow donor	Thymectomized recipient	Thymus	Restriction
(BALB/c × A)F$_1$	(BALB/c × A)F$_1$	None	No killing
(BALB/c × A)F$_1$	(BALB/c × A)F$_1$	BALB/c	BALB/c
(BALB/c × A)F$_1$	(BALB/c × A)F$_1$	A	A

Source: Data from Zinkernagel et al. (1978), J. Exp. Med. 147: 882.

This straightforward experiment has yielded some apparently contradictory results. The first experiments, done by Kindred, suggested that the restriction was for the host (i.e., the lymphocytes and not the thymus). Zinkernagel and his co-workers then repeated this result in a very large series of experiments. In these studies, H-2^b or H-2^d nude mice were implanted with either syngeneic or allogeneic thymus and then injected with virus. The spleen cells were assayed for virus-specific CTL several days later on virus-infected target cells of different haplotypes. Table 6 shows that H-2^b nude mice have restriction for H-2^b targets when they are implanted with thymus of either H-2^b or H-2^k. The same result is seen with H-2^d nudes implanted with H-2$^{k/b}$ or H-2^d—that is, restriction for H-2^d, the haplotype of the host and not the thymus.

In contrast, experiments from Singer's group, using antibody formation as the test system, yielded exactly the opposite result. These studies used the *separated* T cells of thymus-implanted nude mice in a manner similar to that shown in Figure 2. The T cells were incubated with B cells and macrophages in vitro, and their ability to provide help was assessed by the number of antibody-forming cells generated. As shown in Table 7, T cells from H-2^d nude mice implanted with H-2^a thymus gave antibody responses only with B cells and macrophages from H-2^a mice, the haplotype of the implanted thymus.

The difference between these two experiments is that one (Table 6) is looking at the ultimate function of Class I-restricted T

TABLE 6 MHC restriction of cell-mediated response in nude mice with grafted allogeneic thymus.

Nude recipient	Thymus donor	Killing on		
		H-2^d	H-2^k	H-2^b
C57BL/6 H-2^b	C57BL/6 H-2^b	−	−	+
C57BL/6 H-2^b	C3H H-2^k	−	−	+
BALB/c H-2^d	BALB/c H-2^d	+	−	−
BALB/c H-2^d	C57BL/6 H-2^d	+	−	−
BALB/c H-2^d	(C3H × BALB/c)F$_1$ H-2$^{k/b}$	+	−	−

Source: Data from Zinkernagel et al. (1980), *J. Exp. Med.* 151: 376.

TABLE 7 MHC restriction of antibody formation in nude mice with grafted allogeneic thymus.

T cells (from nu/nu)	Thymus (implanted)	B cells + macrophages	pfc
H-2^d	H-2^a	H-2^d	<10
H-2^d	H-2^a	H-2^d	300
H-2^d	H-2^b	H-2^b	1000
H-2^d	H-2^b	H-2^d	0

Source: Data from Singer et al. (1982) *J. Exp. Med.* 155: 339.

ACQUISITION OF THE RESTRICTION REPERTOIRE

TABLE 8 Evidence for an extrathymic site of acquisition of MHC restriction.[a]

Nude recipient	Thymus donor	Responding cells	Percentage of specific lysis[b]		
			b-TNP	d-TNP	k-TNP
BALB/c H-2^d	(BALB/c × B6)F$_1$ H-2$^{b/d}$	Thymus Spleen	37 18	48 28	
(C3H × B6)F$_1$ H-2$^{k/b}$	B6 H-2^b	Thymus Spleen	67 51		−3 67
BALB/c H-2^d	C3H H-2^b	Thymus Spleen	68 57	1	

Source: Data from Singer et al. (1982), *Behring. Inst. Mitt.* 70: 140.
[a] IL-2 added to each culture.
[b] Values printed in color indicate significant lysis.

cells in the generation of CTL and the other (Table 7) is looking at the Class II-restricted T cells that are helper cells in antibody formation. This difference in function may account for the difference in results.

Intrathymic and Extrathymic Acquisition of Class I and Class II MHC Restriction

It was first thought that a resolution to the conflicting results of the two experiments described above lay in the possibility that the thymus controls MHC restriction for Class II (I region) MHC products but restriction for Class I (K/D regions) products is acquired extrathymically. To test this idea, nude mice were implanted with thymus, and the ability to generate CTL of the cells of the thymus and spleen was tested on targets of various MHC haplotypes (Table 8).[3] When the nude recipient is BALB/c (H-2^d) and the thymus is (BALB/c × B6)F$_1$ (H-2$^{b/d}$), both thymus and spleen cells kill targets of H-2^b and H-2^d. When the nude is (C3H × B6)F$_1$ (H-2$^{k/d}$) and the thymus is B6

[3] In these studies a nonspecific T cell helper factor, interleukin-2 (IL-2) was added. IL-2 will be discussed in detail in Chapter 21, but for now it is enough to know that this molecule is a product of the activated T helper cells and allows T cell proliferation. By adding IL-2 to the cultures, Class I-restricted cells (K/D) are able to proliferate even in the absence of Class II-restricted helper cells.

CHAPTER EIGHTEEN

($H-2^b$), the thymus cells are restricted to the MHC of the thymus (kill on $H-2^b$ but not on $H-2^k$). The spleen cells, however, kill equally well on both. This finding supports the conclusion that peripheral CTL do not have the MHC restriction of the thymus.

But these experiments do not answer the crucial question of whether the thymus is the site of acquisition for some cells because of their MHC class restriction (Class I versus Class II), their Lyt phenotype (Lyt 1^+ versus Lyt 2^+), or their function (help versus kill). Singer's group has been able to approach this question by generating Class II-restricted CTL that are Lyt 1^+. These cells have exactly the opposite phenotypes of the usual CTL, so they are the perfect cells to use to determine which of the three parameters the thymic environment influences. They found, using chimeras, that the thymus did *not* influence the MHC restriction of these cells; i.e., the Lyt 1^+ CTL had the MHC restriction of the bone marrow donor and not the recipient thymus.

Thus the current status of the problem is that the thymus is the site of MHC restriction acquisition for helper cells but not for killer cells. The problem now becomes one of determining the factors that influence a cell and what conditions allow a cell to be influenced.

Synthesis: Selection versus Education in the Thymus

The mechanism of the acquisition of MHC restriction, whether in the thymus or in an extrathymic environment, is not known. However, the facts we have just examined make one interpretation the most likely. Because an F_1 has two sets of MHC-restricted T cells and only one of them develops in a P_1 environment, we have the alternative options of one set of the F_1 cells "*learning*"— acquiring some new information (which the MHC then cooperates with)—or of one set of T cells being *selected* (in the Darwinian sense).

Selection is the most attractive alternative because it fits with the general tone of the immune response[4] The ramification of

---

[4] This argument is not the strongest in the world, but it is akin to Copernicus's explanation of why he liked the idea of heliocentricity: it was a theory "more pleasing to the mind."

ACQUISITION OF THE RESTRICTION REPERTOIRE

selection as the process is that the population of cells that will be selected must have members that express the receptors for all of the MHC antigens of the species. In the normal course of events, self-MHC are chosen because the emerging cells see only self. In experimental situations, however, the investigator can choose any MHC and confer MHC restriction upon the animal.

One prediction that follows from this model is that there might be higher numbers of cells reactive to MHC antigens than to ordinary antigens. In fact, this is what is found. The frequency of reactive cells to an antigen such as SRBC or TNP is about 10^{-6}, while the frequency of cells reactive to allogeneic MHC is as high as 10^{-2}.

Summary

1. Macrophages are required for the activation of T cells by antigen. Reacting macrophages and T cells must be of the same MHC haplotype, indicating that this is the site of MHC restriction.
2. A normal F_1 animal has two populations of T cells. One subpopulation has MHC restriction for one parental haplotype and one for the other. All the T cells in the F_1, however, express both parental-type MHC molecules. This fact explains why $F_1 \rightarrow P_1$ bone marrow chimeras display MHC restriction for the P_1 haplotype: the P_1-restricted population of T cells from the F_1 reacted with P_1 accessory cells.
3. The best current explanation of MHC restriction seems to be that it is a "self:anti-self" reaction. The T cell can only recognize foreign antigen when it is seen in the context of self-MHC molecules. In other words, the T cell receptor must somehow be able to recognize self antigens as well as foreign molecules.
4. Studies with thymus chimeras and nude mice yield apparently contradictory results, but the differences are resolved by knowledge of the fact that the experiments were measuring different functions. It now appears that the thymus is the site of acquisition of MHC restriction for helper cells but not for cytotoxic cells, without regard for their Lyt phenotype or class restriction.
5. The MHC restriction repertoire that is acquired in the thymus is acquired by "selection," not by "learning." Those T cells that express a receptor for the MHC antigen expressed in the thymus are selected; T cells displaying receptors for other haplotypes are not. It remains to be discovered how that restriction of CTL is acquired.

CHAPTER EIGHTEEN
Additional Readings

Golding, H., T. I. Munitz and A. Singer. 1985. Characterization of antigen-specific, Ia-restricted, L3T4$^+$ cytotoxic lymphocytes and assessment of thymic influence on their self specificity. *J. Exp. Med.* 162, 943.

Singer, A. and R. J. Hodes. 1983. Mechanisms of T-cell–B-cell interactions. *Annu. Rev. Immunol.* 1, 211.

SECTION III
RECEPTORS AND SIGNALS

> But there is trouble in store for anyone who surrenders to the temptation of mistaking an elegant hypothesis for a certainty.
>
> PRIMO LEVI, *THE PERIODIC TABLE*

In these three chapters we will examine the nature of the antigen-specific receptors used by B cells and T cells to recognize and react with antigen. We will also examine the nature of the molecules that the cells synthesize as a result of these reactions.

We already know that B cells can react with free antigen but that T cells react with foreign antigen only in the context of self-MHC. An understanding of the nature of the receptors and the consequences of cell activation through these receptors is crucial to understanding how the immune system is regulated, the topic to be covered in Section IV.

CHAPTER 19
ANTIGEN-SPECIFIC RECEPTORS ON LYMPHOCYTES

Overview   We already know that B cells and T cells react differently with antigen. T cell reactions are MHC restricted, but B cell reactions are not. Furthermore, one of the first differences ever noted between B and T cells was the fact that T cells were sIg negative. So how can a cell with no surface Ig react with antigen in a specific, MHC restricted manner? This problem has been a source of puzzlement and controversy, but we will now see that advances in methodology have allowed us to approach the solution to it. A very important point, however, is that the question was asked *before* the methodological advances. Thus the problem was defined but it was not amenable to experimental solution. The advances in monoclonal antibody, gene cloning, and sequencing technology allowed the question to be answered. Technology in this case, as it should be in all cases, was the means, not the end.

ANTIGEN–SPECIFIC RECEPTORS
The B Cell Receptor

One of the few things which all immunologists agree on is that the immunoglobulin molecules found at the surface of B cells (sIg) act as receptors for antigen. One could argue that this is a logical assumption, because otherwise nature would have had to invent two different methods of recognizing antigen—one for the receptor on the surface of the cell and one for the antibody that is secreted by the cell. Every scientist knows, however, that what seems logical is not always the way the world is put together. In fact, Stephen Jay Gould has written a wonderful essay arguing that what at times appears to be the very lack of logic in nature is a powerful argument for evolution, because it allows us to see how unique problems were solved in unique ways (*The Panda's Thumb*). The result of this local problem solving can lead to solutions that work for the organism but are far from what one would have predicted by logic. In the case of the B cell, what we assumed to be logical has also turned out to be correct.

Surface Ig Receptors on B Cells

In a now classic series of experiments, Sell and Gell showed in 1965 that anti-immunoglobulin antiserum raised against secreted immunoglobulin could to some extent mimic the action of antigen by causing B cells to undergo blastogenesis. This is indirect evidence that the receptor on the B cell is immunoglobulin, since it assumes that the anti-Ig is activating the cell via the surface immunoglobulin (sIg) in a manner similar to that occurring when antigen binds to the combining site. More direct studies soon followed, and these showed that free antigen binds to the surface of the B cell and this binding can be competitively inhibited by anti-Ig. This finding argues that the antigen is binding to a molecule on the surface of the B cell and also reacts with immunoglobulin.

It had been known for a long time that a B cell displays immunoglobulin on its surface and that the specificity of this Ig is the same as the antigen specificity of the Ig secreted by the cell. If one passes B cells and T cells over a column of immobilized antigen, only a very small fraction of the cells are retained. We know that these cells are B cells that react specifically with antigen, because when the cells are eluted from the column and stimulated with antigen, they respond only to the specific antigen. B cells express the same idiotype as the secreted immunoglobulin, and anti-idiotype (antibody against the antigen-combining site) can stimulate B cells in a manner similar to antigen.

All of this taken together made the nature of the B cell receptor a non-problem. But R. K. Gershon's dictum about the balance of forces in life comes into play very strongly here. Gershon, the discoverer of the suppressor T cell (Chapter 23) and analyzer of the human condition, observed that "what you make on the peanuts you lose on the popcorn." We will see that this is certainly true for receptors on lymphocytes. If the B cell receptor is the peanuts, the T cell receptor is the popcorn.

Isotypes of Surface Immunoglobulin

Although there is general agreement that the sIg molecules on B cells act as antigen-specific receptors, we are only beginning to understand how their reaction with antigen transduces the signal to the cell to proliferate and secrete immunoglobulin. Some of the current notions about signal transduction in general and B cells in particular will be discussed in Chapter 21.

As B cells differentiate, the first Ig expressed on their surface is IgM (sIgM). This sIgM is an 8s monomer, in contrast to the secreted IgM, which is a 19s pentamer. As B cells mature, they begin to express another isotype of immunoglobulin on their surfaces, IgD. Recall from Chapter 4 that IgD is an isotype found in vanishingly small amounts in the serum. The general consensus is that this isotype in some way plays a role as antigen-specific receptor. The sIgM and sIgD both have the same antigen-specificity and idiotype. Other isotypes of immunoglobulin (IgG, IgA and IgE) are also found on a very small number of B cells, but these almost always appear only after antigenic stimulation. In contrast, IgM and IgD appear on resting cells, which argues that they are indeed receptor molecules.

The monomeric membrane forms of immunoglobulin all have a slightly higher molecular weight than the monomers of the secreted forms, probably because the membrane molecules contain a hydrophobic region that is used to anchor them in the membrane. The genetic organization leading to surface or secreted IgM will be discussed in Chapter 20.

ANTIGEN–SPECIFIC RECEPTORS

Mobility of sIg: Patching and Capping

One of the more important developments in cell biology in the past decade has been the realization that the membrane of cells is not a rigid structure but a sea of oil with floating islands of proteins. These floating islands can move in the plane of the membrane, and their movement and reorganization can be of great importance in the economy of the cell. The surface antigens of lymphocytes can move in the plane of the membrane, a fact that can be demonstrated by treating the cells with fluorescein-labeled antibody against a surface component. For example, when labeled anti-immunoglobulin is added to B cells and the pattern of fluorescence is examined at short intervals, a "ring pattern" of fluorescence on the surface of the cells appears immediately. Through the microscope, the outline of the cell appears as a fluorescent ring because the labeled anti-Ig is uniformly distributed over the surface of the cell. Very soon, however, the ring pattern changes and PATCHES of label are seen. After a short time all the patches of label move to one pole of the cell, forming a CAP. This process is called patching and capping (Figure 1).

Although the significance of patching and capping is not completely understood, it is thought that the reorganization of the Ig molecules (i.e., the receptors) in the membrane is important for signal transduction from the surface of the cell to the nucleus (see Chapter 21).

The T Cell Receptor

The T cell receptor has been one of the major unsolved problems of immunology, and in fact our lack of real understanding about its structure and function is a roadblock to further understanding of the regulation of the immune response. Initially there were technical difficulties that accounted for some of the lack of insight (the immunoglobulin molecule is secreted and could be studied, for example, but the T cell receptor is not), but the real difficulty is theoretical, because any solution must address at least three important facts:

1. There is no readily observed Ig on the surface of the T cell. If the T cell uses the same strategy as the B cell (as logic would lead

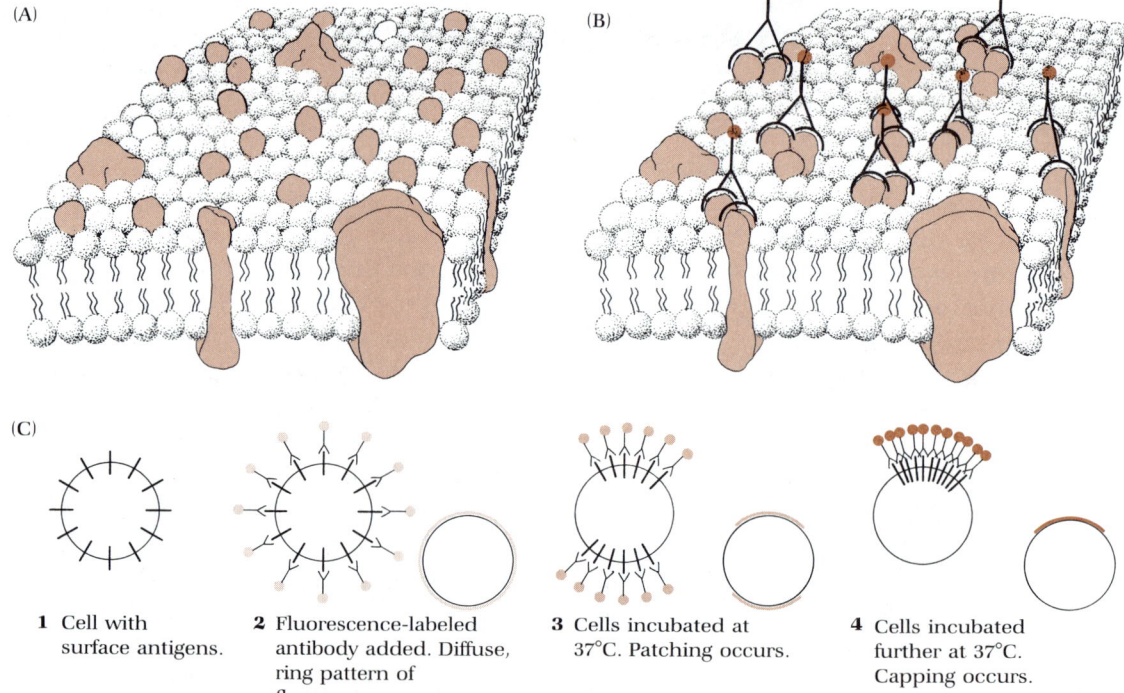

FIGURE 1 PATCHING AND CAPPING

(A) Diagrammatic view of the cell membrane showing the islands of glycoprotein molecules (surface antigens) in a sea of lipid. (B) The antigens are randomly distributed in the lipid bilayer, but addition of antibody causes some of the antigens to be clustered in patches. (C) Schematic representation of patching and capping. **1.** The cell surface antigens are evenly distributed over the surface of the cell. **2.** When fluorescence-labeled antibody is added and the cells examined under the fluorescence microscope, a diffuse staining pattern is visible. **3.** When the cells are incubated at 37°, patching of the antigens occurs. **4.** Further incubation at 37° leads to capping.

us to surmise), then why are we unable to find the molecules at the surface?

2. Even though we know that T cells are antigen-specific, free antigen does not bind to the T cell as it does to the B cell. We will see, however, that T cells can be shown to react with antigen when the antigen is displayed in association with MHC molecules on the cell surface.

3. T cell responses are MHC restricted; and as we have seen, the repertoire of this restriction is acquired during T cell differentia-

ANTIGEN–SPECIFIC RECEPTORS

tion. Why should recognition of self MHC affect the receptor for foreign antigen? And, given the fact that it does, how does it?

In the rest of this chapter, we will show how the story is unfolding to date, but the reader must be forewarned that we do not know the answers. Recent advances in cloning the genes responsible for the structures have added an enormous amount of information, and the answer may be close at hand. But the elegant molecular biology has not yet given us the definitive answers to the biological questions. We might also add that this is a good example of a case where just knowing "the bottom line" would not be of much value to the student of immunology. As new evidence accumulates and new interpretations of that evidence are being made, it will be essential to know the immunobiological context of the questions into which the answers must fit.

Absence of sIg on T Cells

The prehistory of the search for the T cell receptor can be found in the 1960s, when it became generally accepted that the immunoglobulin molecules on the surface of B cells were the receptors for antigen. It seemed logical that immunoglobulin would also be the receptor for antigen on the T cell. A rather acrimonious controversy followed when one group of respectable immunologists found clear evidence for surface Ig on T cells, but another group of equal respectability failed to find it. The data in Figure 2 shows that the differences between the two findings were not subtle. In restrospect one can find any number of reasons for the differences—specificity and absorption of the antibody reagents used, sources of cells, and so on—but support for the idea that there was *not* identifiable surface Ig on T cells continued to increase.[1] When it was discovered that

---

[1] This was an emotional time, and feelings still run high. The whole controversy was treated in an issue of the *Scandinavian Journal of Immunology* in 1983; for that issue Coutinhou and Meo wrote a most scathing (but realistic) introduction to a series of papers by several of the players in the past and the present work on the T cell receptor. They invited several of the investigators who were responsible for much of the early data showing that immunoglobulin was "unequivocally" present on the surface of T cells to submit papers on their current thoughts on the subject. "Three of our contributors who have produced such evidence in the past now appear unanimous in refuting it, one by fairly conced-

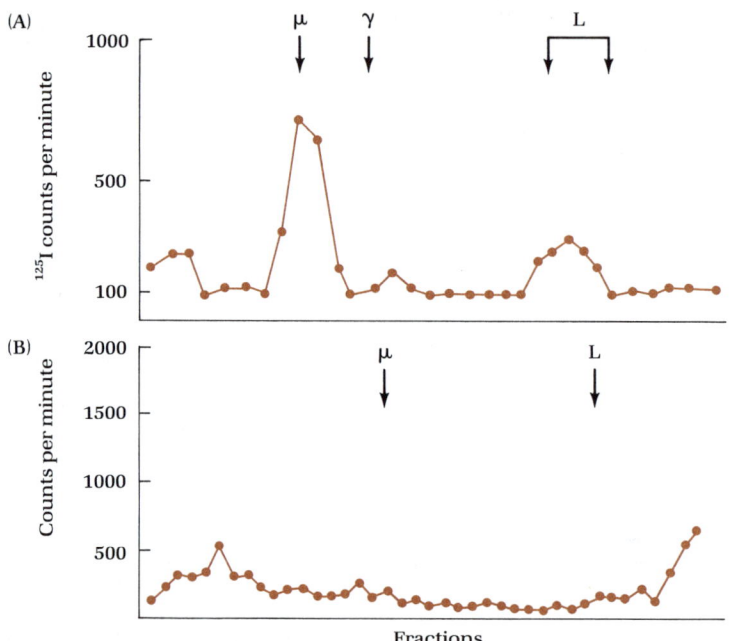

FIGURE 2 IMMUNOGLOBULIN ON THE SURFACE OF T CELLS
The contradictory results of experiments showing presence of immunoglobulin on the surface of T cells. Disc electrophoresis of surface-labeled thymus cells. In (A) immunoglobulin is found [Marchalonis and Cone (1973) *Transplant. Rev.* 14, 3]. In (B) no surface immunoglobulin is found [Vitetta et al. (1972) *J. Exp. Med.* 136, 81]. Heavy (μ, γ) and light (L) chain markers are indicated.

some of the regulation of the immune response was controlled by genes coding for MHC molecules (the Ir genes) there was a mercifully short-lived movement to implicate the MHC products as the T cell receptor.

---

ing a retraction, another by postulating misleading 'homologies,' and the third by ignoring it." [*Scan. J. Immunol.* 18, 79.] So much for high-minded sentiment in science!

ANTIGEN–SPECIFIC RECEPTORS

MHC Molecules and Antigen Binding by T Cells

We already know that T cells are antigen-specific, so the fact that they do not have surface Ig raises questions of how they react with antigen. The problem is confounded even more by the fact that when one incubates lymphocytes with radiolabeled antigen one can show considerable specific binding to B cells but virtually none to T cells. How, for example, can one have TNP-specific CTL that kill TNP-labeled targets (of the appropriate H-2) but do not bind free TNP? Similarly, how does one explain the fact that BGG-primed T helper cells do not bind free BGG?

The lack of binding to free antigen points up one of the more important differences between B cells and T cells. Of the two, only B cells are able to bind free antigen; T cells can only bind antigen when the antigen is *seen in the context of MHC molecules*. An experiment that illustrates this point is diagrammed in Figure 3. In this experiment $H-2^k$ mice were immunized with $H-2^d$ cells, and $H-2^d$-specific CTL were produced, indicating that the $H-2^k$ T cells were able to recognize and react with $H-2^d$ antigens. The spleen cell population that contained these antigen-specific CTL were then *adsorbed* onto monolayers of fibroblasts from either $H-2^d$ or $H-2^k$ animals. After a short time, the cells that had not bound firmly to the monolayer were decanted. The cells that remained bound were either specifically bound via their receptors to $H-2^d$ molecules or were adhering nonspecifically. To determine which of these alternatives is correct, the cells were treated with trypsin, gently removed from the monolayers, and added to ^{51}Cr-labeled $H-2^d$ targets.

If the cells on the $H-2^d$ targets were *nonspecifically* bound, then both the nonadsorbed and the adsorbed cells should have similar abilities to lyse the $H-2^d$ targets. The results given in Figure 3 show that the two populations of cells did not have similar abilities. In fact, the nonadsorbed cells had no killing ability. This means the cells that were adsorbed were *specifically* adsorbed. In contrast, both the adsorbed and nonadsorbed cells that were in contact with the $H-2^k$ monolayer had significant killing, a result indicating no specific binding to that monolayer. The same kind of experiment can be done with hapten-specific CTL, again show-

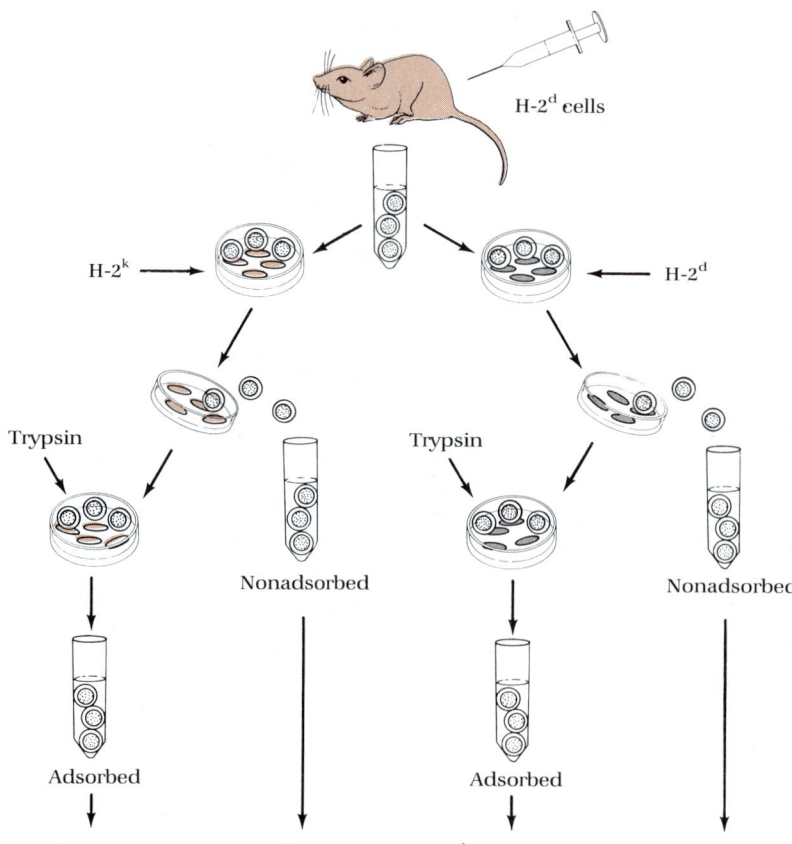

FIGURE 3 SPECIFIC BINDING OF CYTOTOXIC T CELLS

$H-2^k$ mice that have CTL directed against $H-2^d$ antigens are seen to bind to a monolayer of $H-2^d$ cells but not to a monolayer of $H-2^k$ cells. This result shows that T cells do bind antigen, but only when it is on a cell surface. [After Golstein et al. (1971) *J. Exp. Med.* **134**, 1385]

ANTIGEN–SPECIFIC RECEPTORS

ing dramatically that T cells do in fact bind antigen but do so only in the context of MHC at the cell surface.

We have now established the problem: T cells react with antigen only in the context of self-MHC. We already know that the part of the recognition which is MHC-restricted is not by like:like reaction between MHC molecules but involves self:anti-self recognition. What kind of structure can account for reaction to foreign antigens *and* self molecules? As English lawyers in novels always seem to say, "a very pretty problem, indeed."

Models for the T Cell Receptor

Single Receptor versus Dual Recognition

When MHC restriction was first discovered, Zinkernagel and Doherty proposed the two alternative models that still dominate the thinking concerning this question. The first of the models is known as the DUAL RECEPTOR MODEL and postulates a receptor for antigen and another receptor for self-MHC. Binding of one of these receptors with the appropriate ligand (antigen or self-MHC) is insufficient to trigger the cell; only when *both* receptors are occupied does an activation signal get transduced from the membrane to the cell interior. The other alternative is called the NEOANTIGENIC DETERMINANT MODEL. This model postulates that there is a receptor, *not* for antigen or for self-MHC, but rather for the *combination* of the two. This complex of antigen and MHC on the surface of the antigen-presenting cell is seen by the T cell as a new antigen (hence the term neoantigenic determinant). These possibilities are diagrammed in their most simplistic form in Figure 4.

Ruling Out the Two Independent Receptors Model

To test the model of two independent receptors, one of which recognizes antigen and the other self-MHC, Kappler and Marrack and their co-workers in Denver carried out the experiment outlined in Figure 5. They used a cloned, antigen-specific, T cell hybridoma that reacted to ovalbumin presented in the context of $H-2^a$ (OVA:$H-2^a$). Then hybridoma cells were *fused* with normal activated T cells (called "blasts") that responded to KLH in the context of $H-2^d$ (KLH:$H-2^d$). The fused

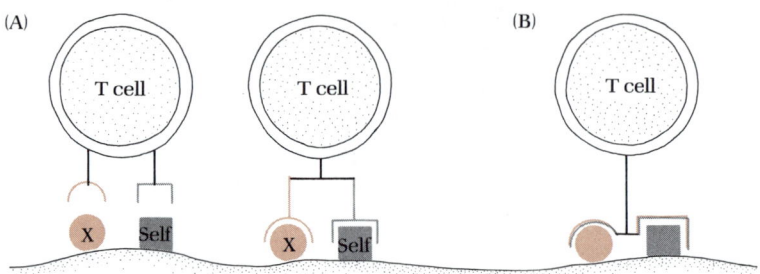

FIGURE 4 MODELS OF THE T CELL RECEPTOR

(A) Dual receptor models. The T cell has a receptor for foreign antigen (X) and a receptor for self MHC (self). These receptors can exist as separate molecules in the membrane or can be joined to a common structure. (B) Neoantigenic determinant model. The T cell has no receptor for either foreign antigen or self, but it does have a receptor for a unique determinant that is formed by the association of foreign antigen and self on the surface of the cell. [After Zinkernagel (1978) *Immunol. Rev. 42*, 224]

cells were shown to respond when presented with the antigen:H-2 combination with which each fusion partner reacted (for example, KLH:H-2^d and OVA:H-2^a). The hypothesis can then be tested by determining whether the fused cells respond to KLH in the context of H-2^a. In other words, when one of the antigen specificities and one of the MHC restrictions from each partner are presented, will the fused cell respond? The answer is no. The cells respond only when the antigen and MHC are presented coordinately (Figure 5). This elegant experiment argues against two *independent* receptors. We are still left with the possibility that the receptors for self and antigen are separate molecules but are linked in the membrane (Figure 4).

Unanswered Questions

The American composer Charles Ives wrote an atonal piece of music called *The Unanswered Question*. The piece requires several listenings and a willingness to let unusual forms take hold of the listener (Ives once said that he did not write for "lazy listeners"). The T cell receptor story is very much like this piece of modern music. The various elements that

ANTIGEN–SPECIFIC RECEPTORS

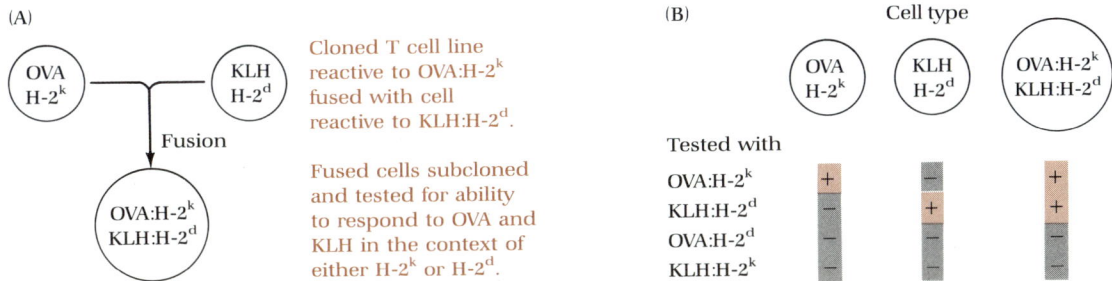

FIGURE 5 TEST OF DUAL RECEPTOR OR SINGLE RECEPTOR MODELS OF THE T CELL RECEPTOR

When cells reactive to an antigen in the context of one H-2 are fused with cells reactive to a different antigen in the context of another H-2 and the fused cell tested with all combinations of antigen and H-2, it is found that the fused cell is reactive to the two antigens but only in the context of the original H-2. This finding argues that if there are separate receptors for antigen and H-2 they function as a single unit. [After Kappler et al. (1981) *J. Exp. Med.* **153**, 1198]

do not come together easily must be dealt with at the same time, and the reader must really work at trying to follow the synthesis of the ideas as they emerge.

How, for example, can the cell recognize *self* if *self* can change to match that of the environment in which the cell differentiated? The Kappler and Marrack experiment seems to rule out two independent receptors; but if a neoantigenic determinant is involved, then we must postulate that the T cell has generated diversity for antigen plus the self of the MHC it "learned" during development. If there is a receptor for self, what prevents autodestructive reactions. Finally, we must be open to the possibilities that we have been looking at the problem in the wrong way and that as the protein chemistry and molecular genetic information comes in we may find new ways of looking at the problem.

An Immunological Approach to the Nature of the T Cell Receptor

Anti-Idiotypic Antibody against the Receptor: The Classical Approach

Just as every sailor knows that if it doesn't move it gets painted and every hunter knows that if it does move it gets shot, every immunologist knows that

CHAPTER NINETEEN

when in doubt, make an antibody against it. The Middle Ages of the saga of the quest for the T cell receptor began in the 1970s with experiments of Ramsier and Lindemann, who made antibodies against the T cell receptor. These investigators used a unique variation on the usual theme of making antibody against everything, a clever plan. They reasoned that, because parental

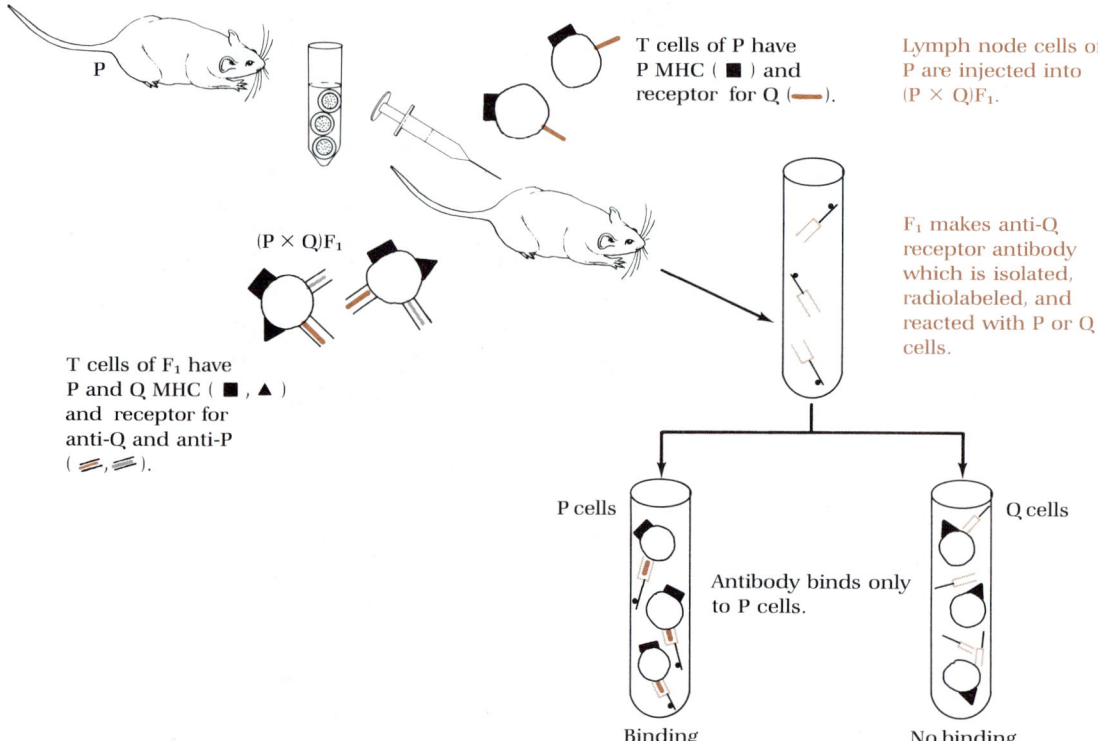

FIGURE 6   GENERATION OF ANTI-T CELL RECEPTOR ANTIBODY: THE CLASSICAL APPROACH

The principle of the experiment is that the F_1, which has MHC *antigens* for P and Q, will not have *receptors* for P and Q but will have receptors for the anti-P receptor and the anti-Q receptor on the parental strains Q and P. By immunizing the F_1 with lymph node T cells of the parental strain P, antibody against the P-anti-Q receptor is generated. [After Ramsier and Lindenmann (1972) *Transplant. Rev.* **10**, 57; and Binz and Lindenmann (1972) *J. Exp. Med.* **136**, 872]

ANTIGEN–SPECIFIC RECEPTORS

cells (P) are not recognized as foreign when injected into an F_1 but can themselves recognize the host as foreign (the basis of the GVH), then the P cells must have *receptors* for the antigens of the other parental strain in the $(P_1 \times P_2)F_1$. The F_1, to be sure, does not recognize MHC antigens on the P_1 cells; but, they reasoned, there is no reason why it should not recognize the *receptors* as foreign. With a little luck, the F_1 should even produce antibody against the receptors, and this anti-receptor antibody might be a useful tool for studying the receptors.

When this experiment was carried out (Figure 6), the F_1 did produce antibody against the receptor molecules on the parental cells. This antibody, when radiolabeled, was found to bind to cells of the P_1 but not the P_2. More important, the antibody could specifically inhibit the reaction of P_1 against P_2, but it did not have an effect on any other reactions that the P_1 cells can carry out. These results are consistent with the idea that the antibody is directed against the receptor on the T cell for a specific antigen.

A variety of experiments then followed, some of great complexity, and all pointing to the conclusion that even though one could not demonstrate immunoglobulin on the surface of the T cell, the antibody against the receptor behaved like an ANTI-IDIOTYPE ANTIBODY—that is, like an antibody against an antibody. This is of course only circumstantial evidence for the idea that the T cell receptor is an immunoglobulin or immunoglobulin-like molecule.[2] The next phase required two technical advances: the use of T cell clones and of monoclonal antibodies.

The Use of T Cell Clones One of the difficulties in doing research on the T cell receptor is that the number of cells with specific receptors for a given antigen is very low. The antibody problem was solved by using myeloma cells, which secreted large amounts of immunoglobulin. It had not been possible to grow antigen-specific functional T cells until the discovery of T cell growth factor (TCGF, or IL-2; see Chapter 21). Initially, long-term

---

[2] For the reader interested in the details of this clever but wrong path, see Chapter 13 of *The Cellular Basis of the Immune Response*, Second Edition (Golub, 1983).

maintenance of both mouse and human T cells had been carried out by maintaining the cultures in constant contact with alloantigen so that the specifically reactive cells were constantly being stimulated. But by adding TCGF to T cells from immunized animals, T cells could be grown in the absence of antigenic stimulation. This development means that one can now have a virtually unlimited supply of antigen-specific cells for experimentation.

Another advance was the production of ANTIGEN-SPECIFIC T CELL HYBRIDOMAS. These cells are produced by using a technology similar to that used for production of monoclonal antibody: fusing an antigen-specific T cell with a tumor. In this case, the tumors are T cell tumors rather than the B cell tumors used in producing monoclonal antibodies. These T cell hybridoma cells are able to grow in continuous culture in the *absence* of TCGF. By immunizing a mouse with an antigen of choice, growing the cells in vitro with TCGF or fusing them to a T cell myeloma, and selecting fused cells of the desired specificity, one can get clones of antigen-specific T cells growing in continuous culture. In other words, the problem of not having enough cells to work with is solved.

Monoclonal Antibody against the Receptor: The Modern Approach

With the availability of antigen-specific T cell clones, several groups independently set about to raise monoclonal antibodies to the receptor. The same basic experiment was carried out successfully with mouse and human T cells. The principle in each case was to immunize a host with the cloned T cells and select monoclonal antibodies directed against a determinant unique to the clone. This CLONOTYPIC DETERMINANT would be a strong candidate for antigen-specific receptor. The cloned cell used as immunogen differed in each of the experiments, ranging from an antigen-specific, MHC-restricted helper cell to a tumor-specific cytotoxic cell to an alloreactive clone of cytotoxic cells. But in each case an antibody directed against the receptor was produced. Of course, other antibodies directed against other components of the cells used as immunogens were also obtained, and in each case very careful specificity controls had to be carried out to assure that the antibody was indeed against the T cell receptor—that is, that it was directed

ANTIGEN–SPECIFIC RECEPTORS

against the clonotypic determinant. The most crucial result of these experiments was the demonstration that addition of the anti-receptor antibody (in the absence of complement) to cultures of the inducing cells prevented the reaction with specific antigen.

Once it was certain that the antibody was directed against the receptor on the cells, it was possible to use the antibody as a specific reagent to *isolate* the receptor molecule. To do this, all of the surface membrane proteins were labeled with ^{131}I. The cells were then lysed and the radiolabeled lysate was incubated with the monoclonal anti-receptor antibody. In this manner the labeled receptor is bound to the antibody in an antigen–antibody complex. These complexes are then isolated by adsorbing them to Staph A (which binds antibody molecules) and analyzed by SDS-PAGE.[3]

A typical result of such an experiment is shown in Figure 7. When the gel is run under *reducing* conditions in which interchain disulfide bonds are cleaved (lane 1), a band at 40,000–45,000 MW is seen. Under *nonreducing* conditions (disulfide bonds remain intact) there is a band at around 80,000 MW (lane 3). In the Figure, lanes 1 and 3 contain the membranes of the

---

[3] Readers who do not have a background in these techniques should consult a textbook such as Alberts et al., *Molecular Biology of the Cell* (Garland, 1983).

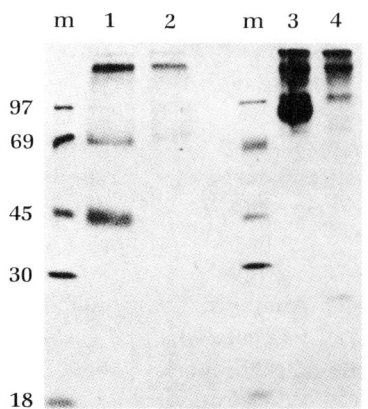

FIGURE 7 IMMUNOPRECIPITATION OF T CELL RECEPTOR

T cell hybridomas were surface-labeled with ^{125}I and the membranes separated by electrophoresis in SDS-PAGE gels. Lanes 1 and 2 were run under reducing conditions and lanes 3 and 4 were run under nonreducing conditions. Lanes 1 and 3 are from the specific cells; lanes 2 and 4 are from cells of another specificity and serve as controls. Under nonreducing conditions a molecule of ca. 80,000 is precipitated by the anti-receptor antibody. [From Haskins et al. (1983) *J. Exp. Med.* 157, 1149; with permission]

specific cells and lanes 2 and 4 are from a clone of another specificity. The crucial point is that the monoclonal antibody against the receptor on one clone does not react with the receptor on another clone.

Two-Chained T Cell Receptor

The fact that the molecular weight of the unreduced molecule was about 80,000 whereas that of the reduced molecule was 40,000 suggests that the 40,000-MW material really consists of subunits joined together in the intact molecule by disulfide bonds. These subunits were resolved by isoelectric focusing. As shown in Figure 8, there was clear evidence of a molecule with a pI of about 5; but there was also an unresolved, more basic molecule with a pI of about 7.0. This second band was resolved by a technique using nonequilibrium pH gradient electrophoresis in one dimension and SDS-PAGE in the second.

Together all these manipulations show that the antigen-specific T cell receptor is a heterodimer of molecular weight 85,000–90,000, which consists of two polypeptide chains (each of 40,000–43,000 molecular weight) linked by disulfide bonds. It is remarkable that a similar structure has been found by at least four independent groups, using both mouse and human cells. The two chains have been named alpha (α) and beta (β).

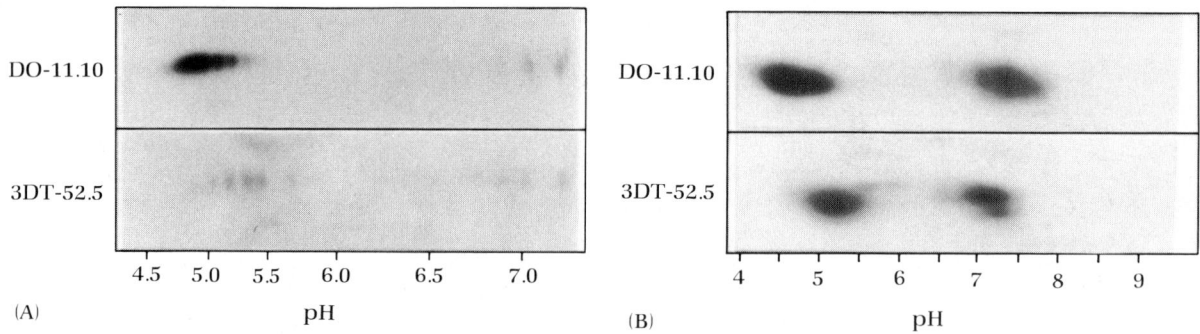

FIGURE 8 SUBUNITS OF THE T CELL RECEPTOR
(A) Isoelectric focusing of surface-labeled proteins of two T cell hybridomas after immunoprecipitation. (B) Nonequilibrium pH gradient electrophoresis of the same preparations. Under these conditions two molecules can be discerned. [From Kappler et al. (1983) *Cell* 34, 727]

ANTIGEN–SPECIFIC RECEPTORS

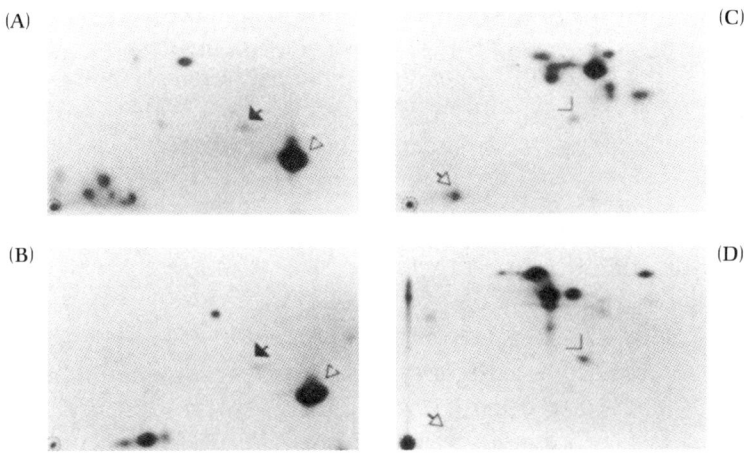

FIGURE 9   PEPTIDE MAPS OF α AND β CHAINS
OF THE T CELL RECEPTOR

(A,B) α Chains of two clones show very few differences. (C,D) β chains from these two clones show many more differences. [From Acuto et al. (1983) *J. Exp. Med.* 158, 1368; with permission]

Resemblance of β Chain to Immunoglobulin

To determine the differences between the peptide structures of the α and β chains, comparative peptide maps were made. The T cell receptor proteins from two clones with different antigenic specificities were isolated, labeled with ^{125}I, and digested with proteolytic enzymes. Two-dimensional peptide maps were then made by subjecting the samples to electrophoresis in one dimension and chromatography in the second dimension (Figure 9).

When we compare the peptide maps of the α chains of the two receptors (A and B in the figure), we see that the chains from both clones are very similar but not identical. In contrast, comparison of the β chains shows that there are many differences. We will see in the next chapter that this is a paradoxical finding, because at the present time it seems that the α chain has the potential for at least ten times more diversity than the β chain.

When the NH_2-terminal amino acid sequence of the β chain was carried out and a comparative protein sequence analysis by computer search was carried out for residues 2 through 12, homology was found between these residues and the variable region of human λ light chains (underlined residues indicate identity):

$$\beta \quad \underline{V} \; I \; Q \; \underline{S} \; \underline{P} \; R \; \underline{H} \; E \; \underline{V} \; \underline{T} \; E$$
$$\lambda \quad \underline{V} \; S \; G \; \underline{S} \; \underline{P} \; G \; \underline{H} \; S \; \underline{V} \; \underline{T} \; T$$

The proteins of the T cell receptor therefore are somewhat similar to immunoglobulins.

T3, a Differentiation Antigen

In Chapter 11 we learned that T3 is one of the differentiation antigens that the human T cell begins to express during intrathymic differentiation. Specialized subsets of T cells express either T4 or T8 molecules, which are associated with MHC restriction specificity, but all functional cells express T3. This 20,000-MW molecule was first thought to be implicated with antigen recognition when it was found that monoclonal anti-T3 antibody blocked all T cell functions, including antigen-induced proliferation. We have just seen that the clonotypic specificity resides in the α and β chains, but the following experiment shows that T3 is associated with these chains of the T cell receptor.

Treating a cloned CTL with anti-T3 in the absence of complement (so that there is binding of the antibody to T3 but not lysis of the cell) causes capping and then selective shedding of T3 from the surface even though other T cell antigens (T1, T11, and T12, for example) are unaffected. A clone of antigen-specific CTL treated with monoclonal anti-T3 in this way was examined to determine whether the α and β chains of the T cell receptor *co-migrated* with T3. It was found that both the α and β chains of the T cell receptor did in fact co-migrate, indicating that they are associated with T3. Treatment of cells with anti-T3 plus complement abolishes *all* immune function. T3 therefore cannot be part of the antigen-specific recognition mechanism of the T cell, but it seems likely that T3 is associated in some way with the α and β chains responsible for specific binding of antigen.

ANTIGEN–SPECIFIC RECEPTORS

Summary

1. Antigen binds directly to B cell receptors, which are surface immunoglobulin molecules. The B cell has two surface isotypes that act as antigen-specific receptors: sIgM and sIgD. These molecules share idiotypic and antigenic specificity. IgM is the first isotype expressed, but as B cells develop they also begin to express surface IgD.
2. The sIg antigen-specific receptors on B cells are mobile within the membrane and can be "patched" and "capped."
3. T cells do not have readily demonstrated immunoglobulin on their surface. They do not bind antigen alone, but only when the antigen is in the context of self-MHC molecules.
4. The use of antigen-reactive T cell clones and monoclonal antibodies against the receptors on these clones has led to the isolation of the clonotypic T cell receptor. It is a two-chained molecule that consists of an α chain and a β chain (a heterodimer) and has a molecular weight of 85,000–90,000.
5. An invariant molecule called T3 is associated with the α and β chains.

Additional Readings

Allison, J. P., B. W. McIntyre and D. Bloch. 1982. Tumor-specific antigen of murine T lymphoma defined with monoclonal antibody. *J. Immunol.* 129, 2293.

Fathman, C. G. and J. G. Frelinger. 1983. T lymphocyte clones. *Annu. Rev. Immunol.* 1, 633.

Hannum, C. H., J. W. Kappler, I. S. Trowbridge, P. Marrack and J. H. Freed. 1984. Immunoglobulin-like nature of the α-chain of a human T-cell antigen/MHC receptor. *Nature* 312, 65.

Immunological Reviews, Volume 81. (1984)

Kronenberg, M., G. Siu, L. E. Hood and N. Shastri. In press. The molecular genetics of the T cell antigen receptor and T cell antigen recognition. *Annu. Rev. Immunol.*

Meure, S. C., O. Acuto, T. Hercend, S. F. Schlossman and E. L. Reinherz. 1984. The human T cell receptor. *Annu. Rev. Immunol.* 2, 23.

CHAPTER 20

GENETIC ORGANIZATION OF RECEPTORS

Overview In the last chapter we saw that the antigen-specific receptor on the B cell is the immunoglobulin molecule and that the receptor on the T cell is a 90-kd heterodimer with immunoglobulin-like characteristics. In this chapter we will examine the genetic organization of the molecules that make up the T cell receptor. We will see that we are closer to the solution to the T cell receptor problem because now the genes for the receptor have been isolated and studied.

The use of cloned lines of functional T cells, an advance that (along with monoclonal antibodies) made the isolation of the receptor protein possible, has also made possible the isolation of the genes that encode the receptor. The T cell receptor uses V–D–J gene rearrangements; thus, even though the structure of the T cell receptor differs from that of the surface immunoglobulin of the B cell, the organization of its genes is similar to those of B cell receptors and products. However, the problem of how the T cell uses the products of those genes to react with antigen in an MHC-restricted manner still remains.

GENETIC ORGANIZATION OF RECEPTORS

Organization of Receptor Genes in B Cells

Because we are accepting the fact that the B cell antigen-specific receptor is an immunoglobulin molecule with structural properties very similar to those of the secreted form of the molecule, we will not have to go into any detail about how the organization of the genetic material leads to the generation of receptor diversity, because we covered the topic of immunoglobulin diversity in depth in Chapter 5. The only question we must examine now is the nature of the differences between the surface, or membrane-associated, form (sIg) of immunoglobulin and the excreted forms of the molecule. Ultimately it will be important to know the features that allow one form of the molecule to remain in the membrane and the other to be secreted.

Synthesis of Surface Immunoglobulin and Secreted Immunoglobulin Two groups of researchers have independently concluded that the membrane form of μ chain and the secreted form are encoded from the same DNA. The difference between the two forms is achieved during the processing of the mRNA. Fred Alt and his colleagues at MIT isolated mRNA from two different B cell lines. One of these lines produced equal amounts of secreted and membrane forms of IgM and one produced almost exclusively membrane form. The mRNA from the line producing both species of μ chain was composed of two species, one with a molecular weight of 64,000 and one of 67,000. The less mature line, which did not produce secreted form, had only the 67,000-MW mRNA. This finding argues that the 64,000-MW mRNA encodes the secreted form and the 67,000-MW the membrane form. When fetal liver (which is a site of embryonic B cell development) was examined, it was found that the only mRNA was identical to the membrane form. The developing B cells in the fetal liver do not secrete any immunoglobulin, but they do have surface IgM.

Rogers and colleagues at UCLA and Caltech prepared cDNA from the two forms of mRNA and found that the sequences are identical through the 3' end of the fourth constant region; that is, the two forms of μ chain use the same gene. They differ only in untranslated segments at the C terminus. Thus the secreted and membrane forms are produced from transcripts of a single gene

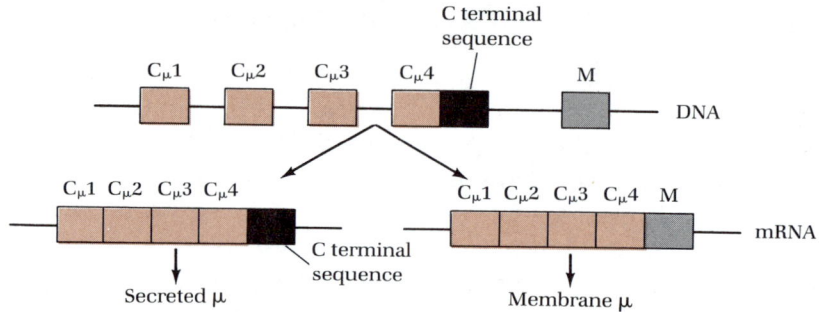

FIGURE 1 MEMBRANE AND SECRETED FORMS OF μ CHAIN
Both μ_s and μ_m are encoded on the same DNA. The mRNA is processed by two alternative pathways. In the pathway leading to the membrane form, cleavage occurs at the boundary of $C\mu 4$ with the μ_s terminal sequence. This reaction eliminates the μ_s C terminal sequence. The M segment then becomes spliced into place on the μ_m. In the pathway leading to the secreted form, the C terminal sequence remains attached to the rest of the molecule. [Redrawn from Early et al. (1980) *Cell* 20, 313]

but are processed by different pathways. The membrane form is produced by two extra mRNA splices resulting in the M segment, which is derived from exons 3' to the $C\mu 4$ exon (Figure 1). The mechanism for the alternative mRNA splicing is not known.

Organization of the T Cell Receptor Genes

The question of how the T cell receptor works is complicated, because we must explain not only how diversity is generated in the 90-kd heterodimer but also how antigen is recognized by T cells. Somehow the T cell receptor must be able to recognize the vast array of foreign antigens but it must also be able to do it in the context of self-MHC.[1]

[1] If by chance the reader has entered the narrative at this point for a quick fix on the T cell receptor, be advised that there are no free lunches. To really understand the organization of the T cell receptor genes and what that organization means to the function of the T cell, you must go back and read (at least) the previous chapter. To those readers who have worked their way to this point, you are better persons for having done so and should hold on to your seats, because what follows is dynamite!

GENETIC ORGANIZATION OF RECEPTORS

Isolation of cDNA Clones: The Subtraction Method

Complementary DNA (cDNA) clones[2] for the T cell receptor were isolated simultaneously and independently by Hedrick, Davis, and their co-workers at the NIH and by Mak and his co-workers in Toronto. The strategies differed slightly, but we will describe only the "subtractive method" of Hedrick and Davis in detail. The basis of the approach was to isolate the genes that encode the T cell receptor from antigen-specific, MHC-restricted T cell hybridomas. In the original work a T helper clone was used, but since that time T cytotoxic clones have also been used.

Several assumptions were made at the outset of the work. *First*, it was assumed that the genes being sought must be expressed in T cells but not in B cells. This means that the mRNA encoding the T cell receptor will not be found in B cells. *Second*, the mRNA for the protein should be found on membrane-bound polysomes and attached to the endoplasmic reticulum by a signal sequence. This notion derives from the extensive work of Blobel and his colleagues, who have proposed the "signal hypothesis" to account for the means by which proteins are transported into and across membranes. Because the T cell receptor will be a membrane-associated protein, it was assumed that it would follow this pattern of behavior. *Third*, the T cell receptor genes will be rearranged. This restriction assumes that there will be a similarity between the mode of recognition of antigen by B cells and T cells. If the T cell receptor is formed by rearranged genes, then the diversity of the receptor should be generated in a manner similar to the generation of diversity in immunoglobulin—that is, there should be variable, constant, and joining regions.

On the basis of these assumptions, cDNA clones were isolated by the "subtractive method" of Mark Davis. This creative and very powerful approach is diagrammed in Figure 2. ^{32}P-labeled cDNA of the membrane-bound polysomal RNA from the hybridoma was made. Next, those sequences that were also expressed in B cells were removed by hybridization to mRNA from B cells. The reasoning here is that even though both T cells and B cells have the

---

[2] What follows assumes a basic knowledge of the principles of DNA cloning. The reader who feels a need for it should review the subject before going on (e.g., J. D. Watson, J. Tooze and D. T. Kurtz, *Recombinant DNA: A Short Course*, Freeman, 1983).

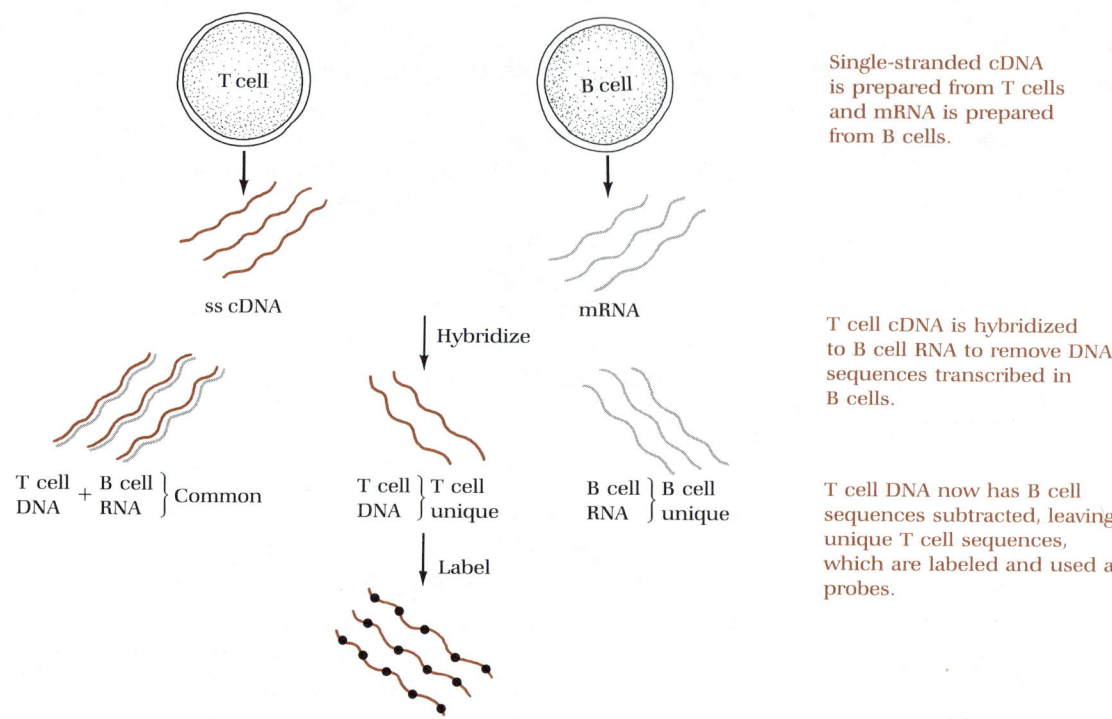

FIGURE 2 THE SUBTRACTIVE METHOD

To obtain a probe for a gene library that is unique to sequences expressed in T cells, the expressed T cell sequences from mRNA are converted into cDNA. This single-stranded cDNA is then hybridized with mRNA from B cells (that is, the expressed sequences in B cells), a procedure resulting in (1) T cell sequences hybridized to B cell sequences, (2) unhybridized T cell sequences, and (3) unhybridized B cell mRNA. After removing the hybridized cDNA (1) and the unhybridized mRNA (3) (this step is not shown in the figure), only expressed sequences unique to the T cell (2) remain. This cDNA can then be labeled for use as a probe.

same DNA, T cell-specific genes will not be *expressed* in B cells.[3] Thus B cell-specific and mRNA transcripts common to T cells and B cells will be removed, leaving a small fraction of the total T cell mRNA unhybridized. Because B cells and T cells differ in only about 2% of their gene expression and only about 3% of lymphocyte mRNA is membrane bound (see assumption 2), one is not looking for a needle in a haystack.

[3] Remember, it is the expressed RNA that is used to bind and remove sequences from the T cell DNA.

GENETIC ORGANIZATION OF RECEPTORS

Having made ^{32}P-labeled cDNA from the polysome mRNA and "subtracted" the sequences that are shared with B cells, they were now in possession of a probe that could be used to probe a cDNA clone library. This library (which had also been constructed by the T-minus-B method just described) consisted of 5000 clones and was 20-fold enriched for T-specific sequences. Screening with the labeled probe produced seven clones from the library that hybridized with the probe, each of which should contain a gene specific for the T cell. With luck, at least one should contain a gene for the T cell receptor.

Evidence of Gene Rearrangement

But how is one to identify a T cell-specific gene as a T cell receptor gene? Recall that assumption 3 is that the T cell receptor gene will be rearranged, so the experimenters examined the seven clones for evidence of such rearrangements. First, labeled probes were prepared from each of the clones. Second, genomic DNAs from T cells, B cells, liver cells, and macrophages were treated with a restriction endonuclease and then hybridized by Southern blotting to the labeled probes. The principle here is the same as we saw in the analysis of gene rearrangements in antibody. If the gene had indeed been rearranged, it very likely will have at least one cleavage site for endonucleases that is different from that in the unrearranged gene. Rearranged and unrearranged genes will therefore give different patterns in the Southern blot. The pattern of the blots showed that there was rearrangement in the DNA from the T cell but not in the DNAs of the B cell, macrophages, or liver cells. All helper and cytotoxic lines and hybrids tested in a similar manner to date shows gene rearrangement (Figure 3). Subsequent sequencing of the cloned T cell-specific genes showed that the β chain gene of the T cell receptor was the gene isolated.

V, C, J, and D Regions in the β Chain

It was also assumed that the T cell receptor genes would have V, D, and J regions similar to those in the immunoglobulin genes. Having already shown that the gene for the β chain is rearranged, Davis and his co-workers screened a thymocyte cDNA library, looking for evidence of these regions. Three thymus-derived clones were selected and their DNA was sequenced and compared with the original clone that

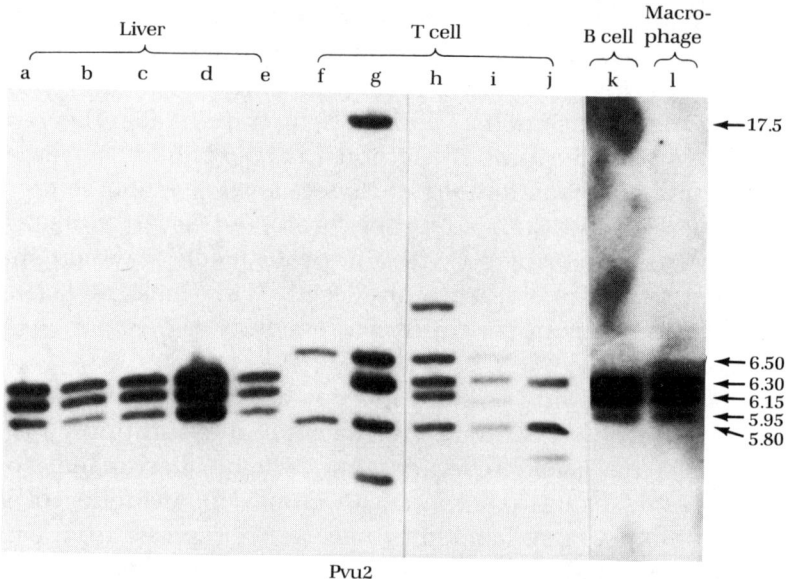

FIGURE 3 GENE REARRANGEMENT IN THE T CELL RECEPTOR
Genomic DNA was prepared from T cell lines, B cells, macrophages, and liver cells. After digestion with the restriction enzyme *Pvu*II, Southern blot analysis was carried out using probes prepared by the method diagrammed in Figure 1. [From Davis et al. (1984) *Immunol. Rev.* 81, 235; with permission]

was used as the probe. From the DNA sequences, the amino acid sequences of the protein could be deduced and compared.

When the Dayhoff bank of known protein sequences was searched, 25 known sequences (of ca. 2300 in the bank) had similarities to the β chain. Of these 25 sequences, 24 were immunoglobulin and 1 was a human Class II MHC molecule. The similarities were in the V, D, J, and C regions. Close analysis of the sequence similarity shows that it is close enough to account for the data which shows the same idiotype on B cells and T cells (Chapter 19) but different enough to explain why so often immunoglobulin was not found on T cells. Thus we see that the pre-

GENETIC ORGANIZATION OF RECEPTORS

diction that the gene for the T cell receptor would resemble immunoglobulin in the manner in which diversity can be generated proved to be correct.

Examination of the DNA sequences of the human T cell receptor gene showed a resemblance to both human and mouse light chains, the location of cysteine residues as well as variable, constant, and joining regions being similar in both.

So in a very short time the mystery of the T cell receptor appeared to be solvable. The receptor molecule was a heterodimer, and the genes for one of the chains was isolated and showed rearrangements of sequences similar to those found in immunoglobulin light chain genes. All that remained, it seemed, was to obtain the gene for the α chain, examine the sequences, and understand the nature of MHC restriction. But the astute reader has no doubt become aware that the immune system always provides surprises.

Three Classes of T Cell Receptor Genes

We have learned that the T cell receptor protein consists of two peptides, the α and β subunits; so when it was realized that the first genes to be isolated were for the β subunit, an intense search began for the gene coding for the α subunit. A gene isolated in Tonegawa's lab was thought to be the gene for the α chain. However, it was quickly realized that there were no sequences for glycosylation sites, and both the α and β peptides were known to be glycosylated. Because it did not encode the α chain, finding this gene, now called γ, was a great surprise. The function of this gene is not known, and no gene product has been found.

The α chain gene was soon isolated by several groups, including Tonegawa's. One indication of the dizzying speed with which this all occurred is the fact that the first report of the β chain appeared in *Nature* in March 1984, and both the γ and α chains were identified by November of the same year. The crucial point is that all of these gene families are homologous to each other and to immunoglobulin genes. All are rearranged, and all have V, D, and J regions (Figure 4).

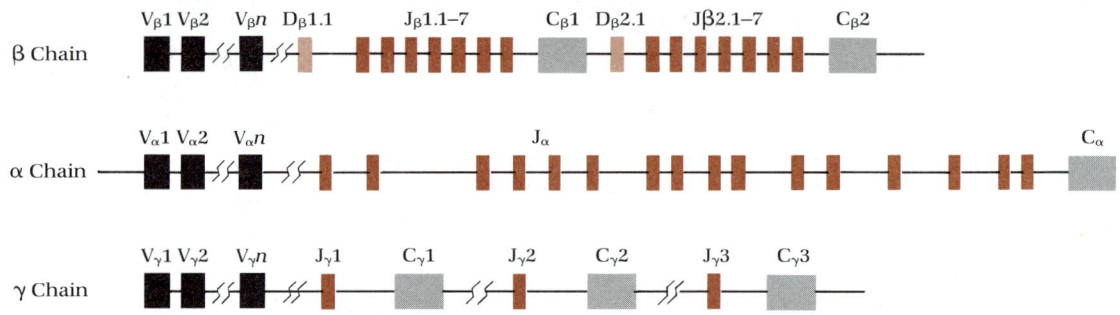

FIGURE 4 ORGANIZATION OF T CELL RECEPTOR GENES

The T cell receptor is composed of two chains, α and β, which are encoded on the genes diagrammed in this figure. A γ product has not been identified, but is encoded on the γ gene shown diagrammatically here. [After Winoto et al. (1985) *Nature* 316, 835]

Chromosome Locations of T Cell Receptor Genes

The chromosome locations of the human α and β genes have been determined by in situ hybridization.

The α gene is found on chromosome 14 in a position proximal to the H chain gene of immunoglobulin. The gene is found on a region of the chromosome (14q11-q12) known to be involved in translocations and inversions in human T cell leukemias and lymphomas. It has been suggested that the locus for the α-chain may participate in oncogene activation of T cell tumors, but, of course, we do not know if this is really the case.

The β chain has been localized to the long arm of chromosome 7 at band q35. The terminal segment of 7q (as well as 7p and 14q) are "hot spots" for chromosome rearrangements.

Generation of Diversity in T Cell Receptor Genes

Figure 4 shows the organization of the three T cell receptor genes as of the winter of 1985. Several points should be noted so that the reader can consult the latest research articles or summaries in *Science, Nature, Cell,* or *The New York Times* to see how things have changed between the writing and the reading.

GENETIC ORGANIZATION OF RECEPTORS

First, the β chain has about 30 V regions (designated Vβ), 6 stretches of D, and 12 J regions ($D\beta_1$, $D\beta_2$, and so on; $J\beta_1$, $J\beta_2$, and so on). These are separated by one of the two constant regions ($C\beta_1$ and $C\beta_2$). Each of the Vβ regions has a highly conserved heptamer, a nonconserved spacer sequence of 12 or 23 nucleotides, and an A/T-rich nonamer. This organization is similar to the joining segments of immunoglobulin. Recall that a 12-nucleotide sequence affords one turn of the DNA helix and a 23-nucleotide sequence two turns. Thus the β chain has all of the elements for generating diversity as well as the joining sequences.

Second, the α chain gene is less well studied but has the potential for even more diversity than the β chain gene has. This may be surprising since we saw in the last chapter that the α chain protein has a peptide map indicative of less diversity than the β chain peptide map. The α chain has at least 200 V segments (V_α), 50 J segments, and an unknown number of D segments. One very strange fact is that the J_α segments are spread over 60 kilobases of DNA, an unusually large spread.

It is clear that an enormous amount of diversity can be generated from the two genes. The following calculation (courtesy of Lee Hood) shows the potential specificities of the T cell receptor.

$30V\beta \times 6D\beta \times 12J\beta = 2 \times 10^3$ arrangements of β chain

$200V\alpha \times 50J\alpha = 10^4$ arrangements of α chain

$2 \times 10^3 \beta \times 10^4 \alpha = 2 \times 10^7$ arrangements of T cell receptor genes

It is clear that there is the potential for as much diversity in the T cell receptor repertoire as there is in immunoglobulins. One striking difference between the two, however, is the greater potential for 3' diversity, because of the large numbers of J and D regions. It is also clear that the α chain has the potential for an order of magnitude more diversity than does the β chain.

Finally, the γ subunit gene has only one functional V segment, an unknown number of D regions, and at least three Jγ and Cγ regions. But the γ gene does not encode sites where glycosylation can occur, and there is no known protein product or function for this gene. We will see below that the γ chain gene is expressed at different times than the α and β chain genes.

CHAPTER TWENTY

The rearrangements of the gene segments in the α and β chains have been shown to follow the same order as those seen in immunoglobulins. The first rearrangement is D to J, giving D–J; this is then joined to V, giving V–D–J.

The Generation of Diversity

Because the β chain has only 30 Vβ segments but 6 Jβ and 12 Dβ segments, one would predict that T cells with different specificities would use common Vβ segments. This is in fact the case. The DNA of two clones of different antigen-specific, MHC-restricted T helper cells were isolated and examined for the nature of their rearranged β genes. One clone was specific for the antigen hen egg lysozyme (HEL) in association with I-A^b (HEL:I-A^b). The other was specific for pigeon cytochrome c (cyt c) in association with I-E^k (cyt c:I-E^k). The antigens do not cross-react, but it could be clearly shown that both clones used the same Vβ gene. However, each clone had rearranged the Vβ gene with a different Dβ and Jβ gene segment. Thus we see that the β chain can use 3′ rearrangements to generate diversity.

A Caution to the Reader and a Disclaimer from the Author

It would be disingenuous to give the impression that it is even possible to write an account of the research that attempts to describe the current status of the organization of the T cell receptor genes which will not be obsolete before this sentence is finished. But by understanding the kind of questions that any explanation must answer and by seeing the strategies that are used to answer them, the reader should be able to follow the unfolding story. The next edition of this book will have an update and the inquisitive reader can compare his/her reading of the literature in the intervening years with that of the author.

Developmental Expression of the Genes

Because T cells differentiate in the thymus, it is logical to assume that the gene rearrangements will occur in this organ. The first lymphoid migration into the fetal thymus occurs on day 11 or 12 in the mouse. Thy 1 is expressed by days 13–14, and immunocompetent cells can be

GENETIC ORGANIZATION OF RECEPTORS

found by days 18–19. The first rearranged T cell receptor gene to be found in the fetal mouse thymus is the γ gene by day 13. In fact, this gene can be found in the rearranged form in the fetal liver, the source of the pre-T cells in the embryo. Neither α nor β genes are rearranged in fetal liver or the 14-day thymus. The β gene is rearranged in the thymus by day 15 and the α gene by day 16 or 17.

Of course we do not know whether the fact that γ is rearranged before α and β is of biological significance, especially since we do not know whether the gene has a function and what its product is. One clue may be that the γ gene is found only in cytotoxic cells and not in helper cells, whereas α and β are found in all helper and cytotoxic cells.

Structure of the Receptor in the Membrane

We do not know the nature of the organization of the subunits of the receptor in the membrane of the T cell. Based on the extensive analogy of the known structures with immunoglobulins, however, it is natural to suppose that the dimer of α and β chains are associated in a manner that allows their variable regions to interact somehow.

Some Alternative Views

We have presented the problem of the T cell receptor in a manner that demands the solution explain why T cells see antigen only in the context of a self-MHC repertoire acquired by selection, primarily in the thymus. Experiments can only be set up when there are hypotheses to test; and some very creative hypotheses about the T cell receptor have been proposed, each of which is testable.

Very recently a model has been proposed by the immunologist Ben Pernis and the molecular biologist Richard Axel at Columbia. Their model uses all of the facts presented up to now, including the mysterious γ chain. Called by Pernis and Axel the "ONE AND A HALF RECEPTOR" model (Figure 5a), it proposes that there are *separate* receptors for antigen and MHC, each composed of two chains. The antigen-specific chain is postulated to be a disulfide-linked dimer of α and β. The MHC receptor is postulated to be a dimer of the *same* β chain linked to a γ chain. The two

CHAPTER TWENTY

heterodimers are then thought to associate to produce the final complex in the membrane, a tetramer with two nonequivalent binding sites.

Lee Hood has taken a different tack (Figure 5b). He argues that there are really no very significant differences between T cell recognition and antibody recognition. The basis of this argument comes first from the intuitive observation that the α and β chains will form in the membrane a dimer very similar to an antibody molecule. We saw from Hood's calculation (page 347) of the amount of diversity that the α:β dimer can generate that comparable amounts of diversity are possible in antibody and T cell recognition systems. Given these similarities, if *antibody* could be shown to function in an MHC-restricted manner, then we could feel justified in arguing that the two are more similar than different, and we would not have to postulate any special cases for T cell recognition. In fact there is evidence that monoclonal antibody against influenza virus can recognize epitopes on the virus in the context of MHC. In these experiments from Norman Klinman's laboratory in La Jolla, tissue culture cells of a given MHC

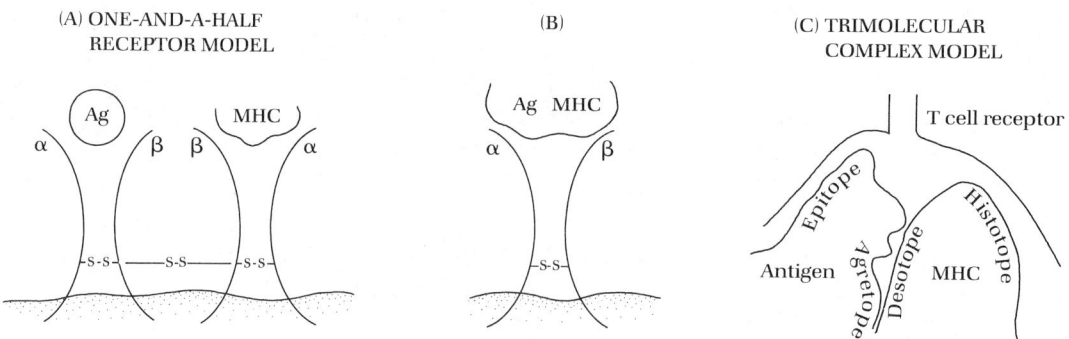

FIGURE 5   ORGANIZATION OF THE T CELL RECEPTOR

Several models of the T cell receptor have been proposed: (A) the one and a half receptor model [Pernis and Axel (1985) *Cell* 41, 13]; (B) an antibody-like model [L. Hood, personal communication]; and (C) the trimolecular complex model [Heber-Katz, Hausberg and Schwartz (1984) *J. Mol. Cell. Immunol.* 1,3].

GENETIC ORGANIZATION OF RECEPTORS

haplotype were infected with influenza virus and injected into mice of the same MHC. Clones of cells producing anti-influenza antibody were tested; and in the majority of cases, the anti-influenza antibody was active only when the influenza epitope was presented on the syngeneic MHC. In this case, then, it could be shown that antibody can behave in an MHC-restricted manner. Because the T cell receptor is antibody-like, has as much diversity as antibody, and can be shown to do all that the T cell receptor does (that is, recognize antigen in the context of self MHC), there is no need to make a more complex theory to explain the function of the receptor. Hood's group is currently testing the theory by transfecting the α and β genes into cells and will test them to determine whether they function in an antigen-specific *and* MHC-restricted manner.

Another, more complex model has been suggested by Ron Schwartz, Ellen Heber-Katz, and their colleagues at the NIH (Figure 5c). This model was originally proposed to account for the genetic control of antibody responses, which are controlled by the I region of the MHC (so-called responders and nonresponders, discussed in Chapter 13), but it also deals with the nature of the T cell receptor. These workers have proposed that the T cell receptor binds to both antigen and MHC molecules to form a trimolecular complex. Four sites determine the interaction: first, the residues on the MHC molecule that react with antigen, called DESETOPES (DEterminant SElection); second, the residue on the antigen that reacts with the MHC, called the AGRETOPE (AntigenRestriction Element); third, the residue on the MHC that reacts with the T cell receptor, called the HISTOTOPE (HISTOcompatibility); and finally, the residue on the antigen that reacts with the T cell receptor, for which the already existing term EPITOPE was retained. In this model (diagrammed in Figure 5) the requirements for activating the T cell are extended to include the need for an association of the antigen with the MHC molecule. Animals that are genetically incapable of responding to a certain antigen (nonresponders) are thought to have MHC molecules that cannot bind to the antigen.

CHAPTER TWENTY

Summary

1. The surface immunoglobulin molecules (sIg) are the B cell antigen-specific receptor molecules. Both sIg and secreted Ig are synthesized from the same DNA but are altered posttranscriptionally.
2. The genes for the T cell receptor were isolated by the "subtractive" method: The mRNA from B cells is hybridized to cDNA from a T cell hybridoma. In this manner, all T cell genes that are shared with B cells are removed. The remaining unique T cell DNA sequences are labeled and used to probe a T cell cDNA library.
3. Genes that encode the α and β chains of the T cell receptor have been isolated. A third gene, called γ (for which no protein product is known), has also been isolated.
4. α, β and γ genes exhibit rearrangements similar to those seen in immunoglobulin genes. Each has V, D, and J regions, used to generate diversity, and each also has C regions. Rearrangements of the variable gene segments can produce enough diversity to account for 2×10^7 different T cell receptor genes.
5. The γ gene is the first T cell receptor gene to become rearranged. This event occurs in the fetal liver and fetal thymus at day 13 in the mouse. β is found in the rearranged form in the thymus by fetal day 15 and α by day 16 or 17. Neither α nor β is rearranged in the fetal liver.
6. The structural basis for MHC-restricted antigen recognition by T cells has not been explained from the genetic information obtained to date.

Additional Readings

Chien Y., N. Gascoigne, J. Kavaler, N. Lee and M. Davis. 1984. Somatic recombination in a murine T cell receptor gene. *Nature* 309, 322.

Chieu Y.-H., D. M. Becker, T. Lindsten, M. Okamura, D. J. Cohen and M. Davis. 1984. Third type of murine T cell receptor gene. *Nature* 312, 31.

Clark, S. P., Y. Yoshikai, S. Taylor, G. Siu, L. Hood and T. Mak. 1984. Identification of a diversity gene segment of human T cell receptor β and comparison with the analogous murine element. *Nature* 311, 387.

Goverman, J., K. Minard, N. Shastri, T. Hunkapiller, D. Hansburg, E. Sercarz and L. Hood. 1985. Rearranged β T cell receptor genes in a helper T cell clone specific for lysozyme: no correlation between Vβ and MHC restriction. *Cell* 40, 859.

Hayday, A. C., H. Saito, S. D. Gillies, D. M. Kranz, G. Tanigawa, H. N. Eisen and S. Tonegawa. 1985. Structure, organization and somatic rearrangements of T cell γ genes. *Cell* 40, 259.

GENETIC ORGANIZATION OF RECEPTORS

Hedrick, S., D. Cohen, E. Nielsen and M. Davis. 1984. Isolation of cDNA clones encoding T cell-specific membrane-associated proteins. *Nature* 308, 149.

Hedrick, S., E. Nielsen, J. Kavaler, D. I. Cohen and M. Davis. 1984. Sequence relationships between putative T cell receptor polypeptides and immunoglobulins. *Nature* 308, 153.

Saito, H., D. M. Kranz, Y. Takagaki, A. C. Hayday, H. Eisen and S. Tonegawa. 1984. A third rearranged and expressed gene in a clone of cytotoxic T lymphocytes. *Nature* 312, 36.

Yanagi Y., Y. Yoshika, K. Leggett,, S. Clark, I. Aleksander and T. Mak. 1984. A human T cell-specific cDNA clone encodes a protein having extensive homology to immunoglobulin chains. *Nature* 308, 145.

CHAPTER 21

INTERLEUKINS

Overview The principal manner by which the cells of the immune system communicate is through the elaboration of soluble factors. These factors (lymphokines and monokines) are hormones made by cells of the immune system (lymphocytes and monocytes or macrophages). Collectively these factors are called cytokines, and they act on other cells of the immune system to regulate their function.

One thing is already clear about T cells: the binding of antigen to the receptor is complex. Because B cells bind antigen directly, it is tempting to treat them as mere spheres with receptors on their surfaces; but this can be a fatal oversimplification. We will see that antigen must act in conjunction with "factors" to activate B cells. Once again the initial reaction of antigen with macrophage will be seen to be important, because one consequence of that reaction is the elaboration of the monokine interleukin-1 (IL-1). IL-1 reacts with T cells, causing them, along with antigen, to elaborate the lymphokine interleukin-2 (IL-2). It is through this interleukin cascade that T cell proliferation is induced and regulated.

The nature of these cytokines is becoming clear, and studies are now beginning to show how these molecules initiate intracelluar events in the cells of the immune system. The emerging picture reveals that very little about the signal transduction from the cell membrane to the nucleus in lymphocytes may be unique, and that studies in a variety of cell systems will prove to be applicable to the cells of the immune system.

INTERLEUKINS

T Cell Activation

Factors Produced by T Cells and Macrophages: Lymphocytes and Monokines

In the 1970s many laboratories carried out experiments showing that soluble factors from spleen cells could be used to augment ConA or PHA mitogenesis or to substitute for helper T cells. Each laboratory used a slightly different assay system, and each laboratory gave its factor a unique name and acronym. The array reached almost comic proportions (see Information Box 1 for a partial list), and it soon

---

INFORMATION BOX 1

The Many Names of Cytokines

Acronyms for IL-1

LAF	Lymphocyte activating factor
MP	Mitogenic protein
HP-1	Helper peak-1
TRF-III	T cell replacing factor-III
TRF_m	T cell replacing factor$_{m\phi}$
BAF	B cell activating factor
BDF	B cell differentiation factor

Acronyms for IL-2

TSF	Thymocyte stimulating factor
TMF	Thymocyte mitogenic factor
TCGF	T cell growth factor
—	Co-stimulator
KHF	Killer cell helper factor
SCIF	Secondary cytotoxic T cell inducing factor

Source: After Garden et al. (1979), *Journal of Immunology* 123: 2928.

became clear that Nature would not be cruel enough to use this apparently endless array of factors to effect proliferation and differentiation. It was also clear that order had to be brought to the near chaotic situation. So, in 1979 a group of investigators actively working in this field met at Ermatigen, Switzerland, and made a systematic comparison of all of the known factors. They concluded that the only differences between most of them were the names and the manner in which they were assayed. In fact, they concluded, the bewildering array really consisted of only two factors. A generic name that had no meaning in any known language (and would therefore have a low probability of offending anyone) was chosen to replace the names that usually described how the factor was assayed. The factors were called INTERLEUKINS because this neologism gives a vague hint of involvement in communication between the cells. The two factors were called INTERLEUKIN-1 and INTERLEUKIN-2 (IL-1 and IL-2). Some biochemical and biological properties of IL-1 and IL-2 are provided in Information Box 2.

INFORMATION BOX 2

Properties of IL-1 and IL-2

	IL-1	IL-2
Molecular weight	12,000–18,000	30,000–35,000
Isoelectric point	Mouse: 4.5–5.5 Human: 6.5–7.5	3.5–5.5
pH sensitivity	pH2 insensitive	pH2 insensitive
Produced by	Macrophages	T cells

INTERLEUKINS

The Discovery of IL-1

In the late 1960s several investigators found that supernatant fluid from cultures of human peripheral blood leukocytes stimulated with alloantigen (i.e., MLR cultures) acted as mitogens when added to unstimulated human leukocytes. It was assumed that the mitogenic factors were produced by lymphocytes, but in 1970 Fritz Bach and his co-workers found that adherent cells were able to produce mitogenic factors. This observation was expanded upon in 1972 when Gery, Gershon, and Waksman at Yale found that a cell-free supernatant fluid obtained from human peripheral blood or from mouse spleen cells that had been stimulated with either phytohemagglutinin (PHA) or lipopolysaccharide (LPS) acted as a potentiating factor for mitogen-stimulated cells. PHA, it will be recalled, acts as a mitogen for peripheral T cells but not for thymocytes. However, in the presence of this factor, thymocytes were able to respond to PHA (Table 1). Most important, they found that adherent but not nonadherent cells produce the factor, which they termed LYMPHOCYTE ACTIVATING FACTOR (LAF), now called IL-1.

Production of IL-1 by Macrophages

We already know that macrophages are required for all immune functions. The experimental results given in Table 2 show that macrophages secrete a soluble factor that can be used in their stead. Part A of the table shows

TABLE 1 Effect of Lymphocyte Activating Factor (LAF) on PHA response.

	Response (cpm)		
Stimulant	Thymus	Lymph nodes	Spleen
None	87	474	1504
PHA	337	39,189	34,491
PHA + supernatant fraction	21,237	41,544	32,291

Source: Data from Gery et al. (1972), *J. Exp. Med.* 136: 128.

TABLE 2 Secretion of soluble factors by macrophages.

A. Macrophage required for proliferative response to mitogen

Cells	Response (cpm)		
	No mitogen	ConA	PHA
T cells alone	94	233	412
T cells + Mφ	279	5900	55,200

B. Macrophage required to activate T cells with surface-bound PHA

Cells	Response (cpm)
T cells alone	142
T cells + PHA-pulsed Mφ	36,251
PHA-pulsed T cells	607
PHA-pulsed T cells + Mφ	32,091

C. Macrophage secretes factor (separate chamber experiment)

Upper chamber		Lower chamber		Response (cpm)
Cells	PHA	Cells	PHA	
T cells	+	None	−	589
	−		−	155
T cells + Mφ	+		−	29,455
	−		−	372
T cells	+	Mφ	−	16,235
	−		−	169

Source: After Rosenstreich et al. (1976), J. Immunol. 116: 131.

INTERLEUKINS

(again) that in the absence of macrophages T cells are not induced to proliferate by the mitogen PHA.

Part B shows what happens if either macrophages or T cells are "pulsed" with PHA so that PHA is bound to their cell surfaces. PHA-pulsed T cells do not proliferate even though the mitogen binds to the surface. Proliferation occurs only when macrophages are added. This result clearly demonstrates that binding of mitogen is necessary but not sufficient to induce proliferation. The macrophage provides something that allows the T cell to proliferate.

Part C explains this last observation by showing that the mitogen-pulsed macrophage elaborates a *soluble factor*, which acts upon the T cell. The cells were separated from each other by a cell-impermeable (but fluid-permeable) membrane, so only a soluble product of the macrophages could act on the T cells to allow them to proliferate. This product is IL-1.

The Discovery of IL-2

In 1976 Morgan, Ruscetti, and Gallo at the NIH discovered that human T cells could be grown in continuous culture in the presence of the supernatant fluid from cultures of PHA-stimulated cells. This discovery, as we have seen (Chapter 19), made it possible to grow normal, nontransformed, functional T cells as clones in culture. The factor was to become known as T CELL GROWTH FACTOR (TCGF). The crucial discovery was made two years later when Steve Gillis, Kendall Smith, and their colleagues at Dartmouth devised a simple, unequivocal assay for TCGF. In this assay, a TCGF-dependent cell line was grown in the presence of various concentrations of TCGF. The ability of the added TCGF to cause proliferation of these cells was then determined by quantifying the incorporation of tritiated thymidine. This situation represents one of those cases where a standard method is needed in order for an advance to be made because, as we have learned, many investigators had been generating "factors" and assaying them in a variety of ways. With the development of this simple, unambiguous assay, a simple and accurate means of quantifying and comparing

CHAPTER TWENTY-ONE

various factors became available. The 1979 workshop mentioned earlier classified the many factors that had TCGF-like activity as a single factor, which they called INTERLEUKIN-2, or IL-2.

Production of IL-2 by T Cells

Diverse pieces of evidence can be marshaled to show that IL-2 is a product of the T cell. First, it is elicited by T cell mitogens such as concanavalin A (ConA) and PHA. Second, when a population of spleen cells is treated with anti-Thy 1 and complement to eliminate T cells, it is unable to produce IL-2. Furthermore, mature T cells are the source of the material, because thymocytes, which contain only a few percent of mature functional cells, are a very poor source of IL-2. On the other hand, cortisone-resistant thymocytes, which are mature T cells, are the best source. Spleen, which contains only 30% Thy 1^+ cells, all of which are mature and functional, is also a good source. Of the mature, functional T cells, it is the Lyt 1^+ subpopulation that is responsible for the production, because treatment with anti-Lyt 1 but not anti-Lyt 2 and complement abolishes the ability to produce IL-2.

Roles of Adherent and Nonadherent Cells in IL-2 Release

We saw above that IL-1 is produced by macrophages and that IL-2 is produced by T cells. With the development of a good IL-2 assay, it was very easily shown that these were two distinct molecules. The picture began to make sense when it was found that the production of IL-2 by T cells required the presence of macrophages. The results of the experiment showing this requirement are given in Table 3A. Spleen cells were divided into adherent and nonadherent populations (macrophages and lymphocytes), and the lymphocyte population was enriched for T cells. Each population was incubated for 24 hours with ConA, and the supernatant fractions were assayed for IL-2 using the IL-2-dependent cell assay. The unfractionated cells produce IL-2, whereas neither the macrophages nor the T cells alone are able to do so. However, combining the macrophages and the T cells resulted in IL-2 production by the T cells.

INTERLEUKINS

TABLE 3 Production of IL-2 by T Cells

A. Production of IL-2 by T cell populations

Cell population	IL-2 activity (U/ml)
Spleen cells	1.1
T cells	0.2
Adherent cells	0
T cells + adherent cells	1.3

B. IL-1 stimulation of T cells in the absence of macrophages

	IL-2 production	Incorporation of tritiated thymidine (cpm)
Medium	0	186
ConA	0.04	5806
IL-1	0	516
ConA + IL-1	1.30	177,920

Source: Data from Smith et al. (1980), *J. Exp. Med.* 151: 1551.

Because it was known that macrophages produce IL-1 after treatment with mitogen, it seemed reasonable to predict that it was the IL-1 released by the macrophages that was causing the T cells to produce IL-2 (Table 3B). To test this, a mixture of ConA and IL-1 was added to T cells. Neither IL-1 nor ConA alone was able to stimulate the production of IL-2, but when the monokine and the mitogen were both added, IL-2 was produced by the T cells. These experiments show that there is an interleukin cascade leading to the activation of T cells.

CHAPTER TWENTY-ONE

The Interleukin Cascade

The scheme of interactions of antigen and the elaboration of IL-1 and IL-2 is shown in Figure 1. Antigen associates with the macrophage, causing the release of IL-1. If the antigen has been able to activate the T cell—that is, react in an MHC-restricted manner—then the IL-1 will activate an Lyt 1^+ T cell, which will elaborate IL-2. The production of IL-2 and the regulation of the IL-2 receptor becomes a crucial regulatory factor in the immune response, and we shall now discuss some aspects of this regulation.

IL-2 Receptors

We have just seen that when T cells are activated by antigen (or mitogen) and IL-1, they produce IL-2. IL-2, in turn, induces T cells to proliferate. It can be shown that during the course of this reaction the IL-2 that is

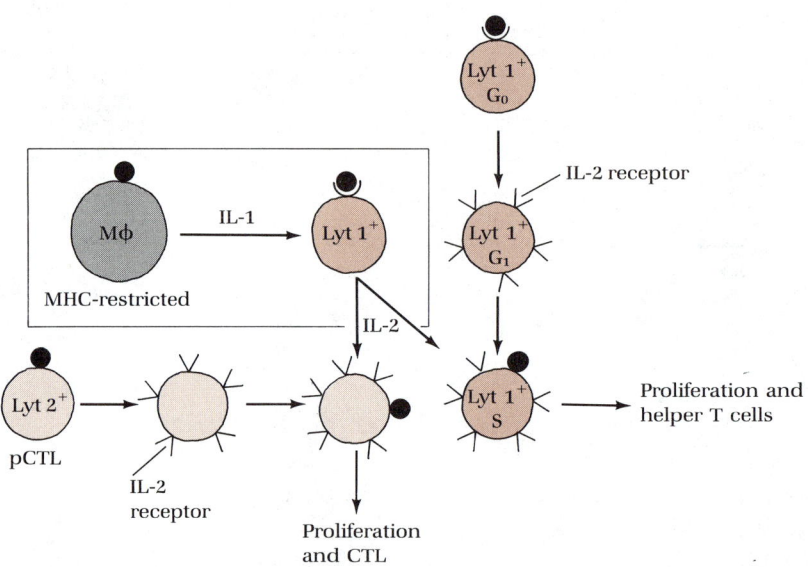

FIGURE 1 THE INTERLEUKIN CASCADE

IL-1, which is released by macrophages, induces a Lyt 1^+ T cell to produce IL-2. This step is MHC-restricted. Antigen also induces T cells to express IL-2 receptors. The combination of IL-2 reacting with the IL-2 receptor and antigen reacting with the antigen-specific receptor induces the T cell to proliferate.

INTERLEUKINS

produced disappears from the medium (the same is true for exogenously added IL-2). Radiolabeled IL-2 can be shown to bind to the activated T cells. These facts strongly suggest that the binding of IL-2 is to a specific *receptor*. In fact, the kinetics of the binding of the labeled material, the saturation curves, and tissue and ligand specificities all suggest that a specific receptor is involved. The binding studies show that IL-2 binds to the receptor with high affinity (K_d = 10 mM) and the saturation studies show that the receptors are saturated at the same concentration of IL-2 that causes T cell proliferation.

By chance, a monoclonal antibody against the IL-2 receptor has been developed. This antibody, called ANTI-TAC, was developed against an unkown molecule on activated T cells. (In addition to its usefulness as a tool, it shows the power of the monoclonal antibody technique. It is extremely difficult to isolate an antibody against a single, unique antigen on the surface of a cell.) Anti-Tac blocks the binding of radiolabeled IL-2 and prevents IL-2-dependent T cell proliferation, which strongly suggests that anti-Tac is directed against the IL-2 receptor.

When anti-Tac was used to *isolate* the receptor from the membrane (using reasoning and methods very much like those that were used to isolate the T cell receptor; Chapter 19), it was found that the receptor molecule is a glycoprotein that consists of a single chain and has a molecular weight of 55,000–60,000. The features of the IL-2 receptor are described in detail in Information Box 3.

Induction of IL-2 Receptors by Antigen or Mitogen

As we saw in Figure 1, the interaction of antigen with macrophage causes the secretion of IL-1, which then reacts with the T cell and causes the synthesis of IL-2. This simplified scheme reveals a problem; the IL-2 that is secreted by the activated T cells could cause the proliferation of *any* T cells in the vicinity. Some control mechanism is necessary, or there would be no specificity in the immune response. The first antigen with which we came into contact could trigger all of our T cells to proliferate. The control mechanism turns out to be rather unique, because it acts at the level of the *expression of IL-2 receptors*.

INFORMATION BOX 3

The IL-2 Receptor

The receptors arise from a peptide precursor of molecular weight 33,000, which is cotranslationally modified to a doublet, whose units have molecular weights of 33,000 and 37,000. The two members of the doublet are joined by an N-linked carbohydrate addition, and this intermediate is modified in the Golgi apparatus to the final 55,000-MW form. Even though there is only one form of IL-2 receptor molecule, there are two IL-2 mRNAs. These two mRNAs differ in their polyadenylation signals. The mature receptor has an extracellular domain of 220 amino acids, a transmembrane domain of 19 amino acids, and a surprisingly small cytoplasmic domain of only 13 amino acids.

The IL-2 receptors are not expressed until the T cell antigen receptor is triggered. The initial evidence for this came from the fact that anti-Tac antibodies only reacted with activated T cells. Because anti-Tac reacts with the IL-2 receptor, this finding must mean that these receptors are only expressed on activated cells. If this is the case, then we immediately see the control mechanism: only cells expressing IL-2 receptors can be induced to pro-

FIGURE 2 KINETICS OF IL-2 RECEPTOR INDUCTION

Human peripheral blood cells were stimulated with phytohemagglutinin, and the rate of expression of IL-2 receptors was determined at 24-hour intervals. (A) Binding of fluorescence-labeled anti-Tac antibodies measured by flow cytometry. The x-axis measures the number of cells and the y-axis the fluorescent intensity of the cells. (B) Relative DNA content of the cells in A is determined by flow cytometry. The appearance of the second peak indicates that new DNA is being synthesized. (C) The number of IL-2 receptors per cell determined by the binding of labeled IL-2 compared with the rate of proliferation of the cells by uptake of tritiated thymidine. There is a steady increase in IL-2 receptors per cell after mitogen stimulation, but DNA synthesis does not begin until around 48 hours. Thus, the expression of the receptors is independent of the cell cycle. [Redrawn from Cantrell and Smith (1983) *J. Exp. Med.* **158**, 1895]

INTERLEUKINS

liferate by IL-2 and only cells that have reacted with antigen can express the receptor. So the IL-2 in the environment is not able to induce all T cells to proliferate, but only those T cells that have been activated by antigen.

An experimental validation of this point is shown in Figure 2. In this experiment cells were cultured in vitro and the level of

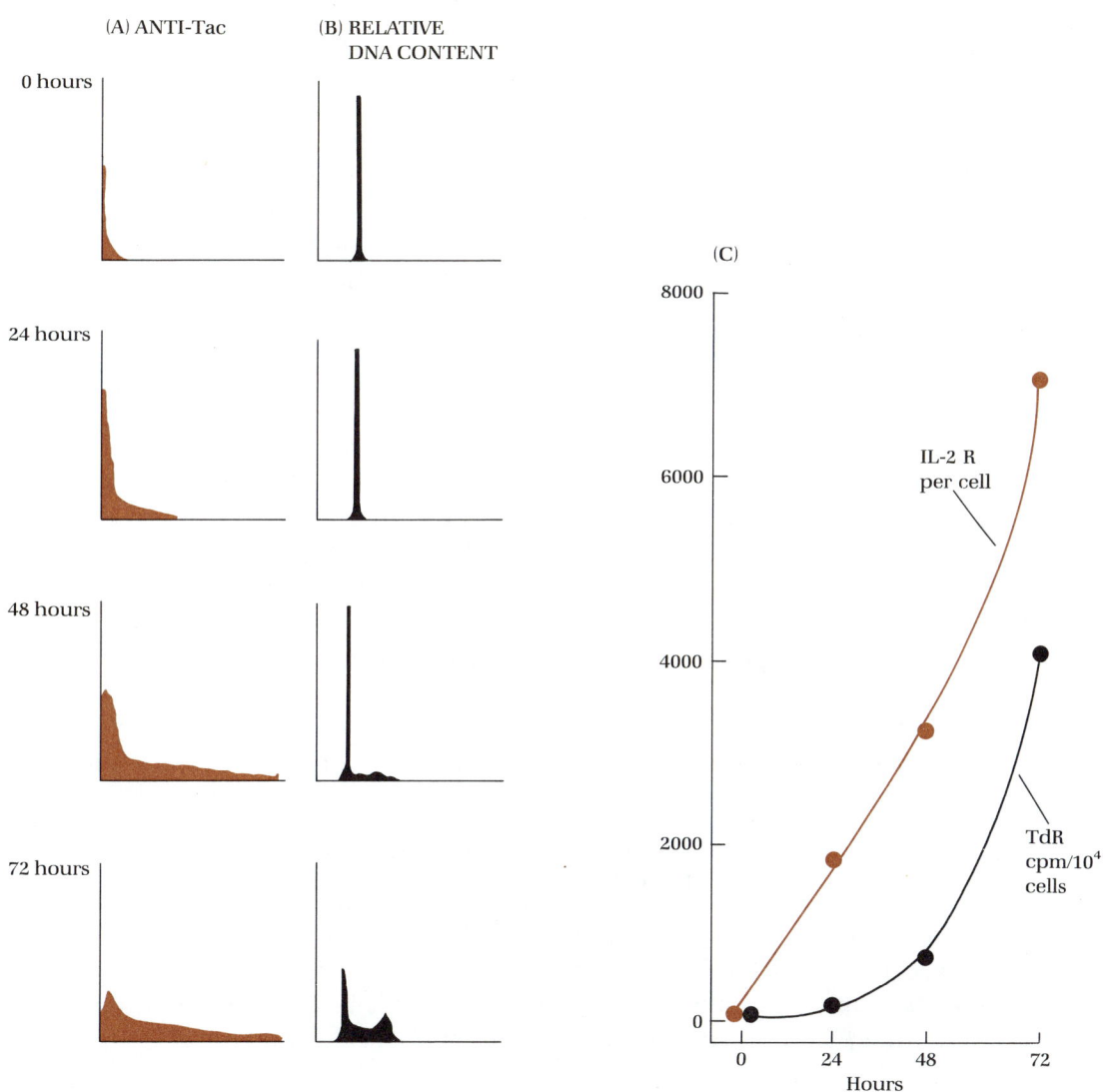

expression of IL-2 receptors (as determined by binding of labeled anti-Tac antibodies or labeled IL-2) was compared to cell cycle stage (as determined by the number of peaks of DNA synthesized in the cell: a single peak indicates the cells are resting, while more than one peak indicates new DNA is being synthesized). The figure shows that resting cells bind little or no anti-Tac or IL-2; but after 24 hours there is significant binding. However, at these times the cells are still arrested in G_0 or G_1 (Information Box 4). Only when the level of IL-2 receptors is high (at day 3) do the cells begin to synthesize DNA in response to IL-2. Because it was already known from saturation studies that the level of bound IL-2 at saturation correlates with the threshold of induction of DNA synthesis (see above), this experiment shows that activation of T cells by antigen (or mitogen) induces the expression of IL-2 receptors. It can even be shown that only the high-density IL-2 receptor-bearing cells enter S phase. Thus we see that the system prevents the promiscuous expansion of T cells by allowing only those cells that have productively reacted with antigen and have become activated to be pushed from the prereplicative stages of the cell cycle into S phase.

One finding worth mentioning is that even though resting mature T cells do not express IL-2 receptors, 30% of the *least* mature cells in the thymus of adults (Thy 1^+, L3T4$^-$, Lyt 2^-) do express IL-2 receptors, and 50% of the cells in the fetal thymus also express them. These receptors are of very low affinity ($K_d =$ 10 pM, in contrast to the receptors on activated mature T cells, which have a $K_d =$ 10 mM), and these cells do not grow in the presence of IL-2. Nevertheless this may be important in the intrathymic events of T cell maturation, where T cell proliferation occurs during selection of the self-MHC repertoire (Chapter 10).

Synthesis: Interleukins and T Cell Proliferation

We know from clonal selection that the antigen-induced proliferation of cells is a crucial part of the immune response. The cascade of IL-1 and IL-2 causes this proliferation of T cells. Furthermore, antigen induces the appearance of IL-2 receptors. So we

INFORMATION BOX 4

The Cell Cycle

We know that proliferation is an essential part of the immune response and that one of the roles of antigen is to initiate cell division. Mitogens are extensively used in immunology because they mimic this role of antigen. Since it was shown that the interleukins are clearly involved in the initiation of cell division, there has been a large amount of work done to determine how these molecules act on cells to cause them to divide.

Cell division requires the replication of DNA as well as of cellular components. DNA is replicated only during a limited portion of interphase called the S PHASE (S for synthesis). Actual cell division occurs in the M PHASE (M for mitotic). The period between M and the start of S is called G_1 PHASE (G for gap). After the S phase there is another gap phase called G_2. The cycle is diagrammed in the accompanying figure. When cell growth is arrested, it always stops in G_1; but once a cell is able to leave G_1, it is committed to complete S, G_2, and M. This fact means that stimulating a cell to move out of G_1 always results in DNA synthesis and division. The point of no return in this process is late in G_1 and is called R (for

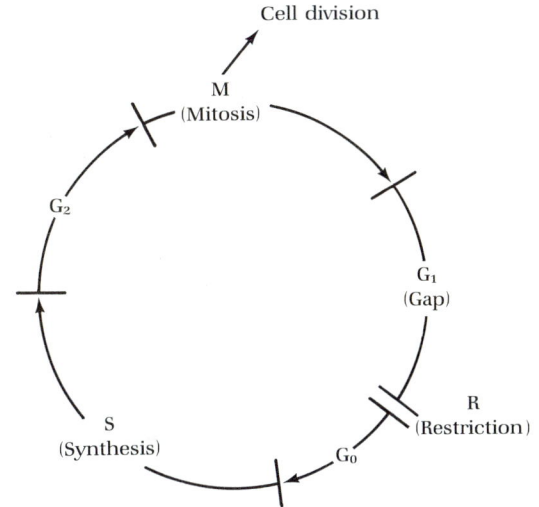

restriction). Cells that are arrested at R are resting cells and are said to be in G_0. Any agent that induces resting cells to become proliferating cells must therefore move them from G_0 into S phase. Antigen or mitogen probably initiates some of the pre-replicative steps of the cell cycle.

can now see how nonspecific initiators of growth can act to induce the proliferation of specific cells: the antigen induces the appearance of the receptor and IL-1 induces the synthesis of IL-2 which reacts with the receptor. Any cell that has not been activated by antigen does not have the receptor, and therefore the IL-2 that is present does not affect these cells.[1]

[1] Cantrell and Smith have devised from this model an autocrine model of cell growth that makes an argument for a more general role for this kind of feedback control.

CHAPTER TWENTY-ONE

B Cell Activation

Up to now we have examined the means by which the antigen-specific, MHC-restricted activation of T cells results in the proliferation of T cells. We will now examine the area of B cell activation.

Need for Receptor Cross-Linking

We have already seen that B cells react directly with antigen, using surface immunoglobulin as the antigen-specific receptor. But the reader has learned by this time to predict that the simple observation in immunology always leads to a more complicated situation. In this case we will see that antigen binding to the receptor is necessary but not sufficient to activate the B cell. In fact, it appears that antigen must *cross-link* the receptor molecules and act in concert with some factors to cause the B cell to become activated.

An example of this need for cross-linking and a soluble factor is shown in Table 4, which is the compilation of the results of several experiments of various designs. In these experiments B cells were treated with anti-immunoglobulin to induce proliferation. Anti-Ig was used instead of antigen because the frequency of antigen-specific cells is so low that it would have been diffficult to study the process using antigen. The anti-Ig thus acts as a

TABLE 4 Role of receptor cross-linking and T cell factors.

Treatment of B cell factors	Addition	Proliferation
Anti-IgM	None	+/−
	T cell factors	+++
Anti-IgM(F(ab')$_2$)	None	+
	T cell factors	++++
Anti-IgM(Fab)	None	+
	T cell factors	+

Source: Based on experiments of Sidman and Unanue (1979), *J. Immunol.* 122: 406; and Yoshizaki et al. (1982), *J. Immunol.* 128: 1296.

INTERLEUKINS

surrogate antigen for B cells, just as the mitogens acted as surrogate antigen for T cells. Because all B cells have sIg, all of them can be induced to proliferate by anti-Ig.

Treatment of the cells with an anti-IgM causes proliferation in the presence of a "factor" from PHA-stimulated T cells (Table 4). Treatment of the B cells with the $F(ab')_2$ fragment of anti-IgM is a more potent inducer of proliferation than treatment with the whole IgM molecule, but treatment with the Fab fragment of anti-IgM is a poor inducer. The best explanation of these data involves a cross-linking model. Although both the Fab and the $F(ab')_2$ fragments bind to the receptors, only the treatment allowing the receptors to become cross-linked produces proliferation. Furthermore, the presence of factors is required, demonstrating that the activation of B cells is a multi-event process.

It must be stated that we do not know why the cells must cross-link their receptors, but we do have the beginnings of an understanding of what the "factors" might be. It has been proposed that the process of B cell activation can be divided into three discrete events: activation, proliferation, and differentiation. Cross-linking is most likely to be important in the activation step.

B Cell Growth Factor

On the basis of the experiments described above, it was not surprising when a T cell factor was isolated and shown to be involved in the proliferation of B cells. This factor, originally called B CELL GROWTH FACTOR, or BCGF (in analogy with TCGF), was isolated from a T cell myeloma line that had been stimulated with the tumor-promoting agent phorbol ester. When added to anti-Ig-stimulated B cells, BCGF augmented the ability of the anti-Ig to induce proliferation. The important point, however, is that this factor is different from IL-2. To show this, the factor was fractionated by column chromatography and each fraction tested for both IL-2 activity and B cell-stimulating activity. The results are shown in Figure 3: there are two distinct peaks, in the ranges of 30,000–35,000 and 16,000–18,000. The former contains all of the IL-2 activity and the latter all of the BCGF activity.

CHAPTER TWENTY-ONE

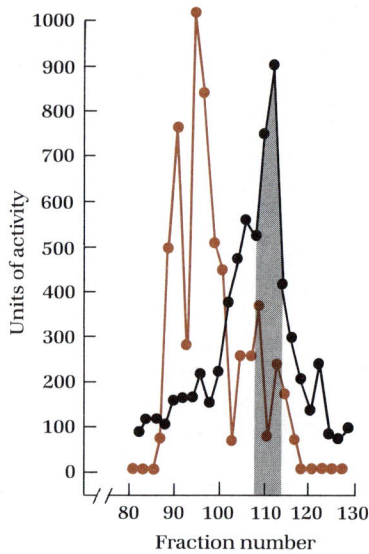

FIGURE 3 SEPARATION OF BCGF AND IL-2
B cell growth factor (BCGF) and IL-2 have been shown to be two distinct entities. The factors that were produced by a T cell myeloma and stimulated B cell growth were separated on a column, and the fractions were tested for IL-2 activity and BCGF activity. BCGF activity was assayed by its ability to augment anti-Ig-stimulated proliferation of B cells. The brown curve is IL-2 activity and the black curve is BCGF activity (the BCGF peak is shaded gray). [Redrawn from Howard et al. (1982) *J. Exp. Med.* 155, 914]

Interleukin 4

On the basis of the preceding experiments, the activation of B cells seemed to require ligand binding antigen-specific receptors, with the resulting cross-linking of the receptors leading to the activation of the B cell. The T cell product BCGF could then be thought to induce proliferation in the activated cells. However, it was soon realized that the factor called BCGF had several effects on B cells, depending upon their state of differentiation.

It could be shown, for example, that BCGF induced *resting* B cells to express Ia molecules and *activated* B cells (activated with anti-Ig or LPS) to proliferate. Two other factors, called B CELL DIFFERENTIATING FACTOR (BCDF) and IgG1 INDUCING FACTOR (IIF) were found to induce *proliferating* B cells to secrete IgG1. The crucial question then was whether all three of these functions were caused by a single molecule or whether they were due to separate factors.

Tasuku Honjo and his colleagues in Kyoto provided the answer. They cloned the IIF gene and used the cDNA as a template to produce mRNA. This mRNA was then microinjected into frog oocytes, where it was translated (Figure 4A). Analysis of the secreted product, which comes from a single gene, showed that it was able to induce all three events in B cell activation (Figure 4B).

Thus we see that the product of a cloned gene is able to carry out the effects that had been attributed to several different factors

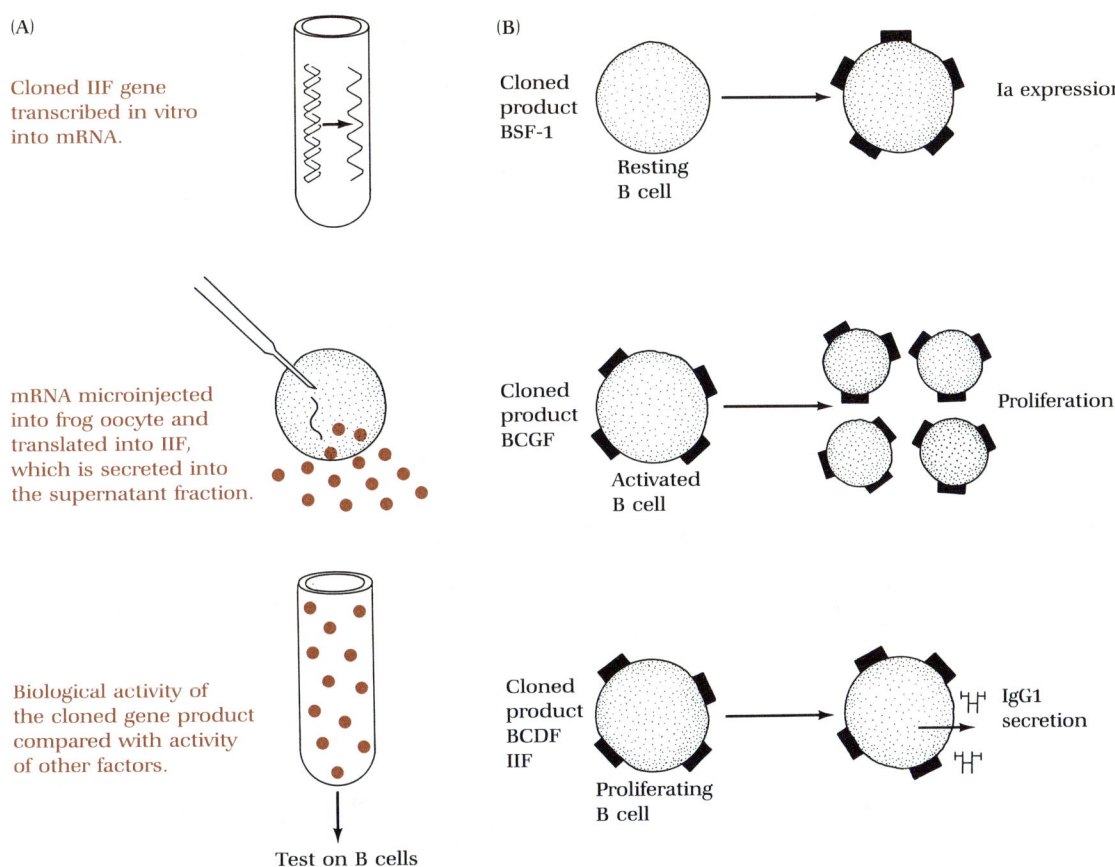

FIGURE 4 CLONING THE IIF GENE
(A) The cloned IIF gene is transcribed into mRNA. The mRNA is microinjected into frog oocytes and translated into protein. (B) The product of the cloned IIF gene carries out the same functions ascribed to the factors BSF-1, BCGF, and BCDF. [After Noma et al. (1986) *Nature* 319, 640]

```
           67                                          78
IL-4      Leu Val Cys Arg Ala Ser Lys Val Leu Arg Ile Phe
                          •   •       •
GM-CSF    Leu Thr Cys Val Gln Thr Arg  -  Leu Lys Ile Phe
           66                                          76

           115                                                              133
IL-4      Thr Met Asn Glu Ser Lys Ser Thr Ser Leu Lys Asp Phe Leu Glu Ser Leu Lys Ser
                          •           •               •           •           •
GM-CSF    Thr Asp Cys Glu Thr Gln Val Thr Thr Tyr Ala Asp Phe Ile Asp Ser Leu Lys Thr
           108                                                              126
```

FIGURE 5 HOMOLOGY BETWEEN GM-CSF AND IL-4

The amino acid sequences of two segments of IL-4 and GM-CSF are very similar. Homologous amino acids are indicated in color; related amino acids are identified with a black dot. [After Noma et al. (1986) *Nature* 319, 640]

(BCGF, BSF-1, BCDF and IFF). This lymphokine has been given the name INTERLEUKIN-4 (IL-4).[2]

The deduced amino acid sequence of IL-4 was compared to known sequences, and significant homology was found between GM-CSF (Chapter 10) and murine γ interferon (see Chapter 25). The homology with GM-CSF is shown in Figure 5.

The Consequences of Activation

For decades immunologists tried to find the unique features of the immune system. So far, they have been able to show that the division of labor, MHC restriction, gene reorganization, and interleukin cascade all have aspects that can be considered to be unique to the immune system. But as we come to this part of the narrative, which deals with the consequences of bringing all of these things together, we must leave the realm of the uniquely immunological and enter the world of general cell biology. Because the events that follow receptor activation by antigen seem

---

[2] The naming of factors is a delicate business. At the time Honjo's group cloned the gene, another group (Lee et al., PNAS, in press) cloned the same gene; and the two groups agreed that the product should be called IL-4. However, they found out after both papers were in press that Sanderson et al. (PNAS, 1986) had proposed the name interleukin-4 for eosinophil differentiating factor.

INTERLEUKINS

to be events common to many, if not all, cell systems, we will not go into much detail. The reader is urged to read the chapters dealing with signal transduction in Alberts et al., *The Molecular Biology of the Cell* or some other good cell biology textbook. Much of the research in immunology in the next decade will be cell and molecular biology that happens to use lymphocytes rather than sea urchins, transformed tissue culture cells, or the retina. The flip side of this, of course, is that facts and concepts garnered from the more traditional cell biology systems can be readily applied to the immune system. Immunologists of the future will have to be very good biologists and may, sad to say, have to give up their identity as fearless pioneers at the frontier of an arcane land and join the ranks of the rest of the biological community.

B Cell Activation

We have learned that antigen causes the antigen-specific receptors on the B cells to become cross-linked, an arrangement triggering cell activation. In a very elegant (and ongoing) series of experiments, John Cambier and his co-workers in Denver have been studying the membrane-associated and intracellular events that follow receptor cross-linking. They have found that one of the earliest events is a *depolarization* of the membrane. This is very reminiscent of the events that follow stimulation of a nerve and the degranulation of the mast cell (see Chapter 25); and, in fact, when the intracellular events of B cell activation, nerve stimulation, and mast cell degranulation are compared, the similarities far exceed the differences.

A very important finding was that the action of antigen or anti-Ig in inducing membrane depolariztion could be mimicked with compounds such as phorbol esters and diacylglycerol, which activate protein kinase C (PK-C). Protein kinase C activity, which has been implicated in a wide range of intracellular regulatory events that involve both proliferation and differentiation, is regulated by the hydrolysis of phosphatidylinositol via the generation of diacylglycerol. The argument that this pathway may be important is consistent with the fact that raising the intracellular levels of cyclic AMP inhibits the hydrolysis of phophatidylinositol and also inhibits the depolarization of B cells. So the suggestion has been made that receptor cross-linking may result in the hydrolysis of phosphatidylinositol, which yields diacylglycerol, which in turn activates PK-C. The activation of this kinase results in the phosphorylation of proteins that may be responsible for regulating growth and differentiation. This scheme and comparative ones for olfaction and vision are shown in Figure 6.

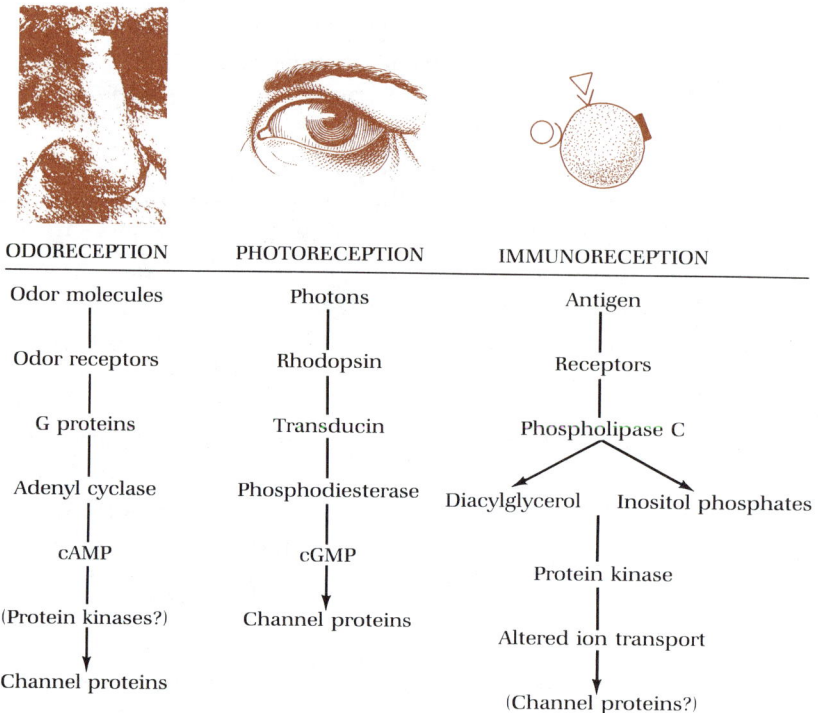

FIGURE 6 HYPOTHETICAL COMMON PATHWAYS IN OLFACTION, PHOTORECEPTION, AND IMMUNORECEPTION

Signal transduction from the surface receptors to the cytoplasm via cyclic nucleotides and protein kinases may be a common mechanism used by cells that must transduce a signal from the environment to the nucleus to bring about rapid responses. [After Sheperd (1985) *Nature* 316, 214, for olfaction and photoreception; and Coggeshall and Cambier (1984) *J. Immunol.* 133, 3382 for immunoreception]

INTERLEUKINS

T Cell Activation

After stimulation with mitogens, T cells have also been shown to exhibit membrane depolarization. In addition they exhibit increased ion flux across the membrane and increased intracellular free calcium. Recently the technique of "patch clamping" has been used to identify in T cells VOLTAGE-GATED POTASIUM CHANNELS that resemble delayed-rectified K^+ channels in nerve and muscle cells. Each T cell has 200–300 K^+ channels, which open when the membrane is depolarized; however, these channels are not sensitive to levels of internal calcium as are many channels in nerve cells. In fact, Ca^{2+} channels have not been detected in lymphocytes. This might mean that the increased free Ca^{2+} has come from the vast store of membrane-bound Ca^{2+} in the cells.

Agents that block K^+ channels (for example, 4-aminopyridine and tetramethyl ammonium) have been shown to block the synthesis of IL-2 but to have no effect on the synthesis of the IL-2 receptor (Table 5). These data indicate a potential avenue of experimentation to examine the control of proliferation of T cells through ion flux or concentration, which regulates the expression of lymphokine.

As the control of intracellular events becomes understood in general terms it will be interesting to see if anything unique to the immune system emerges.

TABLE 5 The effect of K-channel blockers on the expression of IL-2 receptors and the synthesis of IL-2.

PHA	K-channel blocker[a]	Percentage Tac^+ cells[b]	IL-2 activity
−	−	5	0
+	−	80	85
+	+	75	10

Source: Data from Chandry et al. (1984), *J. Exp. Med.* 16: 369.

[a] 4-Aminopyridine and tetramethylammonium.

[b] Based on ability to bind anti-Tac antibody, which binds to IL-2 receptors.

CHAPTER TWENTY-ONE

Summary

1. T cells and macrophages produce factors (lymphokines and monokines, respectively) that act on other cells in the immune system. The generic term for these factors is interleukin.
2. Interleukin-1 (IL-1) is a monokine that augments the ability of T cells to respond to mitogens and antigen. Interleukin-2 (IL-2) is a lymphokine that promotes the proliferation of T cells. Reaction of the T cell with IL-1 is necessary for the production of IL-2.
3. Only cells expressing high-affinity IL-2 receptors are induced to proliferate by IL-2. Activation by antigen induces the expression of IL-2 receptors.
4. B cells react with free antigen but become activated only when the antigen-specific receptors are cross-linked. The lymphokine interleukin-4 is needed for proliferation and differentiation of B cells.
5. The consequences of lymphocyte activation are membrane depolarization, production of second messages, activation of protein kinases and ion fluxes. These appear to be stages common to signal transduction from membrane to nucleus in all cells and not unique to the immune system.

Additional Readings

Alberts, B., D. Bray, J. Lewis, M. Raff, K. Roberts and J. D. Watson. 1983. *The Molecular Biology of the Cell*. Garland, New York.

Cantrell, D. A. and K. A. Smith. 1984. The interleukin-2 T cell system: a new cell growth model. *Science* 224, 1312.

Cohen, S., E. Pick and J. J. Oppenheim (eds.). 1979. *Biology of the Lymphokines*. Academic Press, New York.

Cohn, M. 1985. Why lymphokines? *Lymphokines* 10, 201.

Durum, S. K., J. A. Schmidt and J. J. Oppenheim. 1985. Interleukin-1: an immunological perspective. *Annu. Rev. Immunol.* 3, 263.

Gillis, S., M. M. Ferm, W. Ou and K. A. Smith. 1978. T cell growth factor: parameters of production and quantitative microassay for activity. *J. Immunol.* 120, 2027.

Howard, M. and W. E. Paul. 1983. Regulation of B cell growth and differentiation by soluble factors. *Annu. Rev. Immunol.* 1, 307.

Kishimoto, T. 1985. Factors affecting B cell growth and differentiation. *Annu. Rev. Immunol.* 3, 133.

INTERLEUKINS

Lee, S. C., D. Sabath, C. Deutsch and M. B. Prystowsky. 1986. Increased voltage-gated conductance during interleukin 2-stimulated proliferation of a mouse helper T lymphocyte clone. *J. Cell Biol.* 102, 1200.

Leonard, W. J. et al. 1985. Structure of the human interleukin-2 receptor gene. *Science* 230, 633.

Noma, Y., P. Sideras, T. Naito, S. Bergstedt-Lindquist, C. Azuma, E. Severinson, T. Tanabe, T. Kinashi, F. Matsuda, Y. Yaoita and T. Honjo. 1986. Cloning of cDNA encoding the murine IgG1 induction factor by a novel strategy of using SP6 promoter. *Nature* 319, 640.

Smith, K. A. 1984. Interleukin-2. *Annu. Rev. Immunol.* 2, 283.

SECTION IV
REGULATION OF THE IMMUNE RESPONSE

With such a splendid thesis as that, any fallacy committed by the author becomes insignificant.

JORGE LUIS BORGES

Up to now we have addressed some of the problems of initiating immune responses and have seen that there is a delicate balance of cells and factors involved. It is intuitively obvious that anything as complex as this must have complex regulation. In the next three chapters we will examine what many consider to be the new frontier of immunology: the regulation of the response. We will discuss two distinctly different modes of regulation: the network of idiotype interactions, and suppressor T cells. We will also discuss the ultimate problem of regulation, self–nonself recognition.

CHAPTER 22

THE NETWORK

Overview   Niels Jerne has profoundly changed the thinking of immunology on two occasions. In 1955 he proposed the *natural selection theory* (see Chapter 1) and paved the way for clonal selection, which became the dominant paradigm of immunology. Then in 1973 he proposed the *network theory*, which has come to be one of the two dominant modes of thinking about the regulation of the immune response.[1] The network theory differs from other immunological thinking because it endows the immune system with the ability to regulate itself using only itself. We will see later that this is a profound departure in biological thought and, if correct, gives biological systems a power they had not previously been thought to possess. The theory is based on the fact that antibody not only has the ability to combine with antigen (its traditional function) but also has the ability to *be* an antigen.

Jerne postulated that the antibody molecule can carry out these two functions (acting both as antibody and as antigen) within the *same* animal and that the interplay of these two functions constitutes the makings of a regulatory system. Furthermore, amino acid sequences within the Ig molecules, by chance, share antigenic determinants with all of the antigens to which the animal can respond. These sequences are called the *internal image*, and the idea of the internal image is the crucial philosophical underpinning of the theory.

---

[1] In 1985 Niels Jerne won the Nobel prize. His contributions have been so extensive that it must have been a very difficult task for the committee to decide which of them to cite in the award.

379

CHAPTER TWENTY-TWO

Epitopes, Paratopes and Idiotopes: The Language of the Network

Many immunologists have been put off by the vocabulary of the network, the basis of which is the idea that each member of the immune system is capable of interacting with every other member. This interaction is possible because the antigen-combining site on one antibody molecule is able to recognize an antigenic determinant on another antibody molecule. The language of the network was designed to facilitate this discussion. Accordingly, the antigen-combining site on an Ig molecule is called the PARATOPE. Suppose we immunize an animal with bovine serum albumin (BSA) and raise an anti-BSA antibody. When BSA and anti-BSA combine, the antigen combines with the paratope on the antibody. Although we have been calling this site the antigen-combining site up to now, the reader will find that with a bit of practice paratope rolls more trippingly off the tongue.

The antigenic determinant on a BSA molecule (and on other antigens as well) is called the EPITOPE, a term that has already become an integral part of immunological vocabulary; it was introduced in Chapter 2. Thus an antigen–antibody reaction in the traditional sense is a reaction between the paratope on the immunoglobulin molecule and the epitope on the antigen molecule. In the network, the paratope on one antibody molecule can be recognized by a paratope on another antibody molecule. The first paratope thus is acting as an antigen, or epitope. The part of the combining site of the first antibody that is seen in this manner by the paratope on the second antibody molecule is called an IDIOTOPE. If the paratope has the antibody function of the molecule, the idiotope has antigen function (Figure 1). The reader should keep in mind that the unique structure of the antigen-combining site on any antibody molecule is called the idiotype when it is used as an antigen (see Chapter 4).

Another way of looking at this is the following:

> We know since Landsteiner that practically all molecules in the universe are antigens. The total of all the antigenic determinants of these antigens is the total set of epitopes. No matter how large this set is, *every* member of this set can be recognized

THE NETWORK

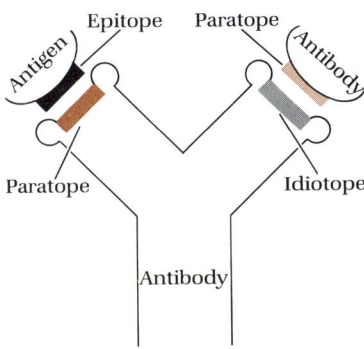

Epitope: Antigenic determinant
Paratope: Combining site
Idiotope: Antigenic determinant on an antibody

FIGURE 1 THE LANGUAGE OF THE NETWORK

Antibody molecules contain antigen-combining sites (paratopes) and antigenic determinants (idiotopes). Antigen molecules contain determinants (epitopes) that combine with the appropriate paratope. The network thus has epitope:paratope and idiotope:paratope interactions.

by a paratope of the immune system of an individual (which possesses an estimated *ten million* antibodies of different specificities). [N. Jerne, personal communication, 1986]

The *vocabulary* of the network is based on the two roles of the antigen-combining site: it combines with antigen (as a paratope, it combines with epitope), and it offers a unique antigenic configuration (it acts as idiotope). The model of the *function* of the network is based on the probability that the paratope of each antibody will recognize the idiotope of some other antibody molecule and react with it. If the idiotope is the receptor on a B cell, reaction with a paratope results in clonal expansion of the cells and the secretion of antibody (which also has the paratope and idiotope of the receptor). The paratope of a second antibody may combine with the idiotope of the first antibody because the idiotope is acting as an antigen. The network postulates that there will be a B cell with a receptor that has a paratope able to combine with the idiotope on the first antibody. In this way there is a network of reactions, as illustrated in Figure 2.

The Internal Image

The concept central to the network theory is that each idiotope is the same as an epitope of one or several antigens. This is another

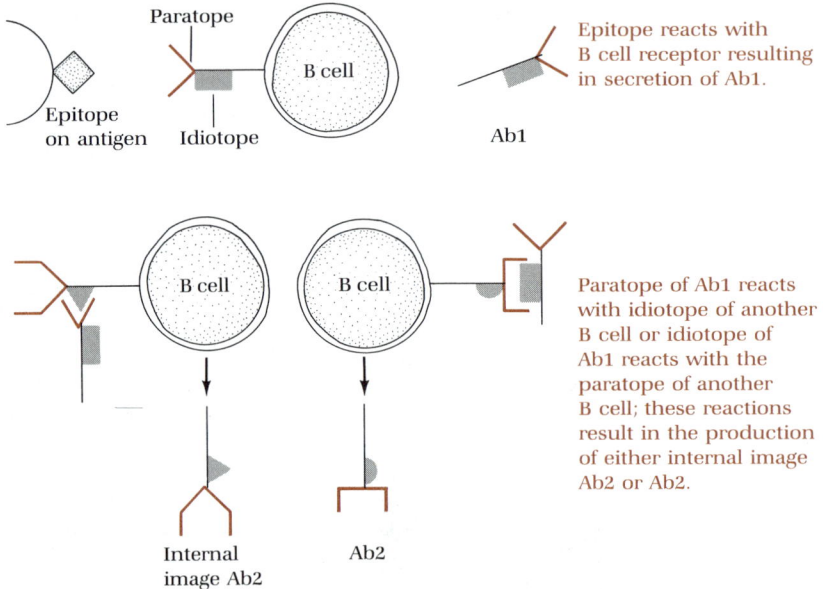

FIGURE 2 THE FUNCTION OF THE NETWORK

(A) Epitope reacts with B cell expressing a receptor with the proper paratope. This surface Ig molecule also has an idiotope. The B cell secretes antibody (Ab1) molecules with the paratope (p1) and the idiotope (i1). (B) Ab1 can react with a B cell expressing *either* an idiotope (i2) that reacts with the p1 *or* with a B cell expressing a paratope that reacts with i1. In both cases the B cells secrete antibody. [Based on W. Paul and C. Bona (1982) *Immunol. Today* 3, 230)

way of saying that several idiotopes would cross-react with a large number of epitopes in nature. These common determinants between paratopes in the animal and epitopes in the world outside of the animal are called the INTERNAL IMAGES of antigens. The network works because all possible antigens are reflected in this cross-reactivity. This being the case, the immune system need only look into itself to see any possible epitope within its own repertoire of paratopes (Figure 3). This is a unique idea, which if correct means that all possible reactions that the immune system can carry out with the epitopes in the world outside of the ani-

THE NETWORK

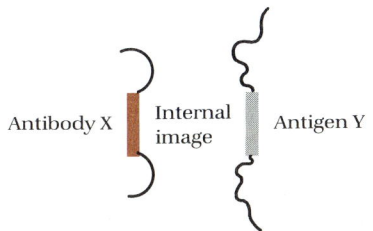

FIGURE 3 THE INTERNAL IMAGE

The idiotope and the epitope are cross-reactive. By chance the structure of the combining site of anti-X (paratope) recognizes the combining site (idiotope) on another antibody.

mal are accounted for in the internal system of paratopes and idiotopes already present inside the animal. The mystical reader may ponder that this is akin to looking at oneself in a mirror and seeing the entire world in the reflection. Jerne in fact began a 1984 review (called "Idiotypic Networks and Other Preconceived Ideas") with a quote from Jean Cocteau: "Mirrors would be well-advised to think twice before reflecting images;" and he ends the review by saying that those who seek exterior pressures on the system "would do well to turn their vision towards the interiors of themselves, and there discover the mystery, perhaps never completely revealed, of the immune system."

Cross-Reactivity Between Paratopes and Epitopes: The Generative Grammar of the Network

Jerne addressed the possible cross-reactivity between paratopes and epitopes in his 1984 Nobel prize address. He likened the immune system to language, and used Noam Chomsky's notion of "deep structure" of language. Note in Figure 4 that a portion of the structure *The production of insulin depends on cells* etc. is also found on the structure *The name of insulinde was given to* etc. and the structure *Diabetes can be a result* etc. Even though they are totally unique structures (both as sentences and as epitopes and paratopes), they by chance share sequences. If these shared sequences are brought into proper position, they can interact with each other.[2]

The idea of the internal image is used in network theory to allow the immune system to regulate itself after initial confrontation with exogenous antigen. The concept is that it does it totally

---

[2] There are two published versions of the Nobel prize address. The version appearing in the *EMBO Journal* 4, 487 (1985) has this illustration. The shortened version, in *Science* 229, 1057 (1985) does not.

CHAPTER TWENTY-TWO

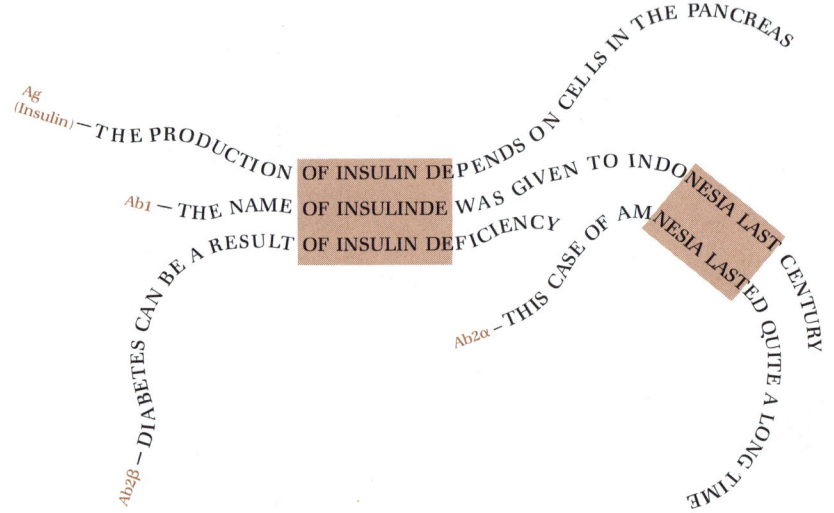

FIGURE 4 THE DEEP STRUCTURE AND GENERATIVE GRAMMAR OF THE IMMUNE RESPONSE

An identical structure can appear on many structures in many contexts and be reacted to by the reader or by the immune system. [From N.K. Jerne (1985) *EMBO Journal* 4, 847]

by its own internal viewing of itself. It can do this, the theory says, because it can see all of the outside world reflected in itself. This is heady stuff and forces us to think about biological systems in general and the immune system in particular in a unique way. We can also see that it is the uniqueness of the vision that necessitates the new vocabulary.

> I see the immune system as continuously seeking a dynamic equilibrium—and by 'dynamic' I mean that a vast number of immune responses are going on all the time, even in the absence of foreign antigen. The old term 'immune response' suggests that the system is 'at rest,' waiting to 'respond,' whereas I think it is continuously active, interacting with self-antigens, idiotopes, factors, etc. [N. Jerne, personal communication]

Testing the Network Theory

A theory of this nature is very difficult to test experimentally, but there are several points that should be immediately testable. One

THE NETWORK

that is crucial to the theory is that it should be possible to generate antibody against the idiotype. Such an antibody is called an anti-idiotype antibody. The theory also predicts that it should be possible to generate antibody against one's own idiotypes—i.e., AUTO–ANTI-IDIOTYPE antibodies. The theory requires that such auto–anti-idiotype antibody be regulatory. We will see below that both of these conditions have been satisfied. In addition to these minimal considerations, the idea of the internal image predicts that under some conditions anti-idiotype antibody should mimic antigen. We will see that this too can be shown to occur.

The Production of Auto–Anti-Idiotype Antibodies

As stated above, the first of the two criteria that had to be met for the network theory to be viable was that it must be possible to generate auto–anti-idiotype antibodies. One of the first experimental demonstrations that this can indeed be done is shown in Figure 5. Scott Rodkey in Kansas immunized rabbits with hapten–carrier conjugate; six months later he collected their serum and purified the anti-hapten anti-

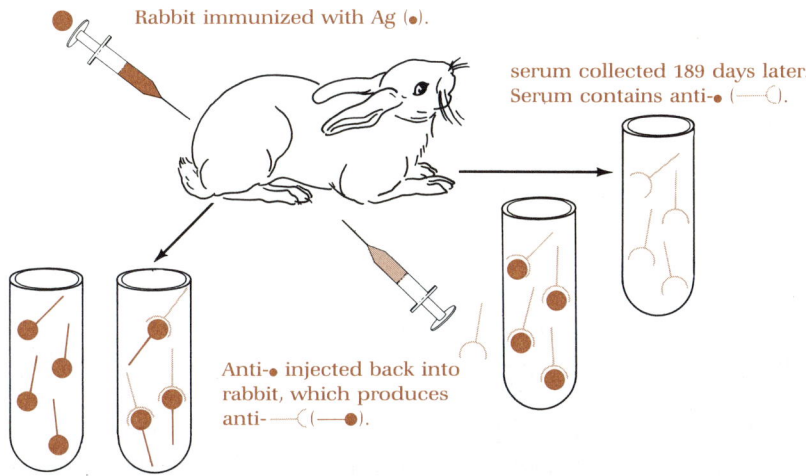

FIGURE 5 PRODUCTION OF AUTO–ANTI-IDIOTYPE ANTIBODY

Antigen is injected into a rabbit, which responds by producing antibody. The antibody is purified and reinjected into the same rabbit, which responds by producing anti-idiotype antibody. [After Rodkey (1974) *J. Exp. Med.* **139**, 712]

bodies. The purified anti-hapten antibodies were then made more immunogenic by polymerization and injected back into the *same* rabbits that had produced them. In a short time these animals began to make antibodies that reacted with their own anti-hapten antibody and with no other immunoglobulin molecules. Thus we see that it is possible for an individual to make a productive antibody response against its own idiotypic determinants.

Similar results have been obtained with molecules that have the properties of lymphocyte receptors and can be found in the urine after presumably being shed from the surface of lymphocytes. In this case the shed receptors had specificities directed against allo-reactive MHC antigen. When these receptors were injected back into the animals, antibodies directed against the idiotypes of the receptors on their own lymphocytes were produced. The production of these auto–anti-idiotype antibodies caused those lymphocytes with the receptors for the allo-reactive MHC to be eliminated. As a result, the animals were not able to mount responses against those MHC antigens.

The Regulatory Role of Anti-Idiotype Antibody

The second criterion the network theory must meet is that anti-idiotype antibody must be shown to be regulatory. The experiment mentioned above, in which auto–anti-receptor antibody causes the elimination of cells with the receptor and hence elimination of the ability to react to a certain MHC, is one example of the possible regulatory role of this antibody.

Anti-idiotype antibody is also able to *suppress* the generation of the immune response (Figure 6). In this experiment spleen cells are incubated in vitro with either of two antigens, phosphoryl choline (PC) or red blood cells (RBC). An anti-idiotype antibody is added to some of the cultures. This anti-idiotype antibody was raised by purifying anti-PC and then making an antibody against the purified antibody. In the cultures that contain anti-idiotype antibody and PC, there is a 90% reduction in cells producing anti-PC. In contrast, the cultures that received the RBC and anti-idiotype made responses comparable to those without anti-idiotype. Remember that in this experiment the anti-

THE NETWORK

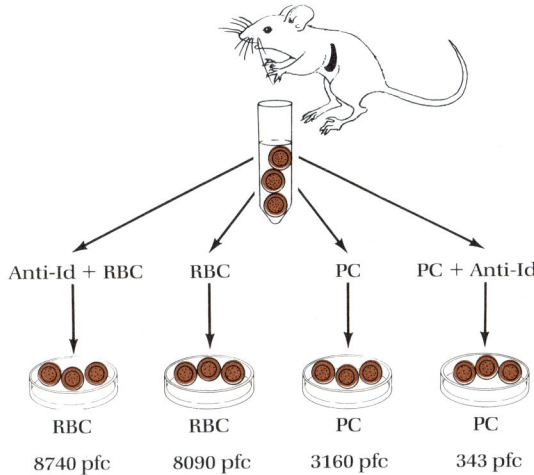

FIGURE 6   ANTI-IDIOTYPE SPECIFICALLY INHIBITS GENERATION OF ANTIBODY RESPONSE

Spleen cells are immunized in vitro with specific antigen (PC) or control antigen (RBC) in the presence or absence of anti-id to PC. Anti-id inhibits production of anti-PC but has no effect on anti-RBC response. [After Cosenza and Kohler (1972) *PNAS* 69, 2701 (in vitro); and Hart et al. (1972) *J. Exp. Med.* 135, 1293 (in vivo)]

idiotype is against the anti-PC antibody, so the RBC immunization is not affected. This experiment shows that an anti-idiotype antibody can *down-regulate* the immune response.

The experiment in Figure 6 shows that anti-idiotypic antibody can act to suppress the immune response, but it is also possible to *enhance* the immune response with anti-idiotype antibody. For example, if an anti-idiotype is produced against an antibody to Group A streptococcus in a guinea pig, it is found that when mice are treated with the IgG1 fraction of this antibody they are primed for a secondary response to the streptococcus even though they have not been injected with a primary injection. There are at least two possible explanations. Either the anti-idiotype was reacting with the receptor, which has an idiotope, and mimicking antigen by stimulating the receptor by its antigen-binding properties (that is, acting as a paratope); or, the anti-idiotype antibody is being seen as antigen because of the internal image. In either case, the end result is that the anti-idiotype antibody acts to enhance the immune response.

Here we have two examples of anti-idiotype antibody behaving in a *regulatory* role, a condition that is essential for validation of the network theory.

The Ability of Anti-Idiotype to Mimic Antigen

Another prediction of the network theory is that the anti-idiotype antibody should under some conditions mimic antigen. This prediction is based on an essential tenet of the theory, namely, that the internal images within the immune system reflect the epitopes outside the system. If this is true, then one should be able to use the idiotopes of antibodies to raise antibodies whose paratopes will bind to other epitopes.[3] This use of the internal image has been done with several antigens, with hormone receptors providing some of the more dramatic examples.

The chain of reasoning for these experiments, which are diagrammed in Figure 7, goes as follows: Hormones bind to receptors. Anti-hormone antibody binds to the hormone. And antibody against the anti-hormone binds to the anti-hormone. Because both receptor and anti-hormone antibody bind to the hormone and because the anti-hormone additionally can bind to the anti-anti-hormone, it follows that the anti-anti-hormone should bind to the receptor. This is a long way of saying that the anti-idiotype should bind to the receptor (Figure 7). If this chain of reasoning is correct, we should be able to raise an antibody against a receptor without ever using the receptor as antigen. The ligand and the internal images should let us end up with anti-receptor antibody. This was first done by Sege and Peterson with insulin in 1978.

An experiment showing that this can be done is diagrammed in Figure 8. In these studies, Erlanger and his co-workers in New

---

[3] The reader should be able to follow this sentence, which is written entirely in networkese. If you can't, do not pass go; return to start and try again.

THE NETWORK

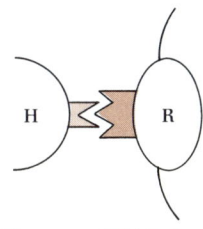

Hormone (H) binds receptor (R).

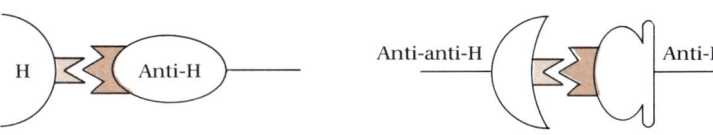

Hormone binds antihormone antibody.

Antihormone antibody binds anti-antihormone antibody.

Since both receptor and antihormone antibody bind to hormone and antihormone binds to anti-antihormone, the anti-antihormone should bind to the receptor.

Therefore, anti-Id of antihormone should bind to receptor of hormone.

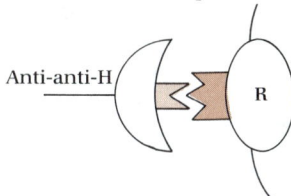

FIGURE 7   GENERATION OF ANTI-RECEPTOR ANTIBODIES

Because both receptor and anti-hormone antibody bind to the hormone, and anti-hormone binds to anti–anti-hormone, then anti–anti-hormone should bind to receptor.

York developed an antibody against the acetylcholine receptor using the principles of the network. As seen in Figure 8A, rabbits were immunized with a molecule called bisQ, a highly active agonist (an agonist is a substance that reacts with the receptor to cause a response) of the acetylcholine receptor (AChR). This anti-bisQ antibody had all of the properties of an anti-acetylcholine antibody; that is, it could react with ACh to prevent its binding to the receptor. The anti-bisQ was purified and used to immunize another set of rabbits to produce anti-idiotype antibodies. The resulting anti-idiotype antibody (i.e., the anti-antibody) had the charactaristics of an anti-receptor antibody. It could bind to the receptor and prevent binding of ACh—the result we would predict from Figure 7.

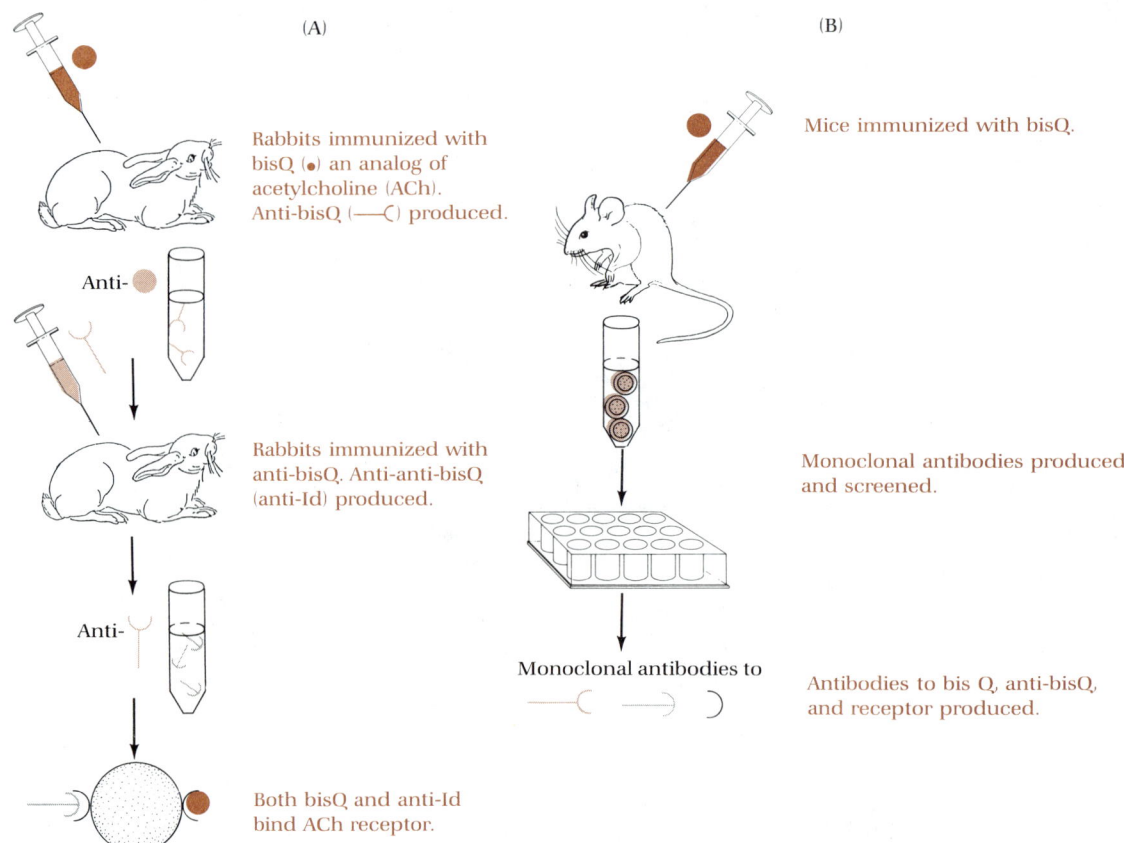

FIGURE 8 ANTI-RECEPTOR ANTIBODIES CAN BE PRODUCED USING THE NETWORK

Two experiments to show that anti-receptor antibodies can be produced using the network. (A) Rabbits are immunized with bisQ and produce anti-bisQ. The purified anti-bisQ is reinjected, and rabbits produce anti–anti-bisQ, which reacts with the acetylcholine receptor. [After Wasserman et al. (1982) *PNAS* 79, 4810] (B) Mice are immunized with bisQ, and monoclonal antibodies are generated. These antibodies can be shown to react to bisQ, anti-bisQ, and the receptor. [After Cleveland et al. (1983) *Nature* 305, 56]

THE NETWORK

Erlanger and his co-workers also showed that animals produce auto–anti-AChR antibody (Figure 8B). First they immunized mice with bisQ and then produced monoclonal antibodies, using the cells in the spleens of these animals. They reasoned here that, if the network theory is correct, the injection of antigen elicits antigen-specific antibody and, subsequently, anti-idiotype antibody. But there should also be antibody against the *receptor*, because the internal image will be reflected in the responding cells. When the clones were screened, it was found that indeed antibodies of all three specificities were produced, namely, anti-bis Q, anti-idioytype, and anti-ACh receptor antibodies.

Experiments like these show that all of the elements of the network are in place and operative during the course of an immune response. The question, of course, remains about their physiological role in the immune response.

Summary

1. The network theory of immune regulation introduces a new concept and a new vocabulary to the immune response.
2. The vocabulary of the network uses the term *paratope* to define an antigen-binding site on an antibody molecule; the term *idiotope* (id) defines the structures on immunoglobulin molecules that are seen as antigenic determinants by other antibody molecules; and *epitopes* are antigenic determinants on other molecules of the universe of antigens.
3. The concept of the network introduces the idea that the idiotopes on an antibody molecule are shared by many antigens and cross-react with a large number of epitopes. Thus a paratope can react with an epitope on a large number of antigens. This results in the whole universe of antigens being reflected in the interacting elements of the immune system. These are *internal images* of the antigen.
4. The immune system is seen as regulating itself through a network of interactions initiated by antigen. An epitope on the antigen reacts with a paratope on a B cell receptor and causes antibody formation. This first antibody is called ab1. Ab1 has a paratope (p1), which binds the epitope and is itself antigenic because it bears an idiotope, i1. Another B cell has a receptor with specificity for i1 and is therefore stimulated to produce antibody. This second antibody is ab2, which has a paratope and idiotope, p2 and i2. The p2 binds i1 on ab1, and the i2 induces a B cell with a paratope for i2 to make ab3. Ab3 has p3 which binds i2 and p3. In

CHAPTER TWENTY-TWO

this way the immune system responds once to an external stimulus and from then on carries out a network of internal responses to regulate itself.

5. Regulatory auto–anti-id molecules can be found in animals undergoing an immune response.

6. The network predicts that anti-id antibody to a hormone should have the internal image of the hormone receptor. Anti–anti-id can be shown to function as anti-receptor antibody.

Additional Readings

Golub, E. S. 1980. Idiotypes and networks. An introduction. *Cell* 22, 641.

Green, M. I. and A. Nisonoff (eds.). 1984. *The Biology of Idiotypes*. Plenum, New York.

Jerne, N. K. 1960. Immunological speculations. *Annu. Rev. Microbiol.* 14, 341.

Jerne, N. K. 1973. The immune system. *Sci. Am.* 229, 52.

Jerne, N. K. 1974. Toward a network theory of the immune system. *Annu. Rev. Immunol.* 125C, 373.

Jerne, N. K. 1984. Idiotype networks and other preconceived ideas. *Immunol. Rev.* 79, 5.

Jerne, N. K. 1985. The generative grammar of the immune system. *EMBO Journal* 4, 847.

Kennedy, R. C., G. R. Dreesman and H. Kohler. 1985. Vaccines utilizing internal image: anti-idiotypic antibodies that mimic antigens of infectious organisms. *BioTechniques* 3, 404.

Paul, W. E. and C. Bona. 1982. Regulatory idiotopes and immune networks: a hypothesis. *Immunol. Today* 3, 230.

Zanetti, M. and D. H. Katz. 1985. Self-recognition, autoimmunity, and internal images. *Current Topics in Microbiol. Immunol.* 119, 111.

CHAPTER 23

SUPPRESSOR CELLS

Overview The immune response also is regulated by suppressor cells. The contrast between regulation by suppressor cells and regulation by the network is an important one at both the biological and philosophical levels. The idea behind the suppressor cell is that the regulation is brought about in a manner compatible with clonal selection; that is, lymphocytes display receptors for the universe of antigens with which the immune system can react, but one function of the T cell is to suppress the immune response. In this system antigen is seen as playing its normal role of selecting cells with the appropriate receptors. These cells then exert a regulatory influence.

In this chapter we will discuss suppressor T cells, although there is evidence that B cells and even macrophages can act as suppressor cells. Suppressor T cells, or T_s, can be antigen-specific or nonspecific, and both types are induced by a complex series of cell interactions. The communication between the interacting cells is carried out by soluble factors. The factors themselves, the mode in which the cells recognize antigen, and the markers on their surfaces all are areas shrouded in mystery and are the subject of controversy. In this sense, the suppressor cell story is a microcosm of cellular and sociological aspects of immunology.

CHAPTER TWENTY-THREE

The Discovery of Suppressor T Cells

By the mid 1960s it was clear to most cellular immunologists that the T cell was crucial in the immune response, because it was able to be both an effector cell in cell-mediated responses and a helper cell in both humoral and cell-mediated responses. At that time Richard K. Gershon at Yale concluded that the T cell could also be a *regulatory* cell that could suppress the immune response. It is important, 25 years after the fact, for the reader to recognize what a creative leap this idea was.[1]

Along with the uniqueness of the idea, the complexity of the original experiments may have been another reason why the idea of the suppressor T cell was not readily accepted. Figure 1 is a figure from the original 1970 Gershon and Kondo paper describing the experiments. The large number of groups and apparent vastness of the experiment worked as a real impediment to immunologists at the time. Groups of adult mice were thymectomized, lethally irradiated, and reconstituted with syngeneic bone marrow. Some of them were injected with thymus cells and others were not. Some groups then received repeated doses of high concentrations of SRBC. The idea here was to induce a state of immunological tolerance.[2] After several weeks of this treatment, half the mice received an injection of thymus cells as a source of helper cells and were challenged with an immunizing dose of RBC. The anti-RBC responses were then quantified and it was found that the groups that had received thymus cells at the time of bone marrow reconstitution did *not* produce anti-RBC antibody.

This result fulfilled Gershon's prediction—that under certain conditions, antigen seen by thymus-derived cells can induce not only helper and effector cells but also cells able to suppress the

---

[1] The idea is now universally recognized as "creative" and Gershon has been called a "genius," but at the time the usual terms were "off the wall" for the idea and "round the bend" for its originator.

[2] This phenomenon will be discussed in detail in Chapter 24, but for our present purposes the reader need only be aware of the fact that immunological tolerance is the phenomenon in which there is a specific loss of ability to respond to an antigen. One way to induce tolerance is to use very high doses of antigen.

SUPPRESSOR CELLS

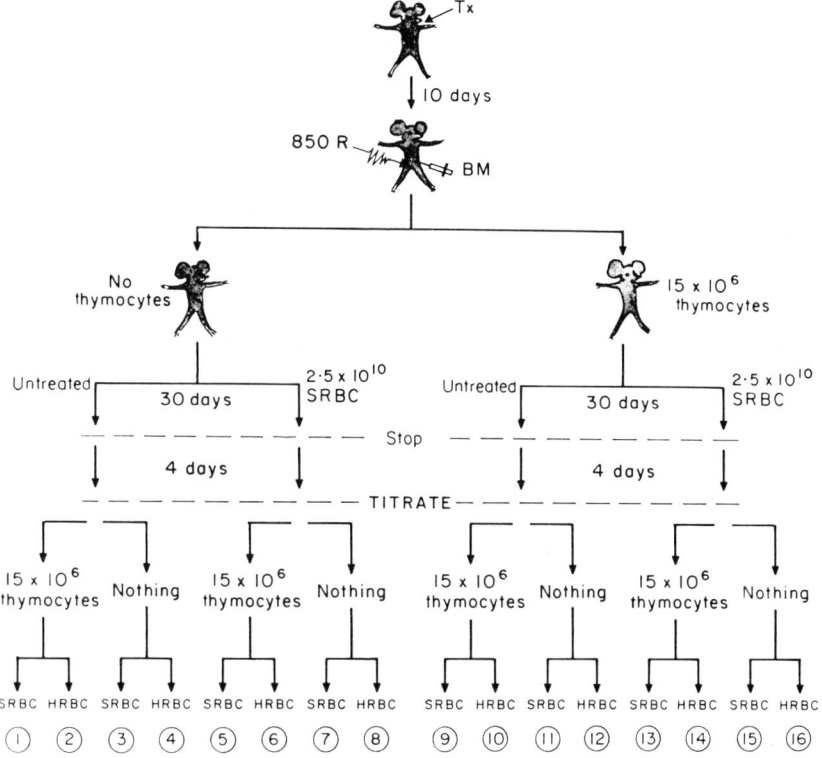

FIGURE 1 PLAN OF EXPERIMENTS

The "plan of experiments" from Gershon's original suppressor paper. [From R.K. Gershon (1970) *Immunology* 18, 723]

immune response. The groups of mice that received the antigen *before* they were reconstituted with thymus (i.e., in the absence of a thymus) made good antibody responses, but the groups that received the antigen while they had thymus cells did not. Thus the presence of a thymus during part of the response prevented the animals from making antibody. The cells responsible for this suppression were found to be T cells (see below) and were termed SUPPRESSOR CELLS.

Nonspecific Suppression   For suppressor cells to exert a regulatory role in the immune response, we would expect that they would be antigen-specific. It is very clear that there are antigen-specific suppressor cells (which will be discussed in detail later), but under a fairly wide range of circumstances it is possible to induce cells which exert *nonspecific* suppression. The physiological role played by nonspecific suppressor cells is not known and current proposals are controversial.

One of the first ways discovered to generate nonspecific suppressor cells was by treatment of a population of spleen cells with the T cell mitogen CONCANAVALIN A (ConA). This phenomenon was first observed when low doses of ConA were added to spleen cell cultures in vitro, and these cultures showed significantly reduced antibody responses after challenge with antigen. To show that there was active suppression, the treated cultures were washed and added to cultures of normal spleen cells. After challenge with antigen, these cultures had reduced responses. Thus, adding cells that were suppressed to a population of normal cells prevented the normal cells from making a response. Treatment of the suppressed cultures with anti-Thy 1 and complement abolished their ability to suppress. *Cell-free supernatant fluid* from the ConA-treated cultures was also shown to induce suppression of normal cells. The suppression by the soluble factors (discussed later) was nonspecific, because the response to any antigen was affected.

The discovery that the *neonatal* thymus is a source of suppressor cells was very important. It had been known for a very long time that newborn animals make poor immune responses and it had been assumed that some cell or cells involved in the response had to mature as the animal developed. The discovery that there are suppressor cells in the newborn now seems to be one of the strongest reasons for the poor response in newborns. Several weeks after birth, the specific time depending upon the strain of mouse, these nonspecific suppressor cells disappear. It is interesting to note that in strains with a high incidence of autoimmune disease these neonatal suppressor cells are either not present or disappear at a very early age.[3]

[3] As an example of how the idea of the suppressor cell was resisted, in my lab in the early 1970s we were attempting to determine which cell in the newborn was immunologically immature. We could not find any immature cell when we separated B cells, T cells, and macrophages but we also could not get responses with unseparated newborn spleen. The suggestion by my closest friend that his recently discovered T suppressor cell was responsible was dismissed as too far-fetched to be considered, even for the sake of friendship.

SUPPRESSOR CELLS

Nonspecific suppressor cells also appear in many instances in animals bearing a tumor. An example of this is the AKR mouse, which develops a spontaneous thymic leukemia at about nine months of age. Once these mice develop the tumor they begin to exhibit nonspecific suppressor cells in their spleens and lymph nodes. Because the general loss of immune responsiveness during tumor growth is a widespread phenomenon, it has been argued that the tumor has induced the suppressor cells and in this manner escapes immune surveillance (Chapter 25).

The mechansim of nonspecific suppression is not understood. One possibility is that under those conditions in which nonspecific suppressor cells are induced, we are really seeing polyclonal stimulation of a vast array of specific suppressor cells. Treatment with ConA, for example, stimulates all T cells, and the suppression seen is the summation of multiple specific suppressor cells. An alternative is that there is a unique nonspecific suppressor mechanism.

Allotype-Specific and Idiotype-Specific Suppressor Cells

When an F_1 neonatal mouse is injected with antibody against the immunoglobulin of one of the parental strains, the production of these immunoglobulins is suppressed when the animal becomes an adult. Recall that allelic exclusion is the phenomenon in which each cell of an F_1 animal produces immunoglobulin of only one of the parental allotypes. An animal that is heterozygous for allotypes *a* and *b* has the genes for immunoglobulins of both allotypes, but each individual cell will produce only *a* or only *b*. If anti-*a* was injected into the animal when it was a newborn, only allotype *b* will be found in the serum of the adult. In the experiments of Mage and Dray, for example, rabbits heterozygous for allotypes *b4b5* were injected at birth with anti-*b4*. These animals had no *b4* immunoglobulin molecules in their serum even a year after treatment, while uninjected littermates had normal levels. This phenomenon is called ALLOTYPE SUPPRESSION.

Allotype suppression is due to suppressor cells. If irradiated BALB/c mice are repopulated with normal (BALB/c × SJL)F_1 spleen cells, then they produce immunoglobulins with the allotypes of both parents. But if they are repopulated with F_1 cells from allotype-suppressed F_1 mice, then they produce only the unsuppressed allotype. If normal F_1 and suppressed F_1 spleen cells are mixed together and injected into irradiated recipients, there is allotype suppression, showing that the suppressed cells prevent the normal cells from expressing one of the allotypes. Treating the suppressed cells with anti-Thy 1 and complement abolishes their ability to suppress the allotype production. This finding is strong evidence for the role of a suppressor T cell in allotype suppression. It should be pointed out, however, that there is no known biological significance to the phenomenon of allotype suppression.

There is also a phenomenon known as IDIOTYPE SUPPRESSION in which an animal can be pretreated with an anti-idiotype antibody so that when it makes an antibody response against a particular antigen, the response lacks Ig molecules with that idiotype because of the pretreatment. Groups of mice can be pretreated either with saline or with an anti-idiotype antibody and then challenged with antigen. When both the *total* amount of antibody and the *proportion* of that antibody bearing the idiotype are determined at a later time, we find that the pretreatment with anti-idiotype antibody reduces the production of antibodies with the idiotype. This suppression is transferrable to irradiated animals by means of the spleen cells of the anti-idiotype–treated mice, and the suppression is abolished by treatment with anti-Thy 1 and complement. From what we know about the possible role of the network of anti-idiotypes as a possible regulatory system, these experiments indicate that there is a possible action of suppressor cells on the network.

Antigen-Specific Suppressor Cells

If suppressor cells are to be of regulatory significance during an immune response, they must be antigen-specific; and there are countless examples of such antigen-specificity. An early example comes from the experiments of Tada and his co-workers in Tokyo (Figure 2). Mice are primed with carrier, and their spleen cells are transferred to unirradiated recipients, which are then challenged with hapten and carrier. The response of the recipients to the hapten is suppressed under these conditions. Treating the cells from the primed donor with anti-Thy 1 and complement before transfer abolishes their ability

SUPPRESSOR CELLS

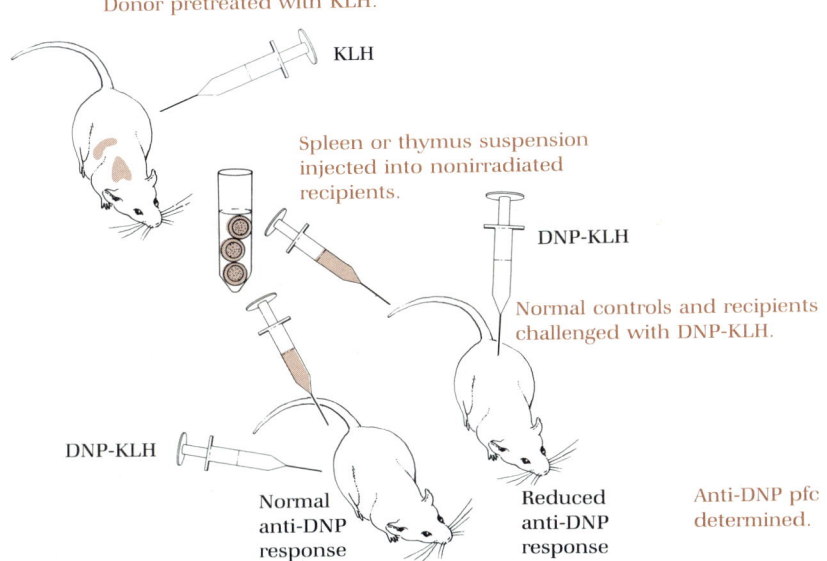

FIGURE 2 GENERATION OF ANTIGEN-SPECIFIC SUPPRESSOR T CELLS
Mice are primed with KLH, and the spleen or thymus cells are injected into unirradiated hosts. After challenge with DNP-KLH, the recipients make a reduced anti-DNP response. [After Tada et al. (1974) *J. Exp. Med.* 140, 239]

to induce suppression of the unirradiated recipients. Treating the donors with a carrier different from the one used in the hapten–carrier conjugate at challenge gives no suppression. These experiments indicate that there is antigen-specific suppression carried out by T cells.

A similar early discovery was made by Benacerraf and his co-workers, using GAT nonresponder mice. Mice of the DBA/1 strain are low responders to the polymer glutamate, alanine, tyrosine (GAT). Gershon had predicted earlier that nonresponder mice might have suppressor cells activated more readily than responder strains. Treating nonresponder strains with GAT and then adding these cells to cultures of responder spleen cells renders the responder cells nonresponsive. Thus the nonresponder strains made cells able to suppress the cells from the responder strain. Treatment of the nonresponder cells with anti-Thy 1 and complement abolishes their ability to suppress, showing that there are suppressor T cells that are responsible for the lack of response.

Properties of Suppressor T Cells

The Lyt Profile

We have already indicated that the suppressor cells we have been discussing are Thy 1^+ and are therefore T cells. This is true for nonspecific as well as antigen-specific suppressor cells. The immediate question that comes to mind (or should at this stage of the game) is, What is the Lyt profile of the cells? The answer to this question originally looked simple, but as often happens, the problem is more complicated than originally conceived. In fact, as we will see below, there are very complex cell interactions involved in the generation of suppressor cells and each of the interacting cells bears a different Lyt phenotype. But it could be shown, at first, that the cell carrying out the suppression (i.e., the suppressor effector cell) is Lyt 1^-, 2^+.

Figure 3 shows that when suppressor cells are generated and treated with anti-Lyt 1 antiserum and complement, their ability to carry out suppressor function is unaffected. However, when the cells are treated with anti-Lyt 2, all activity is removed. This result indicates that *the cells that carry out the suppression* are Lyt 1^-, 2^+.

The I–J Enigma

The finding that T suppressor cells were Lyt 1^-, 2^+ distinguished them from T helper cells but did not allow them to be distinguished from T cytotoxic cells, which are also Lyt 1^-, 2^+. This is important, because one possible explanation for the phenomenon of suppression is that T_s are cytotoxic cells that are killing the helper T cells or the effector cells. However, a cell surface marker unique for the suppressor T cell was discovered in 1976. It was found that an antiserum raised by immunizing the congenic strain B10.A(3R) with cells from B10.A(5R) gave an antiserum that reacted exclusively with T suppressor cells. At first the antiserum could be characterized

SUPPRESSOR CELLS

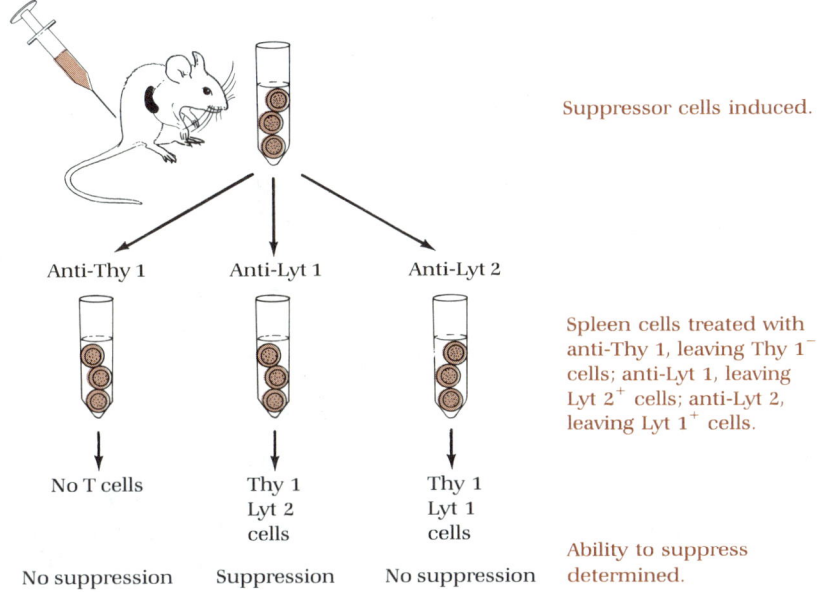

FIGURE 3 SUPPRESSOR T CELLS ARE LYT 2^+

Suppressor cells are induced and the spleen cells are treated with either anti-Thy 1, anti-Lyt 1, or anti-Lyt 2, and complement to kill all T cells, Lyt 1, or Lyt 2 cells, respectively. The remaining cells are then tested for their ability to carry out suppression. Only the Lyt 2 cells suppress.

only by its ability to abolish suppression (i.e., by a functional test), but later it was found that the antiserum could be assayed for cytotoxicity—an assay enabling quantification of the cells expressing the product.

Mapping studies showed that the gene was located in the I region of the MHC. This locus was called I–J and was found to map between I–B and I–E. The presence of a unique surface marker on suppressor cells was cause for jubilation, because it made experiments in which the suppressor cells could be eliminated possible. Indeed, the soluble suppressor product was shown in some cases to react with I–J antiserum. But then events took a sudden change.

The I–B region was defined by the pattern of responsiveness (responder/nonresponder) of two recombinant strains of mice to the enzyme lactate dehydrogenase B and to a myeloma protein.

CHAPTER TWENTY-THREE

Jan Klein's group showed that the control of the antibody response could be explained by the interaction of a helper cell and a suppressor cell. The nonresponder mice were, in fact, able to respond, but they had suppressor cells that made them behave as nonresponders. The regulation was shown to be exerted at the E locus. There was, in fact, no B locus! With the elimination of the I–B locus, the I–J region mapped between the I–E_β and I–E_α. But when the genes of the I region were isolated, cloned, and sequenced, there was not enough DNA between I–E_β and I–E_α to account for the I–J molecule. Thus, the I–J enigma: How can a cell surface marker map to a part of a chromosome where there is not enough DNA for a gene?

There have been several explanations for the obvious presence of a function despite the absence of a gene at the place where the function maps. Klein and his colleagues have concluded that the I–J locus is an "illusion" generated by the appearance of new determinants on a *modified* version of the I–E_β product and in some cases also the I–A_β chain. These workers have predicted that suppressor T cells, in contrast to other T cells, should have the mRNA for only part of the I–E_β chain. Should such mRNA be isolated, the mechanism for the modification in this class of cells would then have to be explained. But should such mRNA not be found, the prediction would be falsified.

Another explanation, put forth by Hayes and her co-workers in Madison, is that the expression of J is controlled by *two loci*. One of these loci is on chromosome 17 (in the MHC) and the other is on chromosome 4. The gene on chromosome 17 is thought to be in I–E and, if the idea is correct, should be a regulatory gene. The gene on chromosome 4 is as yet unstudied, but the prediction is that, barring the appearance of yet another gene involved in the expression of I–J, it should be the structural gene.[4]

---

[4] Feelings are running high in the I–J business. For example, in a recent article in *Immunological Reviews* devoted to the subject, Jan Klein says, "We see very little sense in continuing working as if nothing had happened. Molecular biologists have thrown down a gauntlet and we should accept the challenge. We should not go on using J as a marker for this or that cell, talking further about J restriction, and characterizing further factors with all kinds of reagents. We should try, instead, to see whether there is anything to J at the molecular level. Until we know that, we should perhaps keep quiet about J." [J. Klein et al., 1985, *Immunol. Rev.* 83, 61]

SUPPRESSOR CELLS

Antigen Binding by T_s

We have seen that T cells, in contrast to B cells, can only bind antigen in the context of self-MHC molecules. Suppressor T cells, however, are an exception to this statement. The experiment diagrammed in Figure 4 shows evidence for this. Antigen-specific suppressor cells were induced in mice and then the B cells were removed from the spleen cell population by either passing the cells over a column or incubating them on a petri dish coated with rabbit anti-mouse Ig (RA-

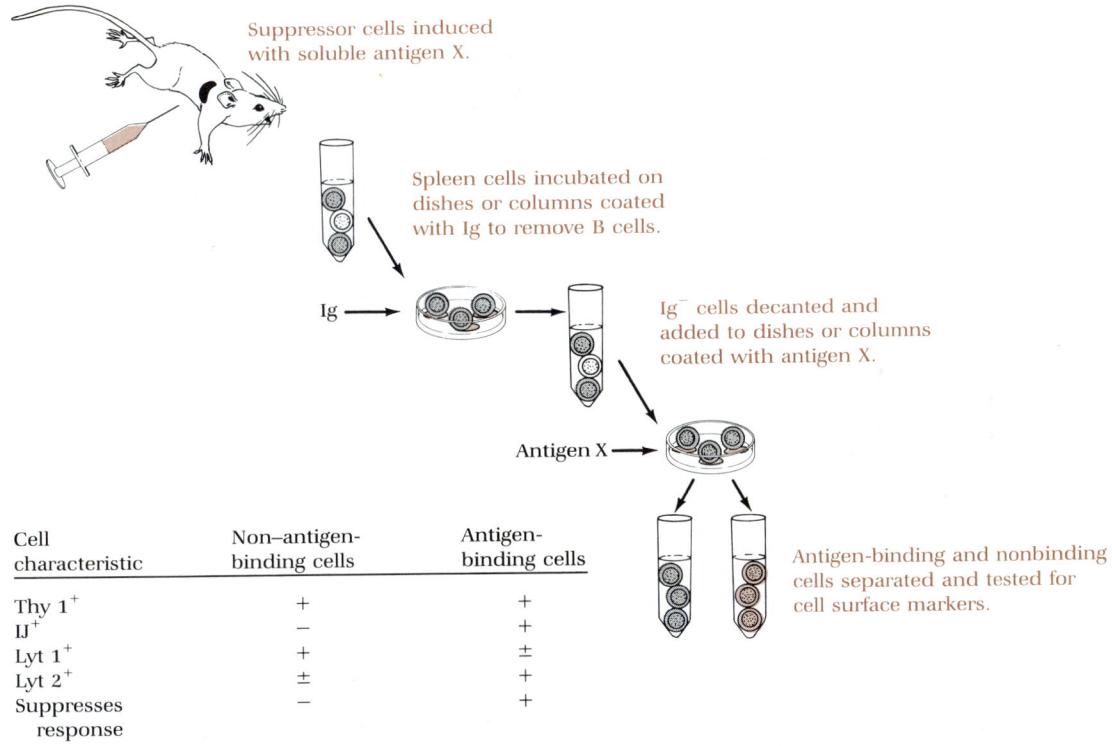

Cell characteristic	Non–antigen-binding cells	Antigen-binding cells
Thy 1^+	+	+
IJ^+	−	+
Lyt 1^+	+	±
Lyt 2^+	±	+
Suppresses response	−	+

FIGURE 4 SUPPRESSOR T CELLS BIND ANTIGEN

Suppressor T cells are induced and the spleen cells tested for ability to adhere to antigen-coated surfaces. Thy 1^+ and Thy 1^- cells bind. IJ^+ cells all bind antigen. Lyt 1^+ cells do not bind antigen, but Lyt 2^+ cells do. All of the suppressor function is in the antigen-binding cells. [After Okumura et al. (1977) *J. Exp. Med.* 146, 1234; and Taniguchi and Miller (1977) *J. Exp. Med.* 146, 1450]

MIG). The B cells, which are Ig$^+$, adhere to the surface; the Ig$^-$ cells, which are T cells, are removed. The T cell population is then passed over a column (or incubated on a plate) coated with the specific antigen used to induce the suppressor cells. A small proportion of the cells adhere to this surface. These cells are gently removed from the surface and compared with the T cells that did not adhere to the antigen-coated surface. As seen in the figure, both populations are Thy 1$^+$, but only the population bound to antigen is I–J$^+$. The I–J$^+$ cells are also strongly Lyt 2$^+$, whereas the I–J$^-$ cells are strongly Lyt 1$^+$. The I–J$^+$, antigen-binding population is able to carry out suppression when incubated with normal cells and antigen.

These experiments show clearly that the effector cell in suppression differs from other T cells in its ability to bind antigen directly. It must be recalled, however, that these cells are not binding antigen by means of a surface immunoglobulin, because neither the antigen-binding nor the nonbinding populations adhered to the Ig-coated surfaces. This result implies that the antigen-specific receptor on the suppressor T cell is different from that on helper and cytotoxic T cells. Indeed, there is molecular evidence for this assertion.

Suppressor T Cell Receptor

When genomic DNAs from cloned T helper, T cytotoxic, and T suppressor cells are probed with a β-chain probe and compared after treatment with the endonuclease *PvuII* (Figure 5), it is found that every helper and cytotoxic clone tested has new bands not seen in the germ line. This indicates that the β chain is in a rearranged form in these cells (Chapter 20). In contrast, suppressor cells have no new bands or germ line β genes, indicating that they do not use the β chain of the T cell receptor. What these cells do use as a receptor is at the moment unknown.

Suppressor and Helper Determinants

Over the past decade Eli Sercarz and his colleagues at UCLA have been carrying out an elegant analysis of the nature of epitopes. Using a variety of antigens—most often β-galactosidase and

SUPPRESSOR CELLS

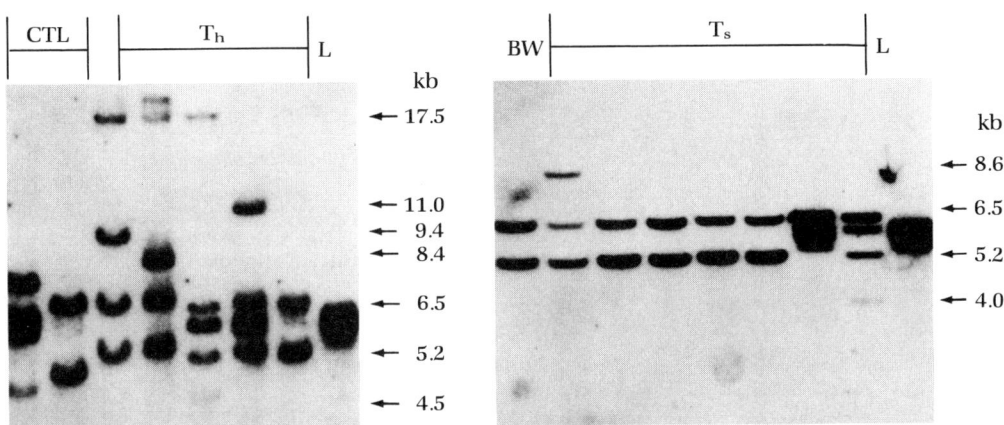

FIGURE 5 ANTIGEN RECEPTOR IN SUPPRESSOR CELLS
Genomic Southern blots of DNA from (A) cytotoxic (CTL) and helper (T$_h$) cells and (B) suppressor (T$_s$) cells. The suppressor cells were from antigen-specific, non–antigen-specific, and idiotype suppressor cell clones. Note that there is no rearrangement of the β chain in the suppressor cells. [From Hedrick et al. (1985) *PNAS* 82, 531]

lysozyme—they have been able to show that some epitopes on an antigen induce help and some induce suppression. For many years it was not clear how one determinant on a molecule could induce suppression that would shut down the response to all of the other determinants, but the picture is now becoming clearer and revealing some of the subtleties of immune regulation.

Induction of Suppressor and Helper Cells

Mice respond to an injection of β-galactosidase by producing successive waves of helper and suppressor cells (Figure 6). When the β-galactosidase molecule is treated with cyanogen bromide (an action that cleaves the molecule at methionine residues) and each fraction is tested for ability to generate either helper or suppressor cells, it is found that some fractions (for example, CB3 and CB10 in Figure 7) induce *either* helper or suppressor cells. But one peptide, CB2, is found to induce *both* helper and suppressor cells. This result can be achieved by varying the experimental conditions under which the animal sees the peptide.

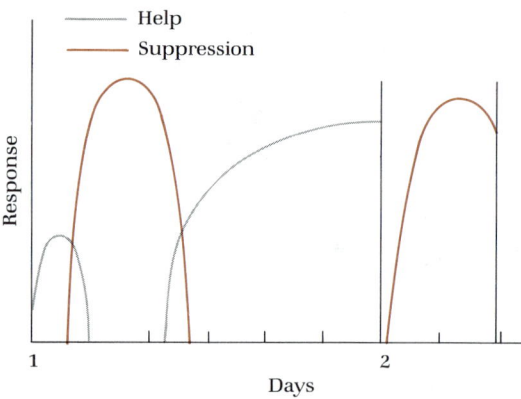

FIGURE 6 HELPER AND SUPPRESSOR PHASES IN IMMUNE RESPONSE

Immunization with β-galactosidase results in successive waves of help and suppression. [After Sercarz et al. (1978) *Immunol. Rev.* 39, 108]

When T suppressor cells are raised with CB2 and tested on T helper cells raised with either CB2 or CB10, it is found that suppression occurs only on the CB2-induced helper cells (Table 1). Similarly, CB3-induced suppressor cells suppress CB3 helper cells but do not suppress helper cells raised with CB10 or CB2. This data shows that the suppressive action is limited to determinants on the same peptide (i.e., those that are physically associated with each other).

TABLE 1 Interaction between T_h and T_s induced with different antigens.

| Inducer | | Percentage |
T_h	T_s	suppression
β-gal	CB2	80
CB2	CB2	80
CB10	CB2	10
β-gal	CB3	90
CB2	CB3	0
CB10	CB3	10

Source: Data from Krzych et al. (1985), *J. Exp. Med.* 162: 311.

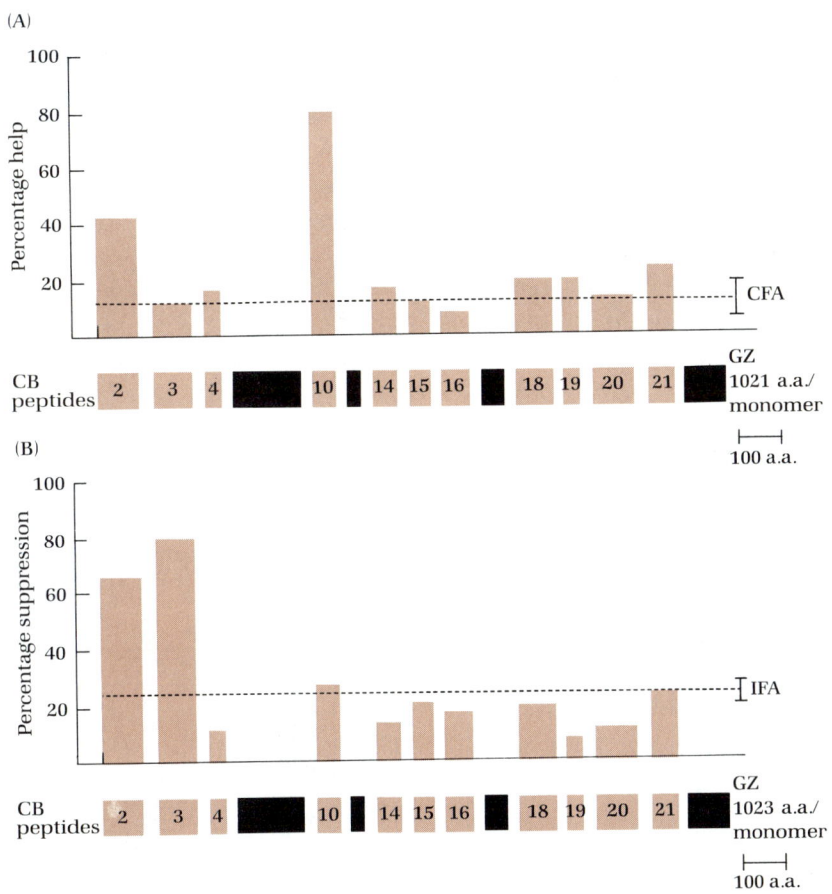

FIGURE 7 INDUCTION OF T_h OR T_s

Peptide fragments of β-galactosidase, which are generated by cyanogen bromide (CB) cleavage, induce either help (A) or suppression (B) of the response to the whole molecule. [(A) after Krzych et al. (1982) *J. Immunol.* 128, 1529; (B) after Krzych et al. (1985) *J. Exp. Med.* 162, 311]

Need for a Triad of Determinants

An approach to the physical organization of the determinants on an antigen has been made with cloned suppressor cells by Richard Hodes and his colleagues at the NIH. We have seen many times how cloned cells have been useful in solving complex problems in immunology, and this finding is true for the suppressor system as well. Clones of helper T cells specific for H-2^b:FGG and clones of suppressor T cells specific for H-2^b:KLH are incubated with H-2^b B cells and accessory cells and challenged with a hapten–carrier system consisting of TNP-KLH, TNP-FGG, or other combinations of these molecules. As shown in Table 2, the specificity controls show that both the T_h clones and the T_s clones are antigen- and MHC-restricted. When mixtures of either TNP-FGG and KLH or TNP-FGG and KLH-FGG are added to the cultures, there is no suppression, even though the molecules that can react with all three of the cell types are present (TNP for B cells, KLH for T_s, and FGG for T_h). Similarly, when TNP-FGG is incubated with KLH and FGG that are covalently conjugated to each other (KLH-FGG) but not to TNP, there is no suppression. However, when the KLH is covalently conjugated to the TNP-FGG, there is suppression.

These experiments have been interpreted to show that a TRIAD OF DETERMINANTS is needed for suppressor cells to function (hap-

TABLE 2 Requirement for a "triad" of determinants in suppression.

T_h	T_s	Challenge antigen[a]	Result
CONTROL			
KLH:H-2^b	KLH:H-2^b	TNP-KLH	Suppression
KLH:H-2^b	KLH:H-2^k	TNP-KLH	No suppression
KLH:H-2^b	KLH:H-2^b	TNP-FGG	No suppression
EXPERIMENTAL			
FGG:H-2^b	KLH:H-2^b	TNP-FGG + KLH	No suppression
FGG:H-2^b	KLH:H-2^b	TNP-FGG + KLH-FGG	No suppression
FGG:H-2^b	KLH:H-2^b	TNP-FGG-(KLH)	Suppression
FGG:H-2^b	KLH:H-2^b	TNP-(KLH-FGG)	Suppression

Source: Data from Asano and Hodes (1984), J. Immunol. 133: 2864.
[a] Antigen was added to cultures of B cells, accessory cells, T_h, and T_s.
Abbreviations: FGG, fowl γ-globulin; KLH, keyhole limpet hemocyanin; TNP, trinitrophenyl-; TNP-FGG-(KLH), TNP-FGG conjugated to KLH; TNP-(KLH-FGG), TNP conjugated to KLH-FGG.

SUPPRESSOR CELLS

ten, helper, and suppressor epitopes). Regulation is thus seen to be exerted at local areas of the molecule. The animal makes a response to an antigen that is characterised by antibody production or suppression, depending on the balance of these local responses. When we speak of an antibody response to a complex molecule such as β-galactosidase, we are speaking of a polyclonal response. To precisely evaluate what is happening, we would have to determine the monoclonal response to each epitope.

These experiments do not address the *mechanisms* of the suppression, which is most probably via the soluble suppressor factors.

Soluble Suppressor Factors

We saw earlier in this chapter that a cell-free supernatant fraction obtained from ConA-induced, nonspecific suppressor cells is able to suppress cultures of normal cells. Antigen-specific suppressor factors have also been found and in fact are generally thought to be a major mode of action of suppressor cell activation in regulatory circuits.

Antigen-Specific Suppressor Factors — One of the first demonstrations of the antigen-specific suppressor factor involved the IgE response to the hapten dinitrophenol (DNP). Tada and his coworkers found that by irradiating rats sub-lethally and immunizing them with DNP conjugated to *Ascaris* (DNP-Asc) plus pertussis vaccine, a good anti-TNP response, which was mostly IgE, occurred.[5] To determine whether a cell-free supernatant fraction could induce suppression, they sonicated thymocytes and spleen cells from these immunized animals and subjected the lysate to ultracentrifugation. They obtained an extract that was able to suppress an ongoing anti-DNP IgE response when injected into rats. The factor was antigen-specific (extracts from normal cells did not work, nor did extracts from cells immunized to other antigens) and had a molecular weight of around 60,000. But, as Tada points out, "In 1973 to 1974, a molecule of less than 60,000

---

[5] It is well known that *Ascaris* and other parasites stimulate IgE responses.

molecular weight with antigen-specific activity was hardly welcomed widely in the immunologic community, inasmuch as the factor was found in the rat and was observed exclusively in the IgE antibody response."

Because of the difficulties involved in working with this system and the inherent conservative nature of scientists, Tada's group went on to develop a soluble suppressor factor in the mouse using KLH, a system that all immunologists felt comfortable with. This second suppressor factor was not only antigen-specific, but also MHC-restricted. If the factor was generated in F_1 mice that were $H-2^{k/d}$, it would suppress each parental haplotype (i.e., $H-2^k$ and $H-2^d$), but not strains of other MHC haplotypes. Upon close examination it was found that the factor would suppress strains that shared the same I–J region of H-2.

Thus by the late 1970s, antigen-specific, MHC-restricted soluble factors that carried out suppression were known. The next advance (as we have seen happen so often) came with the use of cloned T cells. Harvey Cantor's laboratory in Boston generated a series of clones of suppressor T cells that elaborated an antigen-specific suppressor factor. This factor not only suppressed the specific response (to the glycophorin molecule of red blood cells), but also bound the antigen. The factor had a molecular weight of 70,000 and did not bind to columns coated with antibody to either H-2, immunoglobulin, or Lyt antigens.

Nature of Antigen-Specific Suppressor Factors

Many research groups are currently studying suppressor factors, using either cloned lines or in vitro immunizations. Virtually all the factors have been shown to have either an idiotype or an immunoglobulin constant-region determinant that accounts for their antigen specificity. Virtually all of them have also been found to have I–J determinants, although some of the factors are not MHC-restricted. The molecular weights of the factors range from 29,000 to 70,000, and they are composed of either one or two chains. The nature of these suppressor factors will probably continue to be a major research interest in the next few years. The reader should bear in mind that the solution to the I–J enigma may be bound up with the nature of the soluble factors.

SUPPRESSOR CELLS

Regulatory Circuits

Cell Interactions in the Induction of Suppressor T Cells

We saw above that the T suppressor cell expresses Lyt 2 on its surface. In 1978 Dianne Eardly in Gershon's lab found that an Lyt 1^+ helper cell is needed in the induction of T_s. In these experiments (Figure 8) various T cell populations (test cells) were added to cultures of B cells and macrophages (assay cells). As shown in the figure, the addition of either antigen-stimulated or unstimulated Lyt 1^+ cells allowed the cultures to produce antibody. However, when "unselected" T cells were added along with antigen-stimulated Lyt 1^+ cells, the response was suppressed. The primed Lyt 1^+ cells are always needed to get suppression, and the Lyt 1^+ population *induces* a cell in the unselected population to become a suppressor cell.

We know that the cell carrying out the suppression is an Lyt 2^+ cell. This means that either the Lyt 1^+ cell is acting as a helper cell for the Lyt 2^+ cell in a manner analogous to T helper cells in antibody formation and cell-mediated responses, or it is acting as an inducer cell inducing another cell to become a suppressor. Experiments have shown that the latter explanation is correct; that is, Lyt 1^+ cells induce Lyt 1^+, 2^+ cells to become Lyt 2^+ suppressor cells. The Lyt 1^+ cell is called the INDUCER, the Lyt 1^+, 2^+ cell is called the TRANSDUCER, and the Lyt 2^+ cell that carries out the suppression is called the EFFECTOR CELL.

Soluble Factors in the Regulatory Circuit

We saw earlier that there are a variety of soluble factors able to carry out suppression. Work from many labs is beginning to show that the SUPPRESSOR INDUCER CELL produces a factor called Tsif, or T-SUPPRESSOR INDUCER FACTOR. Depending upon the system being studied, some of these factors are composed of I–J molecules, some bind antigen, and some are restricted for Igh genes.

Contrasuppressor Cells

Before his death, Gershon was in the process of developing evidence that had become as controversial as his original idea of the suppressor cell. The germ of the idea came from his older experiments on suppressor cells in which he showed that suppression could be inhibited if the cells that were to be suppressed were stimulated with a *cross-*

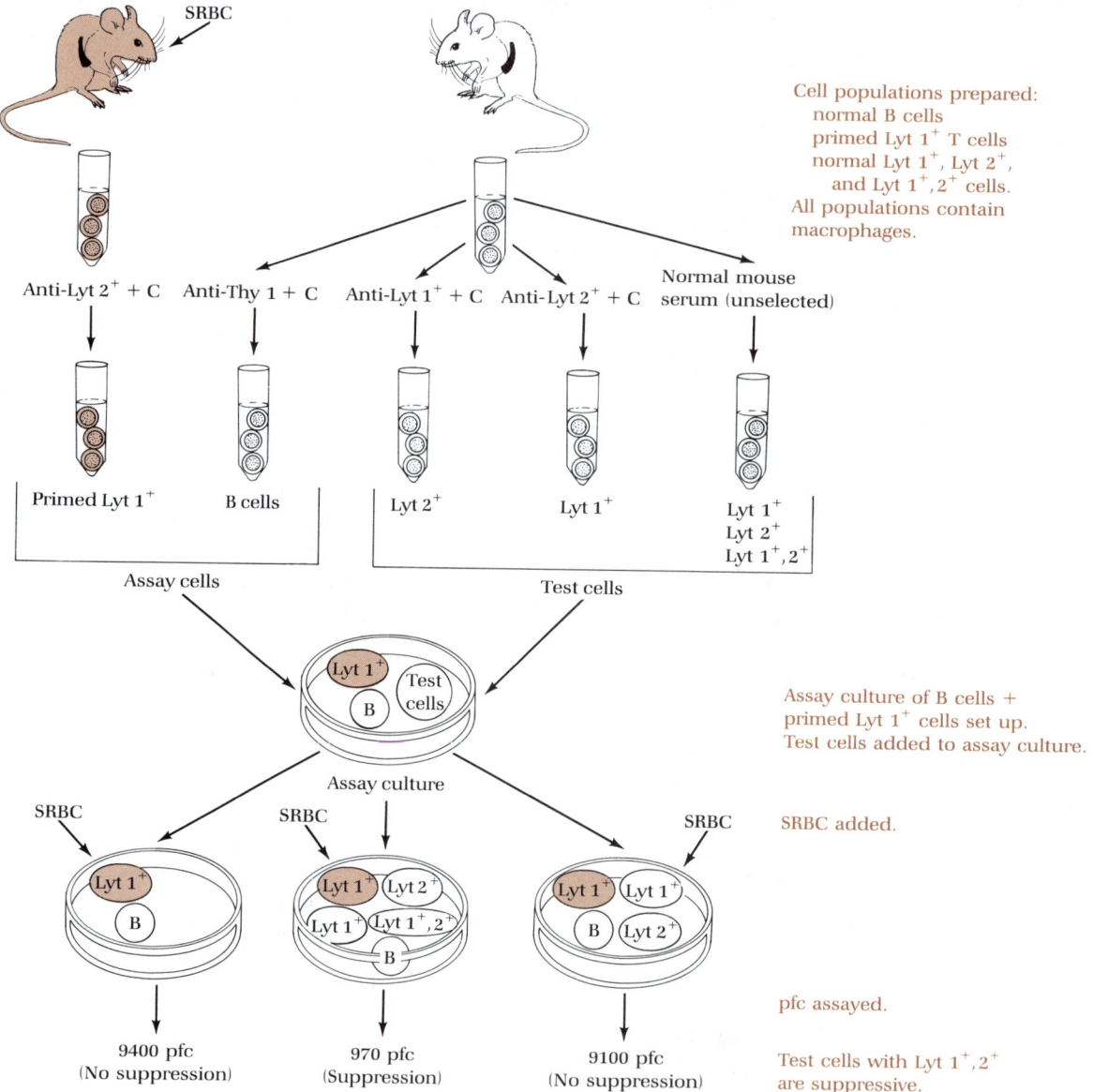

FIGURE 8 CELL INTERACTIONS IN SUPPRESSOR CELL GENERATION
Primed Lyt 1^+ cells and normal B cells are incubated with "test cells" consisting of either unprimed Lyt 1, Lyt 2 or unselected spleen cells. The presence of unprimed Lyt $1^+, 2^+$ cells are needed for the induction of suppression. [After Eardley et al. (1978) *J. Exp. Med.* 147, 1106]

SUPPRESSOR CELLS

reacting antigen. This stimulation did not produce any demonstrable helper effect but it seemed to inhibit the suppressor effect. In essence, it was a suppressor of the suppressor, and he called it the CONTRASUPRESSOR CELL. In a review written in 1984, Doug Green (who was first Gershon's graduate student and then became his trusted young collaborator) states that the contrasuppressor cell, "with the help of hindsight, should have been theoretically predicted to be needed as a homeostatic balance for suppression."

Current evidence seems to suggest that the contrasuppressor cell and the suppressor cell have the same target. If this is correct, it argues that the contrasuppressor may function not by "suppressing the suppressor," but rather by blocking the action of the suppressor cell either by competition or by making the target cell resistant to suppression. What is being competed for or how the target is made resistant is unknown.

A whole regulatory circuit or cascade for the contrasuppressor is envisioned similar to that of the suppressor circuit. The CONTRASUPPRESSOR INDUCER cell differs from the suppressor inducer in that it is Lyt 1^-, 2^+, but both are I–J$^+$. The CONTRASUPPRESSOR TRANSDUCER cell is Lyt 1^+, 2^+, I–J$^+$, and the CONTRASUPPRESSOR EFFECTOR cell is Lyt 1^+, 2^-, I–J$^+$.

Summary

1. There is a subset of T cells, called suppressor T cells (T_s), which functions to suppress the immune response. The suppression can be antigen-specific or nonspecific.
2. T_s are Thy 1^+, Lyt 1^-, 2^+, and express a unique MHC determinant, *i*–J. I–J is an enigma because it maps between E_β and E_α on chromosome 17, but there is not enough DNA in that position to code for the molecule. The structural gene may be on chromosome 4 and a regulatory gene on chromosome 17 in E.
3. Unlike other T cell subsets that bind antigen only in the context of MHC, T_s can bind free antigen. They also do not use a reaaranged β-chain gene as part of their receptor.
4. Suppressor and helper epitopes on antigen stimulate either T_s or T_h. These seem to be organized in a triad with the haptenic determinant on the antigen. Regulation is the balance of responses to these determinants.

CHAPTER TWENTY-THREE

5. T_s probably function via soluble suppressor factors. Factors that bind antigen and express I–J have been isolated.

6. T_s are generated through a regulatory circuit involving inducer, transducer, and effector cells. These cells communicate via soluble factors. A contrasuppressor cell may also play a role in regulation of the immune response.

Additional Readings

Dorf, M. E. and B. Benacerraf. 1984. Suppressor cells and immunoregulation. *Annu. Rev. Immunol.* 2, 127.

Golub, E. S. 1981. Suppressor T cells and their possible role in the regulation of autoreactivity. *Cell* 24, 595.

Green, D. R., P. M. Flood and R. K. Gershon. 1983. Immunoregulatory T cell pathways. *Annu. Rev. Immunol.* 1, 439.

Green, D. R. and R. K. Gershon. 1984. Contrasuppression: the second law of thermodynamics revisited. *Adv. Cancer Res.* 42, 277.

Hayes, C. E., K. K. Klyczed, D. P. Krumb, R. M. Whitcomb, D. A. Hullett and H. Cantor. 1983. Chromosome 4 Jt controls murine T cell surface I–J expression. *Science* 223, 559.

Moller, G. (ed.). 1985. I–J. *Immunol. Rev.* 83.

Webb, D. R., J. A. Kapp and C. W. Pierce. 1983. The biochemistry of antigen-specific T cell factors. *Annu. Rev. Immunol.* 1, 423.

CHAPTER 24

IMMUNE TOLERANCE: SELF–NONSELF DISCRIMINATION

Overview   Because immunology grew out of the study of infectious diseases, the imagery of its language still carries allusions to battle against invading hordes of hostile microbes and the protection of the sanctity of body. Paul Ehrlich was one of the first to write about the fact that in the process of protecting itself from external invaders, the body must take care not to react against itself. He called this bio-taboo against self reactivity *horror autotoxicus*. This was one of those ideas that is so brilliant and obvious that we immediately see that it is correct, wish we had said it first, quote it repeatedly, and then rarely really think about it again. The field of immunological tolerance is the rethinking of this idea.

In this chapter we will examine the experimental approaches to the question of self–nonself discrimination. The condition in which an animal "tolerates" an antigen by not making a response to it is called immunological tolerance. We will see that tolerance can be induced to a wide range of antigens in both the newborn and the adult and that both B and T cells can be rendered tolerant. Furthermore, we will see that the question of how the individual prevents destructive reactions has to be considered in terms of self-recognition of MHC. This raises the question of the difference, if any, between recognition and reaction.

CHAPTER TWENTY-FOUR

Self and Nonself

The central question in immunology has always been, How can the immune system discriminate between "foreign" and "self." Until immunologists were in a position to understand the fundamental processes by which responses to foreign antigens are carried out, there was little hope of understanding how responses to self were prevented. This is not to say that immunologists were not always aware of the question; rather, it shows the need to be able to frame a question that is amenable to the formulation of a testable hypothesis. At the turn of the century Paul Ehrlich stated the problem in Latin (which makes even the most banal content sound imposing) by calling the process of not making autoresponses *horror autotoxicus*. Of course, he was not in a position to predict a mechanism.

The Concept of the Self-Marker

The question of how the immune system prevents (or is prevented from) autoreactions was not seriously dealt with until 1949, when F. M. Burnet and F. Fenner published a monograph called *The Production of Antibodies*. Burnet and Fenner were heavily influenced by the work of Ray Owen at Caltech. Owen is a geneticist who was at that time interested in blood groups of cattle. He noted that the incidence of *monozygotic twins* in cattle as indicated by his blood tests was much greater than farmers and breeders knew to actually be the case. Owen drew upon F. R. Lillie's 1916 observation that *dizygotic twin* fetuses in cattle very often exchange blood because the placentas are so close together. When Owen treated the red cells of cattle that expressed both X and Y blood groups with anti-X antibody and complement, he found that some of the cells were not lysed. The unlysed cells could be shown to be expressing the Y blood group. He concluded that the apparent monozygotic twins were really chimeras—i.e., they were dizygotic twins that had shared the precursors of the blood cells of the other in utero. Because of this sharing, as adults each twin produced the red cells of the other, and each was not making immune responses to the other's red cell antigens. They were, in fact, treating the red cells of the other twin as if they were their own. Somehow the early contact with antigen rendered the animal able to "tolerate" the antigen.

IMMUNE TOLERANCE: SELF–NONSELF DISCRIMINATION

Burnet and Fenner put this very important observation into a theoretical framework by postulating that "self" is distinguished from "nonself" during embryonic development. They postulated a process called SELF-MARKING in which at some point in development the individual *marks* its own tissue in some unspecified manner. After this marking occurs, any antigen that enters the system will lack the self-marker and thus be identified as foreign. In the twin cattle, the precursors of the red cells had been shared and thus were marked. To test the hypothesis experimentally, Burnet and Fenner injected fertilized eggs with influenza virus and then determined whether the chickens that developed from these eggs had the ability to make anti-influenza antibody. Unfortunately, although all of the animals made antibody responses, it was because of the experimental system chosen. Later, in a more appropriate system, it was shown that introduction of antigen into the newborn results in tolerance.

The Experimental Induction of Tolerance in the Newborn

In 1951 Peter Medawar and his co-workers in England showed that a large proportion of dizygotic twin cattle could accept skin grafts from the other twin. Because Burnet and Fenner had cast the question in terms of Owen's discovery that these cattle were blood cell chimeras, Medawar and his group went on to intentionally induce the ability to accept skin grafts by establishing chimeras in laboratory animals. In these experiments, Billingham, Brent, and Medawar injected lymphoid cells from C57BL/6 mice into *newborn* mice of the A strain (Figure 1). When these animals reached maturity (about six to eight weeks), they were grafted with skin from mice of the same strain (A), or from two different strains (C57BL/6 or CBA). The A strain mice that had not been injected at birth rejected the skin from both CBA and C57BL/6. In contrast, those A strain mice which had been injected with the C57BL/6 cells rejected the CBA skin but *did not* reject the C57BL/6 skin (Figure 2). This meant that contact with foreign tissue at a very early stage of life (the experiments were also conducted by injecting mice in utero) allowed them to *tolerate* the specific foreign skin as if it were self. The results were consistent with the Burnet-Fenner hypothesis, and opened the way for the experimental testing of the mechanism of self–nonself discrimination.

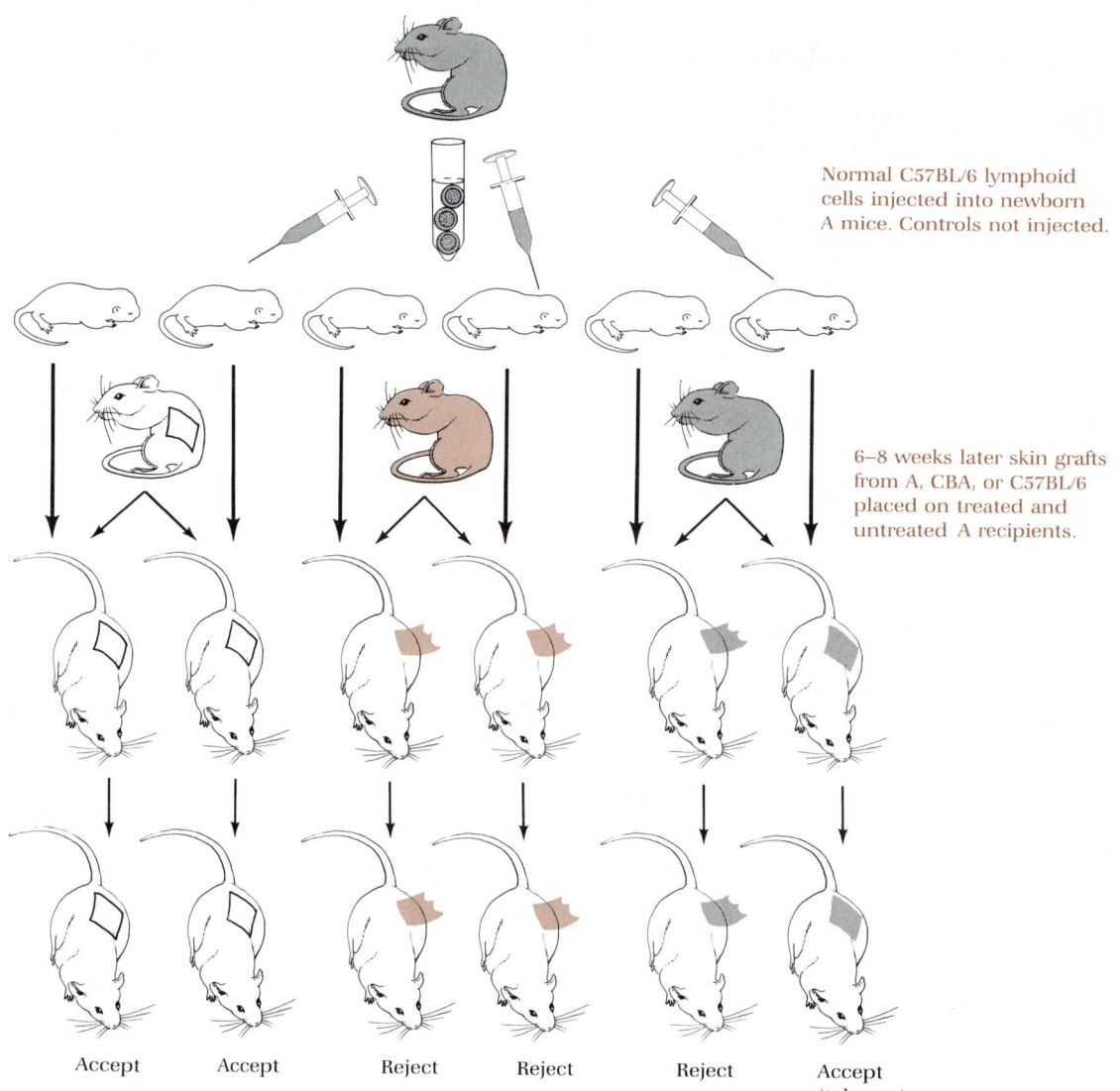

FIGURE 1 INDUCTION OF TOLERANCE IN THE NEWBORN

Lymph node cells from C57BL/6 mice are injected into newborn A mice. When these mice reach 6–8 weeks of age, they, along with normal A mice, are grafted with skin from either A, CBA, or C57BL/6 mice. The A and CBA skin serve as controls (A skin should be accepted and CBA skin rejected). The C57BL/6 skin is rejected by the untreated mice; but those mice receiving the neonatal injection of C57BL/6 tissue are rendered tolerant, and they accept the grafts. [After Billingham, Brent, and Medawar (1956) *Phil. Trans. R. Soc. London* B 239, 257]

IMMUNE TOLERANCE: SELF–NONSELF DISCRIMINATION

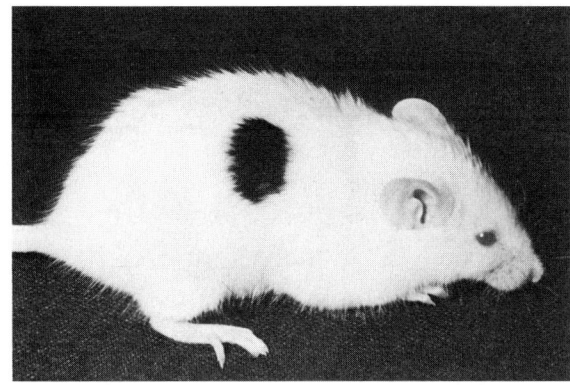

FIGURE 2   TOLERANT MOUSE WITH SKIN GRAFT

"A" strain mouse injected neonatally with lymph node cells from a C57BL/10 mouse. As an adult it received a skin graft from C57BL/10, which grew luxuriantly. [Photo courtesy of P.B. Medawar]

At about the same time, but for quite different reasons, M. Hasek in Prague was carrying out experiments that proved to be a test of the idea in chickens. Hasek had made a deliberate synchorial parabiosis between chick embryos in the shell so that they were exchanging blood. After hatching, the parabionts were separated and found to be incapable of making antibodies to each other's red cells or of rejecting grafts of the other's skin.

The "experiment of nature" that Owens had been astute enough to explain could now be repeated in the laboratory, and the stage was now set for inducing IMMUNOLOGICAL TOLERANCE—the ability to tolerate the presence of an antigen without making a response to it—in the newborn, so that self–nonself discrimination could be studied experimentally. In 1960 Burnet and Medawar shared the Nobel prize for their work. In his lecture Burnet stated that "when Medawar and his colleagues showed that immunological tolerance could be produced experimentally the new immunology was born."

The Triplett Experiment   According to the self-marker theory, all antigens are foreign unless antigen and immune system make physical contact before the functional differentiation of the immune system. This idea was tested by E. L. Triplett in 1961 in one of the more elegant experiments in immunology. Triplett reasoned that if a self component could be removed from the animal before the immune system developed, it would not be marked; then if it were returned to the animal at a later time, it should be recognized as foreign. The frog is a perfect experimental tool for this experiment because all stages of development occur where the experimenter can get at them. Triplett began by removing the pituitary glands from embryonic frogs. As they develop, these hypophysectomized animals are colorless, but they turn dark almost immediately after they receive a pituitary graft. If the graft is accepted, the animals remain dark; but if it is rejected, they revert to the colorless state. This provides a good method for assaying the response, if any, to the replaced pituitary.

Triplett grew the pituitaries that he had removed from individual frogs as implants in the dermis of feeding tadpoles. When the original hypophysectomized (and now colorless) animals grew to the proper stage *their own* pituitaries were re-implanted. The frogs very quickly became dark; but after about 40 days most of the animals became colorless again—they had rejected their own pituitary glands. In other words, they treated their own tissue, which had been temporarily removed, as if it were foreign.

The possibility that the antigens on the frog's pituitary had changed during the time it resided in the intermediate host was tested by performing a partial hypophysectomy, that is, leaving a piece of the pituitary in the animal and growing part of it in a tadpole. If the antigens had changed while growing in the tadpole, then the new piece would be recognized as foreign and rejected when reimplanted. They were not rejected, indicating that they had not acquired new antigens. This experiment very clearly shows that tolerance to an antigen requires that the antigen be present and come into contact with the immune system at a crucial stage of development. This idea has been a basic assumption in all studies of immune tolerance.

Naturally-Occurring Self-Reactivity

We have just developed arguments and evidence to justify the logical idea that the body must not react against itself. However, there are some cases in which there appears to be naturally-occurring autoreactivity without disease. The first thing that comes to mind, of course, is MHC

IMMUNE TOLERANCE: SELF–NONSELF DISCRIMINATION

restriction, whereby foreign antigens must be recognized in the context of self. But there is also a fairly large literature showing that there are reactive cells, both T and B, to tissue components. Normal humans and mice, for example, have cells reactive to thyroglobulin, and many normal individuals have titers of anti-autologous erythrocyte antibody in their serum. But, more convincing, when cells are activated polyclonally with mitogens, both cells and antibodies against a wide range of self antigens appear.

A reaction called the AUTOLOGOUS MIXED LYMPHOCYTE REACTION (A-MLR) is an MLR directed against self MHC antigens. When cells are cultured for an MLR, there is always "background" DNA synthesis, as measured by the incorporation of tritiated thymidine. But it was found that when autologous cells that had been treated with mitomycin and therefore cannot replicate their DNA are added to cultures of lymphocytes an increase in DNA synthesis occurs. This result is surprising, because the mitomycin-treated cells cannot be responsible, so they must be inducing the normal cells to proliferate. When the proportion of non-T cells in a population of normal cells is lowered, the background incorporation also goes down. But the decrease in background occurs in a much greater proportion than can be accounted for merely by the removal of non-T cells. In fact, it can be shown that autologous non-T cells stimulate autologous T cells to proliferate.

The responding T cells in the A-MLR in humans are T4 (and not T8) and are responsive to ConA. The stimulating cells are not clearly defined, and a wide range of hemopoietic cells may be able to stimulate. The stimulating cells express HLA-D and this may be the autoantigen to which the response occurs. The significance, if any, of the A-MLR is not known.

Induction of Tolerance in the Adult

Immunological Paralysis Introduction of antigen into the newborn, an action which results in tolerance, was quite naturally thought to be a means of studying the way the immune system develops "natural" tolerance to self. This seemed reminiscent to some people of a phenomenon known since the mid-1940s and called immunological paralysis. At that time Fel-

CHAPTER TWENTY-FOUR

ton had shown that the injection of a low dose (0.025 μg) of pneumococcal polysaccharide protected mice from a lethal infection of *Pneumococcus* organisms by eliciting anti-polysaccharide antibody. However, when immunization was carried out with a high dose (100 μg), little or no antibody was produced. It was not known whether the high dose of antigen prevented the mice from responding to the antigen, or whether they were making a response but the high concentration of slowly catabolized antigen in the body was absorbing the antibody as it was produced. When the phenomenon was later reexamined, it was found that there was indeed a central failure: the mice were not producing anti-pneumococcal antibody. This result indicates that tolerance can be induced not only to tissues in embryonic development, but also to foreign antigens in the adult.

Induction of Adult Tolerance

We now know that tolerance in the adult can be induced in several ways.

Form of the Antigen A protein antigen such as bovine γ globulin (BGG) can be ultracentrifuged to remove the aggregates. Injection of the aggregate-free antigen into adult mice results in a state of specific tolerance (Figure 3). Similarly, injection of hapten conjugated to a nonimmunogenic carrier results in tolerance to the hapten. For example, DNP conjugated to aggregate-free antigen results in tolerance to the hapten and to the carrier. When the injected hapten is conjugated to a *self* component, such as serum, tolerance to the hapten also is induced (Figure 4). Mice are injected either with autologous serum or a DNP-autologous serum conjugate. After a suitable interval they are challenged with DNP-KLH and the number of anti-DNP antibody-forming cells in the spleen is determined. It is clear from the figure that treatment with hapten conjugated to autologous serum renders the animals tolerant to challenge with the hapten conjugated to the immunogen.

Antigen Concentration Treating animals with extremes of antigen concentration also induces tolerance. Earlier we noted that a very high dose of pneumococcal polysaccharide resulted in im-

IMMUNE TOLERANCE: SELF–NONSELF DISCRIMINATION

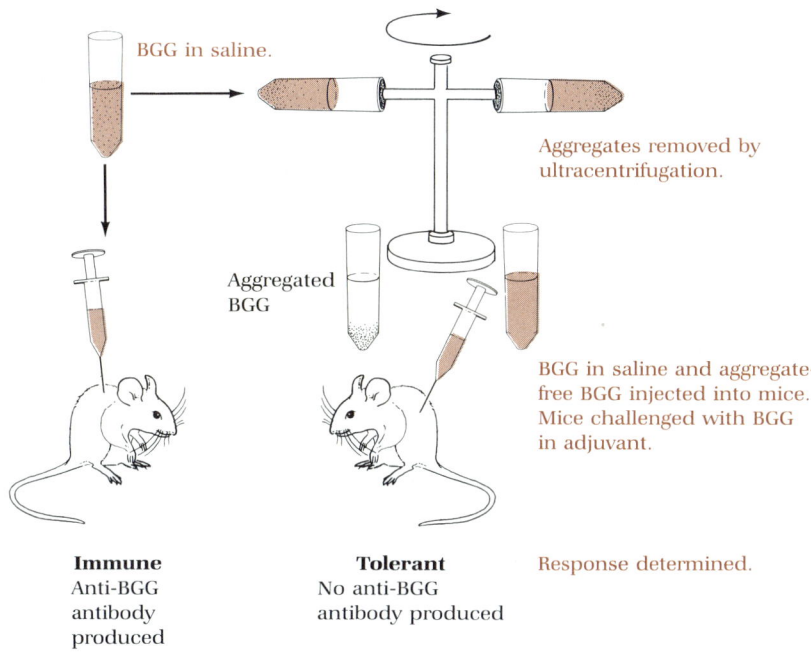

FIGURE 3   EFFECT OF ANTIGENIC FORM ON RESPONSE

The form of the antigen determines whether the response will be immunity or tolerance. BGG in saline is ultracentrifuged to remove aggregates. Injection of aggregate-free BGG induces tolerance (the mice do not make anti-BGG when challenged with BGG in adjuvant). Pretreatment with unfractionated BGG does not result in tolerance. This figure does not show that injection of the aggregates also results in anti-BGG antibody production. [After Dresser (1962) *Immunology* 5, 161]

mune paralysis. A very dramatic example of the effect of low dose as well as high dose can be seen in the now-classic 1964 experiment by Mitchison (Figure 5). Groups of mice were injected with various doses of soluble bovine serum albumin (BSA) three times a week for up to 16 weeks. In this way the effect of dose and time could be determined. The animals were then challenged with an immunogenic form of BSA and the anti-BSA antibody titers determined. When the data were plotted, it was found that high doses

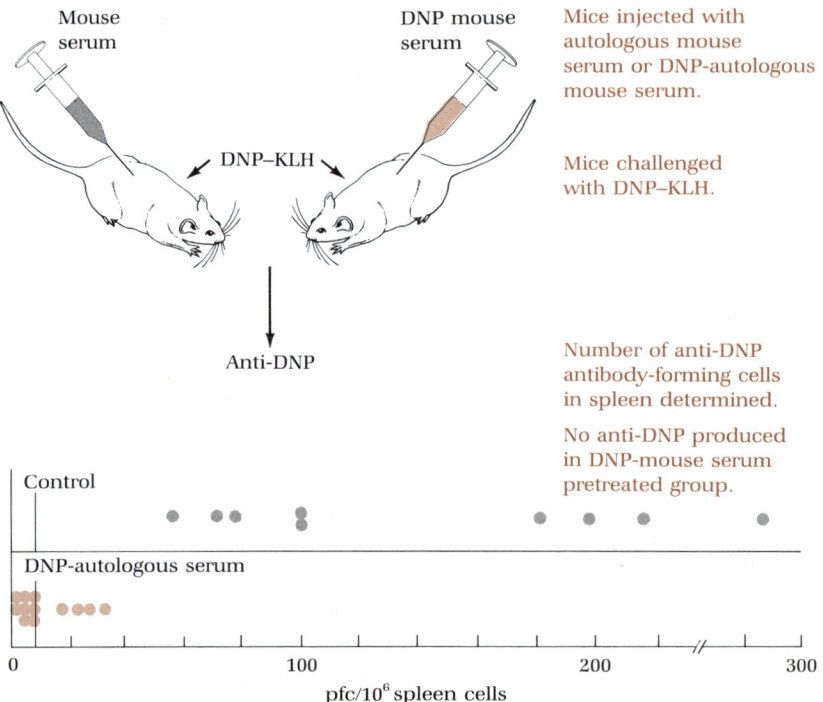

FIGURE 4 TOLERANCE TO HAPTEN

Immunization with DNP conjugated to autologous serum results in tolerance. Groups of mice are pretreated with either untreated autologous serum or DNP-autologous serum. After challenge with DNP-KLH, the DNP–serum-treated group fails to produce anti-DNP antibody; that is, they are tolerant to DNP. [After Borel (1971) *Nature New Biol.* 230, 180]

of tolerogen induced tolerance (as expected). Also as expected, slightly lower doses did not induce tolerance. But the surprise was that very low doses were tolerogenic. This phenomenon is called LOW ZONE TOLERANCE and has been observed with several antigens.

Antibody-Induced Tolerance Tolerance can also be induced by administering antibody. This has been observed in experimental systems both in vivo and in vitro. In this experiment various

IMMUNE TOLERANCE: SELF–NONSELF DISCRIMINATION

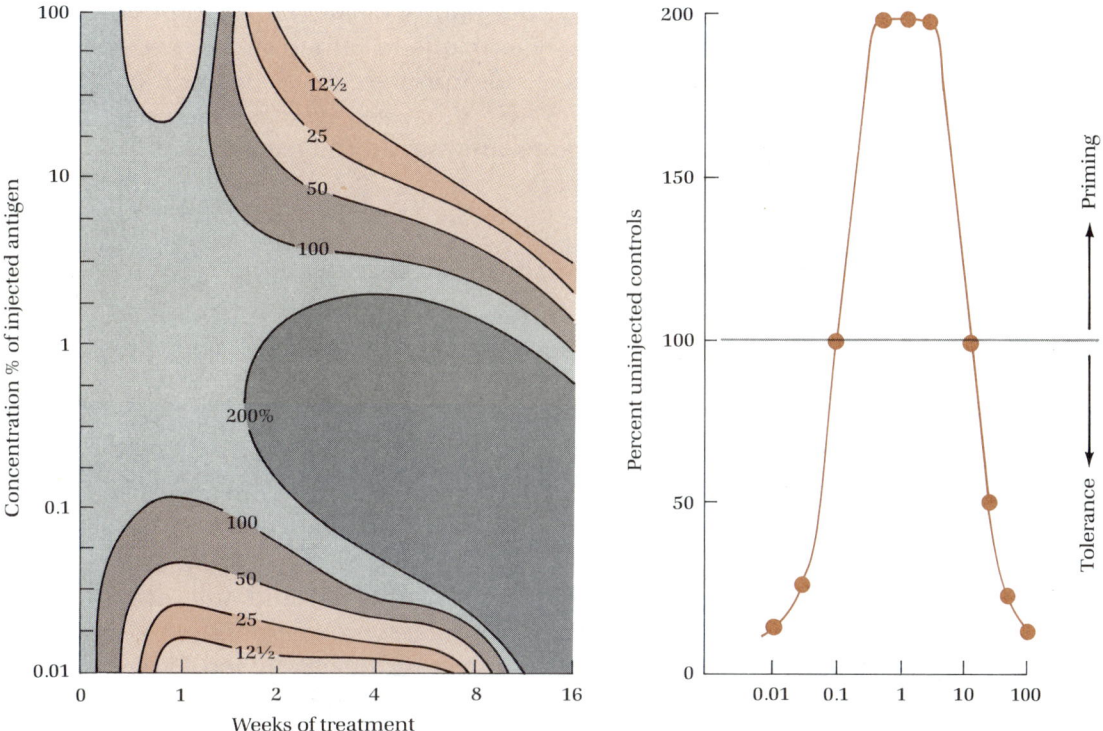

FIGURE 5   HIGH ZONE AND LOW ZONE TOLERANCE

"Contour" map (left) showing that repeated injection with a mid-range dose of antigen for two or more weeks results in immunity (gray) whereas treatment with either a high or a low dose results in tolerance (brown). (Right) Conventional graph of the data. [After Mitchison (1964) *Proc. R. Soc. London* B 161, 275]

amounts of anti-polymerized flagellin (anti-POL) antibody were added to cultures of normal spleen cells. The cultures were then immunized to either POL or sheep red blood cells (SRBC) as a specificity control. It was found that the presence of anti-POL antibody in the cultures inhibits the POL response by the cultures but has no effect on the SRBC response; that is, a state of specific tolerance to POL has been induced by pretreatment with anti-POL.

CHAPTER TWENTY-FOUR

The preceding examples make it abundantly clear that tolerance can be induced to a wide range of antigens in either embryonic, neonatal, or adult animals. As we now prepare to examine the mechanism(s) of tolerance, the reader must ask whether or not all or any of these forms of tolerance are indeed the experimental counterparts of "natural tolerance."

Mechanisms of Immune Tolerance

Induction of Tolerance in B cells and T cells

So far we have established that tolerance can be induced in both newborns and adults to a variety of antigens in a variety of ways. To understand the mechanism (or, almost certainly, the mechanisms) of tolerance induction, it is important to know whether tolerance can be established in both B and T cells. The first approach to this question was carried out by Jacques Chiller and his colleagues in La Jolla (Figure 6). The plan of the experiment was to repopulate irradiated recipients with combinations of normal and tolerant bone marrow and thymus cells to determine which population is tolerant. Tolerance was induced by injecting deaggregated HGG into adult mice. After a suitable interval, bone marrow and thymus cell suspensions were made and used in combination with normal bone marrow and thymus cells to repopulate irradiated recipients. In this manner groups of recipients were repopulated with tolerant thymus and normal bone marrow, normal thymus and tolerant marrow, tolerant thymus and tolerant marrow, and normal thymus and normal marrow. All of the groups were then challenged with antigen in the immunogenic form, and the ability of the recipients to make an anti-HGG response was tested.

As shown in Figure 6A, groups receiving *either* tolerant bone marrow cells or tolerant thymus cells were tolerant, showing that both populations can be rendered tolerant. The experiment was carried out in such a manner that the kinetics of induction could also be investigated. Figure 6B shows that T cell tolerance is acquired quickly and lasts a very long time. In contrast, B cell tolerance appears later and wanes quickly. Originally this was interpreted to mean that T cell tolerance was easier to induce. But when the notion of suppressor T cells gained acceptance, the

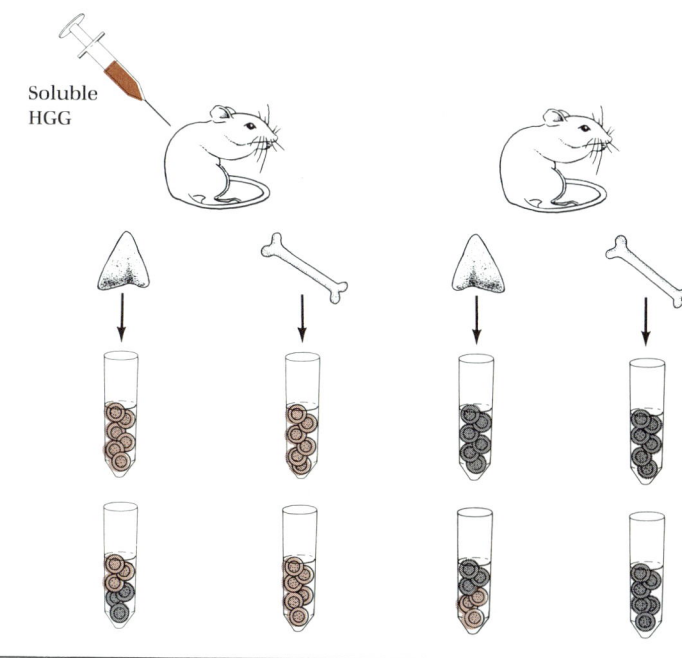

FIGURE 6 TOLERANCE IN B AND T CELLS

(A) Tolerance is induced with deaggregated HGG (DHGG), and bone marrow and thymus cells from the tolerant mice are injected into irradiated recipients along with normal thymus or bone marrow. After challenge with antigen, the mice receiving either tolerant thymus or tolerant bone marrow cells are tolerant. (B) Kinetics of tolerance induction in thymus and bone marrow cells. Thymus cells are tolerant early and remain tolerant. Bone marrow cells become tolerant later and lose tolerance faster. [After Chiller et al. (1971) *Science* 171, 813]

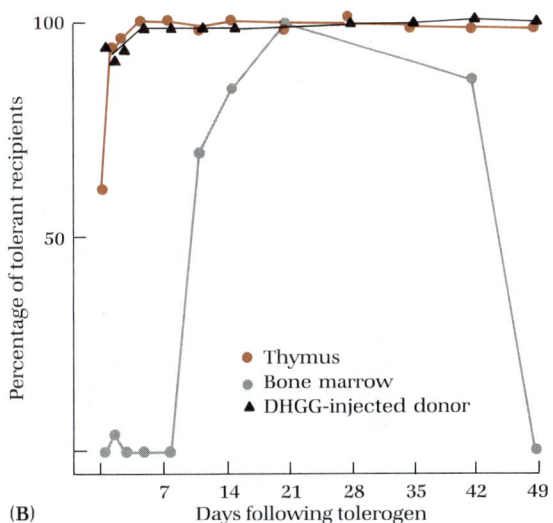

428
CHAPTER TWENTY-FOUR

possibility that the T cell tolerance was due to suppressor T cells became a likely interpretation. The resolution of this question required the development of methods using cloned T cells.

Using cloned T helper cells it has been shown that tolerance can be induced in T cells in vitro. In these experiments (Figure 7), a cloned human T cell line that responds to a peptide antigen from the influenza virus was incubated with various concentrations of the antigen in the absence of B cells or accessory cells. After an interval, the cells were washed and B cells and accessory cells were added to one group. Interleukin-2 was added to another group to show that the cells still had the ability to respond

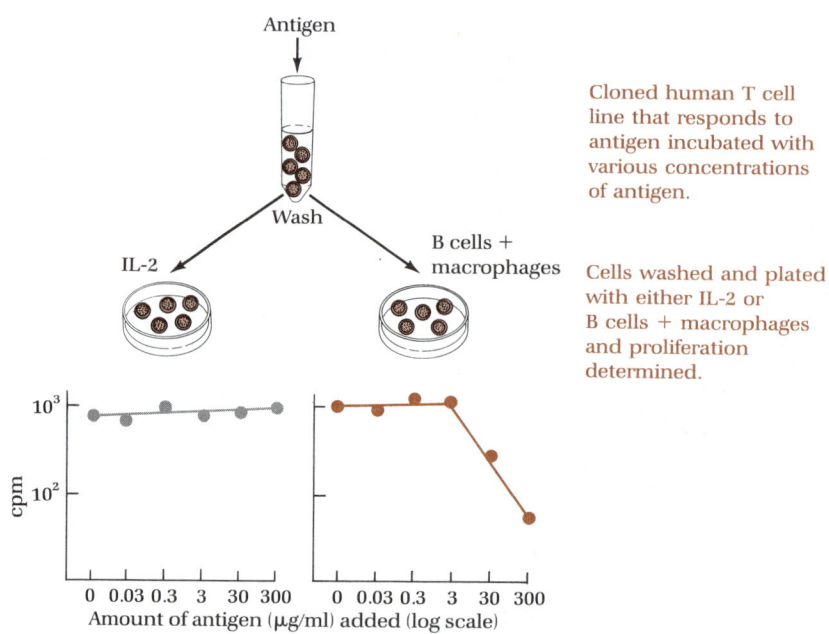

FIGURE 7 TOLERANCE INDUCED IN T CELL CLONES

Cloned T helper cells are pretreated with various concentrations of antigen. After washing, they are incubated with B cells and macrophages (right) or IL-2 (left). Pretreatment does not affect the ability to proliferate in the presence of IL-2 but does prevent antigen-induced proliferation at concentrations of antigen greater than 3 μg/ml of antigen. [After Lamb et al. (1985) *J. Exp. Med.* 161, 897]

IMMUNE TOLERANCE: SELF–NONSELF DISCRIMINATION

to signals. It can be seen that preincubation with antigen did not affect the ability of the cells to respond to IL-2. In contrast, preincubation with antigen above 30 μg/ml did prevent the cells from responding to antigen. This result indicates that this dose of antigen had induced a state of tolerance. Appropriate specificity controls showed that the loss of ability to respond was only for the preincubated antigen. This experiment shows that T cells can in fact be rendered tolerant, but it does not address the question of whether or not there are suppressor T cells in the tolerant state and what the relative contribution of suppressor cells versus some other mechanism may be. This very important but unresolved problem will be discussed later.

Eleanor Metcalf and Norman Klinman, in a very elegant series of experiments (Figure 8), showed that B cells at *early* stages of differentiation are rendered tolerant. Using a spleen microfocus-forming assay they found that immature B cells, in the absence of helper T cells, were rendered tolerant after confrontation with antigen. However, if helper T cells were present at the time of antigen presentation, a productive antibody response was made. More recently, others have shown that similar results are obtained with surface Ig-negative pre-B cells isolated by flow cytometry.

Mature B cells can also be rendered tolerant by direct contact with antigen. In these studies—done by many groups but especially by Gus Nossal in Melbourne—it appears that somehow the antigen-specific receptors (i.e., the sIgM) must be affected so that receptor reorganization cannot be accomplished. (The importance of receptor aggregation was discussed in Chapter 21.) In this form of tolerance induction the receptors become unable to transduce the signal to the cell. For this reason the mechanism is called RECEPTOR BLOCKADE.

Little doubt remains that both B cells and T cells can be rendered tolerant; what remains to be learned is the mechanism of this tolerance.

Clonal Deletion, Clonal Abortion, Clonal Anergy, or Tolerant Cells?

In the original version of the clonal selection theory, Burnet explained the phenomenon of immunological tolerance by postulating the *deletion* of clones. He predicted that lymphocytes that come into contact with antigen

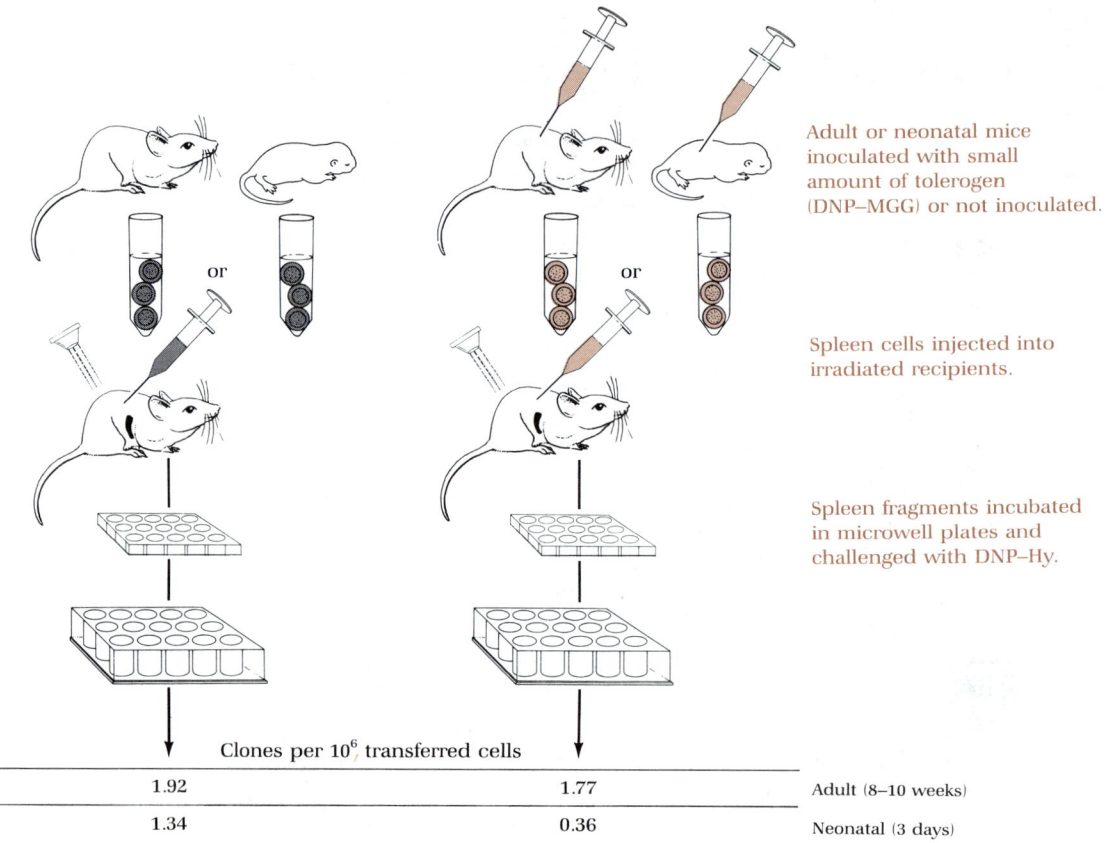

FIGURE 8 TOLERANCE INDUCTION IN NEONATAL B CELLS

Adult and newborn mice are pretreated with DNP-MGG to induce tolerance to DNP, and the spleen cells of these tolerant mice or untreated controls are injected into irradiated recipients. Spleen fragments from the recipients are then cultured in vitro with DNP-Hy to induce anti-DNP antibody. Nontreated spleens give foci of antibody formation, but spleen cells from pretreated newborns do not. [After Metcalf and Klinman (1976) *J. Exp. Med.* 143, 1327]

early in their differentiation would be killed; that is, the clones would be deleted rather than induced to proliferate, as adult lymphocytes are. Nossal and his colleagues have carried out a very large series of experiments over the years addressing this crucial question. The experiments of Metcalf and Klinman have shown that young B cells are rendered tolerant by contact with antigen and the experiments by Nossal's group have shown that

IMMUNE TOLERANCE: SELF–NONSELF DISCRIMINATION

receptor blockade could occur. Nossal has concluded that the sensitivity to loss of function by young B cells after contact with antigen is seen just after the emergence of surface IgM and before the cells express IgD. He postulates that tolerance is the result of an interruption of the differentiation of the cell, an interruption preventing clones of mature B cells of that specificity from developing. He called this phenomenon CLONAL ABORTION, to indicate that the differentiation process had been aborted before the full functional expression of the clone could be achieved.

If tolerance is due to the elimination of antigen-specific clones, then antigen-binding cells for the specific antigen should be absent from tolerant animals. When Nossal tested this point, he found that essentially normal levels of antigen-binding B cells were present (Figure 9). This result led him to conclude that

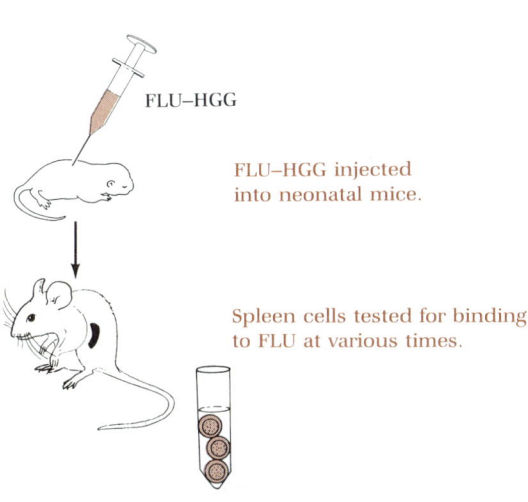

Weeks after injection	Antigen-binding cells per 10^6 cells	
	Control	FLU–HGG
1	119	67
2	146	117
4	147	118
6	161	150

FIGURE 9 **TOLERANT MICE HAVE ANTIGEN BINDING CELLS**

Neonatal mice were rendered tolerant to the hapten fluorescein (FLU) by treatment with FLU-HGG. The number of FLU-binding cells is determined at 1, 2, 4, or 6 weeks later. [After Nossal and Pike (1980) *PNAS* 77, 1602]

tolerance is not due to *physical* elimination of cells but rather to a "recognition and storage of negative signals" that prevents the cells from making responses to the antigen even though they have the receptors. Because the cells are present but not functional, he calls this phenomenon CLONAL ANERGY.

If the idea of clonal anergy is correct then the next experiments in tolerance studies must be an identification of the nature of the anergy. Why do the cells that are capable of binding antigen not respond to it, and what is the nature of the "negative signals"?

The Veto Concept

A possible cellular mechanism for the functional elimination of clones has been proposed by Rick Miller in Toronto. He has introduced the notion of the VETO CELL. As we know, lymph node populations that contain pre-cytotoxic cells (pCTL) give rise to cytotoxic T cells (CTL) when incubated with stimulator cells. But Miller has shown that when spleen cells from athymic nude mice (nu/nu) are included in the initial incubation, the pCTL do not develop into CTL (Table 1). The BALB/c responder lymph nodes develop CTL to either B10 or RNC stimulator cells, even in the presence of BALB/c nude spleen cells. But when the BALB/c lymph node cells are incubated with RNC nude spleen cells, they do not develop CTL to the RNC even

TABLE 1 Veto cell in the nu/nu spleen.

Responder	Stimulator	Target	
BALB/c lymph node	RNC or B10	RNC	Kill
		B10	Kill
BALB/c lymph node + BALB/c nu/nu spleen	RNC or B10	RNC	Kill
		B10	Kill
BALB/c lymph node + RNC nu/nu spleen	RNC or B10	RNC	No kill
		B10	Kill

Source: After Miller (1980), *Nature* 287: 544.

IMMUNE TOLERANCE: SELF–NONSELF DISCRIMINATION

though they develop normal levels of CTL to B10. Thus the inability to respond is specific.

Miller has suggested that the cell in the nu/nu spleen can "veto" a developing clone so that tolerance can be established. According to this model (Figure 10), whenever a pCTL for self is generated, it comes into contact with the "veto" cell, which eliminates it.

Suppressor Cells in Tolerance

When the idea that suppressor cells could be a major mode of regulation of the immune response became established, many groups began to look for the presence of suppressor cells in the tolerant state. There is very clear evidence that they exist in tolerance induced in both adults and newborns to a wide variety of antigens ranging from serum proteins to allogeneic tissues. What we do not know is whether they exist to self antigens or whether they are a major means of maintaining tolerance to self. Even though it is often stated that this is the true role of the suppressor cell, the evidence for such a statement is still not conclusive.

Synthesis: Recognition and Response in MHC Restriction and Tolerance

We have seen that a good case can be made for the existence of the "tolerant cell." Assuming that such a cell exists, we know nothing about the nature of this wonderous condition. Nor do we

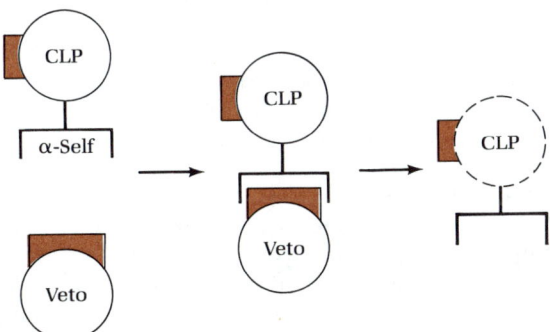

FIGURE 10 VETO CONCEPT
The veto cell eliminates anti-self receptors, using the anti-self cell's receptors.

know the relative contribution of suppressor cells to the tolerant state. If we assume that clones are deleted (either physically or functionally) in some experimentally induced tolerant conditions, can we argue that this is how natural self-tolerance is induced and maintained?

During the next few years these questions should be able to be addressed because we will certainly have learned the nature of MHC restriction. In this text we have been discussing MHC restriction in terms of the system needing to *recognize* self in order to *react* to foreign. If tolerance results from the loss of cells that are able to recognize antigen, then self-tolerance is caused by the absence of cells bearing receptors for self antigens. Should the mechanism of MHC restriction be through recognition of a neoantigenic determinant and not through the simultaneous recognition of antigen and self, then there is no conceptual problem because self, as such, is not being recognized. But should MHC restriction turn out to be due to the simultaneous recognition of self and foreign by separate receptors, then we will have to explain tolerance through a model that retains receptors for self components. If receptors to self components are needed to react to foreign antigen, then tolerance will be a problem of preventing *productive* reactions while maintaining the ability to make *regulatory* reactions.

Summary

1. The question of how the immune system discriminates between self and nonself is the most fundamental question in immunology. The condition in which an animal "tolerates" an antigen by not responding to it is called immune tolerance.
2. Tolerance can be induced in newborn and adult animals to a wide variety of antigens. In the adult, the form and concentration of the antigen are crucial factors in determining whether there will be a response or tolerance.
3. Tolerance can be induced in both B cells and T cells.
4. The mechanism(s) of tolerance induction are not known. Two alternatives are deletion of clones and inability of clones to respond. Deletion could be physical (clonal deletion) or functional (deletion by recep-

IMMUNE TOLERANCE: SELF–NONSELF DISCRIMINATION

tor blockade or by aborted differentiation of a clone, or clonal abortion). The inability of clones to respond to antigen could also be due to negative signals in the tolerant cell (clonal anergy).

4. The suppressor T cell may play a role in maintenance of tolerance, and the veto cell may be important in the induction of tolerance to self.

Additional Readings

Gershon, R. K. and K. Kondo. 1971. Infectious immunological tolerance. *Immunol.* 21, 903.

Golub, E.S. 1981. Immune tolerance and autoreactivity: Do they point to a regulatory role of the immune system for normal cell function? *Cell* 24, 417.

Miller, R. G. 1980. An immunological suppressor cell inactivating cytotoxic T lymphocyte precursor cells recognizing it. *Nature* 287, 544.

Mitchison, N. A. 1978. New ideas about self-tolerance and autoimmunity. *Clinics Rheumatic Dis.* 4, 539.

Nossal, G. V. J. 1983. Cellular mechanisms of immunologic tolerance. *Annu. Rev. Immunol.* 1, 33.

Weksler, M. E., C. E. Moody Jr. and R. W. Kozak. 1981. The autologous mixed-lymphocyte reaction. *Adv. Immunol* 31, 271.

PART THREE
IMMUNITY AND IMMUNOPATHOLOGY

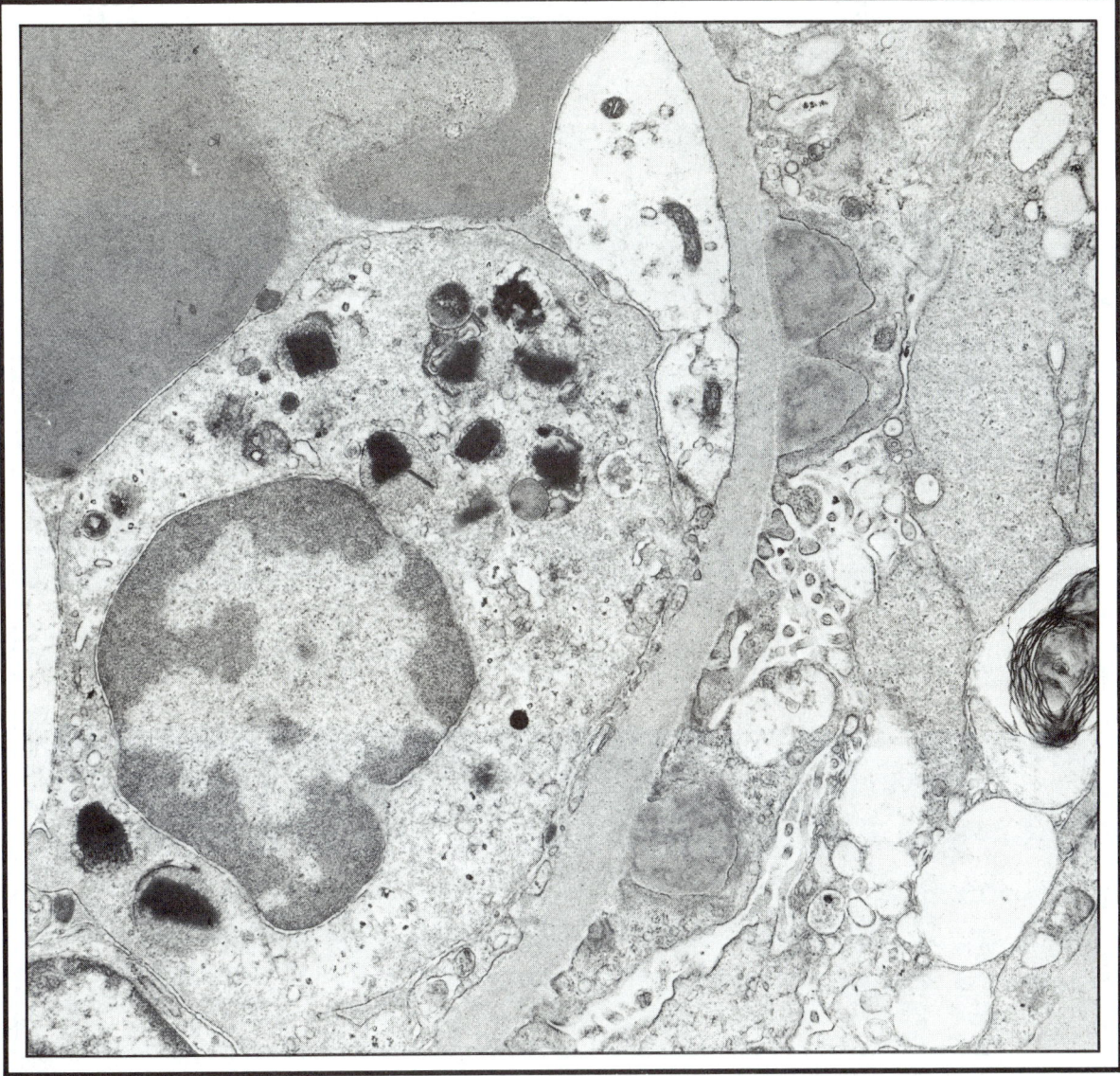

> Diseases desperate grown,
> By desperate appliances are reliev'd,
> Or not at all.
>
> WILLIAM SHAKESPEARE

The purpose of these chapters on immunity and immunopathology is to attempt to put some of the consequences—both good and bad—of the actions of the immune system into a context in which they will be explained by all that has gone before. These chapters are not a catalog of clinical woes, but will let the reader see how the knowledge we have gained about the immune response can be applied to the human condition.

CHAPTER 25

IMMUNITY, INFECTIONS, AND TUMORS

Overview The specific immune response first appeared in the evolutionary tree with the chordates, which means probably 99.999% of the rest of the animals in the world have been doing quite well without it. Their world is as full of potential pathogens as is the world of the animals in the phylum Chordata, so the majority of animals are able to survive with other defense mechanisms. In this chapter we will see that the basic means of achieving immunity are through nonspecific defense mechanisms. These nonspecific mechanisms are also used by the chordates, who have added the specific immune response, thereby making them more efficient.

We will see that the combination of specific and nonspecific immune responses works to protect the organism from external invaders (bacteria, viruses, parasites) and may have evolved in such a manner as to also play a role in the defense against internal invaders such as tumors. Whether the disease is due to external or internal invasion, the invader survives at the expense of the host and is therefore called a parasite. The study of immunity is really the study of the host–parasite relationship. The outcomes of host–parasite relationships depend on factors that allow one or the other to win the battle. The host first uses its nonspecific factors. If this fails, the specific immune response is then used to augment various aspects of nonspecific immunity.

CHAPTER TWENTY-FIVE
The Response to External Invaders: Host–Parasite Relationships

At the outset we defined immunity as the ability to resist infection and remain free from disease. The specific adaptive immune response that we have been studying in this text is one part of the armementarium the body uses to achieve this end. Even the use of the term *armementarium* shows that this process has been visualized as a battle between two opposing forces, one good and one very bad. Because history is always written by the winners, we will be looking at how the good guys do it.

All animals live in a world filled with potentially hostile and harmful species. Perhaps as a result of their neurological development, humans have elevated the natural acts of predation and defense, which the rest of the biological world uses for survival, to the high arts of murder, warfare, and apartheid. But even in the absence of these fine arts, the average member of the biological majority is constantly prey to parasites and predators. We study these in the life cycles of animals and in the interdependence of various species. Public television alone has filled our hours with images of mating moose and predatory panthers in an attempt to personalize nature (or perhaps more correctly, *Nature*). But if one species is dependent upon another for its survival, the only way the first species can maintain itself is to develop a relationship that is beneficial to itself without eliminating the second species. When two species are mutually beneficial and dependent their relationship is called COMMENSALISM. But if one species survives at the expense of the other the relationship is called PARASITISM. Infectious diseases are examples of parasitism. Because the infectious agent benefits at the expense of the organism it has infected, it is the PARASITE. The organism that is parasitized is called the HOST. The "perfect parasite" has evolved a relationship with its host that may be very harmful to the host but still allows enough members of the host species to survive to assure the continued existence of the parasite. The outcome of the infection is determined at several levels by the relationship that is established between the host and the parasite—that is, the host–parasite relationship.[1]

---

[1] The term *parasite* is also used to identify a class of invading organisms, such as trypanosomes and schistosomes, but we will use the term in its general meaning.

IMMUNITY, INFECTIONS, AND TUMORS

Factors Affecting the Host-Parasite Relationship

PHYSIOLOGICAL INCOMPATIBILITY between the two potential interactants is one factor that can affect the potential host–parasite relationship. For example, if a bacterium survives at an optimal temperature of 56°C (a thermophilic bacterium) and the body temperature of the host is 37°C, the host has a NATURAL IMMUNITY to the parasite. Similarly, if the optimal temperature of the invading organism is 37°C but the host is a frog whose body temperature is 26°C, the invader will not grow.

The intact host also has a series of ANATOMICAL BARRIERS that can prevent or deter the infectious agent. The skin is an animal's first line of defense. If the skin remains intact, an invading organism, which requires the temperature, moisture, and nutrients that are inside the body, will be prevented from reaching a compatible environment and will die. Breaks in the skin, therefore, are breaks in the host's defense system because they allow the potential parasite access to a favorable growth environment.

All animals have bacteria that live in and on them, either as perfect parasites or as commensals. These microorganisms constitute the NATURAL FLORA of the host. Mammals, for example, rely on the bacteria of the gut to produce vitamin K, which they are incapable of producing themselves. (The gut is really outside the body, being a lumen around which the body is formed.) In many cases, these organisms of the natural flora act to prevent the growth of invading organisms. But the balance is a very delicate one; and given a change from "normal" conditions, members of the natural flora can become harmful. For example, normal human skin has populations of the bacterium *Staphylococcus aureus*. These organisms cause no harm when they are on the skin, but if the skin is broken and the staph are given access to the inner milieu, they can cause pustules or even severe systemic infections. The common bacterium of the gut, *Escherichia coli*, is a necessary part of our natural flora, but if it leaves the gut and enters the body as a result of trauma to the gut wall, the result can be severe peritonitis.

HOST SECRETIONS can also be a factor in preventing the invading organisms from gaining a foothold. For example, secretions such as saliva, tears, and nasal secretions contain the enzyme LYSOZYME, which cleaves a sugar linkage that is very common in

CHAPTER TWENTY-FIVE

the cell walls of bacteria. The invading organism that lands on a surface bathed by lysozyme-rich secretions is liable to be killed before it can do much harm. Organisms that are ingested and reach the stomach are subjected to extremely low pH, and if they are susceptible to low pH (as many bacteria are), they are killed.

It is likely that under ordinary circumstances these first lines of defense are all that most members of the species need in order to carry on their day-to-day activities of preying upon and being preyed upon. In those instances when these first-line defenses are not enough, another, very powerful, nonspecific defense, called the inflammatory response, has evolved.

The Inflammatory Response

The Cardinal Signs of Inflammation

The INFLAMMATORY RESPONSE is the vascular lymphatic and local tissue reaction elicited in higher animals by the presence of microorganisms or nonviable irritants. This complex response, aspects of which are seen throughout the animal kingdom, has evolved as the most effective defense mechanism in the animal world.

The various aspects of the inflammatory response can be seen by the response to a simple thing like a sliver of wood in the finger. The piece of wood becomes inserted under the skin, and after a few hours the area becomes red. After a while one notices that there is swelling and pain and, if the area is large enough, one notices that it is perceptibly warmer than the surrounding tissue. These are the conditions that have been known since the time of the ancients as INFLAMMATION.[2]

The Greek physician Celcus (ca. 30 B.C. to A.D. 38) described the "Four Cardinal Signs of Inflammation," a phrase that is still used. These four signs are REDNESS (*rubor*), SWELLING (*tumor*), HEAT (*calor*), and PAIN (*dolor*). The first person to write extensively on inflammation was the great Galen (A.D. 130–200), who added a

---

[2] Pus, which we will see is a consequence of inflammatory responses, was described in Egyptian papyri of the second millennium B.C. as being related to the demons of disease. The school of Hippocrates noted the reddening of the skin and called it *erysipelas* (literally, "redness of the skin"). They called the swelling *oidema*, which we now call edema.

IMMUNITY, INFECTIONS, AND TUMORS

fifth sign, LOSS OF FUNCTION. The first of the more modern physicians to write on inflammation was John Hunter (1728–1793).

The redness and heat are caused by an increase in blood flow to the area of trauma and by constriction of the blood vessels that carry blood away from the area. The constriction occurs immediately after the trauma. Capillary permeability increases; consequently both fluids and blood cells leave the capillaries, and cause swelling and pain (a result of increased pressure). From our point of view, however, the most important thing to occur is the exit of phagocytic cells from the capillaries to the extracellular spaces. The most common cell type accumulating at the site of infection is the phagocytic leukocytes, primarily granulocytes (also known as polymorphonuclear neutrophils, or PMNs).

Granulocytes in Inflammation

The GRANULOCYTES are one of the body's most efficient scavenger systems. They are cells that have the ability to engulf particles by the process of phagocytosis and in some cases to destroy them. Thus the inflammatory response acts as a means of bringing scavenger cells to the site of a breach in the first line of defense.

During the inflammatory response the capillary endothelial surfaces become sticky, thus causing the PMNs to attach to the capillary walls. The PMNs then leave the capillaries by migrating between the cells of the capillary walls. Many microorganisms elaborate CHEMOTACTIC FACTORS toward which the cells migrate after leaving the capillaries. The FORMAMYL PEPTIDES, F-met-phe and F-met-leu-phe, are powerful chemotactic agents that are found in many microbes and have been used extensively to study chemotaxis.[3] The complement component C5a, which can be generated either by the classical or the alternative pathway, is also a powerful chemotactic agent. In addition, the complement components C3a and C5a are both ANAPHYLOTOXINS—substances that cause the release of histamine from mast cells, thus causing further increase of vascular permeability.

---

[3] These peptides are found only on prokaryotic organisms, so we may be witness here to two balancing forces in evolution. I thank Larry Draper for pointing this out to me.

CHAPTER TWENTY-FIVE

There are some cases in which the inflammatory response itself can cause the symptoms of the disease. For example, in tuberculosis, the invading organisms (*Mycobacterium tuberculosis*) enter the lung tissue and induce an inflammatory response. The defensive cells that arrive, first granulocytes and then monocytes, ingest the turbercle bacilli, but the parasite in this case has evolved a defense mechanism of its own. *Mycobacterium tuberculosis* has a cell wall that prevents it from being destroyed after it is phagocytized; in fact, it grows inside the monocytes and eventually kills them. Thus there is a chronic inflammatory response going on in the lung, with more monocytes being attracted to the site. Eventually the mass of inflammatory cells causes so much damage to the lung tissue that the symptoms of tuberculosis become manifest: shortness of breath, tiredness, loss of weight, and the classic symptoms of the cough and bloody sputum. In most cases of parasitic invasion, however, the inflammatory response is an efficient and beneficial response.

Phagocytosis

The PMNs that are attracted to the site of infection and inflammation PHAGOCYTIZE the microbes. The notion of phagocytosis as a general defense mechanism was championed by Metchnikoff (1845–1916). This marvelously eccentric man had for complicated reasons resigned his professorship at Messina in 1882 and was relaxing on the shores of the Mediterranean when the whole business of immunity became clear to him.

> I was resting from the shock of the events which provoked my resignation from the University and indulging enthusiastically in researches in the splendid setting of the Straits of Messina.
>
> One day the family had gone to a circus to see some extraordinary performing apes. I remained alone at my microscope, observing the life in the mobile cells of the transparent starfish larva, when a new thought suddenly flashed across my brain. It struck me that similar cells might serve in the defense of the organism against intruders. Feeling that there was in this something of surpassing interest, I felt so excited that I began striding up and down the room and even went to the seashore in order to collect my thoughts.

IMMUNITY, INFECTIONS, AND TUMORS

> I said to myself that, if my supposition was true, a splinter introduced into the body of a starfish larva, devoid of blood vessels or of a nervous system, should soon be surrounded by mobile cells as is to be observed in a man who runs a splinter into his finger. This was no sooner said than done.
>
> There was a small garden to our dwelling, in which we had a few days previously organized a "Christmas tree" for the children on a little tangerine tree; I fetched from it a few rose thorns and introduced them at once under the skin of some beautiful starfish larvae as transparent as water.
>
> I was too excited to sleep that night in the expectation of the result of my experiment, and very early the next morning I ascertained that it had fully succeeded.
>
> That experiment formed the basis of the phagocyte theory, to the development of which I devoted the next twenty-five years of my life. [Quoted in Humphrey and White, *Immunology for Medical Students*, 3rd ed., p. 14]

Metchnikoff, clearly no shrinking violet, soon became embroiled in a controversy over the relative roles of the phagocytic cells and the humoral factors (i.e., antibody) in immunity. We now know that both are important and that the antibody (from the specific immune response) enhances some aspects of the phagocytic process (from the nonspecific response).

The mechanism of phagocytosis is very well studied, and we will go into only enough detail to see how the process is used in immunity. After microbes contact the surface of the PMN, its membrane folds around the particles, bringing them into the interior of the cell. The microbes are now in a vacuole called a PHAGOSOME, whose membrane is formed by the cell membrane of the PMN (Figure 1). One of the characteristic features of the PMN is the presence of large, prominent GRANULES. These granules are in fact LYSOSOMES, which are essentially bags of proteolytic enzymes. DEGRANULATION occurs when the phagosome and several lysosomes fuse, causing the lysosomes to dump the contents of their granules into the phagosome. The lysosomal contents, along with peroxide and superoxides (which are products of the metabolic process during phagocytosis) then aid in the killing of the microbes that have been ingested.

CHAPTER TWENTY-FIVE

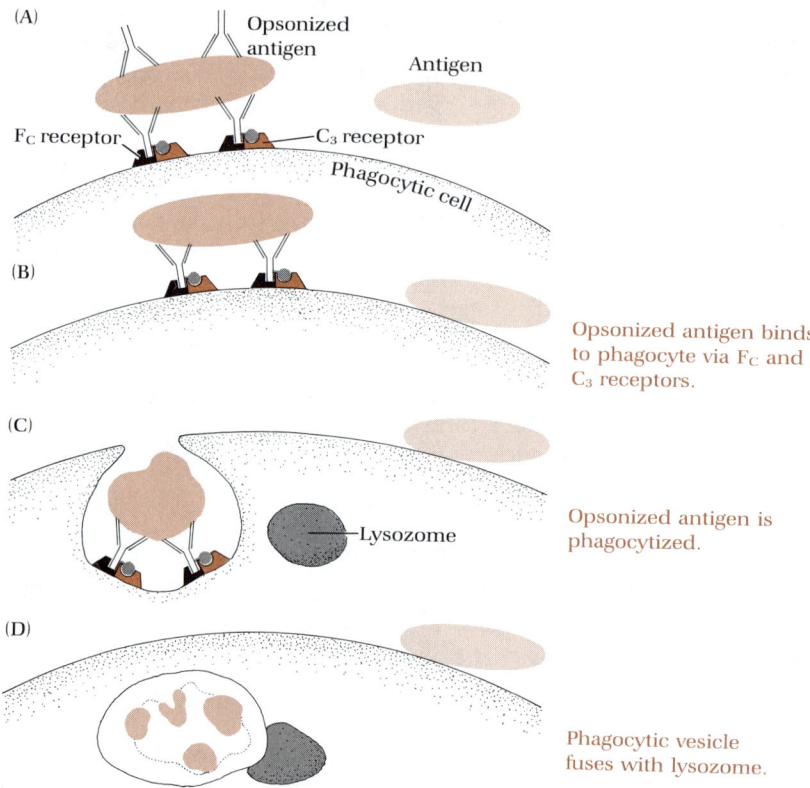

FIGURE 1   THE EVENTS IN PHAGOCYTOSIS
(A and B) Opsonized antigen (reacted with antibody and complement) reacts at the cell surface with Fc and C3 receptors. (C) The particle is brought inside the cell by invagination of the cell membrane, thereby forming a phagosome. (D) The phagosome fuses with a lysosome.

The Interplay Between Nonspecific and Specific Immunity

The events of the inflammatory response, which we have just described, are independent of the specific immune system and are common (with some variations) throughout much of the animal world. Because it has served so many species so well for so long there can be little argument that inflammation and phagocy-

IMMUNITY, INFECTIONS, AND TUMORS

tosis are efficient in evolutionary terms. But as we move further along in evolution, there is greater emphasis on the survival of the individual, and the efficiency of the nonspecific factors has been augmented in the chordates by interaction with the specific immune system.

The realization that the nonspecific and specific immune systems work together in immunity came about only after a rather acrimonious battle between the proponents of the "humoral" school, which argued that antibody and complement could account for all of immunity, and the "cellular" school, which argued that phagocytosis alone was sufficient. It was Almoth Wright in England who eventually brought the two ideas together by showing that the two could work together. Wright coined the term *opsonin* (from the Greek *opsono*, "I prepare food for") for the activity of antibodies that enhance the phagocytic process. As John Humphrey points out in the introduction to his classic textbook (Humphrey and White, *Immunology for Students of Medicine*, 1963), Wright was an enthusiast so well known that he appears, thinly disguised, as Sir Colenso Ridgeon in G. B. Shaw's *The Doctor's Dilemma*:

> Drugs can only repress symptoms: they cannot eradicate disease. The true remedy for all diseases is Nature's remedy. Nature and Science are at one, Sir Patrick, believe me; though you were taught differently. Nature has provided in the white corpuscles as you call them—in the phagocytes as we call them—a natural means of devouring and destroying all disease germs. There is at bottom only one genuinely scientific treatment of all diseases, and that is to stimulate the phagocytes. Stimulate the phagocytes. Drugs are a delusion. Find the germ of the disease; prepare from it a suitable antitoxin; inject it three times a day quarter of an hour before meals; and what is the result? The phagocytes are stimulated; they devour the disease; and the patient recovers—unless, of course, he's too far gone. That, I take it, is the essence of Ridgeon's discovery.

Opsonization

Phagocytic cells can ingest a wide range of particles, from bacteria to polystyrene beads; but the efficiency of phagocytosis is enhanced several fold if the particle that is to be phagocytized has reacted with antibody. The coating of the particle with specific antibody that enhances phagocytosis is called OPSONIZATION. Assume that the sliver of wood that broke the skin in the earlier example of phagocytosis had some bacteria on it. In such a simple circumstance the nonspecific system is almost always able to clear up the local infection caused by the organisms on the wood or pushed from the skin into the tissue. If, however, there are too many microbes, or if they have enough of a counterdefense and are not cleared, their presence induces the formation of a specific antibody. As the antibody is produced, its concentration in the serum increases, and at some point enough antibody is present at the site of inflammation to react with the microbes. The microbes are now opsonized, and the rate at which they are ingested by the PMN increases dramatically.

Phagocytic cells have receptors on their surfaces for the Fc portions of immunoglobulin molecules (Fc RECEPTORS). The antibody reacts with the microbe through its Fab portion, a reaction producing an Ag–Ab complex. This reaction leaves the Fc portions of the antibody exposed. When these Fc portions react with the Fc receptor on the surface of the phagocyte, there is greatly enhanced membrane movement, which is needed to start the process of ingestion and the formation of the phagosome (Figure 1). It should be emphasized that Fc receptors react only with the Fc portion of immunoglobulin that is part of the Ag–Ab complex or has been aggregated in some physical manner. If this were not the case, the receptors would constantly be occupied with the Fc of serum immunoglobulin.

Complement-Mediated Cytolysis

Many gram-negative bacteria are lysed through the action of specific antibody and complement. This reaction has the effect of reducing the number of bacteria infecting the host. But when these organisms are lysed, they may liberate some of their wall components, called ENDOTOXINS, which can then activate the alternative pathway of complement (Chapter 9) and lead to further lysis. Endotoxin also is a pyrogen, and the body temperature can become elevated under these circumstances. Elevated temperature has been thought throughout the years to be one of the body's defenses. In fact, during the last

IMMUNITY, INFECTIONS, AND TUMORS

century it was noticed that syphilis was often cured if the patient contracted malaria. Reasoning that it was the bouts of fever in malaria that cured the syphilis, clinicians attempted to induce fever by inducing "artificial malaria" with mercury. (This led to the adage, "one night with Venus and a lifetime with Mercury.") It is in the realm of the possible that fever may have evolved as another, albeit very dangerous, way of increasing nonspecific immunity.

Patients with inflammatory diseases often have a new β-globulin in their serum called C-REACTIVE PROTEIN. The role of this molecule in the inflammatory process is not known.

Antibody-Dependent, Cell-Mediated Cytotoxicity (ADCC)

A cell that is coated with antibody can be lysed in a reaction called ANTIBODY-DEPENDENT, CELL-MEDIATED CYTOTOXICITY, or ADCC. This reaction is not well understood, and some immunologists have doubts about its importance in host defenses. The effector cells involved are called K CELLS, which have neither B cell nor T cell characteristics, and complement is not involved in the reaction.

Responses to Viral Infections

Interferon

The responses of the host that occur after infection with viruses and lead to a state of immunity are similar to those we have been describing, with the exception of the production of INTERFERON. In 1957 Issacs and Lindenmann discovered that the supernatant fluid obtained from cultures of cells that had been infected with virus, once freed of virus protected other cells from infection. They called the substance that had the ability to interfere with virus infection interferon.

Interferon has been the subject of innumerable review articles and not a few biotech companies. There is reasonable agreement about its role in viral immunity, but because there are several types of interferon, each made by a different cell type, the other roles we can assign to it are controversial. Interferon-α (INF-α) is produced by leukocytes; interferon-β (INF-β) is produced by fibroblasts; and interferon-γ (INF-γ), also called IMMUNE INTERFERON, is produced by stimulated T cells.

It must be remembered that interferon is produced by the host cells infected with the virus. This reaction is a form of biological altruism, because the production of interferon will not save the infected cell. The interferon is exported and used by other cells. When these cells become infected with the virus, the interferon causes cells to produce molecules that prevent the replication of the infecting virus. The events occurring in these cells that react with interferon are only partly understood. Reaction of interferon with an interferon receptor causes what is called the INTERFERON-INDUCED ANTIVIRAL STATE. A sequence of events follows which results in the inhibition of gene transcription through degradation of mRNA. The first event is the induction by interferon of a molecule called 2,5 A POLYMERASE. If a cell that has interacted with interferon (and is now producing 2,5 A polymerase) becomes infected with virus, the virus activates the polymerase to produce 2,5-ADENOSINE (2,5-A). The presence of 2,5-A in turn activates a preexisting, inactive molecule called RIBONUCLEASE L. It is ribonuclease L that degrades mRNA.

In this manner the cycle of virus reproduction is interfered with and the infection is either stopped or the process slowed down enough to enable the specific immune response to eliminate the infecting virus. Interferon-mediated events are nonspecific, because interferon induced by one virus can cause in other cells the appearance of the interferon-induced antiviral state that will protect them from infection by other viruses—namely, the activation of ribonuclease L, which has no specificity for either host or viral mRNA. In theory, *any* transcription events required by the host cell will be inhibited.

Antibodies and Cytotoxic Cells

ANTI-VIRAL ANTIBODIES act by clearing virus from the blood (i.e., reducing viremia) and by viral neutralization, (i.e., preventing the virus from infecting a new cell and initiating a new round of virus production). CYTOTOXIC T CELLS specific for viral antigens are known to be generated in an MHC-restricted manner, and these cells function by destroying

IMMUNITY, INFECTIONS, AND TUMORS

infected host cells that display the viral antigen on the surface. In this manner, the specific immune response eliminates the virus from the system.

Responses to Parasite Infections

Responses of the host to infection with protozoan and metazoan parasites also use the general armamentarium we have been discussing. The unique aspect in these infections is that in many of them the host makes a very strong IgE response. It will be seen in Chapter 26 that IgE is the isotype seen in hypersensitivity reactions. The IgE molecule binds to the surface of mast cells and basophils via an Fcε receptor. When the Fab is bound to specific antigen, the result is degranulation and release of pharmacologically active substances. It is not at all clear why these classes of infectious agents should have evolved in this manner.

The Response to Internal Invaders: The Response to Tumors

Immune Surveillance   Up to now we have been discussing the response of the organism to *external* invaders and have developed the idea that because the specific immune response did not appear in evolution until the chordates, the vast majority of the animal kingdom defends itself against external invaders with nonspecific immunity. This raises the question of why the chordates should have needed the specific immune system. Lewis Thomas addressed this question in 1959 and concluded that the reason probably was not for defense against external invaders. Rather, he reasoned, as organisms grow more and more complex and live longer, the chance for neoplastic growth of cells increases. Thomas introduced the idea that the specific, adaptive immune response may have evolved in response to the need to protect the body from *internal* invaders, specifically neoplasia. Macfarlane Burnet expanded upon this theory, and, as the IMMUNE SURVEILLANCE THEORY, it became the dominant paradigm in tumor immunology.

CHAPTER TWENTY-FIVE

In its most simple form, immune surveillance argues that there are tumor-specific antigens associated with neoplastic cells and that the immune system acts as a surveillance system to identify and destroy any cells that begin to express these new antigens.[4]

Tumor-Specific Antigens We saw much earlier in this book that the discovery of the major histocompatibility complex was intimately associated with the experimental models of tumors. It had been noted at the beginning of this century that when animals were inoculated with tumors they often rejected them and they rejected a second injection of the same tumor even more rapidly. The logical explanation for this was that the host was responding to something unique on the tumor, perhaps a tumor-specific antigen, and mounting an immune response to the tumor. But, as we will see in the chapter on transplantation immunity, with the development of inbred strains of mice the reason for the rejection could be shown not to be due to responses to tumor-specific antigens but to normal antigens encoded in the MHC. Even so, the idea that the immune system is involved in the defense against tumors is an attractive one. But if the immune system really does play a role, the basic requirement is that there be TUMOR SPECIFIC ANTIGENS—that is, antigens that are present on tumors but are not found on normal cells and tissues. It would be to these antigens unique to the tumor that the immune response would react.

In the 1950s, the results of some experiments strongly indicated the existence of tumor-specific antigens. The basic design of these classic experiments (Figure 2) is to remove a tumor from an animal and then rechallenge the animal with the same tumor. If there are tumor-specific antigens, the animal should have made an immune response to them while the tumor was growing. When the tumor is *reintroduced*, the immune response

---

[4] "The thesis is that when aberrant cells with proliferative potential arise in the body they will carry new antigenic determinants on their cell surfaces. When a significant amount of new antigen has developed, a thymus-dependent immunological response will be initiated and eventually eliminates the aberrant cells in essentially the same way as a homograft is destroyed." [Burnett (1970) *Prog. Exp. Tumor Res.* 13, 1]

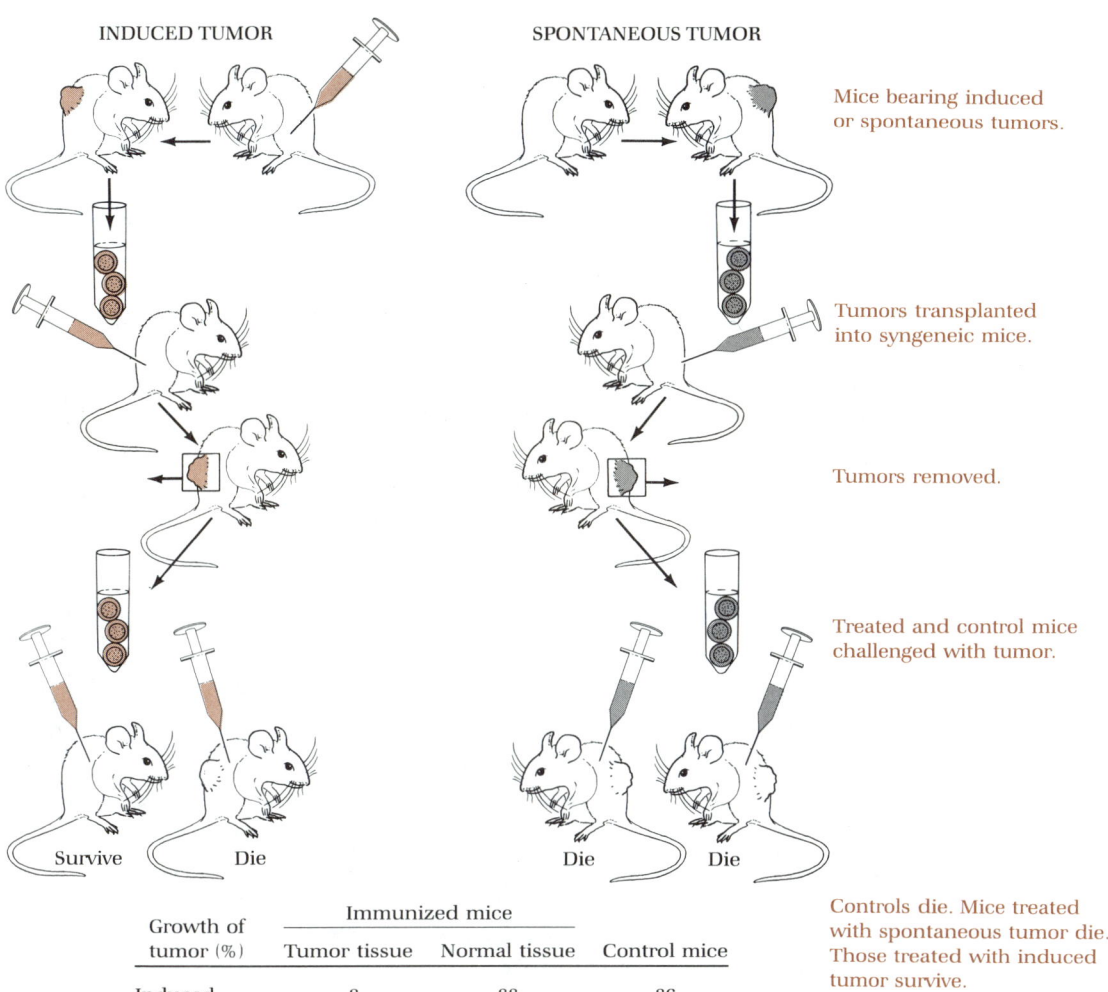

FIGURE 2 IMMUNITY TO INDUCED AND SPONTANEOUS TUMORS

An induced or spontaneous tumor is removed from the animal and "stored" in a syngeneic mouse. Later the tumor is removed from the host mouse and reimplanted into the mouse in which it originated. Normal mice are inoculated with tumor at the same time as controls. The controls die, showing that the tumor is still active. Reintroducing the induced tumor into the original animal does not lead to death, but reintroduction of the spontaneous tumor into the original animal shows that there is no protection. [After Foley (1953) *Cancer Res.* **13**, 835; Prehn and Main (1957) *J. Natl. Cancer Inst.* **18**, 769; Klein et al. (1960) *Cancer Res.* **20**, 1561]

CHAPTER TWENTY-FIVE

should cause it to be rejected. In the experiments by Foley, for example, tumors were induced in C3H mice with methylcolanthrene (MCA; see below) and then caused to regress by looping some surgical thread around the base of the tumor and "strangling" it by drawing the knot tight. Deprived of its vascular supply, the tumor "dried up" in a few days and disappeared. When the mice were later challenged by implanting the same tumor, it was found that they were able to reject it. Untreated controls all died of the tumor. However, when the same experiment was attempted with spontaneous mammary tumors, it was found that these tumors grew. Thus the response to spontaneous tumors differed from the response to induced tumors. We will return to this fact later.

This basic experiment was repeated and then modified by Prehn and Main, who used surgical excision (as well as the strangulation) and obtained the same result as Foley. In addition they added another control: they injected groups of mice with normal tissue and showed that the tumors grew in these mice at the same rate as in the uninjected controls. This showed that there must be something on the tumor that is different from its counterpart on normal tissue. Finally, Klein and his co-workers in Sweden carried out similar experiments in which the tumor was induced and the leg with the tumor was amputated. These mice were able to reject the tumor when it was later reimplanted.

Figure 2 shows that for the induced tumors there was clearcut TUMOR IMMUNITY, which was not seen with the spontaneous tumors. Thus the crucial experiments had been done, and the stage was now set for developing the idea that the immune system plays a role in the host response to tumors.

The fact that under some conditions tumor-specific antigens can be demonstrated is a strong point in favor of the theory. But the theory raises the question of why animals develop cancer. The answer, according to immune surveillance in its purest form, is that either the tumor overpowers the immune system or it develops when the immune system is not functioning well. The prediction would be that as the animal ages its immune function, like other bodily functions, operates at lower efficiency; so one would expect to see more cancer in older animals. This is well

IMMUNITY, INFECTIONS, AND TUMORS

> ### INFORMATION BOX 1
>
> ## Cancer Terminology
>
> NEOPLASM Any abnormal growth of tissue; literally, "new thing formed"
>
> MALIGNANT TUMOR A neoplasm that replaces surrounding normal tissue
>
> BENIGN TUMOR A neoplasm that grows discretely and does not invade surrounding tissue
>
> METASTASIS Neoplastic growth that leaves the main growth and travels to another part of the body
>
> CARCINOMA Neoplasm derived from epithelial tissues; terms bronchocarcinoma, hepatocarcinoma, adenocarcinoma, and so on indicate the organ from which the neoplasm has arisen (lung, liver, gland, etc).
>
> SARCOMA Neoplastic growth of mesodermal origin; the terms lymphosarcoma, osteosarcoma, and so on indicate the tissue of origin (lymphoid, bone, etc.)

known to be the case. One might also expect to see more tumors early in life, when the system is just beginning to function. Childhood leukemias are a well-known disease of the young. How then does the theory handle the tumor that is overpowering the immune system? The prediction is that tumors are either immunosuppressive or arise when the animal is in a state of impaired immune function.

Immune Suppression and Cancer The literature abounds with examples of tumor-bearing experimental animals and humans having depressed immune function. These cases led to a general acceptance of the immune surveillance theory. But in 1975 Osias Stutman at the Sloan Kettering Cancer Center in New York did an extensive analysis of the literature and concluded that "there are almost as many exceptions as there are positive associations between immune deficiencies and increased risk for tumor development" [O. Stutman (1975) *Adv. Cancer Res.* 22, 261].

Furthermore, since the theory postulated that the T cell response would eliminate the tumors as they developed, the prediction would be that the athymic nude mouse should have a very high incidence of tumors. In fact, these animals are essentially free of spontaneous tumors. Originally it was argued that nude mice do not live long enough to develop tumors, but when these mice are maintained under germ-free conditions so that their life span is increased, they develop tumors at roughly the same rate as euthymic nu/+ heterozygous littermates of the same age do.

It should also be remembered that in the original experiments protective responses to tumor-specific antigens were demonstrated only on induced tumors and not on spontaneous tumors. This finding raises the possibility that the responses that were observed and the protection that the responses afforded are laboratory artifacts. Induced tumors or spontaneous tumors that have been passaged for many generations may have antigens that are more potent than those on spontaneously arising tumors.

Natural Killer Cells in Tumor Immunity

If the evidence for the two basic requirements of the immune surveillance theory (unique tumor antigens and impaired immune function) is open to question, is there *any* evidence that the immune system plays a role in defense against tumors? In the course of looking for specific cytotoxic T cells that lyse chromium-labeled tumor target cells, it was noticed that normal individuals have high levels of cells cytotoxic for some tumor targets. These were called NATURAL KILLER CELLS, or NK cells, because they exist, apparently, in the absence of immunization with the antigens on the tumor cells (Figure 3).

NK cells are a subpopulation of lymphocytes, which are identified morphologically as LARGE GRANULAR LYMPHOCYTES (LGL) and can be enriched by centrifugation through a discontinuous gradient of Percoll. The LGL are sIg$^-$ and complement receptor-negative but Fc receptor-positive. This fact allows NK to carry out antibody-dependent cellular cytotoxicity (ADCC) in addition to the lysis of targets in the absence of antibody. Interferon enhances their cytotoxic activity.

NK cells are able to lyse a fairly wide range of cells, both tumor and normal. They do this with no known MHC restriction, and, as mentioned, in the absence of known prior contact with

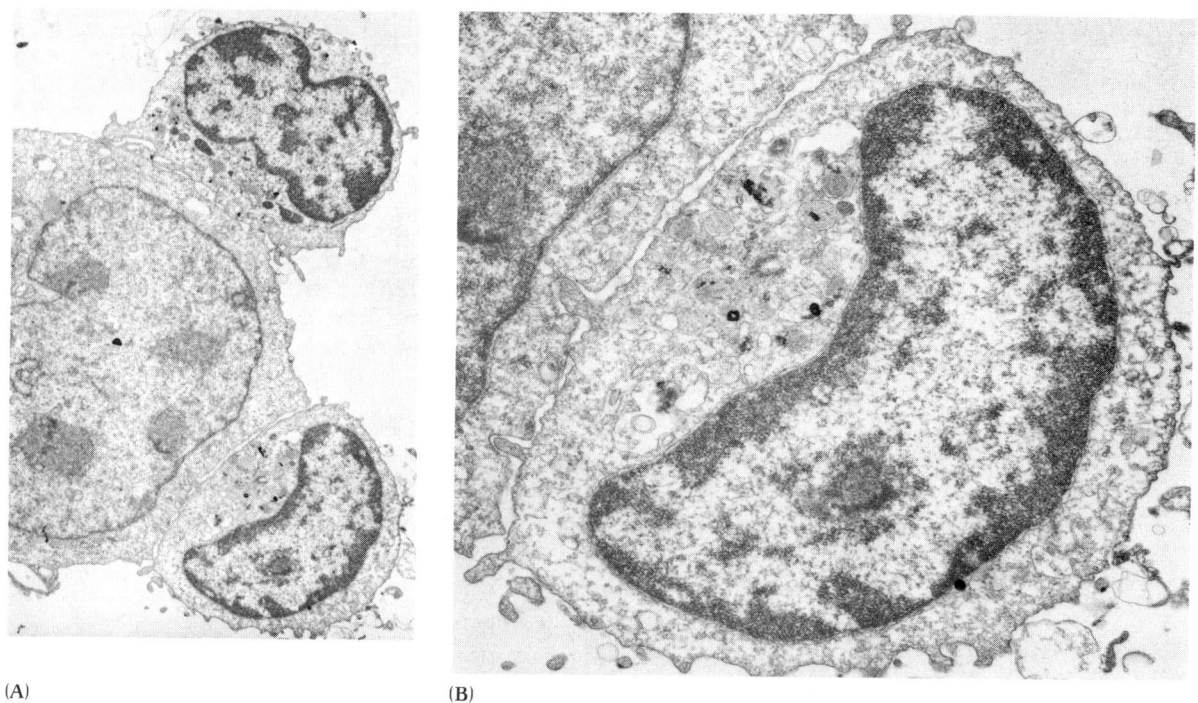

FIGURE 3 NK CELL KILLING TUMOR

It is not known how NK cells kill their targets, but contact is necessary. (A) Two NK cells conjugated to a melanoma tumor cell target seen at low magnification (×5300). (B) The NK cell on the bottom of A seen at higher resolution (×16,000). Projections of the NK cell push deeply into the target cell. [From Zucker-Franklin, Grusky, and Yang (1983) *PNAS* 80, 6977; courtesy of Dr. D. Zucker-Franklin]

antigen. Little is known about the nature of the structures on the surface of the target cells with which the NK cells react. The possible role of NK cells in tumor immunity is a much-discussed question. We do not know the range of specificities possessed by these cells, so we cannot even begin to predict the range of structures on newly emergent tumor cells that would be recognized and reacted with.

CHAPTER TWENTY-FIVE

Tumor Immunotherapy

The reader has concluded from the above that at the present time it is very difficult to assign relative weights to the importance of nonspecific and specific asspects of immunity. Richmond Prehn, whose work was so instrumental in the initial formation of the immune surveillance theory, has argued as follows:

> The evidence overall seems to suggest that immunological surveillance of nascent tumors, as originally conceived, may not exist in most tumor systems. On the other hand, there is a late acting and inefficient immunological defense mechanism. Hopefully, this mechanism may be subject to augmentation for purposes of immunotherapy. [R. Prehn, *Clinical Immunobiology*, Vol. 2, F. H. Bach and R. A. Good, eds., p. 191]

Based upon the assumption that the immune system can play an important role in the destruction and elimination of tumors, much effort has been put into attempts to enhance the ability of the immune system to carry out these ends. A great deal of the effort has gone into attempts to nonspecifically increase the activity of the system. The most commonly used system uses the idea of ADJUVANTS—nonspecific amplifiers of immune function. The organism used to vaccinate against tuberculosis is called BCG (bacillus Calmette-Guérin). For reasons poorly understood, this bacterium enhances phagocytosis, antibody formation, and cell-mediated responses. It was hoped that by treating patients with this organism both the nonspecific and antigen-specific mechanisms would be increased. Unfortunately, there has been only limited success with this method.

Another method which has had some success is the intentional painting of a hapten onto skin tumors so that when antigen-specific cytotoxic T cells are generated they will kill the tumor cells to which the hapten is conjugated. This method has had some success with melanomas and may act by reducing the tumor load so that the immune system can cope with the remaining cells.

A potentially promising area that is receiving much attention is the use of IMMUNOTOXINS. Immunotoxins are antibody molecules to which a toxin has been covalently conjugated. The rationale is that if one has an antibody, especially a monoclonal antibody,

IMMUNITY, INFECTIONS, AND TUMORS

directed against a tumor antigen, it can serve as a vehicle to deliver the toxin to the tumor cells and kill them. Ricin (a plant toxin) and diphtheria toxin are two very commonly used agents. The toxins consist of a toxic polypeptide (called the A chain) that is disulfide-bonded to a cell surface-binding polypeptide (called the B chain). The most potent immunotoxins are composed of the A chain of the toxin linked to the antibody molecule. Several immunotoxins are undergoing clinical trial.

Summary

1. Immunity, the ability to resist and remain free from disease, is achieved by a variety of specific and nonspecific means. A parasite is an organism that functions at the expense of another, and the host–parasite relationship is determined by a delicate balance of factors.
2. The host may have natural immunity because of physiological incompatibility with the potential parasite. Natural physical barriers such as the skin and mucosa also prevent potential pathogens from invading the host. In addition, host secretions may destroy invaders.
3. When an invader penetrates these first lines of defense, the host uses the inflammatory response as a potent nonspecific defense. The inflammatory response ultimately leads to the accumulation of phagocytic cells at the site of infection. Phagocytes ingest and kill the invading organisms.
4. There is an interplay of the nonspecific immune system and the specific reactions to antigens on the parasites. When an organism is coated with antibody the efficiency of phagocytosis is enhanced. Cytotoxic T cells also are important.
5. Interferon is produced by virus-infected cells and may be of importance in viral immunity.
6. The immune system may play a role in the response to tumors. The immune surveillance theory states that neoplastic cells that express tumor-specific antigens will be recognized by the immune system and removed. Cancer would develop only when the immune system fails. It is not clear whether this system plays a major role or whether natural killer cells are important in tumor immunity.

CHAPTER TWENTY-FIVE

Additional Readings

Bach, M. K. 1982. Mediators of anaphylaxis and inflammation. *Annu. Rev. Microbiol.* 36, 371.

Doherty, P. C., B. B. Knowles and P. J. Wettstein. 1984. Immunological surveillance of tumors in the context of major histocompatibility complex restriction of T cell function. *Adv. Cancer Res.* 42, 1.

Drutz, D. J. and J. Mills. 1982. Immunity and infection. In *Basic and Clinical Immunology*, 4th ed., D. P. Stites et al. (eds.). Lange Medical, Palo Alto.

Ortaldo, J. R. and R. B. Herberman. 1984. Heterogeneity of natural killer cells. *Annu. Rev. Immunol.* 2, 359.

Stutman, O. 1975. Immunodepression and malignancy. *Adv. Cancer Res.* 22, 261.

Vitetta, E. S. and J. W. Uhr. 1984. The potential use of immunotoxins in transplantation, cancer therapy, and immunoregulation. *Transplantation* 37, 535.

CHAPTER 26

HYPERSENSITIVITY

Overview Up to now we have been focusing on the mechanism of the immune response and the protective effect of the response. In this chapter we will see that the normal functioning of the immune system can have harmful effects. We will examine a series of reactions known as hypersensitivity or allergy. The discovery of hypersensitivity came at the time when the protective effects of antibody were discovered; the two have grown up together. A conceptual advance in the study of hypersensitivity was the classification of the various forms of disease into four groups, based on the immune mechanism that causes the symptoms. We will see that antibody-mediated hypersensitivity is brought about by the fixation of IgE to mast cells and the subsequent reaction of that bound IgE with the allergen, causing degranulation of the cells; or by the fixation of complement antigen–antibody complex, a reaction causing lysis of cells; or by the disruption of normal functions by immune complexes. A fourth type of reaction is caused by effector T cells.

CHAPTER TWENTY-SIX

The Nature of Hypersensitivity

Origins of the Idea That an Immune Response Can Be Harmful

The immune response has undoubtedly evolved into its complicated and diverse state because it has survival value to the species. However, like all good things, there are aspects of the immune response that can be harmful to the individual. The original discovery of the immunological nature of the harmful effect of antibody came in the early 1900s by the French physician Paul Richet. His description of the discovery is of interest not only because it shows how the "prepared mind" works but also because it gives us a glimpse of science in the Grand Style of a lost era.

> During a cruise on the yacht of Prince Albert of Monaco, the Prince advised me to study Physalia[1] poison, together with our friends Georges Richard and Paul Portier. We found that it is easily dissolved in glycerol and that by injecting this glycerol solution, the symptoms of Physalia poisoning are reproduced.
>
> When I came back to France and had no more Physalia to study, I hit upon the idea of making a comparative study of the tentacles of Actinia which can be obtained in large quantities, for Actinia abound on all the rocky shores of Europe.
>
> Now Actinia tentacles, treated with glycerol, give off their poison into the glycerol and the extract is toxic. I therefore set about finding how toxic it was, with Portier. This was quite difficult to do, as it is a slowly acting poison and three or four days must elapse before it can be known if the dose be fatal or not. I was using a solution of one kilo of glycerol to one kilo of tentacles. The lethal dose was of the order of 0.1 liquid per kilo live weight of subject.
>
> But certain dogs survived, either because the dose was not strong enough or for some other reason. At the end of two, three or four weeks, as they seemed normal, I made use of them for a new experiment.
>
> An unexpected phenomenon arose, which we thought extraordinary. A dog when injected previously even with the smallest dose of 0.005 liquid per kilo, immediately showed serious symptoms: vomiting, blood diarrhoea, syncope, unconsciousness, asphyxia and death. [Charles Richet, Nobel lecture, 1913. In *Nobel Lectures in Physiology and Medicine, 1901–1921*, p. 475.]

---

[1] The Portugese Man of War.

HYPERSENSITIVITY

Richet termed this phenomenon ANAPHYLAXIS. In his Nobel lecture he tells why he coined the term.

> First I feel I must explain and indeed justify the use of the word itself, for it may seem somewhat barbarous at first glance. This neologism I invented twelve years ago on the assumption, which I think is still valid, that a new idea calls for a new word in the name of scientific precision of language.
>
> *Phylaxis*, a word seldom used, stands in the Greek for protection. *Anaphylaxis* will thus stand for the opposite. Anaphylaxis, from its Greek etymological source, therefore means that state of an organism in which it is rendered hypersensitive, instead of being protected. [p. 471]

Richet soon established that this "hypersensitivity" was transferable by serum and that the active material(s) were the same as antibodies. This fact is important in the historical context because the first Nobel prize, given in 1901, was to Emil von Behring for his work on the serum therapy of diphtheria—that is, on the *protective* effect of antibody. Indeed, the period was full of the excitement and hope that the combined efforts of two new sciences, bacteriology and immunology, would end the scourge of infectious diseases through immunization and serum therapy. Richet was astute enough to recognize that even though antibody could be protective, it also could be destructive.

We will see in this chapter that anaphylaxis has come to be used for only one type of harmful immunological reaction and that the term *hypersensitivity* (which Richet used in the quotation above) has become the generic technical term for harmful reactions.

The Need for Sensitization There are many manifestations of hypersensitivity, none of them pleasant and all having in common the fact that they are initiated by an immune reaction to an antigen and occur in or on a host who has become SENSITIZED (i.e., has previously made an immune response to that antigen). Thus hypersensitivity in all of its many and varied forms is the result of *restimulation* with the offending antigen. In common parlance, these reactions are called ALLERGIC REACTIONS and those antigens involved in a hypersensitive or allergic response are called ALLERGENS.

CHAPTER TWENTY-SIX

Because hypersensitivity reactions occur to a wide variety of allergens and at any number of areas and organs of the body, they come in what at first appears to be a bewildering variety. For years this catalog of dread was the realm of the allergist, who treated the particular symptoms as well as the times allowed. However, as more was learned about the mechanisms of the immune response, both in experimental animals and in humans, it became clear that there were some unifying principles. In the 1950s Gell and Coombs devised a classification system based upon the *nature of the immunological reactions* rather than on the symptoms.

The Gell and Coombs Classification

The GELL AND COOMBS CLASSIFICATION divides hypersensitivity reactions into four groups based upon the features which they have in common. The characteristics of the groups are presented below and shown in diagrammatic form in Figure 1.

Type I: Type I reactions are those caused by the fixation of IgE to mast cells with the subsequent release of pharmacologically active substances which produce the symptoms. Examples of Type I diseases are anaphylaxis, atopy, and urticaria.

Type II: Type II reactions are caused by the action of antibodies —usually IgG and IgM—on target cells and the activation of complement, a reaction that leads to lysis of the cells. Examples of Type II diseases are certain drug allergies and erythroblastosis fetalis.

Type III: Type III reactions are those in which antigen–antibody complexes form and cause damage by their presence in a vital organ. An example of this type of reaction is glomerulonephritis, which can be induced by immune complexes.

Type IV: Type IV reactions are cell-mediated reactions (induced by T cells) called DELAYED-TYPE HYPERSENSITIVITY (DTH) reactions. Allergic contact dermatitis is the principal example of diseases of this type.

HYPERSENSITIVITY

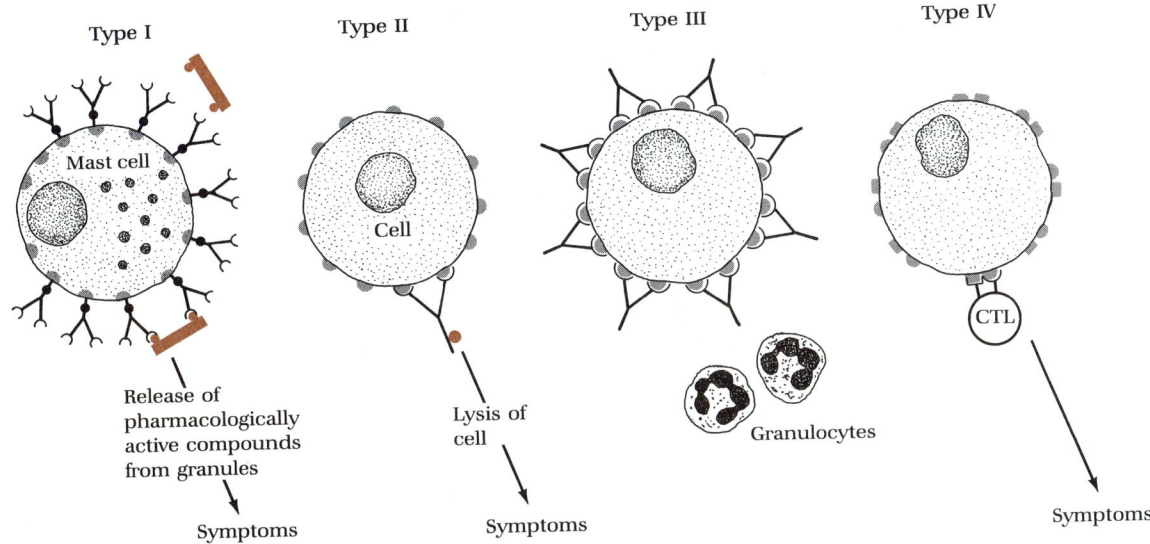

FIGURE 1 THE CLASSIFICATION OF HYPERSENSITIVITY REACTIONS

Type I reactions: Allergen reacts with IgE bound on mast cells, causing degranulation and release of granule contents, which produce the symptoms. Type II reactions: Antibody binds to antigen on the cell surface. Complement is fixed and cell lysis occurs, a reaction producing the symptoms. Type III reactions: Immune complexes form on the surface of cells, causing loss of function or accumulation of granulocytes. Type IV reactions: Delayed-type hypersensitivity. T cells react with antigen in the context of MHC and cause the symptoms. [After Gell and Coombs (1969) *Clinical Aspects of Immunology*, 2nd ed. Oxford: Blackwell]

Type I Reactions: Immediate Hypersensitivity

Atopic Diseases

Allergic rhinitis, or HAY FEVER, is the most common form of immediate hypersensitivity or ATOPIC DISEASE. Even though 10% of the U.S. population suffers from hay fever, the nonallergic individual often has trouble realizing the extent of the misery which hay fever and similar syndromes inflict on the sufferer.

CHAPTER TWENTY-SIX

I am suffering from my old complaint, the hay-fever (as it is called). My fear is, perishing by deliquescence; I melt away in a nasal and lachrymal profluvia. My remedies are warm pidiluvium, cathartics, topical application of a watery solution of opium to eyes, ears and the interior of the nostrils. The membrane is so irritable, that light, dust, contradiction, an absurd remark...sets me sneezing; and if I begin sneezing at twelve, I don't leave off till two o'clock, and am heard distinctly in Taunton, when the wind sets that way—a distance of six miles. [Sidney Smith to Dr. Holland, 1835]

A less frequent form of atopic disease is bronchial asthma and atopic dermatitis. A rarer form is gastrointestinal food allergy.

Atopy

It has been known for a long time that these clinical manifestations were due to antibody that somehow caused the mast cells to release histamine and other vasoactive amines. The released agents cause the contraction of smooth muscle and the other symptoms described by poor Sidney Smith. The antibody was known to have the ability to fix to the skin and (for convoluted historical reasons that we will not go into, dealing with the reagin of the old syphilis tests) was called *reaginic* antibody. What made reaginic antibody so special was not known until the Ishizakas showed that the property of fixing to tissue, specifically to mast cells and basophils to cause their degranulation, was unique to the IgE class of immunoglobulins. The route they took to this discovery was discussed, along with the properties of IgE, in Chapter 4.

Mast Cell Degranulation

MAST CELLS are basophilic cells found in connective and subcutaneous tissues. They have been called "sentinel cells" because they are located around venules and near mucosal surfaces and can effect rapid physiological changes by releasing the contents of their granules (Figure 2). Mast cells contain a large number of granules, which contain an array of pharmacologically active mediators (Figure 3). In atopic disease the reaction of IgE and allergen on the surface of the mast cell results in DEGRANULATION and release of these mediators.

In an especially elegant series of experiments the Ishizakas showed that IgE bound to the mast cell via the C_H3 and C_H4

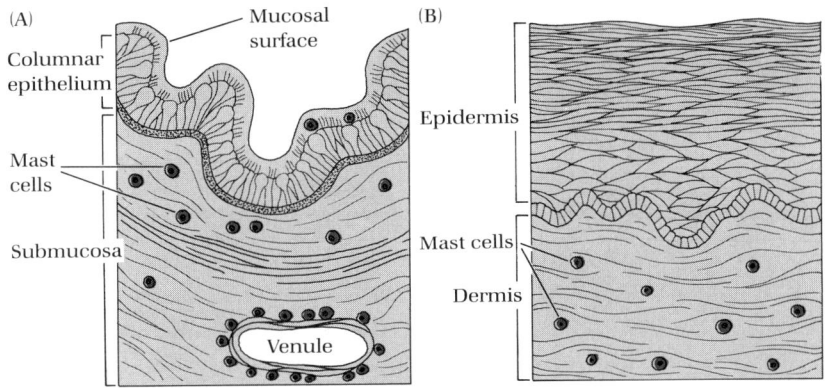

FIGURE 2 MAST CELL DISTRIBUTION

(A) In the bronchial tissue, mast cells are found near the mucosal surfaces and in the submucosa, as well as around venules. (B) Skin mast cells are in the dermis. It can be seen that these "sentinel cells" are near interfaces with the external environment or between venous and arterial circulations. [From Austen (1983) Tissue mast cells in immediate hypersensitivity. In Dixon and Fisher, eds. *The Biology of Immunologic Disease*, p. 224; with permission]

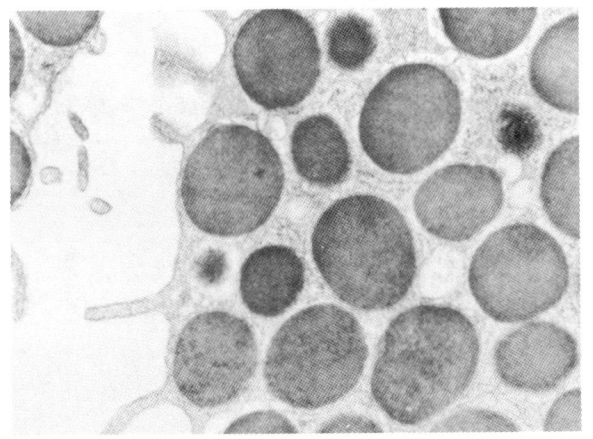 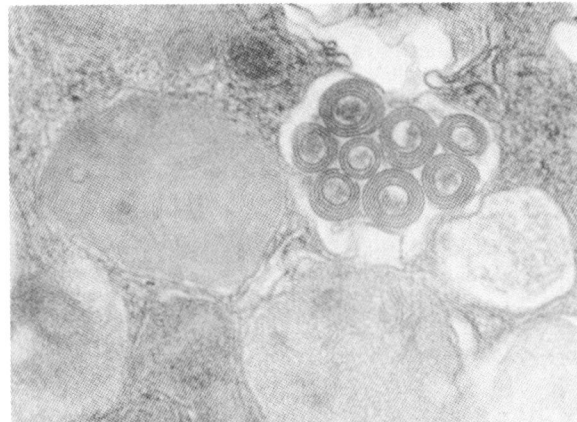

FIGURE 3 INTERNAL STRUCTURE OF MAST CELLS

Rat peritoneal mast cells (*left*; ×50,000) and human mast cells (*right*; ×174,000). [From Austen (1983) Tissue mast cells in immediate hypersensitivity. In Dixon and Fisher, eds. *The Biology of Immunologic Disease*, p. 224; with permission]

domains of the Fc and that the reaction of the mast cell-bound (or fixed) IgE after reaction with allergen caused the receptors to aggregate. Somehow this receptor reorientation results in the mast cell degranulation. This classic experiment is shown in Figure 4. (The nature of the receptor is discussed below.) When IgE is allowed to react with mast cells (Figure 4A) there is binding; but this binding alone does not result in degranulation of the mast cells. Degranulation requires both binding of the IgE to the cell and binding of allergen to the Fab portion of the IgE (Figure 4B). Thus, if the IgE is not specific for the allergen, there will be no degranulation.

Why should the reaction of allergen at the antigen-combining site of molecules whose Fc portion is attached to the cell have this effect? Because it was known that the membrane of the cell is a fluid mosaic with floating islands of proteins, many of which are receptors, and that antibody to the "islands" could move them in the plane of the membrane (patching and capping), it was postulated that degranulation was the result of movement and reorientation of some molecule in the mast cell membrane. The membrane molecule involved must be a receptor for the IgE Fc. To test this idea, IgE was allowed to react with mast cells in the absence of allergen (as in Figure 4A); but instead of allergen, anti-IgE antibody was added. If the degranulation was due to the reorientation of the receptors, the anti-IgE should have the same effect as allergen—that is, moving the receptors. This is exactly the result obtained (Figure 4C). The anti-IgE reacting with the receptor-bound IgE caused degranulation.

This finding suggested that the crucial event is the binding of the Fc portion to the mast cells and that the function of allergen is merely to reorient the receptors. To further test this idea, Fc fragments of IgE (with no Fab attached) were allowed to react with the mast cells (Figure 4D). Once the Fc fragments had bound to the receptors, anti-IgE was added. Remember, the class-specific antigens on Ig H chains are in the Fc portion, so the anti-IgE bound to the Fc fragments. This also resulted in degranulation. In contrast, when allergen was added to the bound Fc, there was no degranulation.

The argument was made even more convincing (Figure 4E, F, and G) by showing that an antibody to the Fc receptor of the

HYPERSENSITIVITY

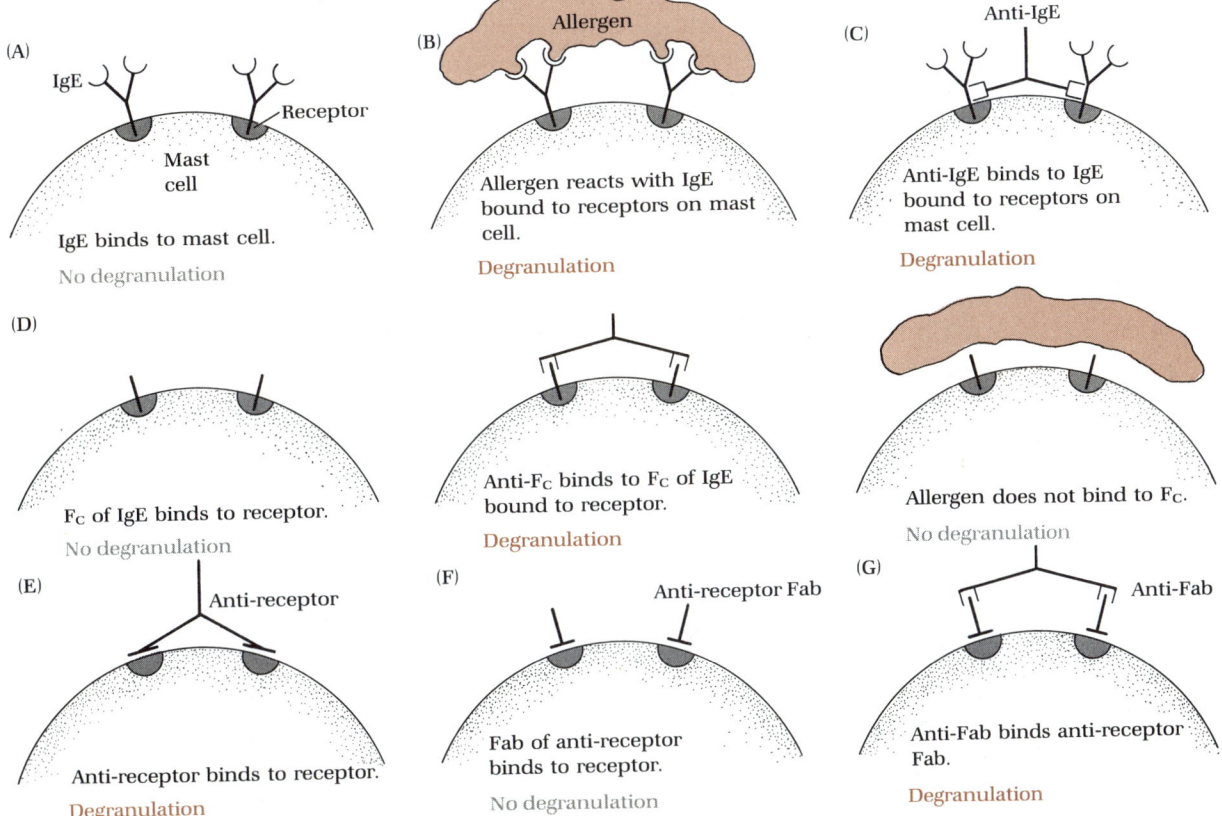

FIGURE 4 IgE-INDUCED MAST CELL DEGRANULATION
(A) IgE binds to mast cells via IgE receptor but does not cause degranulation. (B) Allergen binds specifically to the IgE, causing degranulation. (C) Treating mast cell-bound IgE with anti-IgE causes degranulation. (D) Fc of IgE binds to receptor but does not cause degranulation. Adding anti-Fc to the bound Fc causes degranulation in contrast to allergen which does not. (E,F,G) Anti-Fc receptor antibody causes degranulation but Fab fragment does not. Adding anti-Fab to the bound Fab causes degranulation. [Based on the experiments of Ishizaka and Ishizaka (1975) *Prog. Allergy* 19, 60]

mast cells bound to the surface caused degranulation. However, an Fab fragment of the anti-receptor antibody (which is monovalent and cannot cause cross-linking), even though it bound to the cell, did not induce degranulation. When an anti-Fab was added to the surface-bound Fab, there was degranulation.

The conclusion from these experiments is that reorientation of the receptor for IgE on mast cells leads to the production of a signal for the granules to lyse. Under natural conditions, the reorientation is induced by the reaction of allergen with the IgE that is attached to the mast cells. An allergic individual therefore is one who has responded to the allergen by producing anti-allergen antibodies of the IgE class. The IgE is bound to that person's mast cells via the Fc receptors on the mast cells. This is like turning the mast cell into an armed bomb waiting for the firing pin to be detonated. Contact with the allergen is the triggering device.

Why does degranulation cause the symptoms? As seen in Table 1, the granules of the mast cells are an armory of pharma-

TABLE 1 Contents of the mast cell granules.

Active agent	Activity
Histamine	Increases vascular permeability; elevates level of cyclic AMP
Heparin	Anticoagulation
Serotonin	Increases vascular permeability
SRS-A (slow-reacting substance of anaphylaxis)	Increases vascular permeability; causes contraction of human bronchioles
Chymase	Proteolysis
Hyaluronidase	Increases vascular permeability
Eosinophil Chemotactic Factor	Chemoattraction of eosinophils
Neutrophil Chemotactic Factor	Chemoattraction of neutrophils
Platelet Aggregating Factor	Aggregates platelets

Source: Modified from Austen (1978), *J. Immunol.* 121: 793.

HYPERSENSITIVITY

cologically active materials. The opening of this Pandora's box causes alteration in capillary permeability, smooth muscle contraction, and so on, depending upon the surface that is affected (skin, lung, etc.)

The biochemical events that occur after receptor binding have been studied extensively and present a very complicated picture. The main events involve the activation of the adenylate cyclase system, which converts ATP to cAMP. However, several interconnected systems are known to be involved, so that phospholipid metabolism, protein phosphorylation, prostaglandin production, and intracellular pH all come into play.[2] The complex picture is illustrated diagrammatically in Figure 5. The intracellular level of cAMP is affected by β-adrenergic compounds such as epinephrine. The mast cell, in fact, has receptors for both α- and β-adrenergic compounds, so they can be used in therapeutic strategies.

The IgE Receptor and Its Regulation

From all of the above, it is clear that the crucial event initiating the process leading to degranulation is the binding of IgE to the mast cell. The IgE receptor on the mast cell has been studied extensively. The availability of both human and rat mast cell tumors has made these studies possible. The receptor is a four-chain molecule. Two α chains, each with a molecular weight of 50,000, are associated with two β chains (molecular weight 30,000–35,000). The molecule is very hydrophobic, indicating that most of it is buried in the membrane. The α chains are the sites of IgE binding.

Since it became clear that an IgE response to an allergen with IgE results in allergy, the central question in allergy research has been, "Why is it that some individuals respond in this manner and others do not?" There is clearly a *genetic* component because atopic diseases such as hay fever can be a familial trait. For example, although 38% of atopic individuals have no parental history of atopy, there is a 75% chance that if both parents are atopic, the child will suffer the same fate. If only one parent is

---

[2] All of this should sound familiar from Chapter 21. Once again we see that the uniquely immunological events act to trigger a system common to many phenomena.

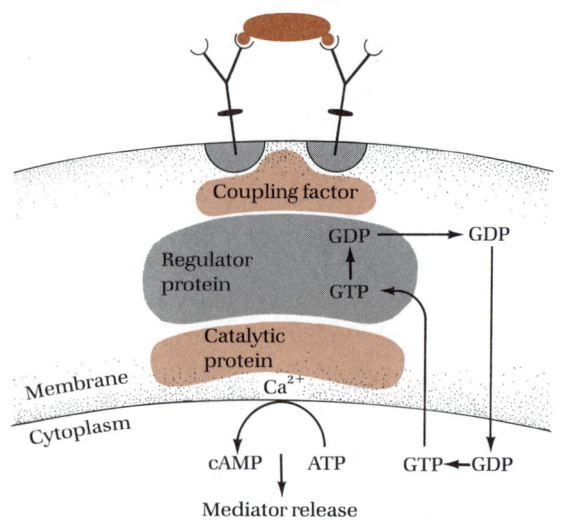

FIGURE 5 MAST CELL DEGRANULATION
The intracellular consequences of receptor reorientation in mast cell degranulation. The reorientation causes the catalytic subunit to activate the GDP-GTP system and the cAMP system, resulting in mediator release [Based on Winslow and Austin (1982) *Fed. Proc.* 41, 22]

atopic, there is a 50% chance of the child also being atopic. Even though no single HLA haplotype has been associated with atopy, within a family the atopic individuals tend to have the same haplotype.

It is known that certain adjuvants promote the production of IgE in experimental animals, converting what would be an IgG response into an IgE response. The most effective promoters are the parasites *Nippostronglylus brasiliensis* and *Ascaris suum*. Conjugating haptens to these agents or injecting ordinary antigens along with them results in a preferential IgE response. But even though this technique allows one to study the response in experimental systems, it does not answer the question about the natural response.

One avenue of approach that is being pursued is the notion that a balance between IgE inducing and suppressing factors occurs in all individuals. In allergic individuals there is an "allergic breakthrough" because the suppressive factors have become less potent than the enhancing factors. This model is illustrated in Figure 6.

Several groups have been able to generate factors that affect the IgE response. The Ishizakas, for example, have isolated IgE B

HYPERSENSITIVITY

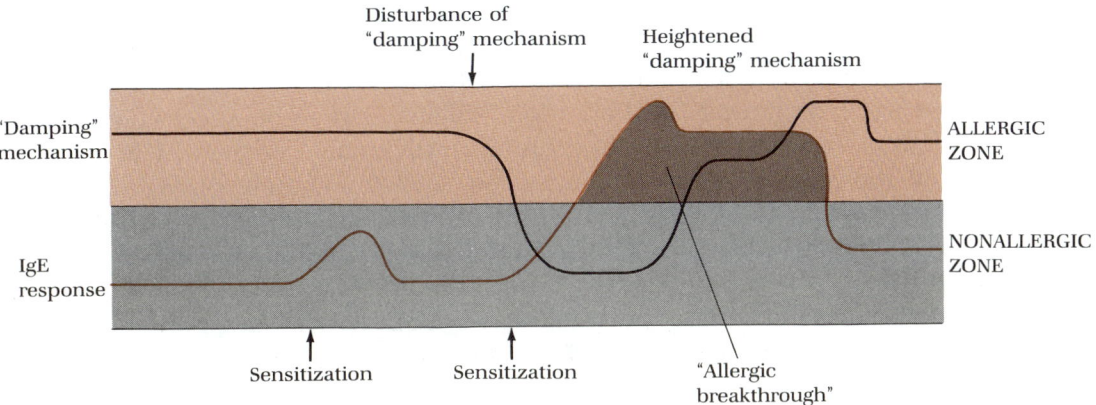

FIGURE 6 ALLERGIC BREAKTHROUGH
When the magnitude of the IgE response is below line A, there are no allergic symptoms. When it crosses the line, allergic symptoms occur. In normal (that is, nonatopic) individuals, the response remains in the lower section because of a "damping" mechanism that prevents the conversion of the response to IgE (a net balance of suppressive factors and enhancing factors). A disturbance of the damping mechanism causes the IgE response to cross the line and produce an "allergic breakthrough." When the "damping" mechanism corrects itself, IgE production falls below the line. [Redrawn from Katz et al. (1979) *J. Immunol.* 122, 2191; with permission]

CELL GENERATING FACTOR, which induces an increased number of IgE-bearing B cells, and IgE POTENTIATING FACTOR. Both of these are made by T cells. These enhancing factors are balanced by IgE-SUPPRESSIVE FACTOR. Katz and his colleagues have isolated two factors, SUPPRESSIVE FACTOR OF ALLERGY (SFA) and ENHANCING FACTOR OF ALLERGY (EFA). As the nature of these factors becomes clear, they may be of great usefulness in the down-regulation of allergic responses.

The mast cell has receptors for adrenergic compounds, and these alter the intracellular levels of molecules involved in degranulation; therefore, one strategy for control of the symptoms is to decrease the rate of degranulation. Epinephrine, for example, has been used for over 40 years for this purpose. If the release of the active molecules cannot be prevented, the symptoms can be treated with drugs that block the action of the molecules, for example, antihistamines.

One strategy that has had a long history and some success is the attempt to DESENSITIZE the atopic individual. Sufferers of allergy have known that they can get "shots" for their diseases. Many nonimmunologists assume the "shots" contain some wonder drug, but in fact they contain small amounts of purified allergen. The strategy is to inject as pure a form of the allergen as possible in small doses and attempt to convert the immune response from one producing IgE to one producing predominantly IgG. In this way it is hoped that the IgG will compete for the allergen before it can react with any mast cell-fixed IgE. With the discovery of the enhancing and suppressing factors, the rationale has changed; according to the current model the purified allergens may induce the production of suppressive factors. The methods of quantifying IgE are seen in Methods Box 1.

Type II Reactions: Cytolytic Reactions

Type II allergic reactions are those brought about by antibody reacting with antigen on the surface of a cell; these reactions cause the activation of the complement cascade and ultimately the lysis of the cell. The specific manifestation of the reaction depends upon the cell type on whose surface the reaction is occurring, although the result of the reaction is always the destruction of the cell and hence the loss of the function the cell carries out, with all the attendant difficulties which follow.

ERYTHROBLASTOSIS FETALIS is a Type II reaction that can now be controlled through immunologic means. When an Rh^- mother delivers an Rh^+ fetus, she may become sensitized to the baby's Rh^+ erythrocytes during delivery. In such cases she will produce anti-Rh antibodies, which may cross the placenta and destroy the fetal erythrocytes of her next child if it too has Rh^+ red blood cells. This fetal hemolysis results in the overproduction of immature erythrocytes, or ERYTHROBLASTS (hence the name of the disease). This disorder can result in a variety of difficulties, including an aborted fetus or damage to the child's central nervous system

HYPERSENSITIVITY

because of the release of bilirubin and other factors. An Rh^- mother is prevented from becoming sensitized by receiving an injection of anti-Rh antibodies at the time she delivers her first Rh^+ child. This form of immunoregulation has proved remarkably successful.

On occasion, an individual makes an antibody response to a drug that results in hemolysis because the drug interacts with red blood cells. This response and subsequent red cell destruction can result in HEMOLYTIC ANEMIA. Another form of drug-related Type II reaction is an "innocent bystander" phenomenon. Some drugs such as sedormid or quinine and quinidine induce antibody responses that result in drug–antibody complexes which become adsorbed onto circulating platelets. When complement reacts with the complex, lysis of the platelets ensues and produces THROMBOCYTOPENIA.

Type III Reactions: Antigen–Antibody Complex Diseases

In Type III hypersensitivity diseases, the deposition of antigen–antibody complexes results in tissue damage. The prototype reaction is the ARTHUS REACTION. In the experimental form of this reaction, antigen is introduced into the skin of an immunized animal. After a few hours an inflammatory reaction is discernible at the site, followed in 12 hours by induration. The reaction can develop to such a point that the area becomes necrotic. Histological examination of the site shows that the area has been infiltrated by a large number of PMNs.

We now know that the mechanism of the reaction is as follows: the deposition of antigen into the skin of the immune animal causes antigen–antibody complexes to form at the site of injection. These complexes fix complement and the split products of complement act as potent chemotactic factors for PMNs. The Ag–Ab complexes are then ingested by the PMNs that have been attracted to the scene. The ingestion of the immune complex causes them to degranulate, and the contents of the PMN granules then cause tissue damage. In humans, several conditions are known to be due to the Arthus reaction. Hay fever

METHODS BOX 1

Determining IgE Levels

Radioimmunoabsorbent test (RIST) for presence of IgE

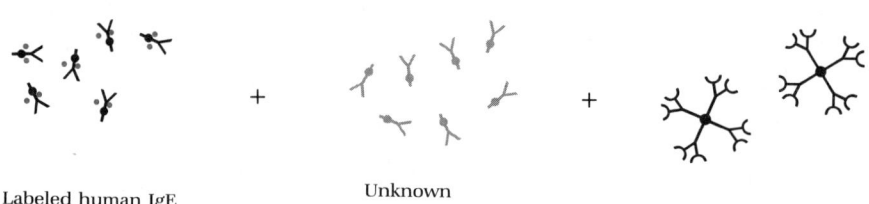

Rabbit anti-human IgE   Agarose beads

1. Rabbit anti-human IgE is conjugated to agarose beads.

Labeled human IgE   Unknown serum sample

2. Radiolabeled human IgE and unknown serum sample are added to the anti-human IgE–agarose complex.

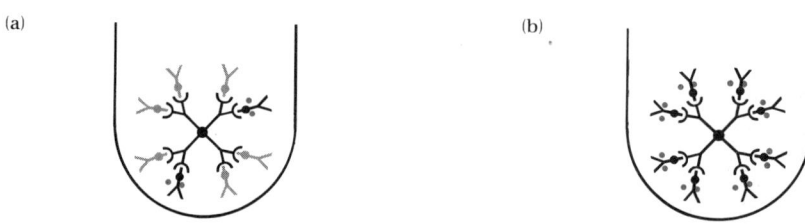

3. (a) The IgE present in the unknown serum competes with the labeled IgE for sites on anti-IgE.

    (b) No IgE is present in the unknown serum, so all the labeled IgE is bound.

4. Centrifuge and count label in pellet. A low count (a) indicates competition for sites and therefore presence of IgE in the unknown serum. A high count (b) indicates a low level of competition and therefore a low level of IgE in the unknown.

METHODS BOX 1

Radioallergosorbent test (RAST) for presence of specific IgE

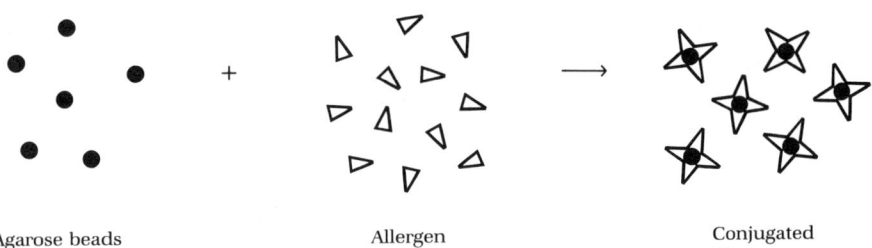

Agarose beads   Allergen   Conjugated allergen

1. Allergen is conjugated to agarose beads.

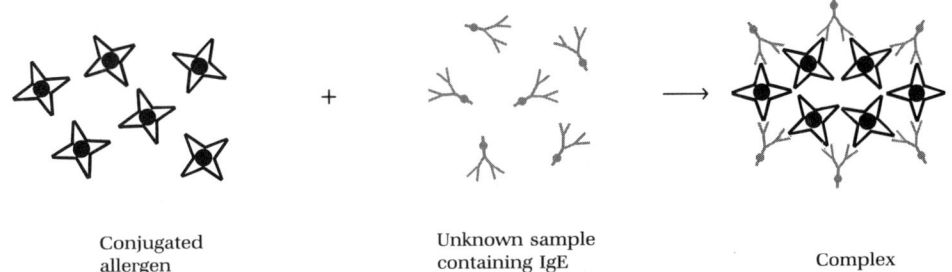

Conjugated allergen   Unknown sample containing IgE   Complex

2. Unknown serum and conjugated allergen are mixed. If specific antibody to the allergen is present, it will form a complex with the conjugated allergen.

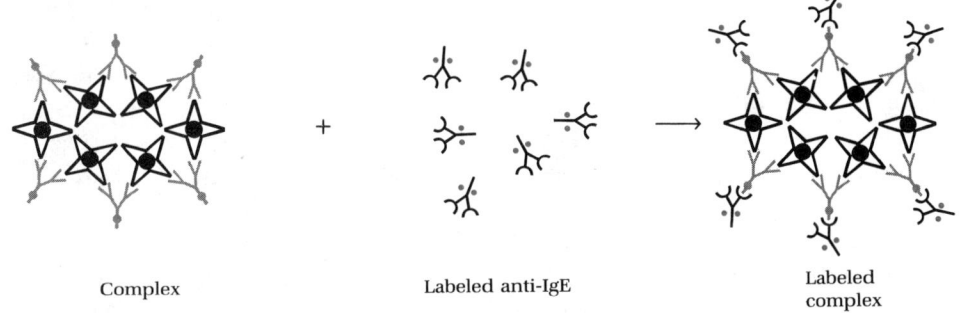

Complex   Labeled anti-IgE   Labeled complex

3. Allergen–antibody complex is mixed with labeled anti-IgE. The complex is centrifuged and the amount of radioactivity is measured. The labeled antibody binds only to antigen-specific IgE.

conjunctivitis, while usually a Type I reaction, does have a severe form that is caused by the Arthus reaction. Hypersensitive pneumonitis is also caused by this reaction.

SERUM SICKNESS is a classical form of Type III allergic disease. This was discovered when serum therapy for diphtheria was commonly used. The antitoxin was produced in a horse and administered to humans. If an individual received multiple injections of the passive antibody, they often became sensitized and produced antibodies to components in the horse serum. The result was a severe form of arthritis and glomerulonephritis caused by deposition of the antigen–antibody complexes.

ALLERGIC GLOMERULONEPHRITIS is a very well studied allergic disease. In this case complexes are formed between either exogenous antigen and antibody that the sensitized individual has produced or, in some cases, it is an autoimmune disease in which the complexes are formed between glomerular basement membrane and anti-glomerular basement membrane.

Type IV Reactions: Delayed-Type Hypersensitivity

The final type of hypersensitivity reactions are those called the DELAYED-TYPE HYPERSENSITIVITY or DTH reactions. These reactions are mediated not by antibody but by T lymphocytes. Historically the first delayed hypersensitivity reaction was seen by Robert Koch when he injected a small amount of fluid from tubercle bacilli cultures and found that an area of induration developed after 48 hours. This test is now used as a clinical screening procedure to determine whether an individual has come in contact with *Mycobacterium tuberculosis* (the tuberculin test). It has also been modified for use with another mycobacterium, *M. leprae*. The most common form of DTH disease is CONTACT DERMITITIS such as that caused by poison ivy and allergies to clothing. These reactions begin at about 24 hours and reach a maximum at 48 or even 96 hours. This response is in sharp contrast to that of the immediate-type reaction, which can occur within minutes.

DTH reactions are initiated by T cells, which react with antigen that either has been deposited in the skin or has become

HYPERSENSITIVITY

covalently attached to skin cells. In the latter case, haptens such as dinitrobenzene, when painted onto the skin, can cause severe reactions. The reaction of the T cells with the antigen results in their activation and the release of lymphokines, some of which are probably chemotactic for monocytes and macrophages. It is the accumulation of these cells that results in tissue damage. It will be recalled from Chapter 15 that in the mouse the effector T cell for DTH (T_{DTH}) expresses Lyt 1 and that the effector cells that carry out delayed-type hypersensitivity and cytotoxicity are different cells.

Summary

1. Hypersensitivity reactions are reactions in which antibody or T cells react with antigen on surfaces of cells, causing the release of pharmacologically active substances that damage the cells.
2. Type I reactions are those mediated by IgE. IgE fixes to mast cells via an Fc receptor for IgE on the mast cell. When the fixed IgE reacts with allergen, a complex series of reactions occurs, culminating in the degranulation of the mast cells. The granules contain active substances that cause the symptoms of allergy.
3. Type II reactions occur when antibodies bind to antigens (allergen) and complement is fixed to the complexes. If the allergen associates itself with the surface of a cell and the antigen–antibody complex forms, the binding of complement causes lysis of the cell.
4. Type III reactions are those in which antigen–antibody complexes form and cause damage by affecting the function of the organ in which they are deposited.
5. Type IV reactions are those caused by effector T cells, which in the mouse are Lyt 1^+ and therefore different from cytotoxic T cells. These reactions are called delayed-type hypersensitivity because they reach a maximum at 48 hours. T cells initiate the response, but monocytes are attracted to the site.

CHAPTER TWENTY-SIX
Additional Readings

DeWeck, A. 1983. Regulation of IgE responses. In *New Trends in Allergy*, J. Ring and G. Burg (eds.). Springer-Verlag, Berlin.

Ishizaka, K. 1983. Structure and biological activity of immunoglobulin E. In *The Biology of Immunologic Disease*, F. J. Dixon and D. W. Fisher (eds.). Sinauer Associates, Sunderland, Mass.

Metzger, H., S. A. Wank and B. Rivnay. 1982. The receptor for immunoglobulin E: taking it apart—putting it back together. Monographs in *Allergy* 18, 1.

Rose, N. R. and H. Friedman. 1980. *Manual of Clinical Immunology*, 2nd ed. American Society for Microbiology, Washington D. C.

CHAPTER 27

AUTOIMMUNITY

Overview The central problem of the immune system is to respond to foreign antigen while not making reactions to self components. But an apparent paradox is raised, because we know that the recognition and the response to foreign antigen is MHC-restricted—that is, foreign antigens are somehow recognized in the context of self. We saw in the chapter on immune tolerance that we do not know how nonreactivity to self is maintained. It is intuitively obvious that a breakdown in the mechanisms that prevent self-reactivity can have dire consequences, and in this chapter we will examine some autoimmune diseases that come from destructive self reactions.

We will divide the autoimmune diseases into those in which antibody is involved and those in which T cells are the agents of destruction. Among the antibody-initiated diseases, we will examine those involving organ-specific antibody and those involving antibodies to a wide range of tissues and components. We will see that a humoral or cellular immune response to self tissue can have wide-ranging and serious consequences.

CHAPTER TWENTY-SEVEN

Horror Autotoxicus Revisited

Recognition versus Reaction

In Chapter 24 we discussed immune tolerance in terms of the mechanisms by which the immune system prevents itself from making responses against self in the context of MHC restriction—the immune system must *recognize* self in some manner in order to react to something foreign. The situation appears to be paradoxical. On one hand we have shown that self-recognition is needed, but on the other hand we know that self-reaction can be suicidal. The crucial point is that recognition and reaction are not the same, a point that is often overlooked in discussions of the immune response. For the purposes of continuing the analysis of the immune response along the path we have been following, the reader should keep this distinction in mind. Maintaining a state of not *reacting* to self while continuing to *recognize* self is really a problem of maintaining a state of not making *destructive* reactions to self. This means that, finally, tolerance and autoimmunity are problems of immune regulation.

Ehrlich termed the need not to react to self *horror autotoxicus*. He designed experiments in which he deliberately attempted to immunize animals against their own tissues and, in general, failed to do so. This confirmed, in his mind, the obvious correctness of his idea of *horror autotoxicus*. However, over a period of time many investigators, including Ehrlich, began to find that under certain conditions it was possible to induce reactions to self components, and that in many diseases there were antibodies to self tissues. The question then became very much like the question General Custer asked at Little Big Horn when he first saw all the Indians: How did they get there and are they really dangerous? Because of the traditional orientation of immunology toward infectious diseases, there was a tendency to think in terms of a single cause—probably an infectious organism—as the etiological agent of those diseases in which it could be shown that there was reaction to self. Because we knew how to deal with them, it was not only logical but also comforting to think that a bacterial or viral agent had produced the damage to the tissue, resulting in disease, and that the antibody to self components (autoantibody) was a secondary event. But slowly the awareness that the antibodies might be the cause of the symp-

AUTOIMMUNITY

toms grew; even if the initial insult was from external sources, the pathogenesis was immunological.

In recent years we have become aware that most things do not have one simple cause. The interconnection and interdependence of various systems have made us aware that the symptoms seen in any particular disease are likely to be due to an interplay of causal agents, some of which may be external. The price the immune system may have paid for its ability to react quickly to any external insult is that its delicate regulatory mechanisms are liable to be upset by many factors, both external and internal. Because of this, in the modern era we are likely to think of autoimmune diseases as diseases of regulation. In fact, we do not know the relative importance in most autoimmune diseases of external factors, genetic predisposition, and internal malfunctions.

Organ-specific and Non–Organ-specific Autoimmune Diseases

Table 1 lists several autoimmune diseases and characterizes them in terms of the distribution of the autoantigens. Some diseases occur at a specific site; for example, in Graves disease there is an antibody against the receptor for thyroid-stimulating hormone. The primary site of the disease is the thyroid gland and the symptoms of the disease are all attributable to the actions of these antibodies. In contrast, some diseases—for example, systemic lupus erythematosus—are non–organ-nonspecific, and in these disorders there are antibodies to a large range of tissues and symptoms affect many systems. But for these diseases it is difficult to know whether an antibody is the initiating event of the pathology or a by-product of tissue damage.

Antibody-Mediated, Organ-Specific Autoimmune Diseases

Anti-Receptor Diseases There are several diseases in which the pathology is known to be caused by anti-receptor antibodies. The point we want to make in this section is that the effect of the reaction of the antibody with the receptor can have

CHAPTER TWENTY-SEVEN

TABLE 1 Antigens in autoimmune diseases

Disease	Antigen type[a]					
	A	B	C	D	E	F
Systemic lupus erythematosus	+		+		+	
Sjögren's syndrome	+				+	
Scleroderma	+					
Polymyositis	+		+			
Chronic active hepatitis	+				+	
Mixed connective tissue disease	+					
Insulin-dependent diabetes	+	+				+
Primary biliary cirrhosis	+					
Pernicious anemia	+					+
Autoimmune thyroiditis	+	+				+
Idiopathic Addison's disease	+					
Vitiligo	+					
Gluten-sensitive enteropathy	+					
Chronic active hepatitis	+					
Graves disease	+	+				
Myasthenia gravis		+				
Autoimmune hemolytic anemia			+			
Autoimmune neutropenia			+			
Idiopathic thrombocytopenia purpura			+			
Rheumatoid arthritis			+		+	
Cirrhosis			+			
Multiple sclerosis			+			
Pemphigus vulgaris			+	+		
Autoimmune infertility			+			
Goodpasture's disease				+		
Bullous pemphigoid				+		
Discoid lupus				+		
Dense deposit disease					+	

Source: Modified from Smith and Steinberg (1982), *Annu. Rev. Immunol.* 1: 175.

[a] A, intracellular; B, receptors; C, cell membrane components; D, extracellular; E, plasma proteins; F, hormones.

AUTOIMMUNITY

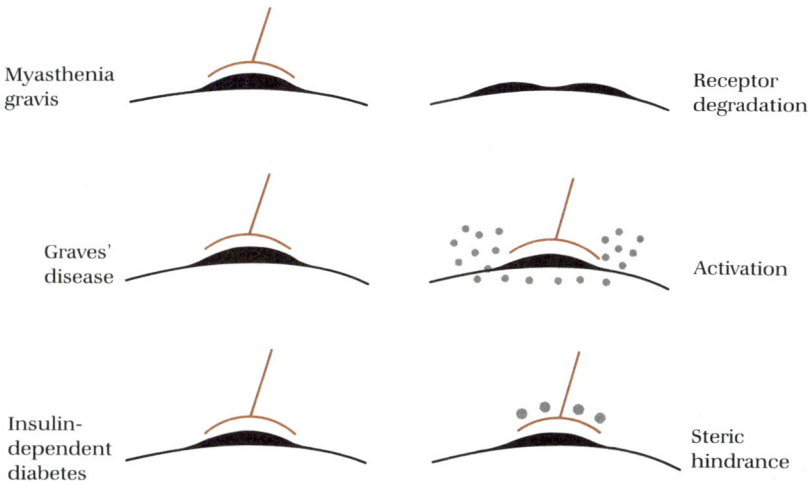

FIGURE 1 MECHANISMS OF ANTI-RECEPTOR AUTOIMMUNE DISEASES

Auto-anti-receptor antibody reacting with a receptor can result in disease by several mechanisms. (A) Myasthenia gravis: Anti-acetylcholine receptor (AChR) antibody causes degradation of the receptor; as a result acetylcholine fails to stimulate the cell. (B) Graves disease: Anti-thyroid stimulating hormone (TSH) antibody binds to the receptor and activates the cell. This reaction causes an unregulated production of TSH. (C) Insulin-dependent diabetes: Anti-insulin receptor antibody blocks the receptor and thus prevents insulin from acting.

very different results. Some of these results are illustrated in Figure 1.

MYASTHENIA GRAVIS (MG) is a neuromuscular disorder of humans which is characterized by weakness and easy fatigability of skeletal muscles. The clinical features of the disease were first noted in 1672 and were thoroughly described by 1900, when it was noted that there was great similarity between the symptoms of MG and curare poisoning. In the 1930s it was noted that patients treated with anticholinesterase drugs showed great improvement. Because cholinesterase is known to be involved in nerve impulses at the neuromuscular junction, it was concluded

CHAPTER TWENTY-SEVEN

that the disease was due to some malfunction at that site. In the 1960s it was found (using microelectrode techniques) that the amplitude of miniature endplate potentials (MEPPs: the amount of depolarization at the presynaptic nerve terminal) was reduced by 80% at the neuromuscular junction in MG patients. This finding led to the conclusion that there was a *presynaptic* defect in the disease. The most likely explanation was a reduced number of acetylcholine (ACh) molecules as a result of some unknown defect in the motor nerve terminals.[1]

In the 1970s it became possible to study the ACETYLCHOLINE RECEPTOR (AChR). Because α-bungarotoxin (α-BuTx) binds specifically and irreversibly to the AChR of skeletal muscle, it can be radiolabeled and used to quantify the number of AChR. When this was done, it was found that the neuromuscular junctions in MG patients bind only 11–30% of normal amounts. Furthermore, treatment of experimental animals with α-cobra toxin, a procedure that reduces the number of AChR, causes the characteristics of human MG in these animals. These findings indicated that the defect in MG is not presynaptic but *postsynaptic*, and that the events involved are not those preceding the release of ACh but those that follow.

The *autoimmune* nature of MG was inferred from the finding that in MG patients there is a high incidence of thymus abnormality (an association also found in other autoimmune diseases), reduced levels of complement, and the presence of anti-skeletal muscle antibody. These facts led to a search for antibody reactive with the acetylcholine receptor; and in the 1970s several groups independently identified such anti-AChR antibodies in MG patients.

The fact that MG patients have anti-AChR antibody in their serum and the fact that there are fewer available receptors in the disease might lead to the conclusion that the effect of the antibody is merely a steric blocking of the receptor site. This is not the case. Drachman and his colleagues at Johns Hopkins have

---

[1] Readers interested in the structure and function of the synapse are directed to Kuffler, Nicholls, and Martin (1984), *From Neuron to Brain*, 2nd ed.; and to Hille (1984), *Ionic Channels of Excitable Membranes*, both published by Sinauer Associates, Sunderland, Mass.

AUTOIMMUNITY

shown that the anti-AChR antibody acts in this disease by causing an *accelerated degradation* of AChR (Figure 2). The anti-AChR antibody, either as the intact IgG or as Fab_2, when bound to the receptor causes degradation of the receptor (Figure 2A and B). In contrast, Fab can bind to the receptor but cannot cause degradation (Figure 2C). Treating the bound Fab_2 with anti-Ig causes

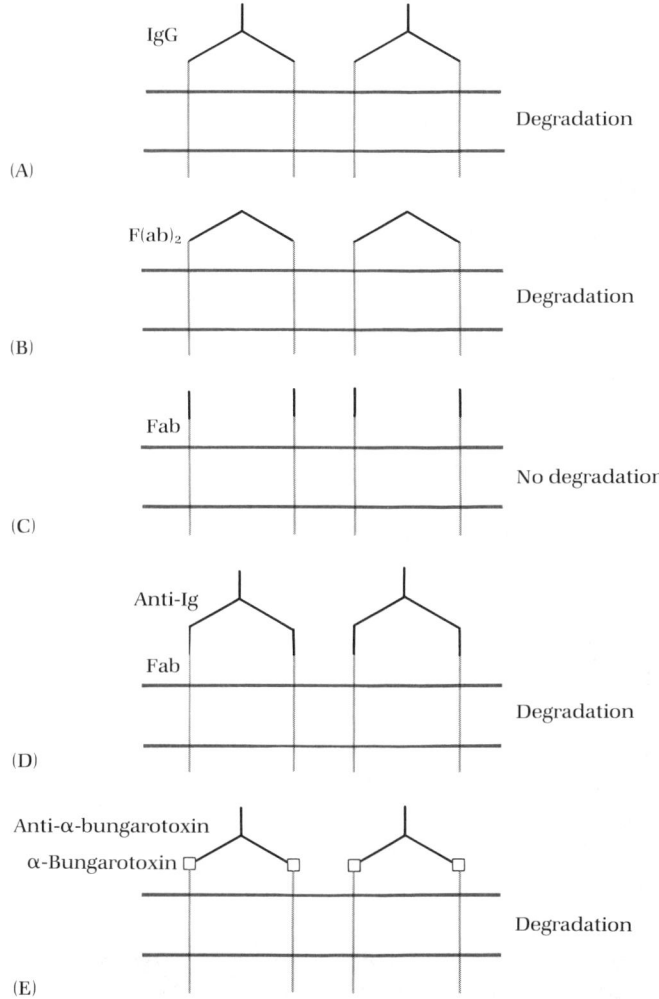

FIGURE 2 DEGRADATION OF THE ACETYLCHOLINE RECEPTOR BY ANTIBODY

(A,B) Either intact antibody or Fab_2 causes degradation of the acetylcholine receptor (AChR). (C,D) Monovalent Fab does not cause degradation, but the addition of anti-Fab does. (E) Bungarotoxin does not cause degradation, but the anti-bungarotoxin does so. These findings imply that cross-linking of receptors is crucial for their degradation. [After Drachman (1978) *N. Engl. J. Med.* 298, 120]

degradation. The similarity between these experiments and those of the Ishizakas on the degranulation of mast cells by IgE will not be lost on the reader, and the interpretations are similar. When reaction of antibody with the receptor produces cross-linking of receptors, degradation occurs. In an analogous manner, when the ACh receptors are cross-linked by treatment with α-bungarotoxin, degradation also occurs (Figure 2E). So we see that anti-AChR antibody can cause degradation of receptors and that the symptoms of the disease result from the loss of AChR.

GRAVES' DISEASE is another autoimmune disease in which anti-receptor antibodies play a role in the pathogenesis. Patients with Graves' disease suffer from overproduction of the thyroid hormones thyroxine and triiodothyronine. In normal individuals the pituitary secretes the hormone THYROID-STIMULATING HORMONE (TSH), which binds to TSH receptors on thyroid cells. This binding activates the adenylate cyclase system and causes the thyroid cells to produce thyroxine and triiodothyronine. As with most hormone systems, there is a very delicate feedback control of the amount of TSH produced and consequently of the amount of thyroid hormone released. Patients with Graves' disease produce *antibodies to the TSH receptor*. The binding of these anti-receptor antibodies, however, has an effect very different from that produced by the binding of anti-AChR antibodies to the ACh receptor. In this case, binding of antibody to the receptor has the same effect as the binding of TSH—the production of thyroid hormone. In other words, the antibody acts like the agonist and triggers the cell to produce the hormone. Of course, the anti-receptor antibodies are not under the same hormonal feedback control, so the thyroid keeps producing, and then overproducing, hormones. The symptoms of this disease, then, are due to the antibody-stimulated overproduction of thyroid hormone.

In some cases of INSULIN-RESISTANT DIABETES there are anti-insulin receptor antibodies that react with the insulin receptor and partially block it. This competition prevents the insulin molecule from reacting with the receptor resulting in the symptoms of the disease.

Thus these three autoimmune diseases are caused by anti-receptor antibodies but in each case the antibody has a very different mechanism of pathogenesis.

AUTOIMMUNITY

Autoimmune Thyroiditis

Another organ-specific disease associated with antibody is autoimmune thyroiditis, or HASHIMOTO'S DISEASE. But unlike the anti-receptor diseases discussed above, it is not clear whether the antibody is the cause or the effect of this disease. The thyroid in Hashimoto's disease is filled with inflammatory cells; and antibodies to thyroglobulin, cytoplasmic antigens, and cell-surface antigens of the thyroid can be found in the serum. The role, if any, of these antibodies, however, is not known.

The OBESE CHICKEN is an experimental model of autoimmune thyroiditis. In this model neonatal thymectomy accelerates the disease and neonatal bursectomy prevents it. Even though there are many questions to be answered the research seems to be pointing toward a breakdown of the regulatory interaction between suppressor T cells and antibody forming cells.

Hemolytic Anemia

There are many reasons for the development of anemia in an individual, only one of which is due to autoimmunity. Even in cases of autoimmune hemolytic anemia, it is important to determine if the disorder is one of the sequelae of another disease (even another autoimmune disease such as lupus erythematosus; see below) or is due to an autoimmune response to the patient's erythrocytes.

The autoimmune hemolytic anemias are divided into WARM ANTIBODY TYPE and COLD ANTIBODY TYPE. In the warm type, which is the more common, the patients have antibody on their red cells. This condition can often be diagnosed by the addition of anti-immunoglobulin which causes agglutination of the red cells. This assay is called the COOMBS TEST. Cold agglutinin disease is associated with very high titers of agglutinating IgM antibodies, which react optimally in the cold. The specificity of this IgM is usually to the I or Ii red cell antigen. Clinically, hemolysis occurs in the patients when they become cold and the treatment consists of keeping the patients warm and waiting for a spontaneous resolution. The symptoms associated with warm autoantibody hemolytic anemia are anemia; fever, jaundice, and splenomegaly associated with hemolysis; and congestive heart failure. Very commonly these signs are associated with other autoimmune disorders or leukemia. When the disease is not associated with another disease, it often follows viral infection.

There are a whole class of autoimmune hemolytic anemias that are known to be *drug induced*. A wide range of drugs, from insulin to sulfonamides to chlorinated hydrocarbons, are implicated. In these cases the pathology may be caused by circulating immune complexes of drug and anti-drug antibody, which bind to the red cells and allow them to be lysed by complement. This sequence is called the "innocent bystander effect." In other cases, the drug may become bound to the red cell, which acts as a carrier and allows an anti-drug response to be made. It will be recalled from Chapter 24 that this is not a normal phenomenon, because self components usually do not act as carriers.

Non–Organ-Specific Autoimmune Diseases Associated With Antibody

Systemic Lupus Erythematosus

SYSTEMIC LUPUS ERYTHEMATOSUS (SLE) is an autoimmune disease which is widespread and non–organ-specific. It is characterized by fever, skin rashes, polyarthritis, effusions in the pleural, pericardial and peritoneal cavities, and central nervous signs. SLE patients have reduced complement levels and high levels of immune complexes in their serum and glomeruli. In fact, the life-threatening lesion is often a progressive IMMUNE COMPLEX-MEDIATED GLOMERULONEPHRITIS. Deposits of autoantibody and complement can be found in the glomeruli as immune complex deposits which may be focal, membranous, or diffuse.

Antibodies to intracellular components, cell-surface membrane components from various cell types, serum components, and *nucleic acids* are seen in SLE patients. Because of the great variety of antibodies and the spectrum of symptoms, SLE is another autoimmune phenomenon in which it has proved difficult to tell which of the antibodies are the cause of the disease and which are the result of tissue damage.

AUTOIMMUNITY

Animal Models of SLE

The availability of several animal models for SLE has been useful in the attempt to analyze the importance of the immune abnormalities and autoantibodies seen in human lupus. However, even with these models it is still not clear which are the most important factors in this multifactor disease.

In New Zealand, M. and F. Bielschowsky observed that New Zealand Black (NZB) mice died with widespread and diverse symptoms of hemolytic anemia, glomerulonephritis, and vasculitis, all very reminiscent of human lupus. Another mouse, New Zealand White (NZW), did not develop autoimmune disease; but the F_1 [(NZB $\times$ NZW)F_1] developed severe disease. Backcrosses and extensive genetic studies have shown that the disease is not inherited as a single dominant trait. From these genetic studies it has become clear that some of the factors that contribute to the disease are susceptibility factors. For example, NZW mice contribute at least two genes to the susceptibility to disease of the (NZB x NZW)F_1 and NZB contributes one. At least one of these three genes is in H-2, and one is linked to H-2. The nature of the genes or their influence is not known.

The NZB model of SLE has been studied very extensively; but like the human disease, it has been difficult to analyze for either cause and effect relationships or for the relative importance of the pathological changes. The late E. Murphy and J. Roths at the Jackson Laboratory in Bar Harbor have developed two strains of mice, called MRL/1 and BXSB which develop lupus-like disease and are aiding the analysis, but to date the problem is far from solved.

All of the strains that develop lupus-like disease have several features in common. In all of them it is very difficult to *induce immunological tolerance* to serum protein in adult life. In all of them there is *increased immunoglobulin production*, although the class varies in different strains. All strains have *lymphoid abnormalities* such as lymphoid hyperplasia and increases in T cell or B cell numbers. As in the human disease, *glomerulonephritis* is a prominent feature of the experimental disease in all of the strains.

CHAPTER TWENTY-SEVEN

As previously stated, it is not clear which antibodies are the initiators of the pathology in lupus and which the result of the initial tissue damage. Moreover, the disease is clearly the result of several factors. The autoantibody that is responsible for the immune complexes could be the result of nonspecific activation of B cells. The inability to induce tolerance in NZB could indicate that the mechanism for maintenance of self-tolerance is impaired. The thymus disorders and T cell defects could result in a loss of suppressor T cells, which would allow the polyclonal activation of T cells. Many or all of these could be correct, but we do not know the reason for the initiation of the events that bring them all together.

Rheumatoid arthritis One of the most common diseases is the autoimmune disease RHEUMATOID ARTHRITIS, commonly known as rheumatism. It is a disease associated with advanced age, and it is estimated that as much as 80% of the population experiences some form of rheumatic discomfort at some time in their lives. The disease is characterized by a chronic inflammation of the joints, which is caused by autoantibodies against the Fc portion of the patient's IgG. These antibodies are called RHEUMATOID FACTOR (RF), and are either IgM or IgG. They form immune complexes with IgG molecules, and the complexes produce synovitis and vasculitis, the major symptoms of the disease. However, it is not known what causes the production of RF. There is some genetic disposition to the disease because people with the HLA types DRW3 and DRW4 have a significantly higher incidence of the disease. It is also not known why the synovia of the joints should be the point of deposition of the immune complexes.

Another form of the disease, *rheumatic fever*, is known to be initiated following infection with group A streptococci. These organisms have cross-reactive antigens with heart, cartilage, muscle and kidney. In some patients, often children, the sequelae of a "strep throat" are heart disease ("rheumatic heart"), kidney disease due to immune complexes, or arthritis. Why some patients respond to the cross-reactive antigens by producing antibody, that is, breaking tolerance, is not known. In some rare cases of

AUTOIMMUNITY

rheumatic fever, there is the neurological disorder known as ST. VITUS DANCE. This syndrome occurs primarily in females and after recovery there is no permanent neurological damage (although religious fame may have been achieved).

T Cell-Mediated Autoimmunity: Autoimmune Demyelinating Diseases

Multiple Sclerosis

MULTIPLE SCLEROSIS (MS) was described as a clinical entity in 1868 by Charcot. Clinically it is a highly variable disease, which usually begins between the second and fifth decades of life. The common signs are sensory and visual motor dysfunction. In the *chronic form* the patient has periods of remission. But with each remission there is greater neurological dysfunction. A *benign form* exists and is characterized by mild exacerbations followed by a complete recovery.

The pathology of MS is confined to the nervous system. Macroscopic lesions of 1–4 cm called PLAQUES are scattered throughout the white matter. The term *multiple sclerosis* was initially used to describe the wide distribution of the lesions in the white matter. Microscopically the disease is characterized by a *breakdown of the myelin sheath*. The demyelinated lesions have a perivenous distribution and contain macrophages and lymphocytes. There is loss of myelin basic protein in the area of the lesions.

The etiology of MS is unknown. Both chronic infectious agents and autoimmunity have been invoked, and in fact both might be important. An altered suppressor:cytotoxic T cell ratio is seen in the disease and has led to the idea that a decrease in suppressor cells allows clones of autoreactive cells to become activated. MS patients have been shown to have immune complexes; but these are considered to be secondary, because levels are low compared to those seen in SLE. Similar levels are seen in the demyelinating diseases amyotrophic lateral sclerosis (Lou Gehrig disease) and subacute sclerosing panencephalitis. These facts have led to the general conclusion that MS is a T cell-mediated autoimmune disease. The similarity between the human disease and the murine disease, experimental autoimmune encephalitis, has strengthened this belief.

CHAPTER TWENTY-SEVEN

Experimental Autoimmune Encephalitis

Injection of experimental animals with CNS tissue emulsified in complete Freund's adjuvant (an oil–water emulsion containing mycobacteria) results in characteristic lesions of the central nervous system. As stated above, the experimental disease mimics MS in so many ways that it is considered the best experimental model of the human disease. The fact that the symptoms can be transferred to normal animals by lymphoid cells but not by serum from a diseased animal has strengthened the conclusion that the disease is a cell-mediated one.

The antigen in brain that is responsible for the disease has been studied extensively. When the basic protein component of myelin, called MYELIN BASIC PROTEIN, is injected into animals in adjuvant, all of the symptoms are produced. Analysis of the basic protein has shown that there are ENCEPHALITOGENIC PEPTIDES but a peptide that is encephalitogenic in one species may not be in another. Encephalitogenic peptides not only may initiate the disease, but they also may regulate it, because circulating basic peptide has been shown to reduce the activity of the effector T cells in the disease.

Self-Reactivity in the Absence of Pathology

We have just developed arguments and evidence to justify the logical idea that the body must not react against itself. However, there are some cases in which there appear to be naturally occurring auto-reactive cells and antibody without disease. The first thing that comes to mind, of course, is MHC-restricted T cell responses in which foreign antigens are recognized in the context of self. And there is a fairly large literature showing that there are reactive cells, both T and B, to normal thyroglobulin in normal humans and mice and that many normal individuals have titers of anti-autologous erythrocyte antibody in their serum. Perhaps more convincing, if cells are activated polyclonally with mitogens, both cells and antibody against a wide range of self-antigens appear. All of this is in the absence of pathology, so it may be that responses to certain antigens do not lead to pathology.

AUTOIMMUNITY

A reaction called the AUTOLOGOUS MLR (A-MLR) is directed against self-MHC antigens. When cells are cultured for an MLR, there is always background DNA synthesis, as measured by incorporation of tritiated thymidine. It was found, however, that when mitomycin-treated *autologous* peripheral blood cells are added to cultures of lymphocytes, there is an increase in DNA synthesis. This result is surprising because the mitomycin-treated cells cannot be responsible for the increased DNA synthesis—because mitomycin inhibits new DNA synthesis. The autologous cells must therefore be inducing the normal cells to proliferate. When the proportion of non-T cells in a population of normal cells is reduced, the incorporation is reduced to a much greater extent than can be accounted for by the proportion of cells removed. The conclusion: autologous non-T cells stimulate autologous T cells to proliferate. The responding T cells in the A-MLR are T4 (and not T8) cells which are responsive to concanavalin A. The nature of the stimulating molecules is not defined, although, in humans, the stimulating cells express HLA-D. The significance of the A-MLR is not known.

Summary

1. The immune system must recognize self to respond to foreign antigens (MHC restriction) but must not react against itself. In those cases where there are reactions against self-tissue or self-components, the result is autoimmunity.
2. Autoimmune diseases can be brought about by antibody or by cell mediated mechanisms.
3. There are autoimmune diseases in which the reactions are organ-specific or tissue-specific and those in which the specificity is not obvious, either because of many sites of reaction or because of secondary effects.
4. In many cases there is difficulty in determining whether the antibody is the cause or the result of the disease.

CHAPTER TWENTY-SEVEN

Additional Readings

Paterson, P. Y., and E. D. Day. 1981. Current perspectives of neuroimmunological disease: multiple sclerosis and experimental allergic encephalomyelitis. *Clin. Immunol. Rev.* 1, 581.

Samter, M. (ed.). 1971. *Immunological Diseases*, 2nd ed. Little, Brown and Company, Boston.

Smith, H. R. and A. D. Steinberg. 1983. Autoimmunity—a perspective. *Annu. Rev. Immunol.* 1, 175.

Weigle, W. O. 1980. Analysis of autoimmunity through experimental models of thyroiditis and allergic encephalomyelitis. *Adv. Immunol.* 30, 159.

Weksler, M. E., C. E. Moody and R. W. Kozak. 1981. The autologous mixed-lymphocyte reaction. *Adv. Immunol.* 31, 271.

CHAPTER 28

TRANSPLANTATION

Overview The ability to respond to foreign antigen undoubtedly is important in the survival of the species (or else why would there be immunologists?). However, the response can be an impediment to surgical intervention when we wish to replace parts of the body. Surgeons have made the necessary technical advances that allow them to hook up the plumbing for kidneys, hearts, and livers. But these procedures would all be doomed to failure, because of the immune response of the host, if adequate tissue matching and immunosuppression were not available. These advances are not of sufficient public interest to warrant television interviews, but the surgeons and transplant immunologists who have carefully worked out these methods have brought us to the point where transplantation of vital organs is the medical procedure of choice in many diseases.

It is amazing to think that within the lifetimes of some of the more mature readers of this book there was still a question about whether or not foreign tissue could be transplanted and what the nature of the rejection mechanism could be. We will see that the immunological basis of rejection is now firmly established and the success of clinical transplants has come about through our ability to control these phenomena.

CHAPTER TWENTY-EIGHT

Graft Rejection as an Immune Phenomenon

For many years surgeons had been faced with a dilemma when treating burn patients needing such large amounts of new skin that skin from the patient would not be sufficient to cover the area. They could either use "pinch grafts" to make one piece of skin do the job of two or three or use skin from another individual. Although Lexner in 1911 had shown clearly that skin cannot be transferred from one individual to another, many surgeons continued the practice. As Peter Medawar pointed out in his 1957 Harvey lecture, "Holding their critical faculties in abeyance, [these surgeons] had convinced themselves that the skin of rabbits or dogs could flourish on human soil. The problem of whether or not skin grafts could survive transplantation from one person to another was still thought to be worth debating as recently as fifteen years ago [that is, 1942]."

In 1943, in fact, Medawar had done an experiment showing convincingly that foreign skin was rejected by "a mechanism of active immunization."

> A 22 year old burn patient was treated with 52 pinch autografts from her own thigh and 50 homografts from her brother's. A second set of 28 pinch homografts from her brother were transplanted 15 days after the first. The autografts grew and formed a continuous sheet. In contrast, the first set of homografts started growing, but by biopsy could be seen to be degenerating by 15 days and degeneration was complete by 23 days. The second set of homografts were in an advanced state of degeneration by day 8. [Gibson, T., and P. B. Medawar (1943) *J. Anat.* 77: 299.]

It was clear to Medawar that the second set of grafts was being rejected at the same time as the original. He concluded that the patient had made an immune response to the first set of homografts and this caused the accelerated rejection of the second set of grafts. In other words, graft rejection was an immune phenomenon.

In a classic paper in 1945 ("A Report to the War Wounds Committee of the Medical Research Council") Medawar summarized his experiments with the transplantation of skin of rabbits. "Resistance to homologous grafted skin therefore belongs to the general category of actively acquired immune reactions." [P. Medawar (1945) *J. Anat.* 79, 157]

TRANSPLANTATION

In 1954 Medawar's student, N. A. Mitchison, showed that immunity to a tumor could be transferred from one mouse to another with lymph node cells from an immunized animal but not with serum. This was so similar to the transfer of delayed-type hypersensitivity, which Chase had shown many years before, that the idea that tissue rejection was the result of an immune response became firmly established. It will be recalled from Chapter 13 on the MHC that at about this same time Peter Gorer was showing that tumor rejection and homograft rejection had the same mechanism. The stage was now set to understand graft rejection in terms of a cell mediated immune response.

The Laws of Transplantation

Since the fate of a graft depends upon the ability of the host to respond to foreign antigens, the use of inbred mice was crucial for carrying out careful studies to determine the factors involved. From these studies, the LAWS OF TRANSPLANTATION were developed (Figure 1).

Law I. Autografts survive. An AUTOGRAFT is the grafting of tissue from one area of the body to another area of the body on the same individual. There may be anatomical barriers to such a procedure, but there are no immunological barriers because the recipient's immune system is seeing no new antigens.

Law II. Syngeneic grafts survive. Syngeneic animals are animals of the same inbred strain. This "law" is really a truism, because in inbred strains of mice each member is as genetically close to any other as identical twins.

Law III. Allografts are rejected. Members of the same species but with different genetic composition are allogeneic. The grafting of tissue from one strain to another is called an ALLOGRAFT. An allograft introduces genetic differences, which the recipient sees and responds to. Allografts are therefore rejected unless some means of preventing the host's immune system from responding to the foreign antigen is used.

	Law	Donor antigens	Recipient Receptors	Reaction

I. Autografts survive

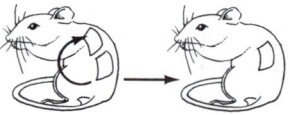 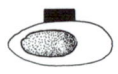 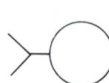 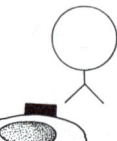

II. Syngeneic grafts survive

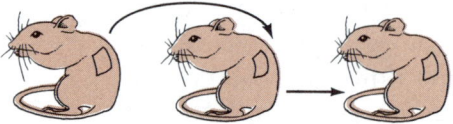 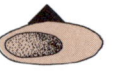 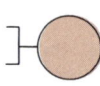 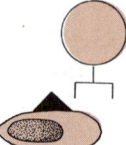

III. Allogeneic grafts are rejected

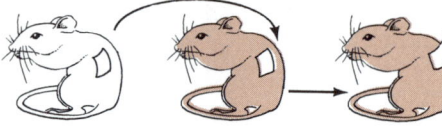 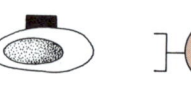 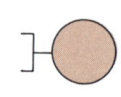 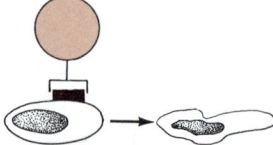

IV. Parent→F_1 grafts survive

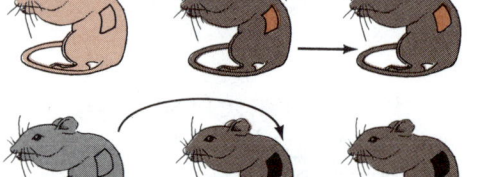 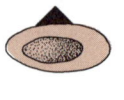 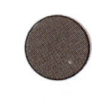 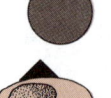

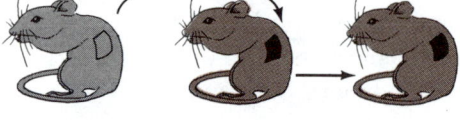 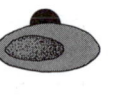 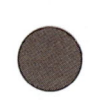 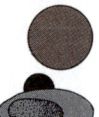

V. F_1→parent grafts are rejected

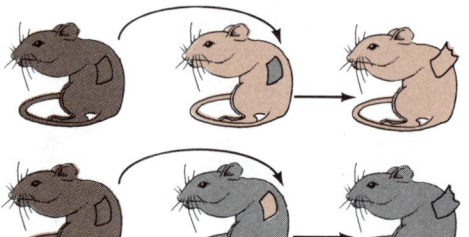 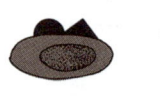 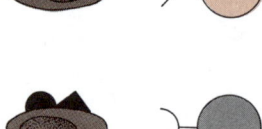 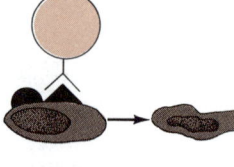

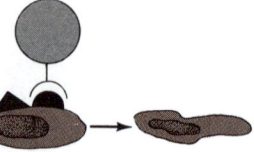

TRANSPLANTATION

Law IV. Parent-to-F_1 grafts are accepted. Given two strains of mice, P and Q, the $(P \times Q)F_1$ will express the antigens of both parental types. Thus when parental tissue is grafted to the F_1 which has both P and Q antigens, the F_1 host will not see any foreign antigens on the parental graft. The graft will therefore succeed. In cases where the graft is immunologically competent the graft itself may respond to the foreign antigen of the recipient or host. This is called a graft-versus-host reaction (GVH) and was discussed in Chapter 15.

Law V. F_1-to-parent grafts are rejected. In this case the F_1 has the antigens of both parental strains, P *and* Q. The recipient is one of the parental types, P *or* Q. The parental recipient P will therefore see the antigens of Q as foreign on the $(P \times Q)F_1$ graft and will respond to them. The graft will therefore be rejected.

Problems in Human Transplantation

Matching Donor and Recipients and Immunosuppression

Given the fact that antigenic differences determine the outcome of a graft, it follows that the fewer the differences the greater the chance of acceptance. Thus, in choosing a donor of an organ for a prospective recipient, the transplant team will seek a donor who most closely matches the recipient. Experience has shown that the matching of the Class I antigens are the most crucial. It will be recalled that in humans the Class I antigens are A, B, and C (DR was considered a Class II antigen but may be Class I). However, the D antigens (Class II) are known to play a role.

FIGURE 1 THE LAWS OF TRANSPLANTATION

I and II. Autografts and grafts between syngeneic recipients survive because there are no T cells that are able to recognize the self-syngeneic antigens on the graft. III. Allografts are rejected because the recipient has T cells that are reactive to the antigens on the graft. IV and V. Parent-to-F_1 grafts survive because the F_1 host has antigens of the parent and therefore has no reactive T cells against these antigens. In contrast, F_1-to-parent grafts are rejected because the parent has reactive T cells to the other parent's antigens.

Figure 2A shows the results of renal transplants at the University of Minnesota, a major transplant center, from the early years of transplantation (1963 to 1968). Note that the two-year survival rate was slightly less than 60% when the donor and recipient were related but was zero when donor and recipient were unrelated. Cadaver kidneys had less than 20% survival rate after two years. Compare this to Figure 2B, which shows transplants in the same center in the modern era, that is, the era of immuno-

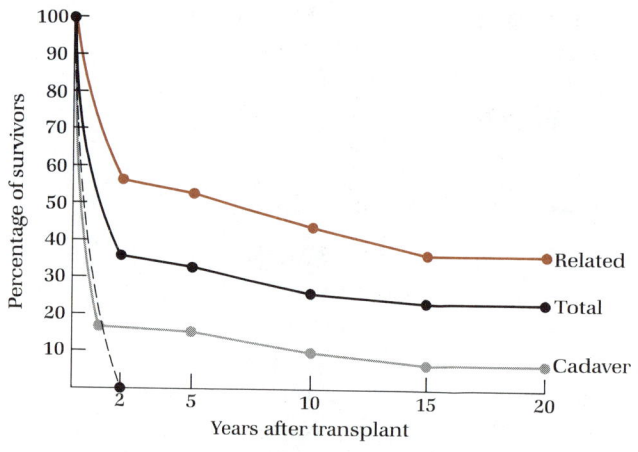

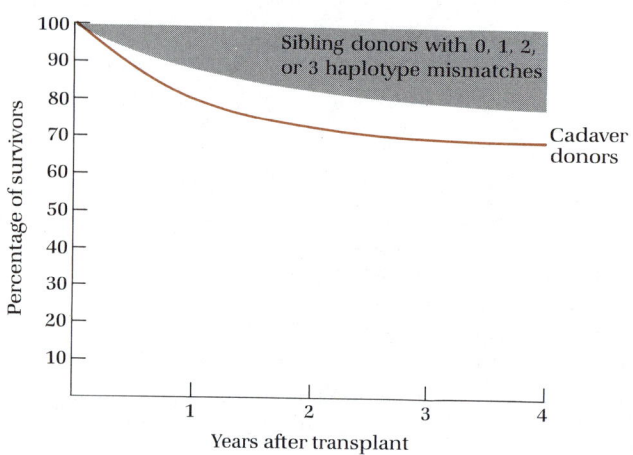

FIGURE 2 SURVIVAL RATES FOR KIDNEY TRANSPLANTS

(A) Survival rates from 1963 to 1968. With tissue typing, a 50% survival rate was achieved. Cadaver kidneys could not be properly matched and so had a very low survival rate. (Of the 123 cases documented here, 59 were between relatives, 4 between unrelated persons, and 60 used cadaver kidneys.) (B) Survival rates from 1970 to 1984. Use of immunosuppressive drugs allowed survival rates to approach 90% with good matching and 70% with cadaver kidneys. [Based on data from Sutherland et al. (1985) *Transplant. Proc.* 17, 110]

TRANSPLANTATION

suppression. The four-year survival rate for cadaver kidneys is 70% and for sibling donor:recipients it is over 80%. Clearly, matching of donors and recipients is important, but the major improvement has been in immunosuppression.

A variety of immunosuppressive regimens have been used over the years. At present four "modalities" are used: the purine analog azathioprine, the corticosteroid prednisone, anti-lymphocyte globulin, and the antibiotic cyclosporin A. Used in judicious combination, these agents serve to suppress the ability of the recipient to reject the graft. Of course, they also reduce the ability of the recipient to respond to any other antigen and so must be used with great care.

AZATHIOPRINE is an analog of purine and is metabolized by the body to 6-MERCAPTOPURINE. These agents probably work by being incorporated into newly synthesized DNA where, because they are analogs and not the proper base, they disrupt DNA synthesis and prevent the cell from proliferating.

PREDNISONE is a corticosteroid. Cortisone and other corticosteroids have many physiological functions and at varying doses they have various effects on the immune system. Earlier we discussed the fact that nonfunctional cells in the thymus are cortisone-sensitive. The corticosteroid that has had the most recent use in transplant immunosuppression is prednisone, because it is a very effective immunosuppressant and has the fewest side effects.

ANTI-LYMPHOCYTE GLOBULIN (ALG) is a commonly used adjunct to drug immunosuppression. Because the graft is rejected through the action of T lymphocytes, it was reasoned that injecting the recipient with anti-lymphocyte antibody would reduce the number of lymphocytes and increase the survival time of the graft. In experimental situations this is certainly the case, and ALG has proved to be a very useful method used in conjunction with immunosuppressive drugs and splenectomy (see below). More recently monoclonal ALG has been used.

CYCLOSPORIN A is perhaps the greatest advance in immunosuppression in recent years. Figure 3 shows how the introduction of this fungal antibiotic as an immunosuppressant has dramatically improved graft survival. The evidence suggests that

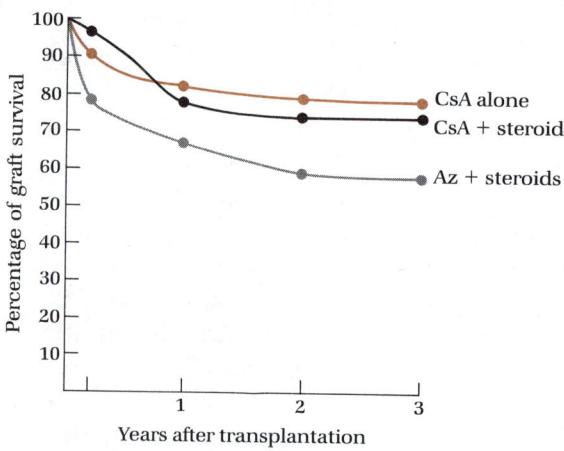

cyclosporin A acts by blocking the release of IL-2 by T lymphocytes. B cells and macrophages, as well as other cells in the hemopoietic series, are not affected by the drug.

Pretreatment of the Recipient

A fortuitous observation that transplant patients who have received a BLOOD TRANSFUSION a day or two before the transplant surgery have better acceptance rates than nontransfused patients has led some surgeons to include pretransplant transfusion as a routine part of kidney transplantation procedures. The reasons for this effect are not known and may not even be immunological.

Another pretransplant procedure used by some transplant teams is SPLENECTOMY. The rationale for splenectomy is that by removing a large sequestering site for graft antigens, the onset of rejection can be delayed.

TOTAL LYMPHOID IRRADIATION (TLI) is used by some transplant teams. In this procedure the recipient receives a large dose of X ray (over 3000 r) directed at the thymus, spleen, and cervical, axillary, inguinal, and mesenteric lymph nodes. This procedure has been shown to lead to tolerance of grafted tissue in experimental animals and has been of some value in heart transplantation.

TRANSPLANTATION

The Mechanism of Graft Rejection

Acute Rejection. Acute rejection is the most common type of rejection seen in allografts. It begins between one and three weeks after transplant and has a variety of symptoms, the swelling of the graft, chills, and fever being the most common. The exact mechanism of the rejection is not known, but it is known that T lymphocytes are the major factor. The cellular infiltrate to the graft contains many cell types including macrophages and B cells along with the T cells; but it is the T cells that initiate the rejection process and probably play the major role as effector cells. The exact role of "killer" cells and DTH cells is not clear. The infiltrating mononuclear cells and serum antibody may play augmenting roles in the actual destruction of the graft. These cellular rejection episodes are managed clinically with high-dose corticosteroid therapy.

Hyperacute Rejection. A rarer form of rejection occurs within a few days of transplant and is called HYPERACUTE REJECTION. These cases are due almost exclusively to the presence of antibodies in the recipients' serum that are cytotoxic to donor lymphocytes which are present in the graft— so-called PASSENGER LYMPHOCYTES. Examination of the graft shows deposition of immunoglobulin and complement (Type II hypersensitivity) as well as PMN infiltration (Type III hypersensitivity). Because of this problem, many transplant teams screen the recipient for cytotoxic antibodies to the prospective donor's lymphocytes.

Chronic Rejection. In some cases a slow rejection phase begins many months or even years after transplantation. This CHRONIC REJECTION appears to be due to the slow buildup of antigen–antibody complexes.

Types of Transplants

Organ transplantation is becoming a commonplace event and with the advent of cyclosporin A, many of the rejection phenomena can be controlled. The reader is referred to the Proceedings of the Tenth International Congress of the Transplantation Society in *Transplantation Proceedings* 17, 1985, to get the latest clinical advances in immunosuppression and the success rates for the various organs.

Kidney   Kidney transplants are the most successful transplants in clinical medicine. The surgical procedures have been perfected to the point that the operation itself is no longer an experimental procedure, and the organ seems to lend itself to transplantation (number and kinds of antigens, vascularization, and so on). With the recent advances in immunosuppression (see above), long-term survival is routine. In addition, the availability of dialysis machines to maintain the patient until a suitable donor is found means that most candidates for renal transplants are in reasonably good health (considering their kidney disease) at the time of the transplant.

Heart and Heart-Lung   Heart transplants are perhaps the most dramatic of the transplants. The procedure is technically extremely difficult and is still experimental, used only as a last resort. This fact means that the recipients are very sick at the time of the rigorous surgery. Within the last few years the artificial heart has shown promise of becoming the equivalent of the dialysis machines that maintain renal allograft patients in reasonable condition before transplant. The artificial heart has raised many scientific and ethical questions, but its short-term use in keeping patients alive until a suitable heart is available for transplantation seems to be gaining in acceptability.

It is not yet clear whether the antigen number and distribution on heart and lung will present special immunological difficulties because not enough transplants have been done and those that have been done have lacked the careful matching that precedes renal grafting.

Liver   Liver transplants have become as common as kidney transplants in some centers such as Pittsburgh. With the advent of cyclosporin, the survival rate of these grafts has reached approximately 70% even though there is very little chance to prematch donor and recipients.

TRANSPLANTATION

Skin Skin is the most extensively studied organ for transplantation in experimental systems. It is therefore ironic that the only transplantation of skin used in clinical situations is that in autografts. Even when patients are well matched, rejection is common; and aside from autografts, only grafts between identical twins have a reasonable chance of being accepted.

Bone Marrow Bone marrow transplantation is unusual because the recipient is immunoincompetent, but the graft often contains immunocompetent cells. This arrangement leads to graft-versus-host reactions. Bone marrow transplants are used in a variety of diseases, especially leukemias and some immunodeficiency diseases. The recipients are given high doses of X irradiation (>1000 r) before transplantation and then are given the usual immunosuppressive regimen.

Because the GVH is brought about by T cells a recent innovation has been to remove the T cells in the bone marrow by agglutination with a lectin such as soybean agglutinin before transplantation. This procedure has improved the survival rate of the transplants dramatically (Figure 4).

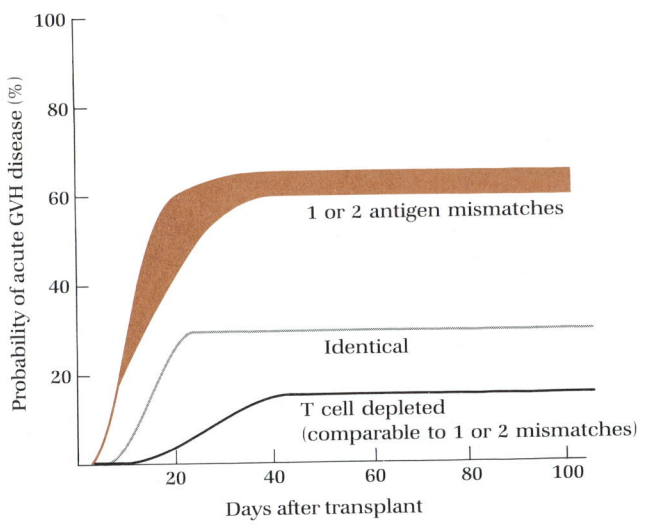

FIGURE 4 GRAFT-VERSUS-HOST DISEASE

After bone marrow transplantation, HLA-matched donor and recipient have a 30% probability of acute GVH. There is a 60% probability with HLA mismatches, but this is reduced to less than 20% if the bone marrow is depleted of T cells. [Data from Clift et al. (1985) *Transplant. Proc.* 17, 445; and Martin et al. (1985) *Transplant. Proc.* 17, 486]

CHAPTER TWENTY-EIGHT

Summary

1. Tissue from one individual cannot survive in another because the antigens are recognized as foreign and the host mounts a cell-mediated immune response against the graft.

2. The "laws of transplantation" say that syngeneic grafts will survive but allogeneic grafts will be rejected. Parental grafts into F_1 are accepted because the F_1 shares the same antigens as each of the parental types. F_1 grafts into parental strains are rejected because each parent recognizes the antigens of the other on the graft.

3. In cases of human transplantation matching of HLA antigens in donors and recipients improves the chances of graft survival because these are the major antigens that are responded to in rejection.

4. The advent of powerful immunosuppressants, especially cyclosporin A, has improved the chances of graft acceptance even in the face of a HLA mismatch.

Additional Readings

Najarian, J. S. 1983. Immunologic aspects of transplantation. In *The Biology of Immunologic Disease*, F. J. Dixon and D. W. Fisher (eds.). Sinauer Associates, Sunderland, Mass.

O'Reilly, R. J. 1983. Allogeneic bone marrow transplantation: current status and future directions. *Blood* 62, 941.

Shevac, E. M. 1985. The effects of cyclosporin A on the immune system. *Annu. Rev. Immunol.* 3, 397.

CHAPTER 29

IMMUNODEFICIENCY AND IMMUNOPROLIFERATIVE DISEASES

Overview Perhaps the most serious forms of pathology involving the immune system are those conditions which result in a loss of function of all or part of the system. These conditions are called immunodeficiency diseases. Immunodeficiency diseases are usually congenital but some are acquired. In the latter group, AIDS is of course the disease of greatest interest. In this chapter our emphasis on the congenital immunodeficiency diseases will be an attempt to analyze the point in the differentiative pathway of lymphocytes at which the defect has occurred so that we can understand the cellular manifestations of the defect. In fact, these tragic "experiments of nature" are very often important tools in defining the normal differentiative pathway.

In immunodeficiency diseases the defect is manifest in all of the cells of the type involved. The other malfunction which we will consider in this chapter presents the opposite problem. In immunoproliferative diseases, a single cell, in the course of differentiation, undergoes a malignant transformation and begins to proliferate rather than continuing along its differentiative pathway. This results in lymphoma or leukemia, diseases in which there is an accumulation of cells of the lymphoid or myeloid series. We will discuss these disorders in terms of the cells involved and the consequences to the patient.

CHAPTER TWENTY-NINE

Immunodeficiency Diseases

The immunodeficiency diseases which we will now describe all have in common the fact that all or some part of the immune system is not functioning. Patients affected by these deficiencies present a range of symptoms, but the underlying symptom is always inability to resist infection. These diseases were originally discovered because the patients had recurring infections. Over the years, as the defects became more clearly identified, it became clear that there were many forms of immunodeficiency diseases. Given the complexity of the immune response, it is not surprising that things can go wrong at many sites. What follows is to some extent a catalog of immunodeficiency diseases, with an attempt to identify where in hemopoietic differentiation the congenital defects occurred and to identify the cells affected in the acquired diseases.

Congenital Immunodeficiency Diseases

Immunodeficiency Disease as Defects in Differentiation

In Chapter 10 we saw that the cells of the immune system derived from the multipotent STEM CELL. Figure 1 shows this pathway as well as the stage of differentiation at which various immunodeficiency syndromes are thought to originate (dotted lines). From the practical point of view, if these conditions are going to be corrected it is imperative that we know where the defect has occurred.

Table 1 is a list of immunodeficiency disorders classified according to the site of the defect.

Defects of Stem Cells and Progenitor Cells

These diseases, most of which are very severe, are due to a malfunction very early in differentiation of the lymphoid system. Because the defect is so early in the differentiative pathway, both the humoral and cell-mediated limbs of the response are affected.

Reticular dysgenesis This is a rare and fatal disease in which there is no lymphoid or myeloid development (PMN and monocytes). However, erythroid and thrombocyte development contin-

IMMUNODEFICIENCY AND IMMUNOPROLIFERATIVE DISEASES

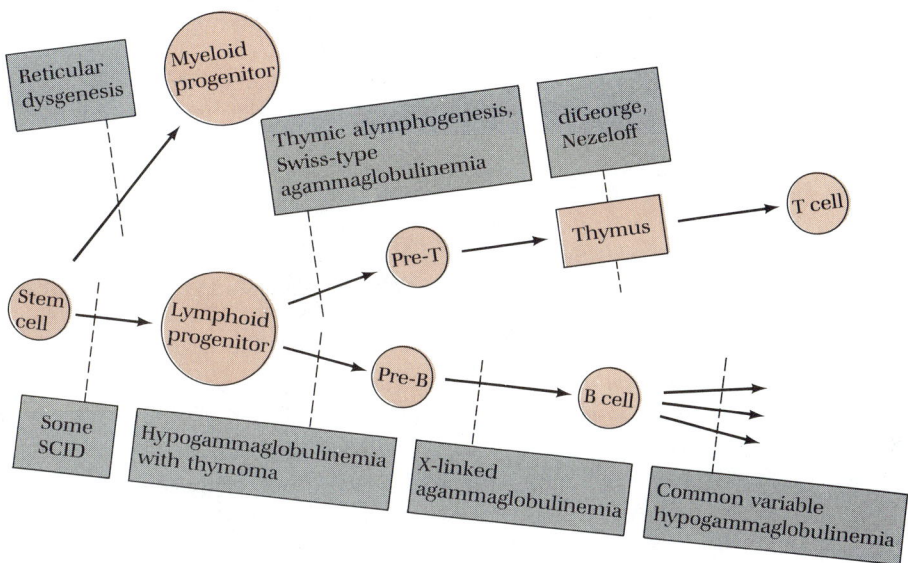

FIGURE 1 SITES OF CONGENITAL DEFECTS IN IMMUNODEFICIENCY DISEASES

The differentiation of lymphoid cells is shown with the disease associated with defects at various stages of the process indicated. [Based on Hammerling (1981) *Prog. Allergy* 28, 40; Wall and Keuhl (1983) *Annu. Rev. Immunol.* 1, 353; Kincaid (1981) *Adv. Immunol.* 31, 177]

ues. Thus the defect must be at a very early stage in lineage establishment (but one at which erythroid and megakaryocyte progenitors have already been determined).

Severe Combined Immunodeficiency Diseases (SCID) There is a fairly wide range of diseases that seem to have their basis in defects in early differentiation of cells along the lymphoid pathway. The term *severe combined immunodeficiency* is very descriptive, because in these diseases both the B cell and T cell lineages are affected (sometimes in varying degrees). SWISS-TYPE AGAMMAGLOBULINEMIA or AUTOSOMAL RECESSIVE ALYMPHOPENIC AGAMMAGLOBULINEMIA was first described by the Swiss physician W. H. Hitzig. It is an autosomal recessive disease (thus affecting both

TABLE 1 Classification of immunodeficiency disorders according to function affected.

Classification	Diseases
Antibody (B cell) immunodeficiency diseases	X-linked (congenital) hypogammaglobulinemia Transient hypogammaglobulinemia of infancy Common, variable, unclassifiable immunodeficiency (acquired hypogammaglobulinemia) Immunodeficiency with hyper-IgM Selective IgA deficiency Selective IgM deficiency Selective deficiency of IgG subclasses Secondary B cell immunodeficiency associated with drugs, protein-losing states B cell immunodeficiency associated with 5′-nucleotidase deficiency
Cellular (T cell) immunodeficiency diseases	Congenital thymic aplasia (DiGeorge syndrome) Chronic mucocutaneous candidiasis (with or without endocrinopathy) T cell deficiency associated with purine nucleoside phosphorylase deficiency
Combined antibody-mediated (B cell) and cell-mediated (T cell) diseases	Severe combined immunodeficiency disease (autosomal recessive, X-linked, sporadic) Cellular immunodeficiency with abnormal immunoglobulin synthesis (Nezelof's syndrome) Immunodeficiency with ataxia-telangiectasia Immunodeficiency with eczema and thrombocytopenia (Wiskott-Aldrich syndrome) Immunodeficiency with thymoma Immunodeficiency with short-limbed dwarfism Immunodeficiency with adenosine deaminase deficiency Episodic lymphopenia with lymphotoxin GVH disease
Phagocytic dysfunction	Chronic granulomatous disease Glucose-6-phosphate dehydrogenase deficiency Myeloperoxidase deficiency Chédiak-Higashi syndrome Job's syndrome Tuftsin deficiency "Lazy leukocyte syndrome" Elevated IgE, defective chemotaxis, eczema, and recurrent infections
Complement abnormalities and immunodeficiency diseases	C1q, C1r, and C1s deficiency C2 deficiency C3 deficiency (type I, type II) C4 deficiency C5 dysfunction, C5 deficiency C6 deficiency C7 deficiency C8 deficiency C9 deficiency

Source: From Altman and Fudenberg (1982), in Stites et al. (eds.), *Basic and Clinical Immunology,* 4th ed.

IMMUNODEFICIENCY AND IMMUNOPROLIFERATIVE DISEASES

sexes) in which all classes of immunoglobulin are depressed, the clotting system malfunctions, and there is a severe decrease in the number of lymphocytes. Numbers of other blood cell types are normal. The thymus is atrophic, and the few circulating lymphocytes that the patient has are not reactive to T cell mitogens. The symptoms, which manifest themselves shortly after birth, are recurring severe infections. The only treatment is bone marrow transplantation. PRIMARY LYMPHOPENIC IMMUNOLOGIC DEFICIENCY is a disease whose symptoms are similar to those of Swiss-type agammaglobulinemia, but it is sex linked, occurring only in males. SCID WITH ADA-DEFICIENCY patients also exhibit symptoms similar to Swiss-type agammaglobulinemia, but there is also an additional bone defect, and a very unusual defect in the enzyme adenosine deaminase (ADA). The relationship between the ADA deficiency and the immunodeficiency is not clear because members of the !Kung tribe in the Kalahari desert and some Arabian horses have the ADA defect without the immunodeficiency. ATAXIA-TELANGIECTASIA is an immunodeficiency disease that has its onset by two years of age. It results in abnormalities in both T and B cells. The defect is thought to be in the endoderm or endoderm–mesoderm interaction. The thymus is atrophic and Ig levels are reduced. Aside from recurring infection, this disease also exhibits cerebral ataxia and oculocutaneous telangiectasia (loss of ability to control the muscles controlled by the cerebellum, and dilation of the vasculature of the skin of the face and eyeball).

Deficiencies of B cell Origin

A group of congenital immunodeficiencies are due to a defect in the differentiation of B cells. Patients with these diseases suffer from recurrent infections but the infections are predominantly bacterial. Because much of viral immunity is due to T cells, these patients very often are able to defend themselves against virus infections.

X-Linked Infantile Hypogammaglobulinemia (Bruton) Bruton-type hypogammaglobulinemia is thought to be the first clinical description of an immunodeficiency disorder. The symptoms, first described in 1952 in a male child, are recurrent pyogenic infections beginning at about six months, severely depressed IgG levels, absence of IgM, IgA, IgD, and IgE, as well as an absence of peripheral B cells. The disease is X-linked so only boys develop it. Because the disease is limited to B cell function, γ-globulin therapy is successful, but survival into the second or third decade is rare.

Immunodeficiency with Thrombocytopenia and Eczema (Wiscott-Aldrich Syndrome)   This is another X-linked disease, affecting only boys. Lymphocytes and thrombocytes are decreased, resulting in both recurring infections and bleeding.

Selective Immunoglobulin Disorders   There are a variety of disorders showing selective decreased levels of one or more classes of immunoglobulin. Examples include selective IgG, IgM, and IgA deficiency. In these patients the other levels of immunoglobulin are normal, as is T cell function.

Deficiencies of T cell Origin

Defects in T cell development have far-reaching consequences because the T cell population contains helper, effector, and regulatory cells. Because the thymus is the hemopoietic inducing microenvironment for T cell development, it is possible in some cases to pinpoint the defect to the absence of the entire organ or to the reticular cells within it.

Thymic Aplasia (DiGeorge)   Immediately following birth, children with DiGeorge syndrome exhibit the symptoms; characteristic facial features, hypoparathyroidism, congenital heart disease, and immunological defects. These children are born without a thymus. The syndrome reflects a defect that occurs in the twelfth week of intrauterine life. At that time the thymus and parathyroid have already developed from the third and fourth pharyngeal pouches and the philtrum of the lip, the ear tubercule, and aortic arch structures are becoming differentiated. This developmental sequence accounts for the grouping of the symptoms. DiGeorge patients have an absence of T cells and T cell functions, with

IMMUNODEFICIENCY AND IMMUNOPROLIFERATIVE DISEASES

some impairment of B cell function. Thymus transplantation is of value in correcting the immunological disorder but the patients often have such severe heart disease that survival is threatened.

Thymic Dysplasia (Nezeloff) Unlike DiGeorge in which the thymus is absent, this is an autosomal disease in which the thymus is vestigial and devoid of lymphocytes. This deficiency probably indicates a defect in the reticular elements of the thymus, which are necessary for the organ to act as a hemopoietic inducing microenvironment.

PNP Deficiency This is a disease with a T cell defect, but it is also characterized by a deficiency in the enzyme purine nucleoside phosphorylase. The connection between the enzyme and the immune malfunction is not known, and it appears that the disease may affect only some subsets of T cells. The point of origin of the defect is not known.

Disorders of Granulocytes   There are a few diseases that affect the differentiation of granulocytes and are manifested by GRANULOPENIA or NEUTROPENIA. Infantile genetic agranulocytosis, familial neutropenia, and cyclic neutropenia are examples of these defects. In all these cases the lymphoid tissue is normal, but the patients have decreased resistance to infection because of loss of granulocyte function.

Acquired Immunodeficiencies

The deficiencies in the immune system discussed in the preceding section are all congenital. There are a few known syndromes in which immunodeficiency is acquired. The two most common are acquired hypogammaglobulinemia, a syndrome that is not too common and not catastrophic in results, and acquired immunodeficiency syndrome (AIDS). Because AIDS is of such importance, we will devote almost the entire discussion of acquired immunodeficiency to this disease.

CHAPTER TWENTY-NINE

Common, Variable Unclassifiable Immunodeficiency (Acquired Hypogammaglobulinemia)

This disease is an acquired form of immunodeficiency, but the origin of the disease is unknown. It has its onset when the patients are 15–35 years old and affects both males and females. The patients have the symptoms of recurrent infection and are usually found to have detectable, but very low levels of total immunoglobulin. T cell numbers and function are usually normal; but there are cases with T cell defects, and these may grow more severe as the disease progresses. Treatment is similar to X-linked hypogammaglobulinemia—that is, γ-globulin therapy—but patients can survive into the seventh and eighth decades. Women with the disease deliver normal infants, but the newborn is deficient in maternal Ig.

Acquired Immune Deficiency Syndrome: AIDS

The diseases discussed above have been known for several decades as identifiable clinical entitites, but they have no doubt always been with us. In the last few years a new and catastrophic disease affecting the immune system has become known. ACQUIRED IMMUNE DEFICIENCY SYNDROME or AIDS is before us every day in the newspapers, television, and scientific journals. Had this disease appeared a decade ago, we would not have known enough about the working of the immune system to understand it and to begin to apply the advances in basic science to clinical medicine to devise treatments.

The First Appearances of AIDS

In 1981 three papers appeared in *The New England Journal of Medicine* describing immunodeficiency in previously healthy homosexual men. The disease was characterized by an increased incidence of *Pneumocytsis carinii* pneumonia and herpes simplex infection. Shortly after that it was noted that there was an unusually high incidence of disseminated Kaposi's sarcoma in male homosexuals. By the middle of 1982 it was clear to the medical community and to the gay communities of New York and San Francisco that a disease of epidemic proportions was spreading through the community and that it was fatal. By the end of the year the entire world knew of AIDS. By

IMMUNODEFICIENCY AND IMMUNOPROLIFERATIVE DISEASES

1985 AIDS was a feared, misunderstood and controversial disease.[1]

The number of AIDS cases has been increasing at an exponential rate since 1982 (Figure 2); and, as we will see, public health officials are not able to predict whether the numbers will level off or continue to rise at this rate. As a comparison, the number of paralytic polio cases in 1952, the worst year, was 21,000.

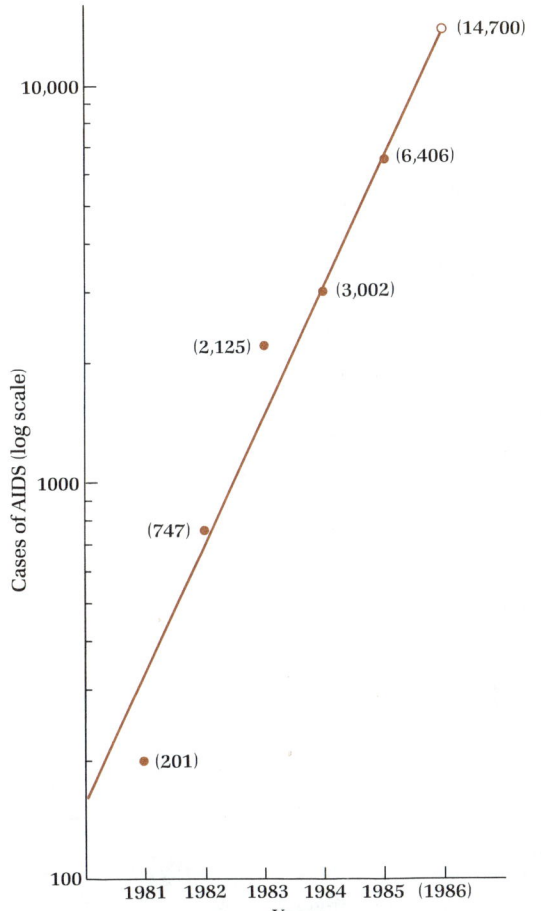

FIGURE 2 CASES OF AIDS IN THE UNITED STATES

Cases for 1986 are projected. [From Center for Disease Control, January 1986]

[1] The best description of the sociological, ethical and political aspects of the disease have been discussed by Jonathan Lieberson in *The New York Review of Books*, January 16, 1986.

CHAPTER TWENTY-NINE

Immunology of AIDS

AIDS, as the name describes, is an acquired failure of the immune system. Table 2 lists the characteristic abnormalities of the immune system in the disease as well as those most consistently observed. The important point is that the symptoms show a wide-ranging failure of the immune system but are all due to an elimination of the T helper cells. It will be recalled from Chapter 11 that in humans the helper subset of T cells is characterized by the CD4 antigen and the suppressor subset of the CD8 antigen. AIDS patients have a quantitative reduction of CD4 cells and a concomitant increase in the proportion of CD8 cells.

Examination of Table 2 reveals that lymphopenia, absence of DTH, in vitro proliferative responses, and decreased antibody responses are exactly the list of defects we would expect from an absence of T4 cells. The explanation for elevated IgG and IgA and increased spontaneous Ig secretion from B cells are not so obvious, and tell us that these B cell functions may be under subtle control of T cells. However, we will see below that the immunology of the disease presents some very challenging problems whose solution will be important not only for the control of the disease, but in understanding some aspects of T cell control of normal function.

TABLE 2 Immunological abnormalities in AIDS.

Characteristic abnormalities	Lymphopenia
	Quantitative reduction of CD4 cells
	Decrease or absence of DTH
	Elevated serum IgG and IgA
	Increased spontaneous Ig secretion by B cells
Consistently observed abnormalities	Decreased in vitro proliferative response to mitogens, antigen, and alloantigen
	Decreased cytotoxic activity of cytotoxic T cells and NK cells
	Decreased antibody response to new antigens
	Altered macrophage function
	Elevated serum levels of immune complexes

Source: Modified from Seligmann et al. (1984), *N. Engl. J. Med.* 311: 1286.

IMMUNODEFICIENCY AND IMMUNOPROLIFERATIVE DISEASES

The dramatic loss of T4 cells is seen in Figure 3. This reduction in the absolute number of T4 cells results in the increased percentage of T8 cells, thus altering the T4:T8 ratio. In normal individuals this ratio is approximately 1.2 to 1.5. It can be seen in Table 3 that AIDS patients have a ratio of 0.34. Moreover, AIDS *prodrome* patients (those individuals who did not have the symptoms of the disease when studied but who developed them during the course of the study) have a severely reduced T4:T8 ratio. Those patients with what is called the AIDS-RELATED COMPLEX (ARC), which is characterized by lymphadenopathy, also have a significantly reduced ratio. In contrast, healthy subjects who are at risk to AIDS (see below) or have sexual contact with AIDS patients have normal levels. From the point of view of distinguishing between AIDS and congenital immune deficiency, patients with common variable immune deficiency (see above) have a normal *ratio* of T cell types, even though the absolute number of their lymphocytes may be decreased.

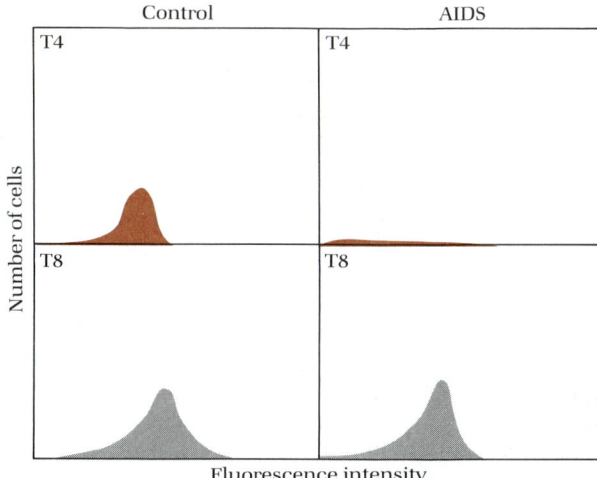

FIGURE 3 FLUORESCENCE-ACTIVATED CELL SORTER ANALYSIS

Fluorescence-activated cell sorter analysis of peripheral blood monocytes from a patient with AIDS and a normal control subject, showing the concentrations of T4 and T8 cells. Cells were incubated with monoclonal anti-T4 or anti-T8 and then fluorescence-labeled goat anti-mouse Ig. Values on the X axis represent fluorescence intensity; values on the Y axis represent the number of cells with that intensity. [Redrawn with background fluorescence subtracted, from Facui et al. (1984) *Ann. Int. Med.* 100, 92]

TABLE 3 Helper : suppressor ratio and viral antibodies in AIDS.

Patient category	$T_h:T_s$ [a]	LAV$^+$ (%) [b]
AIDS	0.34	68
Risk group		
Prodrome	0.58	100
Lymphadenopathy	0.77	100
Controls		
Healthy; AIDS risk	1.20	0
Sexual contact with AIDS patient	1.09	40
Common variable immune deficiency	1.52	0

Source: Based on Laurence et al. (1984), *N. Engl. J. Med.* 311: 1296.

[a] The $T_h:T_s$ ratio is the T4:T8 ratio.

[b] Note that anti-AIDS virus antibody is found in all the groups associated with AIDS except the healthy at-risk group. Other studies have begun to show that the incidence of antibody may be significant in this group. The group with congenital immunodeficiency has neither the antibody nor a reduced CD4:CD8 ratio.

Risk Groups and Modes of Transmission

Since its discovery in the male homosexual population, two other groups have been identified as high risk groups. These are intravenous drug users and hemophiliacs who receive either blood or blood fractions.[2]

The common denominator of these groups was the opportunity for an infectious agent to be transmitted via blood. The intravenous drug users were at risk because of the possibility of using a contaminated needle, and the hemophiliacs because they relied on intravenous injection of blood and blood products, either of which could be contaminated with the agent. Among male homosexuals, the disease could be spread during anal intercourse,

[2] Originally Haitians in the United States were designated a risk group. This was rather mysterious, because these cases did not seem to fall into the homosexual, intravenous drug user, or hemophiliac categories and the disease was not identified in Haiti. This group has since been removed from the risk group category.

IMMUNODEFICIENCY AND IMMUNOPROLIFERATIVE DISEASES

during which blood vessels may be torn, thereby allowing the agent to be transmitted. So, based on the risk groups involved, it seemed that the etiological agent would be bloodborne. Because hemophiliacs receive blood products that are filtered and free of bacteria and fungi, a virus was the most likely candidate.[3]

Etiology

By early 1984 the virus that causes the disease was independently isolated by the group headed by Gallo at the NIH and by Montagnier and his colleagues at the Institut Pasteur in France. The disease is caused by a retrovirus related to human T-lymphotropic virus (HTLV). The NIH group has termed the virus HTLV III (human T cell leukemia virus III) and the Institut Pasteur group has called the virus LAV (lymphadenopathy-associated virus).[4] A somewhat controversial proposal to call the agent human immunodeficiency virus (HIV) has been put forward.

The AIDS virus (HTLV-III/LAV) has been shown to have a tropism for activated CD4 cells. Viral infection of resting lymphocytes does not result in either virus replication, cytopathic effect, or the expression of surface antigen. When these cells are activated with either lectin or antigen, replication, antigen expression, and the cytopathic effect are seen. The CD4 molecule itself has been shown to be the receptor for the virus.

---

[3] This accounts for the fact that the disease cannot be spread by casual contact. However, a September 1985 CBS poll showed that 47% of the people polled thought it was possible to contract AIDS from a drinking glass; 32% thought it possible to contract it by kissing, and 28% from a toilet seat. A Harris poll at about the same time found that 50% thought that one could get the disease by living in the same house with an AIDS patient and a third by "going to a party where someone has AIDS." In the USSR, the chief of a Black Sea sanitarium has said that AIDS might be the result of "genetic mutations" caused by "mixed marriages." In the wilds of Indiana, the author, while waiting in line at the local supermarket, keeps up on the advances in the hysteria associated with the disease by reading articles, in tabloids, all by "top docs," telling how movie stars are at risk because of kissing with their mouths open and that AIDS is a form of germ warfare.

[4] A battle has been raging over precedence for the discovery and patent rights for the test for anti-viral antibody since that time. We will not enter into this interesting offshoot of the scientific life, but readers are referred to a series of articles in *Science* by Colin Norman, appearing during 1985.

CHAPTER TWENTY-NINE

Some Important Questions

We noted above that the AIDS virus has a tropism for T4 cells. But it has been found that only 10% of the total population of T4 cells is susceptible to infection. If this is true, why is there such a drastic loss of helper function and loss of the immune response?

The second question is one of epidemiology. At present we do not know what proportion of individuals infected with the virus will eventually display the symptoms of the disease. Estimates range from a very small number (5–10%) to a very high number (40–50%). Time alone will tell, and the few studies that have been done so far give disparate results. For example, from studies of the male homosexual population in New York City, two studies show 25 and 34% of infected individuals contracting the disease, but six other studies show 8–15% percent. From a public health point of view, the answer to this question, which will become known over the next years, is of extreme importance. Another aspect of this question is whether the risk of the infection becoming disease declines in an individual with time after infection. This is totally unknown at this time. There has been a great deal of speculation about the factors that determine whether an infected individual will contract the disease; factors ranging from gastrointestinal infection to the general health of the individual have been implicated.[5]

Therapy for AIDS

Drugs that destroy the virus and virus-infected cells are being tested. The drugs HPA23, suramin, and ribavirin have been shown to reduce or eliminate virus in the blood of patients as long as the drug is administered, but the virus reappears at the end of the treatment. There has been no clinical improvement in patients receiving these drugs. Treatment with interleukin-2 or interferon have not had any reported beneficial effects in restoring the immune response of an AIDS patient. Recently some French clinicians held a news conference to report that treatment of AIDS patients with the *immunosuppressive* drug cyclosporin (see Chap-

---

[5] For a provocative discussion of this question see D. L. Archer and W. H. Glinsmann (1985) Enteric infections and other cofactors in AIDS. *Immunol. Today* 6, 292.

IMMUNODEFICIENCY AND IMMUNOPROLIFERATIVE DISEASES

ter 28) resulted in a rise of T4 cells from 9 to 250 cells per microliter (normal is around 900). Unfortunately, the patient died two weeks after the announcement. Nonetheless, Montagnier's group has raised the possibility that some aspects of the disease are similar enough to autoimmune disease to merit further investigation along this line.[6]

Finally, there is, of course, the possibility of immunizing against the virus. There is preliminary evidence that there will be a vast array of serotypes of AIDS virus, a situation that may make finding the protective antigens as difficult as has been the case in other viral diseases (see Chapter 2) and in parasite diseases (see Chapter 25). But more recently antibodies have been raised to a synthetic peptide on the virus envelope by using the techniques and strategy for producing antisera against synthetic antigens (Chapter 2). It is assumed that for retroviruses, as for other enveloped viruses, that the antigenic determinants are associated with surface glycoprotein. In the AIDS-associated viruses, two glycoproteins are suspected of being strong immunogens; these are 120,000- and 41,000-MW molecules called gp120 and gp41. Computer analysis of the amino acid sequences of the envelope protein of HTLV-III showed a highly hydrophilic (and therefore exposed) area that seemed to have a conserved sequence when compared to LAV and to be associated with gp41. The sequence of 17 amino acids was synthesized using solid-phase methods, and the peptide conjugated to keyhole limpet hemocyanin. Rabbits were then immunized and the antibody tested for its ability to react with both the synthetic peptide and native proteins associated with HTLV-III. The antibodies bound to the synthetic peptide as expected and also precipitated a band from the virus with a molecular weight of 160,000. It is known that gp41 is a cleavage product of gp160 so there is strong suggestive evidence that this antibody may be against gp41. As of this writing there have been no reported attempts to immunize humans with this peptide, but it seems safe to assume that these will be carried out in the near future.[7]

---

[6] See a very informative "News and Views" article by Klatzmann and Montagnier (1986) *Nature* 319, 10.

[7] This paper should be of interest to the reader, not only for its importance to AIDS research, but because it shows the application of methods that have been discussed earlier in the text. Kennedy et al. (1986) *Science* 231, 1556.

CHAPTER TWENTY-NINE

Lymphoproliferative Diseases

Leukemias and Lymphomas

In the last chapter we saw some of the consequences of defects in the differentiation pathways of hemopoietic cells, defects that lead to the failure of the stem cells to establish certain lineages and result in the absence of the end cells. These defects affect *all* of the cells that differentiate along the affected pathway. Another form of pathology is the loss of regulatory control of an *individual cell* at some point in its life history. The disease that results from this is the excessive proliferation of the cells resulting in the clonal expansion of the progeny of the affected cell. When these diseases occur in the lymphoid system they are called LYMPHOPROLIFERATIVE DISEASES.

The result of excess proliferation, of course, is an increase in the number of cells above the normal level. When this proliferation occurs, a tumor (called a NEOPLASM) develops at the site. In lymphoid tissue, excessive proliferation in an organ such as a lymph node or the thymus is called a LYMPHOMA. When the proliferation of cells is manifest as an increase in the number of cells in the blood it is called LEUKEMIA. In practice the two terms are often used interchangeably.

Leukemias and lymphomas are classified according to the symptoms they cause and the tissue in which they arise. One of the practical benefits of the work on cell surface markers of lymphocytes has been the ability to classify and identify leukemias and lymphomas.

Leukemias

LEUKEMIA is the accumulation of white blood cells in the circulation. The leukemias are classified as either acute or chronic on the basis of both the clinical course of the disease and the hematological features, especially the maturation of the accumulating cells. The leukemia, either acute or chronic, can be of either the lymphoid or the myeloid cell lineages.

ACUTE LEUKEMIA is characterized by a block in maturation early in the differentiation process (either in the lymphoid or myeloid cells). This defect causes the progeny of the cell with the defect

IMMUNODEFICIENCY AND IMMUNOPROLIFERATIVE DISEASES

to proliferate and accumulate first in the bone marrow and then, in the peripheral blood. CHRONIC LEUKEMIA is similar, except that the cells that accumulate are farther along the differentiative pathway, and therefore partially functional.

Because leukemias can involve cells of either lymphoid or myeloid cell lineages, there can be acute lymphoid leukemia, acute myelocytic leukemia, chronic lymphoid leukemia, chronic myelogenous leukemia, and a disease called hairy cell leukemia which is a leukemic reticuloendotheliosis. Table 4 lists the leukemias as classified according to the cell type involved. This decision is most often made on the basis of cell surface markers.

The symptoms of leukemia are fever, malaise, spontaneous bleeding in the skin and subcutaneous tissues, frequent infections, and enlargement of the lymph nodes and spleen. The diagnosis is made by observing increased numbers of leukocytes in the

TABLE 4 Leukemias and lymphomas classified by cell surface marker.

Marker	Disease
T cell	Acute lymphocytic leukemia Lymphoblastic lymphoma Sézary syndrome Mycosis fungoides
B cell	Chronic lymphocytic leukemia Waldenström macroglobulinemia Multiple myeloma Burkitt's lymphoma
Null cell	Acute lymphocytic leukemia Some non-Hodgkin's lymphomas
Histiocyte-monocyte	Acute monocytic leukemia Malignant histicytosis
Controversial	Hodgkin's disease Hairy cell lymphoma

Source: From Wells (1982), in Stites et al. (eds.), *Basic and Clinical Immunology*, p. 460.

circulation. Very often there are large numbers of immature cells and often there is anemia and thrombocytopenia due to a reduction in erythrocytes and platelets.

Acute Lymphoblastic Leukemia (ALL)   ALL is the most frequent neoplasm of children. Immature lymphocytes, called blast cells, are found in the blood. The disease is often rapidly progressive and death can occur in a few months if the patient is not treated.

The disease is divided into four types (Table 5), according to the pattern of markers expressed on the surface of the cells. COMMON-ALL cells have neither B cell nor T cell antigens but express a COMMON-ALL ANTIGEN (CALLA). NULL-ALL cells express neither B cell, T cell antigens nor CALL antigens. This is the most common form of the disease, comprising close to two-thirds of all cases of ALL. About 20% of ALL cases have cells that do not express B or CALLA markers but do express a T cell marker.

At the time of diagnosis, the tumor mass in patients can be 10^{12} cells. With multiple drug therapy, the number of leukemic cells can be reduced by 99.9%. This results in a remission of all symptoms but still leaves a tumor load of ca. 10^9 cells. In recent years multiple drug therapy has resulted in primary remission in 95% of children with the disease. Because of the blood-brain barrier that impedes the entry of the drug into the brain, patients are then often treated with cranial irradiation as prophylaxis to eliminate more of the remaining tumor cells and are then given maintenance levels of the drugs for several years.

TABLE 5   Classification of Acute Lymphocytic Leukemia (ALL).

Type	Frequency (%)	Surface antigen
Common ALL	50–65	CALLA
Null ALL	15–40	None
T ALL	20	T cell antigens; SRBC Rosettes
B ALL	2–5	Ig

IMMUNODEFICIENCY AND IMMUNOPROLIFERATIVE DISEASES

Chronic Lymphocytic Leukemia (CLL) Chronic lymphocytic leukemia is a disease of adults and is characterized by the progressive accumulation of small lymphocytes in blood, bone marrow, lymph nodes, and other organs. In over 95% of the cases the lymphocytes are B cells. Because the disease is monoclonal, that is, almost always arising from the transformation of a single cell, the serum of these patients very often displays a single "spike" of immunoglobulin when subjected to electrophoresis. This immunoglobulin is of one isotype, most usually IgM. This can often be a slowly progressive disease with an unusually high incidence of autoimmune hemolytic anemia and tumors (over 15% of the patients develop malignant solid tumors).

Myeloid Leukemias There are several diseases of myeloid cells that are both chronic and acute. CHRONIC MYELOGENOUS LEUKEMIA (CML) results in the overproduction of PMN. This disease is of scientific interest because it is associated with the "Philadelphia chromosome." Chromosome 22 is shortened, and half of its longer arm is translocated to chromosome 9. The Philadelphia chromosome also is present in the erythroid and thrombocyte series of cells, as well as in the granuloid series, but it is not present in lymphoid cells.

There are two forms of ACUTE MYELOGENOUS LEUKEMIA (AML) called acute *monocytic* leukemia and acute *melomonocytic* leukemia.

HAIRY-CELL LEUKEMIA is a rare but increasingly diagnosed disease affecting older adult males. The cells involved have a mixed series of markers on their surfaces, including some lymphoid, but they are glass-adherent and phagocytic.

Lymphomas

Transformed cells that continue to reside in the lymphoid organ in which they arose are called LYMPHOMAS. Lymphomas are divided into two classes, *Hodgkin's* and *non-Hodgkin's*.

Hodgkin's Disease Hodgkin's disease (which is named after Thomas Hodgkin who described it in 1822) is characterized by painless enlargement of the lymph nodes, fever, skin eruptions, and anemia. The enlarged nodes show HODGKIN CELLS—large (40 μm) cells with a single nucleus and one large eosinophilic nucleolus. These cells give rise to REED-STERNBERG CELLS, which are cells with multiple nuclei and prominent nucleoli. Hodgkin's patients show impaired immune function, with reduced DTH and graft rejection ability and an increased susceptibility to infection. The origin of the Reed-Sternberg cells is not known, although current evidence seems to favor the monocyte–macrophage lineage. Because there is no immunological classification, the standard classification is based on histology. The Rye Conference classification of Hodgkin's disease is shown in Table 6.

Non-Hodgkin's Lymphomas: T Cell Tumors

Thymomas These tumors of the thymus are rare and may be lymphoid or epithelial in nature, or mixed.

Lymphoblastic Lymphoma This lymphoma is a rare childhood disease in which the tumor cells spread from the thymus-dependent zones of the lymph nodes and spleen. Leukemia is often the terminal phase of this disease.

Mycosis Fungoides and Sézary's Syndrome Mycosis fungoides begins in the skin and is characterized by a dermatitis that may last for years before giving rise to gross tumors. Sézary's syndrome is a leukemic form of the disease.

TABLE 6 Rye Conference classification of Hodgkin's disease.

Histological classification	Frequency (%)
Lymphocyte predominance	10–15
Nodular sclerosis	40–70
Mixed cellularity	20–40
Lymphocyte depletion	5–10

IMMUNODEFICIENCY AND IMMUNOPROLIFERATIVE DISEASES

Non-Hodgkin's Lymphomas: B Cell Tumors

Multiple Myeloma This disease is characterized by the presence of tumor cells in the bone marrow and high levels of serum immunoglobulin. Bence-Jones proteins are light chains excreted in the urine. Waldenström's macroglobulinemia is characterized by monoclonal serum IgM.

Burkitt's Lymphoma Found originally in Africa, this disease is associated with the Epstein-Barr virus. The American version of the disease seems to be more virulent than its African counterpart. The E-B virus is also associated with INFECTIOUS MONONUCLEOSIS, which, although not a form of cancer, does show a lymphocytosis of both T and B cells and lymphadenopathy. Antibodies to EB virus are present in this disease and are used as a diagnostic tool. The public health control of this "kissing disease" is part of the informal education of most college students and although the disease rarely results in severe complications, it is well known that it can severely impair the social life of the average undergrad.

Summary

1. Immunodeficiency diseases are syndromes in which all or part of the immune system does not function. Congenital immune deficiencies are a result of a defect at some stage in the differentiation of the B cell, T cell or macrophage.
2. Congenital immunodeficiencies of the T cell line can be due to the failure of the thymus to form, failure of the reticular cells to develop, or failure of lymphocytes to develop and function. B cell defects are less well identified because of the lack of an identifiable hemopoietic inducing microenvironment.
3. The most important acquired immunodeficiency is AIDS. In this disease the helper T cells (T4 subset), are infected with the AIDS virus, a situation resulting in an almost complete shutdown of the immune system. The symptoms are recurrent infections, leading to death.
4. Immunoproliferative diseases are the result of a single cell losing its proliferative regulatory mechanisms. These cells are trapped at some early stage of differentiation, and the diseases that result from this accumulation of lymphoid or myeloid cells are called leukemias or lymphomas.

5. Leukemias are the accumulation of early forms of blood cells in the blood. Lymphomas are the accumulation of these cells at a single site. The leukemias can be of either lymphoid or myeloid origin and can take the form of an acute or chronic disease.

6. Lymphomas are divided into either Hodgkin's disease or non-Hodgkin's types.

Additional Readings

Altman, A. J. and H. Fudenberg. 1982. Immunodeficiency diseases. In D. P. Stites, J. D. Stobo, H. H. Fudenberg, and J. V. Wells. *Basic and Clinical Immunology*, 4th ed. Lange Medical Publishers, Los Altos, Calif.

Cline, M. J. et al. 1979. Acute leukemia: biology and treatment. *Ann. Int. Med.* 91, 758.

Holborow and W. G. Reeves. 1983. *Immunology in Medicine, A Comprehensive Guide to Clinical Immunology*, 2nd ed. Grune and Stratton, London.

Kaplan, H. S. 1981. Review: Hodgkin's disease: biology, treatment, and prognosis. *Blood* 57, 813.

Koeffler, H. P., and D. W. Golde. 1981. Chronic myelogenous leukemia: new concepts. *N. Engl. J. Med.* 304, 1201 and 1296.

Lane, C. H., and A. S. Fauci. 1985. Immunologic abnormalities in the acquired immune deficiency syndrome. *Annu. Rev. Immunol.* 3, 477.

APPENDIX A
Richard Gershon and the Immunological Orchestra

> To be a great scientist, you have to be a mental athlete. You have to think until it hurts, and then you have to keep on thinking *through* the pain. Then maybe you'll find some new answers. When you get up to bat, swing for the fences.
>
> R. K. GERSHON, QUOTED BY DOUG GREEN

One of the great immunologists of our time was Richard K. Gershon, the discoverer of the suppressor T cell and the regulatory circuits. Early in his career Gershon conceived of "The Immunological Orchestra," and for the next 15 years the orchestra was a mainstay at meetings and gatherings of cellular immunologists. Gershon died of lung cancer in July 1983, at the age of 51. While all of immunology is poorer for his absence, for his generation of immunologists science will never be the same again.

Just before his death Gershon was awarded the Gairdner Award by the Gairdner Foundation of Canada. Below is the introduction to a lecture entitled "An Appreciation of R. K. Gershon," which I presented at the award ceremony. I include it here to give young scientists a glimpse of what the full scientific life can (and, I think, should) be like. Gooch brought the same excitement to science that he brought to all of life.

> In this lecture, I want to attempt to convey to you the essence of both the work and the character of my dearest friend, Dick Gershon. You will see, I hope, that the work is complex, sometimes elegant, sometimes confusing, but always exciting. Exactly the same can be said of the man.
>
> The photograph shows "Gooch" in a typical pose; smiling and at ease, but with an underlying, ever-present intensity. Note that he wears a vest, no tie (he was inducted into the National Academy of Sciences in similar attire) and stands in front of one of the wine racks in his office at Yale. Great wine, great ideas, great passion about life and immunology were always with him.

APPENDIX A

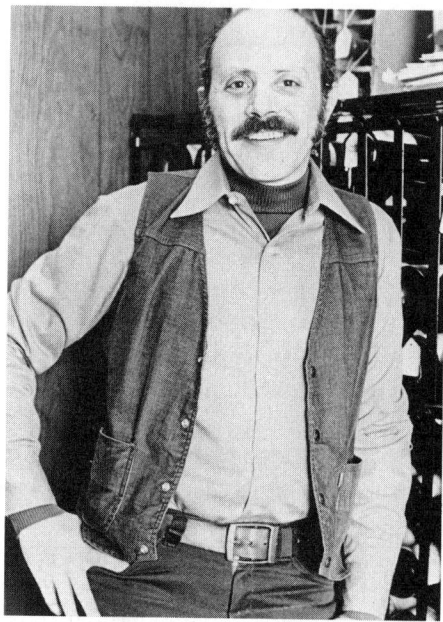

RICHARD K. GERSHON

He suffused himself with the beauty of the world; he was a collector of art, a connoisseur of wine, an energetic traveler (he was fluent in French and proficient in Japanese) and knew more limericks than any six other men. And intertwined in all of this was his unflagging enthusiasm for the beauty of the immune response. He gloried in the layer upon interconnected layer of its complexity. He thrilled at seeing a layer of that complexity which no one had seen before. In this, he must have had what the earliest explorers had, an insatiable desire to be the first person to see something, to know that you are where no man has been before. At his funeral someone said, "He had champagne in his veins." I disagreed; it was his beloved Burgundy—complex, subtle, intense, interesting, and important—that flowed through him.

I start this way not as another funeral oration but rather to set the tone for the understanding of his work. Because ultimately, Gooch, the suppressor cell, and the regulatory circuits are inseparable. There are many smart immunologists, but few could have seen into the complexities of the immune response as he did because no one else brought the energy and passion which he had for so much of life so constantly to the story of the immune response.

GERSHON'S IMMUNOLOGICAL ORCHESTRA

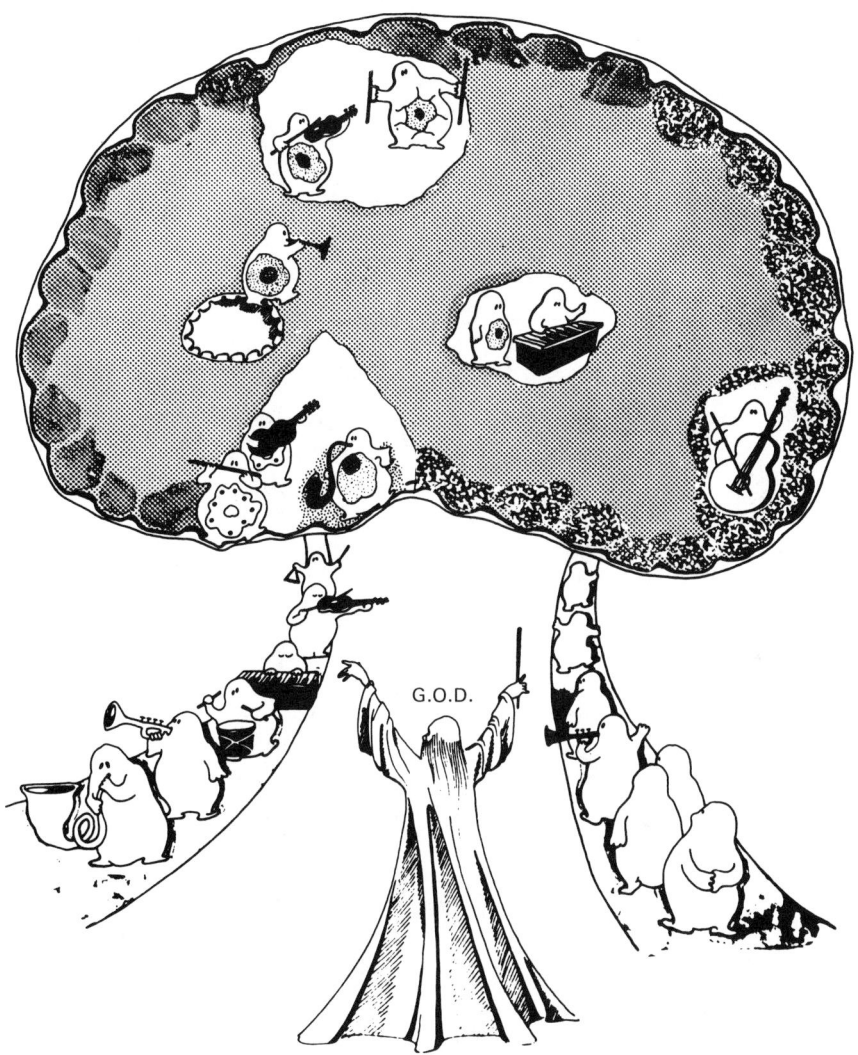

The immunological orchestra in 1968. The focus was on cell cooperation. The players are B cells, T cells, and macrophages conducted by the generator of diversity (G.O.D.).

APPENDIX A

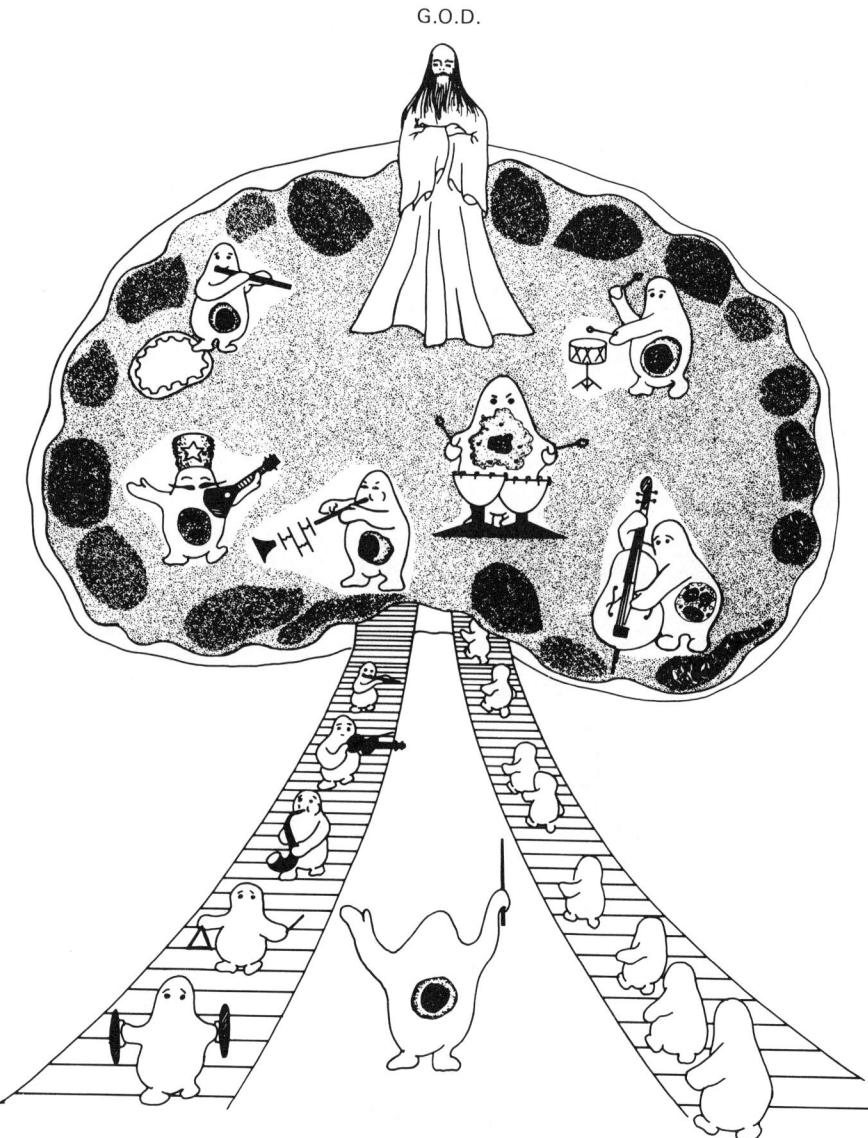

The immunological orchestra in 1974. The role of the thymus as helper, cytotoxic, and suppressor cell is known and Gershon has made the T cell the conductor.

535
GERSHON'S IMMUNOLOGICAL ORCHESTRA

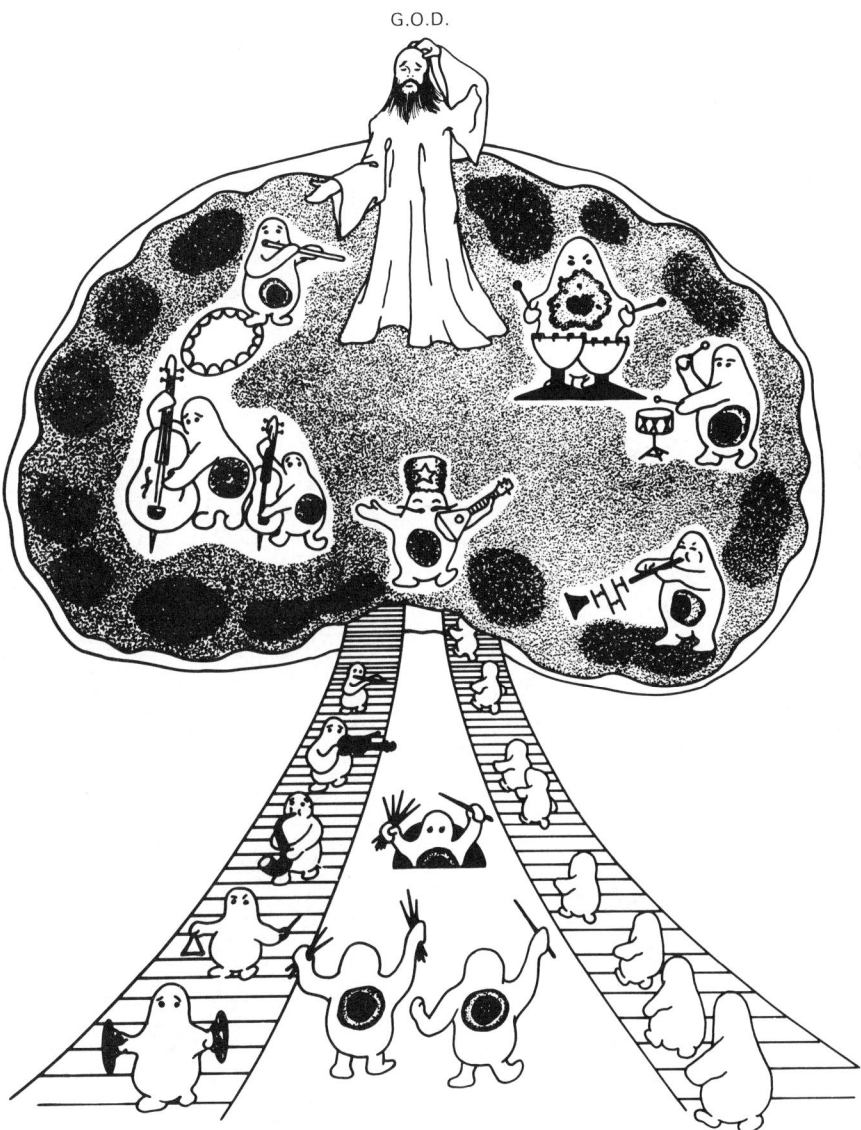

The immunological orchestra in 1977. With the discovery of subsets of T cells Ly 1 and Ly 2,3 cells become joint conductors and Ly 1,2,3 becomes the prompter. This complicated situation clearly has distressed the generator of diversity.

APPENDIX A

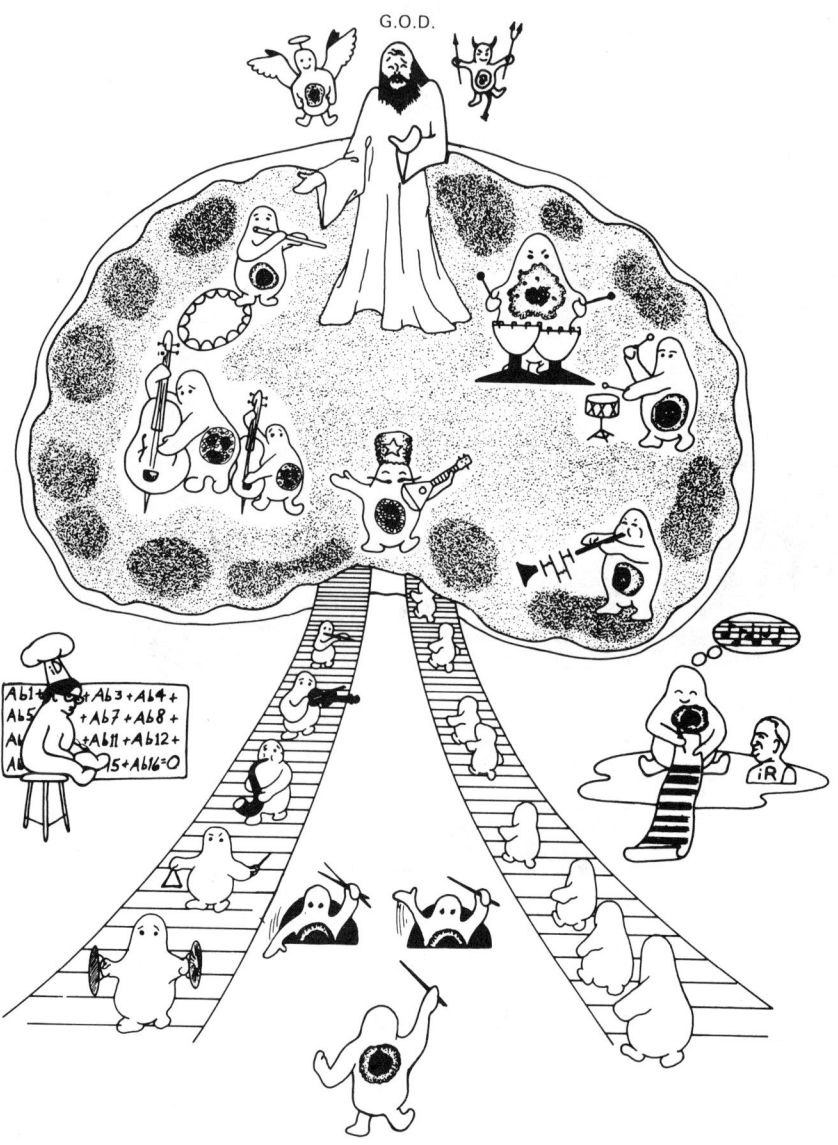

The immunological orchestra in 1982. The T cell is the conductor and the Lyt 1^+ (helper) and Lyt 2^+ (suppressor) cells are prompters, each urging its own interpretation. The generator of diversity seems resigned to the conflicting calls of the angels of help and suppression. At the sides sit the idiotype network and Ir gene (as impresarios?). The caricatures are of Niels Jerne and Baruj Benacerraf.

APPENDIX B
Chromosome Locations of Some Genes of Immunological Importance

Structure encoded	Human	Mouse	
Immunoglobulins			
H chain	14		12
κ chain	2		6
λ chain	22		16
MHC	6		17
T cell structures			
Surface markers: Thy 1	11	Thy 1	9
T8, CD8	2	Lyt 2	6
T4, CD4	12	L3T4	?
T3, CD3	11	T3	9
Receptors: α chain	14		14
β chain	7		6
γ chain	7		13
Complement components			
C2, C4, Factor B	6 (MHC-linked)		17
C3	19		?
C1q (B chain)	1		?
Factor H	?		2

Sources: Fitch, F. (1986) *Microbiol. Rev.* 50, 50; Campbell, R. D., M. C. Carroll, and R. R. Porter (1986) *Adv. Immunol.* 38, 203.

Index

ABO system, 25
Accessory cells
   macrophages, 238, 245
   MHC restriction and, 300–307
Acetylcholine receptor (AChR), 486–488
   anti-AChR antibody, 487
   degradation of, 487
Acquired immunodeficiency syndrome (AIDS)
   AIDS-related complex (ARC), 519
   elimination of T helper cells, 518, 520
   HTLV-III/LAV virus, 521
   immunological abnormalities in, 518
   T4 cells and, 519, 521–522
   therapy for, 522–523
Acute lymphoblastic leukemia (ALL), 526
Adaptive differentiation, 303, 306
   MHC restriction, 295–297
   thymus as site of, 309
Adherent cells
   macrophage, 245–246
   produce mitogenic factors, 357
Adjuvants, 458, 494
Adoptive transfer, 270–271, 273
Affinity of reaction
   AgAb reaction, 104–107
   defined, 105
   equilibrium constant, 105
   equilibrium dialysis, 105–106
AgAb, see Antigen–antibody complex
Aggamaglobulinemia, Swiss-type, 511
Agglutination reactions, 122–123
AIDS, see Acquired immunodeficiency syndrome
Allelic exclusion, 67
   defined, 89, 397
   regulated model, 90
   stochastic model, 90
Allergens, 463
Allergic rhinitis, 465
Allergy, see Hypersensitivity
Alloantibodies
   defined, 185
   differentiation antigens and, 185
Alloantigens, 185
Allogeneic effect, 275–276, 282
Allograft rejection
   acute, 505
   defined, 238, 499
   host rejects graft, 240
Allotype suppression, 397
Allotypic determinants, 69
Alternate pathway, 141
   activation of, 148
   AgAb not required, 148
   amplification loop, 148
   C5 convertase, 149–150
   factor B and C3.B complex, 148
   factor D, 148
   fluid phase, 147
   properdin, 147, 149
   stabilization of C3bBb, 149
Aminopterin, 95–97
Amplification loop, 148
Amyotrophic lateral sclerosis (Lou Gehrig disease), 493
Anaphylaxis, 463
Anaphylotoxins, 553
Antibodies of predetermined specificities, 32–35
   amino acid sequences, 34
   nucleotide sequences, 33
Antibodies to proteins
   antigenicity, 26–27
   multideterminant hypothesis, 29
   segmental mobility, 28–29

INDEX

tobacco mosaic virus (TMV), 28
Antibody, *see also* Immunoglobulin
   affinity and valence, 107–109
   structural basis of diversity, 42–45
Antibody-dependent, cell-mediated
   cytotoxicity (ADCC), 449
Antibody formation
   hapten–carrier conjugates, 18, 268
   specificity, 19–23
Antibody labeling
   electron-dense labels, 127–128, 131–133
   enzyme labels (ELISA), 125–126
   fluorescence, 127, 130
   primary and secondary methods, 123–124
   radioactive labels (RIA), 125
Antibody response
   B–T cell cooperation, 260
   immediate hypersensitivity reactions, 237
   in vitro studies, 245–248
Antigen
   antigenic determinant, 22
   cross reactions, 22–24
   initiates cell division, 367
   nature of, 17–35
   T cell proliferation and, 301
Antigen–antibody complex (AgAb)
   affinity of the reaction, 104–107
   agglutination reactions, 122–123
   avidin and biotin, 134
   C1,C4,C3,C2 reactions, 141
   heterogeneity of binding, 109–110
   kinetics of reactions, 110
   labeled antibody techniques, 123–135
   measuring, 112–135
   precipitin reaction, 113–115
   protein A, 134
Antigen–antibody complex diseases
   (Type III reactions), 475–478
   allergic glomerulonephritis, 478
   Arthus reaction, 475
   serum sickness, 478
Antigen-combining site
   complementarity-determining surface, 53
   Fab fragments and, 51, 53
   immunoglobulin fold, 51
   shape, 49
   size, 48–49
Antigenic activation, 300
Antigenic determinants
   cross reactivity and, 22
   define Ig class, 55
   isotypic determinants, 67
   molecular mapping of, 29–30
Antigenicity
   amino acid sequence and, 26–28
   conformation and, 26–27
   defined, 17–18
   segmental mobility and, 28–29
Antigen pulsing, 300, 302
Antigen-specific T cell hybridomas, 332
Anti-lymphocyte globulin (ALG), 503
Antiserum
   complement and, 140
   γ globulins in, 37
Anti-Tac, 363
Arthritis, *see* Rheumatoid arthritis
Arthus reaction, 475
Ataxia-telangiectasia, 513
Autoantigens, 483
Auto–anti-idiotype antibody
   network theory and, 385
   production of, 385–386
Autoimmune demyelinating diseases
   experimental autoimmune encephalitis, 493–494
   multiple sclerosis (MS), 493
Autoimmune diseases
   antigens in, 484
   non-organ specific, 490–493
   organ-specific, 483–490
Autoimmune encephalitis, experimental, 494
Autoimmune thyroiditis, 489
Autologous MLR (A-MLR), 495
Autosomal recessive alymphopenic SCID, 511
Avidin, 134
Azathioprine, 503

Background strain, 220
BCDF, *see* B cell differentiating factor
B cells
   antibody-forming, 183

INDEX

bind free antigen, 325
bursapoietin, 193
complement receptor-bearing lymphocytes (CRL), 192
Fc receptor, 192
hapten-primed, 296
immediate hypersensitivity reactions, 238
mitogen response, 193–194
surface immunoglobulin (sIg), 191
B cell activation
  BCGF, 369–370
  consequences of, 372–375
  depolarization of membrane, 373
  receptor cross-linking, 368–369, 374
B cell differentiating factor (BCDF), 370
B cell growth factor (BCGF)
  IL-2, separation from, 370
  T cell factor, 369
B cell receptor, *see also* Surface immunoglobulin
  blastogenesis of B cell, 319
  genes, 339
B cell tumors, 89
BCGF, *see* B cell growth factor
Bence–Jones proteins
  antibody light chains, 43
  multiple myeloma, 529
"Beta barrels," polypeptide chains and, 30–31
BFU-E (burst-forming unit, erythroid), 170
Blood group antigens, 25
Bone marrow
  chimeras, 292–294, 304, 309
  -thymus reconstitution experiments, 252, 255
  transplants, 240, 507, 513
Breinl, Friedrich, template theory, 7–8
Burkitt's lymphoma, 529
Burnet, Macfarlane, 416–417, 419, 429, 452n
  clonal selection theory, 10
Burnet–Fenner hypothesis, 417
Bursa of Fabricius
  bursectomy, 243–245
  lymphoid differentiation in birds, 181, 193

Cancer
  immune suppression and, 455
  terminology, 455
Capping, 321–322
Carrier effect
  adoptive transfer, 270–271, 273
  cellular basis of, 273
  described, 268–269
  helper T cells and, 273
Carrier priming, 270–272
Cell cooperation
  in CTL, 265
  in GVH, 254
Cell cycle, 367
Cell interaction molecules (CI), 289
Cell-mediated lympholysis (CML), 242
Cell-mediated responses
  allograft rejection, 238
  CTL reaction, 242
  defined, 237
  delayed-type hypersensitivity, 237
  effector cells, 261
  graft-versus-host reaction, 240–241
  helper cells, 261
  lymphocytes, 236
  mixed lymphocyte reaction, 243
  T cell as effector cell, 263
  varied nature of, 261
β-Chain probe, 404
Chargaff palindrome, 83–84
Chemotactic factors
  Arthus reaction, 475
  formamyl peptides, 443
Chimeras
  allophenic or tetraparental, 290
  blood cell, 417
  bone marrow, 292–294
  defined, 290
  $F_1 \rightarrow P_1$, 303–304
  MHC restriction, 295
  primed with carrier, 296
  production of, 291
  T cells, antibody response of, 307–308
  thymus, 309
Chomsky, Noam, 383
Chromosome markers
  CFU-S and, 164
  lymphocyte origins and, 180–181

INDEX

"Chromosome walk," 225
Chronic lymphocytic leukemia (CLL), 527
Claman experiment, 252, 281, 282
Classical pathway, 141–147
    activation unit: C4,C2, 144, 146
        C3 convertase or C4C2 complex, 146
        C5 convertase, 147, 150
    recognition unit, 142, 145
Class switching, 87
Clonal abortion, 430
Clonal anergy, 432
Clonal selection theory, 10
    as paradigm, 11
    tolerance and, 429
Clonotypic determinant, 332
Cluster of differentiation (CD), 188, 190
CML, see Cell-mediated lympholysis
Colony forming unit (CFU)
    assay of, 159–160
    erythrocyte (CFU-E), 170
    single-cell origin, 160–161
    spleen (CFU-S), 159–165
Colony forming unit-spleen (CFU-S)
    characteristics and lineage, 164
    chromosome markers, 162
    lymphocytes and myeloid cells, 181
    multipotent hemopoietic stem cell, 162–165
Colony stimulating factor (CSF), 170
Commensalism, 440
Complement cascade, 141
    pathways, 152
    synonyms for products, 144
Complement fixation (CF) test, 138
Complement receptor-bearing lymphocytes (CRL), 192
Complement system
    alternate pathway, 141, 147–149
    anti-complementary effects, 138
    C1,C2,C3,C4, 141
    C1q, 143
    classical pathway, 141–147
    common pathway, 149–151
    components, 151
    discovery of, 138–141
    Fc of antibody and, 137, 143
    lysis and, 140–142
    membrane attack complex (MAC), 147, 149, 151
Concanavalin A (ConA)
    IL-2 from T cell, 360
    suppressor cell, 396
    T4, responsive to, 421
Congenic mice, 211, 276
    defined, 220
    production of, 220–221
Constant region, 42–44
Cooperation
    allogeneic T and B cells, 294
C-reactive protein, 449
C region, see Constant region
Cross reactions
    albumins of different species, 23–24
    immunofrequent, 23n
CTL, see Cytotoxic lymphocyte
Cyclosporin A, 503, 505–506
Cytokines, 354, 355
Cytolytic reactions (Type II reactions), 474–475
    erythroblastosis fetalis, 474
    hemolytic anemia, 475
    thrombocytopenia, 475
Cytotoxic cells
    class I antigens, 286
    MHC restriction, 286–288
Cytotoxic lymphocyte (CTL), see also Killer cells
    CTL reaction, 242
    effector cell, 247, 279
    macrophage required, 247
    viral infections and, 450

Dayhoff bank of protein sequences, 344
Delayed-type hypersensitivity (DTH) (Type IV reactions)
    contact dermititis, 478
    defined, 479
    tissue rejection and, 499
    T lymphocytes and, 478
    tuberculin test, 237, 478
Differentiation
    committed cell, 166
    determination, 166

INDEX

hemopoietic inducing factors, 169
pathways in blood, 167
stem cells to progenitor cells, 168
Differentiation antigens
alloantibodies and monoclonal antibodies, 185
human T cells and, 186, 188–190
murine T cells and, 187
Diphtheria toxin, 459
Diversity
germ line, 74, 82
somatic, 74, 82–86
DNA
cDNA clone library, 343
transfection, 98

Effector cells
antigen-induced, 18
bone marrow-derived, 260
cell-mediated responses and, 261
K cells, 449
Lyt $2^+, 3^+$, 266
T cell as, 263
Effector molecules, 59
Ehrlich, Paul
complement and, 140
horror autotoxicus, 415, 416, 482
side chain theory, 5–6
Electron-dense labels
colloidal gold, 127
ferritin, 127
immunogold, 127, 131
immunoelectron microscopy, 128
ELISA, *see* Enzyme-linked immunosorbent assay
Endotoxins, 448
Enhancer element, 88
Enhancer sequences, 88
Enhancing factor of allergy (EFA), 473
Enzyme-linked immunosorbent assay (ELISA), 125–129
horseradish peroxidase (HRP), 125
inhibition method, 128
screening hybridomas, 98
sensitivity, 128
Epinephrine, 473
Epitope
cross-reactivity with paratope, 383

defined, 380
nature of, 404–405
network and, 382
suppressor, 409
T cell receptor, 351
Epstein–Barr virus, 529
Equilibrium dialysis, 105–106
Erythropoietin, 170
Exon–intron relationships, 41, 76, 224

Fab
degranulation and, 469
hybrid antibody production, 100
parasite infections and, 451
phagocytosis, 448
proteolysis of Ig, 37
Fc
amino acid sequences compared, 59
complement and, 137, 143
hybrid antibody production, 100
IgE, 65
proteolysis of Ig, 37
subclasses and, 57
Fc receptor
Fcε, 451
mast cells and, 470
phagocytic cells, 448
Flow cytometry, 134–135
Fluorescence quenching, 107
Fluorescent labels, 127
fluorescence microscopy and, 130
Follicular dendritic cell (FDC), 206
Framework regions, 45
Freund's adjuvant, 494

Gell and Coombs classification, 464–479
Generative grammar, 383–384
Gene transfer therapy, 174, 177n
Germ theory, of disease, 4
Glomerulonephritis, 490–491
Gorer, Peter, tissue transplantation and, 210
Graft rejection, 498–499, 505
Graft-versus-host (GVH) reaction, 292
bone marrow transplantation, 240, 507, 513

INDEX

cell-mediated response, 240–241
  spleen index, 240
  splenomegaly, 240
Granulopenia, 515
Graves disease, 483, 488

Haplotype, 216–217
Hapten
  antibody responses, 19
  anti-hapten antibodies and, 20
  defined, 18, 268
Hapten–carrier systems, 18–23
  conjugates (H–C), 268
  suppressor T cells and, 408
Hashimoto's disease, *see* Autoimmune thyroiditis
Hassall's corpuscles, 198
HAT (hypoxanthine, aminopterin, thymidine) selection, 97
Haurowitz, Felix, template theory, 7–8
Hay fever, 465
H chain
  antigenic determinants on, 55
  defined, 39–40
  immunoglobulin fold, 51
Heart transplant, 506
Heart-lung transplant, 506
Heavy chain, *see* H chain
Helper T cells (T_H)
  antibody formation and, 261
  Class II antigens, 288
  CTL, 262–263
  β-galactosidase-induced, 405–407
  GVH, 262
  Lyt 1^+, 266
  MLR, 262
  suppressor T cells and, 405–406
  thymus and MHC restriction, 314
Hemolytic anemia, autoimmune, 489–490
Hemopoiesis, 157–177
  defined, 158
  inducing factors, 169–172
Hemopoeitic differentiation, 181
Hemopoeitic-inducing microenvironments (HIM)
  lymphoid differentiation, 172, 179
  myeloid differentiation, 172

Hemopoeitic stem cell
  differentiation, 166
  low proliferation, 165
  new genes into, 173–177
  progenitor cells, 168, 170
  self-renewal, 166
  sickle-cell anemia and, 173–174
  "tritium suicide" experiments, 165
Heterogeneity index, 103, 109–110
High endothelial venules (HEV), 203–206
Hinge region, 40
Histamine
  immediate hypersensitivity, 466
  inflammation and, 443
Histocompatibility (H-2) antigens
  defined, 210
  fused tail (*Fu*) gene, 211
  genes, 210–211
HLA, *see* Human lymphocyte antigens
Hodgkin's disease, 528
Homologous sequences
  C_H regions, 47–48
  structural domains, 48
Host–parasite relationships, 439–442
Human Leukocyte Differentiation Antigens, First Workshop on, 188
Human lymphocyte antigens, nomenclature, 218–219
Human rhino virus (HRV), 30
Human T cell differentiation, 188–191
Humoral response, *see* Antibody response
Hybrid antibody molecules
  DNA transfection, 98
  hybrid Ig genes, 99
  mouse and human, 100
  production of, 98–99
Hybridomas
  monoclonal antibody production, 94
  screening of, 97
Hypersensitivity
  allergic reactions, 463
  anaphylaxis, 463
  classification of reactions, 464–479
  harm of antibodies, 462
  nature of, 462–464
  sensitization, 463

INDEX

Hypervariable regions, 44–45
Hypogammaglobulinemia
    acquired, 515–516
    X-linked infantile, 514

^{125}I, T cell receptor label, 335
^{131}I, surface membrane protein label, 333
Idiotype
  antigen-combining site, 380
  anti-idiotype antibody, 386–387
  anti-idiotype enhances responses, 387–388
  anti-idiotype mimics antigen, 388–389
  anti-idiotype suppresses responses, 386–387
  auto-anti-antibody, 385–386
  network theory, 385–386
  suppression, 398
Idiotypic determinants
  anti-idiotype antibody (anti-id), 69–71
  cross reactive, 70–71
  defined, 69
  inheritance of, 70
  major, 70–71
  markers of antigen-combining sites, 69
  public, 70
IEP, see Immunoelectrophoresis
IgA
  J chain, 63, 64
  secretory IgA, 63–64
  serum IgA, 62–63
IgD
  B cells, 320
  function, 65
  properties, 64
IgE
  B cell generating factor, 472–473
  Fc portion, 65
  hypersensitivity, 466–474
  parasite infections and, 451
  potentiating factor, 473
  properties, 65
  reagenic antibody, 65
  suppressive factor, 473

IgE receptor, 471
IgG, 61
IgG1 inducing factor (IIF), 370
  IIF gene, cloning of, 371
IgM
  B cells, 320
  clasp model, 61
  J protein, 62
  properties, 61
IIF, see IgG1 inducing factor
IL, see Interleukin
IL-1
  adherent cells and, 357
  discovery of, 357
  macrophages and, 357
  properties of, 356
IL-2
  BCGF and, 370
  discovery of, 359–360
  production by T cells, 360–361
  properties, 356
  T cell helper factor, 313n
  T cell proliferation, 363
IL-2 receptors
  anti-Tac antibody, 363
  expression of, 363
  features of, 364
  induction of, 363
  kinetics of induction, 364–365
  T cell activation, 366
IL-3, 170
IL-4, 370–372
Immediate hypersensitivity (Type I reactions), 464–474
  antibody, 237
  atopic disease, 465–466
  degranulation, 466–470
  epinephrine, 473
  hay fever (allergic rhinitis), 465
  histamine, 466
  IgE, 466–474
  reaginic antibody, 466
Immune surveillance theory, 451–458
Immunity, disease and, 2–4
Immunocompetent cell, 236, 238
Immunodeficiency diseases, acquired
  acquired hypogammaglobulinemia, 515–516
  acquired immunodeficiency syndrome (AIDS), 516–523

INDEX

Immunodeficiency diseases, congenital
  classification by function, 512
  granulopenia or neutropenia, 515
  PNP deficiency, 515
  reticular dysgenesis, 510–511
  selective immunoglobulin disorders, 514
  severe combined immunodeficiency diseases (SCID), 511, 513
  sites of, 511
  thymic aplasia, 514
  thymic dysplasia, 515
  Wiscott-Aldrich syndrome, 514
  X-linked infantile hypogammaglobulinemia, 513–514
Immunoelectrophoresis, 119–120
Immunogen, 32–33
Immunogenicity, 17–18
Immunoglobulin (Ig), *see also* Antibody; specific class
  allotypic variation, 66–68
  chain dissociation studies, 39–40
  chain structure of, 37–40
  class, 55–65
  constant regions, 42, 74–76
  Fab, 37, 100, 448, 451
  Fc, 37, 57, 65, 100
  framework regions, 45
  genetic variation, 66–71
  heavy chains, 40, 51, 55
  hinge region, 40
  homologous sequences, 47–48
  human, 60
  hypervariable regions, 44–45
  idiotypic variation, 67
  inter- and intrachain disulfide bonds, 40–41, 57
  light chains, 40, 51
  myeloma protein, 39
  non-specific binding to, 134
  physical heterogeneity, 55
  sIg versus secreted, 339
  subclasses, 56–58
  variable regions, 42, 74–76
Immunoglobulin fold, 51
Immunoglobulin genes
  allelic exclusion, 89–90
  class switching, 87–88
  cloning, 77
  coding for V and C regions, 75
  constant region, 86–88
  D segments, 80
  gene reorganization, 79–86
  heavy chain genes, 81, 87
  J segment, 79
  leader sequences, 79
  transcription enhancement, 88–89
  V–D–J joining, 80–81
  V–J joining, 79
Immunoglobulin superfamily
  domain structure and sequences, 48
  MHC, Ig, Thy 1, 227–228
Immunological paralysis, 421
Immunology, Fifth International Congress of, 188
Immunophotoelectron microscopy
  electron-dense labeling, 128
  fluorescence compared, 133
Immunosuppression, 497, 503
Immunotoxins, 459
Inducing factors in hemopoiesis
  concentration effects, 171
  GM-CSF, 169–171
  physiological inducers, 169
  "surrogate inducers," 169n
Inflammatory response, 442–445
  cardinal signs of, 442
  chemotactic factors, 443
  C-reactive protein, 449
  granulocytes (polymorphonuclear neutrophils, or PMNs), 443
  phagocytic leukocytes, 443
  phagocytosis and, 444–446
"Innocent bystander" phenomenon, 475, 490
Insulin-resistant diabetes, 488
Interdigitating cell (IDC), 206
Interferon
  2,5-adenosine (2,5-A), 450
  immune interferon, 450
  induced antiviral state, 450
  natural killer cells, 456
  ribonuclease L, 450
  viral immunity and, 448
Interleukins, *see also* specific factor
  properties of, 356
  T cell proliferation and, 366–367

INDEX

Interleukin cascade, T cells and, 361–362
Internal image, 379, 381–384, 391
Introns, 76
Ir genes
  control of immune response, 229
  MHC, 214
Isoantibodies, 185
Isoelectric focusing, 334
Isotypic determinants, 55, 68–69

Jerne, Niels
  dynamic equilibrium of immune system, 384
  natural selection theory, 9–10
  network theory 379, 383
Jerne plaque assay, 257n, 259
J protein, 62

K cells, 449
Kidney transplants
  survival rates, 502
  success of, 506
Killer cells, *see also* Cytotoxic lymphocytes
  CML, 242
  thymus and MHC restriction, 314
Kuhn, Thomas, 1, 11

Landsteiner, Karl, 6, 380
  ABO system and, 25, 209
  hapten–carrier systems and, 18–23
  nitrophenyl isomers as antigens, 7
  The Specificity of Serological Reactions, 19
Langmuir absorption isotherm, 107, 109
L chain, 40, 51
Leukemia, 524–525
  lymphocytic, 239
Light chain, *see* L chain
Like:like interactions, 289–290
Lipopolysaccharide (LPS), 357
Liver transplants, 506
Lupus, *see* Systemic lupus erythematosus

Lymphatic vessels, 202
Lymph nodes, 202
Lymphoblastic lymphoma, 528
Lymphocyte activating factor (LAF), *see* IL-1
Lymphocytes
  circulation of, 203–206
  lymphoid progenitor cells, 182, 184
  origins of, 180–183
  primary and secondary lymphoid organs, 182, 196
Lymphocytic leukemia, 239
Lymphoid-inducing microenvironments, 181, 184, 192
Lymphoid organs
  B and T cell regions, 206–207
  structure of, 197–202
Lymphokines, 354, 372
Lymphomas
  classified by cell type, 525
  defined, 524
  Hodgkin's, 527–528
  non-Hodgkin's, 528–529

Macrophage
  role of, 245–248
  secretion of soluble factors, 358
  T cell activation, 300
Major histocompatibility complex (MHC)
  cell-mediated responses and, 211
  Class I, 214–215
  Class I antigens, 222
  Class I genes, 225
  Class II, Ia antigens, 214, 217
  Class II molecules, 223–224
  Class III, 214
  discovery of, 209
  exon–intron relationship, 224
  expression of, 226–227
  H-2 (mouse), 208
  HLA (human), 208
  mapping, 213–214
  multiple alleles and genes, 215
  organization of genes, 224–226
  polymorphisms of, 214–222
  recombinant Class I–Class II, 225–226

INDEX

self versus nonself, 214
traits controlled by, 212
Malaria
  antigen and vaccine, 34
  syphilis and, 449
Mancini assay, 116–117
Mast cells
  contents of granules, 470
  degranulation, 472
  IgE, 470–472
  "sentinel cells," 466
  structure, 467
Medawar, Sir Peter, 417, 419
  graft rejection, 498
  tolerance induced, 417–419
Melanomas, 458
Membrane attack complex (MAC), 147, 149, 151
MHC, see Major histocompatibility complex
MHC restriction
  adaptive differentiation, 295–297
  allophenic mice and, 291
  antibody formation, 281–284
  bone marrow chimeras, 280, 292
  cell interaction molecules, 289
  cell mediated responses, 284–290
  changed or "learned," 295, 298
  chimeras and, 290–293
  cooperation of T and B cells, 294
  cytotoxic cell and target, 286–288
  Lyt 1^+ and Lyt 2^+, 186
  nude mice, 281
  self:anti-self, 307–308
  site of, 286
  thymus and acquistion of, 309–310
  Zinkernagel-Doherty-Sherer phenomenon, 285
Mitchell-Miller experiment, 255–257, 281, 282
Mitogens, 183
  defined, 193
  B and T cell, 194
Mixed lymphocyte reaction (MLR)
  cell-mediated, 243
  helper cells, 279
  one-way MLR, 243
  stimulation index (SI), 277
  tolerance and, 421

Moloney leukemia virus, 33
Moloney sarcoma virus, 176
Monoclonal antibodies
  cell fusion, 94–95
  cell surface markers and, 184–185
  defined, 93
  IL-2 receptor and, 363
  mapping antigenic determinants, 29
  production, 94–98
  spleen and myeloma cells, 94
  T cell receptor and, 332
Monokines, 354, 361
Morphogenesis, 166n
Mosier experiment, 306
Multiple myeloma, 529
Multiple sclerosis (MS), 493
Murine T cell differentiation antigens, 186–187
  Lyt, 187
  Thy 1, 187
  TL, 187
Myasthenia gravis (MG), 485–488
Mycosis fungoides, 528
Myeloid inducing factors, 170
Myeloid leukemias, 527
Myeloma cells
  culture of, 94
  major synthetic pathway, 96
  salvage pathway, 96
Myeloma protein, 39

Natural killer cells (NK), 456–457
Natural selection theory, 9–10
Neoplasia, 451
Network
  anti-receptor antibody, 389–390
  auto–anti-idiotype antibody, 385–386
  function, 381–382
  generative grammar of, 383–384
  testing of, 384–391
Neutropenia, 515
Nonadherent cells, 245–246
Non-Hodgkin's lymphomas, 528–529
Nude mice
  defined, 281
  MHC restriction and thymus, 310–313
  repopulation failure, 281

INDEX

Opsonin, 447
Opsonization
   antibody-dependent, cell-mediated cytotoxicity (ADCC), 449
   complement-mediated cytolysis, 448
   defined, 448
   phagocytosis, 446–448
Ouchterlony assay, 116–117

Paradigm, 1, 11, 451
Parasite, see Host–parasite relationship
Parasitic infections, 451
Paratope
   antigen-combining site, 380, 382
   cross-reactivity with epitope, 383
Passenger lymphocytes, 505
"Patch clamping," 375
Patching and capping
   degranulation and, 468
   mobility of sIg, 321–322
Pauling, Linus, direct template theory, 8
Peyer's patches, 204, 206
PHA, see Phytohemagglutinin
Phage Group, 9–10
Phagocytosis
   events in, 446
   granules, 445
   lysosomes, 445
   mechanism, 445
   opsonization, 447–448
   PMNs, 444–445
Phagosome, 445, 448
Phytohemagglutinin (PHA), 357
Picorna viruses, "beta barrels" and, 30
Pillemer, Louis, 147, 149
Plasma cell, 236
PMNs (polymorphonuclear neutrophils), 443–445
PNP deficiency, 515
Polyclonal antibodies, 93
Precipitin reaction
   cross linking, 114
   equivalence zone, 114–115
   gels, 116–121
   IEP, 118–119
   Mancini assay, 116–117
   Ouchterlony assay, 116–117
   quantitative, 115, 117
Prednisone, 503
Primary lymphopenic immunologic deficiency, 513
Private specificities, 216
Progenitor cells
   BFU-E, 170
   CFU-E, 170
   growth factors and, 168
   of hemopoietic stem cells, 168, 170
   lymphoid, 182, 184
   mutant mice and cloned tumor lines, 172–175
Protein A, 134
Protein kinase (PK-C), 373–374
Proteins, see Antibodies to proteins
Public specificities, 216
Pulsed T cells, 359

Radioimmunoassays (RIA), 125–126
Raff experiment, 273–274
Reaginic antibody, 65, 466
Recombinant antibodies, 98
Reed–Sternberg cells, 528
Regulated model, 90
Reticular dysgenesis, 510–511
Rheumatic fever, 492
Rheumatoid arthritis, 492–493
Rhino virus, 30
Ricin, 459
Rocket immunoelectrophoresis, 119–120

Scatchard plot, 107, 108
SCID, see Severe combined immunodeficiency diseases
Secretory component, 64
Selective immunoglobulin disorders, 514
Self-marker theory, 419
Self–nonself discrimination, 416–421
   MHC restriction, 420–421
   self-marking, 417
   tolerance induction, 417
   Triplett experiment, 419–420

INDEX

Self-reactivity, 494–495
Serological antigens, 212
Severe combined immunodeficiency diseases (SCID), 511, 513
Sézary's syndrome, 528
Side chain theory, 5–6, 10
sIg, see Surface immunoglobulin
"Signal hypothesis," 341
Sips distribution function, 109
  plot of AgAb binding, 110
Skin transplants, 507
SLE, see Systemic lupus erythematosus
Smallpox, vaccination and, 3–4
Snell, George, 210–211
Somatic diversification
  combinatorial, 82–83
  D–J recombination, 85
  junctional site, 83–84
  somatic mutation, 84–86
  V–J joining, 84
Southern blot, 120, 343
Southern hybridization, 177
Specificity
  acid groups and, 20
  defined, 19
  glycoside bonds and, 23
  group position and, 22
  non-ionic groups and, 21
Spleen
  B- and T-dependent areas, 201, 206
  capsule of, 200
  central arteries, 202
  colony-forming unit, 159–165
  functions of, 200
  pulp, 200
  sinuses, 201
  trabeculae, 200
Splenectomy, 503–504
Splenomegaly, 240
Stem cell, see Hemopoietic stem cell
Stochastic model, 90
Structural domains, 48
St. Vitus dance, 493
"Subtractive method," 341–342
Suppressive factor of allergy (SFA), 473
Suppressor T cells (T_S)
  allotype-specific, 397
  antigen binding, 403–404

antigen-specific, 398–399, 404, 409–410
cloned, 407
ConA-induced, 396–397
contrasuppressor cascade, 411, 413
cytotoxic T cells and, 400, 404
discovery of, 394–400
effector, 411
β-galactosidase-induced, 405
helper cells and, 405–409
idiotype specific, 398
I–J enigma, 400–402, 410
inducer, 411
Lyt $1^-,2^+$, 400–401
neonatal thymus, 396
nonspecific suppression, 396–397
properties of, 400–404
receptor, 404–405
regulatory circuits, 411–413
soluble factors, 409–410
surface marker, 400
thymus reconstitution and, 395
transducer, 411
triad of determinants, 408
T-suppressor inducer factor (Tsif), 411
tumors and, 397
Surface antigens, 183
Surface immunoglobulin (sIg), see also B cell receptor
  B cell hallmark, 191
  fluorescein-labeled, 321
  isotypes of, 320
  mobility of, 321
  secreted Ig versus, 339–340
Swiss-type agammaglobulinemia, 411
Syngeneic thymus cells, 281
Systemic lupus erythematosus (SLE), 483
  glomerulonephritis, 490–491
  models of, 491
  thymus disorders, 492

Talmage, David, 10
Target cells, 242, 248, 286
T cell(s), see also Effector cell; Helper T cell; Suppressor T cell
  accessory cells, 308

INDEX

activation by antigen, 300, 365–366
antigen binding, 325–326
carrier-primed, 296
differentiation antigens, 184–190
gene library, 342
K^+ channels and, 375
macrophage activation, 300
MHC restriction, 302
mitogen response, 193–194
myeloma and BCGF, 369
PHA-pulsed, 359
regulatory cell, 394
sIg-negative, 323
subpopulations, 303–304
T cell:T cell interaction, 263, 275
types of, 183
T cell activation
  membrane depolarization, 475
  voltage-gated K^+ channels, 375
T cell growth factor (TCGF or IL-2)
  antigen-specific T cells and, 331–332
  assay for, 359
T cell inducing factors, 193
T cell receptor
  agretope, 351
  antibody against, 330–331
  anti-idiotype antibody, 331
  cDNA clones for, 341, 343
  α- and β-chain, 337, 347
  classical approach, 329–330
  desetope, 351
  dual receptor model, 327, 329
  epitope, 351
  gene rearrangement, 343–344
  gene resembles Ig, 345
  histotope, 351
  homology with Ig, 336–337
  immunoprecipitation of, 333
  models for, 327–329
  monoclonal antibodies to, 332
  neantigenic determinant model, 327
  "one and a half receptor" model, 349–350
  peptide maps, 335
  self-MHC and, 340
  structure, 349
  T3 chain, 337
  T cell clones used, 331

T cytotoxic classes, 341
T helper clone, 341
trimolecular complex model, 350
two-chained, 334
T cell receptor genes, 340–351
  α-chain gene, 345
  β-chain gene, 343
  γ-chain, 345–349
  chromosome locations, 346
  developmental expression, 348–349
  generation of diversity, 346–351
  organization of, 346
TCGF, *see* T cell growth factor
Template theory, 7–8
"Three-cell experiment," 278
Thymectomy
  immune response depressed, 243–245
  neonatal, 239, 241, 243–244, 255–257
Thymic aplasia, 514
Thymic dysplasia, 515
Thymic humoral factor, 193
Thymocytes, 198–199
Thymomas, 528
Thymopoietin, 193
Thymosin, 193
Thymus
  atrophy of, 198
  capsule, 198
  chimeras, 309
  cortex, 198
  gene rearrangement, 348
  helper cells, 258
  maturation in, 199–200
  medulla, 198
  selection versus education, 314–315
  T cell differentiation and, 183–184, 186
  T cell inducing factors and, 192–193
T locus, 228–230
Tolerance
  adult, 421–426
  antibody-induced, 424–425
  antigen-binding cells, 431
  antigen concentration, 422–424
  autologous mixed lymphocyte reaction (A-MLR), 421
  B cells, 427–451
  chimeras, 291

INDEX

clonal abortion, 430
clonal anergy, 432
cloned T_H cells, 428
defined, 419
deletion of clones, 429
form of the antigen and, 422–423
hapten, 424
high and low zone, 424–425
MHC restriction, 420–421, 434
mechanisms of, 426–433
"negative signals," 432
neonatal, 417–418
receptor blockade, 429
suppressor cells, 394, 426–428, 433
T cells, 426–429
tolerogen, 424
veto cell, 432–433
Total lymphoid irradiation (TLI), 504
Transfection experiment, 174–176
"Transgenic mice," 177n
Transplantation
allografts, 499
autografts, 499
blood transfusion, 504
Class I antigen matching and, 501
human, problems of, 501–504
laws of, 499–501
parental grafts, 501
splenectomy and, 504
syngeneic grafts, 499
total lymphoid irradiation (TLI), 504
types of, 505–507
Transplantation antigens, 212
Triplett experiment, 419–420
"Tritium suicide" experiments, 165
Tuberculin test, 237, 478
Tuberculosis, 444

Tumors
adjuvants, 458
immune surveillance theory, 451–458
immunotherapy, 458
immunotoxins, 458
melanomas, 458
natural killer cells and, 456–457
spontaneous versus induced, 453–454
tumor immunity, 454
tumor-specific antigens, 452–454
Two-gene, one-polypeptide hypothesis, 73, 75
testing of, 76–79

Variability ratio, 44
Variable region, 42–44, 74–76
Veto cell, 432–433
Viral infections, 449–450
V region, *see* Variable region

Western blot, 120–121
Wiscott-Aldrich syndrome, 514
Wu–Kabat plots, 44–47

Xenoantibodies, 185
X-linked infantile hypogammaglobulinemia, 513–514

Zinkernagel-Doherty-Shearer phenomenon, 285

About the Book

This book was set at DEKR Corporation on the Linotron 202, using typefaces of the Zapf family. The book was copy edited by Jodi Simpson. Joseph Vesely designed the book and coordinated artwork and other aspects of production. Artwork was produced under the direction of John D. Woolsey. Sandra Redemske designed the cover, which was printed at Lehigh Press Lithographers. The book was manufactured at R. R. Donnelley & Sons.